Therapeutic Immunosuppression

Immunology and Medicine Series

VOLUME 29

Series Editor:

Professor Keith Whaley, *Kuwait University, Safat, Kuwait*

A list of titles in the series can be found at the end of this volume.

Therapeutic Immunosuppression

Edited by

Angus W. Thomson

University of Pittsburgh,
Pittsburgh, PA, U.S.A.

SPRINGER-SCIENCE+BUSINESS MEDIA, B.V.

Library of Congress Cataloging-in-Publication Data

Therapeutic immunosuppression / edited by Angus W. Thomson.
     p. ; cm. -- (Immunology and medicine ; v. 29)
     Includes index.
     ISBN 978-94-010-3821-8   ISBN 978-94-010-0765-8 (eBook)
     DOI 10.1007/978-94-010-0765-8
     1. Immunosuppressive agents. 2. Immunosuppression. I. Thomson, Angus W. II.
Immunology and medicine series ; v. 29.
     [DNLM: 1. Immunosuppression. QW 920 T398 2001]
     RM373 .T475 2001
     615'.37--dc21

                                                               2001020373

ISBN 978-94-010-3821-8

Printed on acid-free paper

In Memory of Graham Bird

Graham Bird, my co-editor for this series, died on 14th January 2000 after a short illness. His outstanding career in clinical immunology has been reviewed in a number of obituaries and appreciations. Graham elected to co-edit the "Immunology in Medicine" series with me 2 years ago and applied his knowledge and enthusiasm for clinical immunology to the task. He made an immediate impact on the range of topics covered and the quality of the final products. Hopefully further books in this series will continue to foster the same degree of enthusiasm for this fascinating discipline.

Keith Whaley
Kuwait, June, 2001

CONTENTS

PREFACE

Therapeutic immunosuppression has very broad applications in clinical medicine, ranging from prevention and treatment of organ and bone marrow transplant rejection, management of various autoimmune disorders (e.g. rheumatoid arthritis) skin disease, and asthma. Whereas traditionally, only a small repertoire of immunosuppressive agents was available for clinical use, recent discoveries have significantly increased the number of approved agents, resulting in numerous trials to further evaluate their potential. In addition, products of the biotechnology industry, - monoclonal antibodies, cytokines, cytokine antagonists and other products of genetic engineering that target key molecular pathways in disease pathogenesis, have either already made, or are on the verge of making an important impact on treatment. There is also considerable interest in the potential of cell-based therapies (particularly hematopoietic stem and dendritic cell therapy) of allo- and autoimmunity. Important recent advances in the immunotherapy of allergic diseases are also covered in this book. Gene therapy offers considerable promise for suppressing pathogenic processes in either transplantation or autoimmune disorders. The possibility of combining these important new advances to maximize benefit to the patient, and to minimize possible untoward effects (that are also given extensive coverage in this book) is one of the most exciting challenges of contemporary medicine.

This volume is intended both for practicing physicians and surgeons and for biomedical scientists at the graduate/postdoctoral levels, and is designed to provide the theory behind these various approaches to immunosuppression, and to provide state-of-the-art reviews of current developments in each area. Each chapter is contributed by an expert(s) in the field. There was a need to bring this information together in a single volume, as much of the key recent developments have been dispersed throughout the biomedical literature, largely in specialized journals. Since, as in the past, important developments in immunosuppressive therapy in one branch of medicine (i.e. transplantation) are likely to benefit another (e.g. dermatology, rheumatology, gastroenterology), cross-disciplinary coverage of the mechanistic basis of the various therapeutic strategies in a single volume is likely to convey the potential of advances in therapy in the most coherent manner possible. I extend my thanks to the many contributors who have so generously given of their valuable expertise and time, and without whom, this volume would not have been possible.

Angus W. Thomson
University of Pittsburgh
Summer, 2000

CALCINEURIN-TARGETED INHIBITION OF IMMUNE REACTIVITY

1

Lina Kung and Philip F. Halloran
Division of Nephrology & Immunology
University of Alberta
Edmonton, Alberta, Canada

INTRODUCTION

The modern era of transplantation began with the emergence of a potent immunosuppressive drug, cyclosporine (CsA). This drug had features unlike any previous drugs. CsA was soon joined by FK506 (FK), later named tacrolimus, an unrelated agent with many similar properties. The exploration of the actions of these drugs revealed new aspects of signal transduction in the T cell and many other cells. A third drug, rapamycin (sirolimus) differed in important ways from CsA and FK, but shared some properties and also elucidated a remarkable new pathway. These three drugs are derived from fungi and target intracellular proteins that are highly conserved through evolution, reflecting their important biological functions. The proteins targeted by these drugs include the binding proteins named immunophilins and the drug targets calcineurin (CN) and target of rapamycin. The ubiquity of these proteins raises the question of why these drugs affect the immune response relatively selectively. This chapter will review inhibition of the immune response by CsA and FK, drugs that inhibit CN phosphatase activity.

CYCLOSPORINE AND TACROLIMUS

Drug Discovery

CsA (as shown in Figure 1) is a hydrophobic, cyclic peptide isolated in the

1

A. W. Thomson (ed.), Therapeutic Immunosuppression, 1–30.
© 2001 *Kluwer Academic Publishers*.

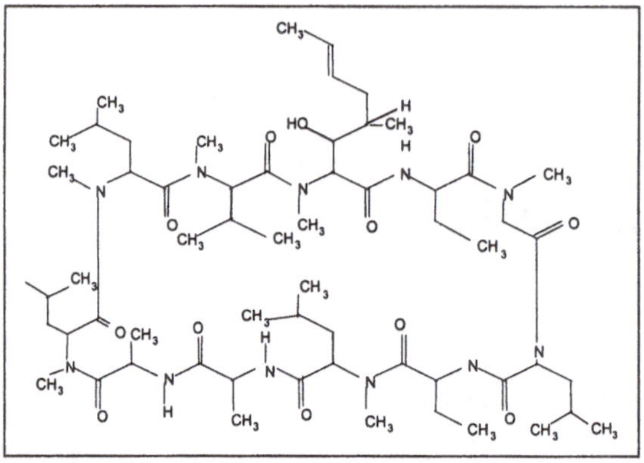

Figure 1
Cyclosporine

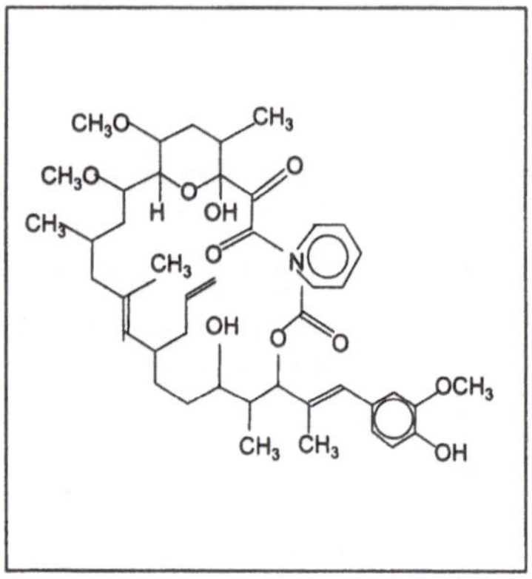

Figure 2
Tacrolimus

early 1970s from culture broths of fungi *Tolypocladium inflatum* and *Cylindrocarpon lucidum*. The antilymphocytic properties of this 11 amino acid, 1202.6 kDa fungal metabolite were described by Borel *et al* working in Basel, Switzerland [1]. The introduction of CsA for organ transplantation in the early 1980s led to significant increases in graft survival. FK, an 822.05 kDa immunosuppressive macrolide (as shown in Figure 2), was discovered in Tsukuba, Japan by Kino *et al* [2] in 1987 in the fermentation broth of *Streptomyces tsukubaensis*, and was introduced into clinics in 1989. Structurally dissimilar, FK and CsA have similar immunosuppressive effects, although FK has greater molar potency than CsA *in vitro* and *in vivo*.

Inhibition of the immune response

The *in vitro* and *in vivo* immunosuppressive effects of CsA were first reported by Borel *et al*. CsA suppressed both humoral and cellular immunity in animals. CsA administered to mice inhibited direct and indirect hemolytic plaque-forming cells and hemagglutinin formation in a dose-dependent manner. CsA also prolonged survival of skin allografts in mice as well as decreasing the incidence and symptoms of experimental allergic encephalomyelitis and Freund's adjuvant arthritis [1]. The immunological characterization of FK in comparison with CsA showed suppression of mixed lymphocyte reactions, antibody production, delayed-type hypersensitivity response, interleukin (IL)-2 secretion [2]. Inhibition of IL-3 and 4, interferon (IFN)-γ, granulocyte-monocyte colony stimulating factor (GM-CSF), and tumor necrosis factor (TNF)-α production have also been demonstrated [3]. CsA blocks progression from the G_0 resting phase to the G_1 activation phase in T cells, thus acting early after T cell stimulation. Treatment following expression of these early cytokine mRNAs fails to inhibit cytokine production.

An important step was the recognition that CsA blocked the induction of IL-2 mRNA and indeed inhibited the activation of transcription of many cytokines in T cells [4,5]. Subsequently CsA was shown to bind to a ubiquitous and abundant set of proteins called cyclophilins (CyP) [6], and FK was shown to bind to an unrelated set of ubiquitous proteins called FK506 binding proteins (FKBPs) [7]. Both CyPs and FKBPs were found to have rotamase or proline isomerase activity [7,8]. The most surprising finding was that both CsA:CyP and FK:FKBP complexes bound to and inhibited CN phosphatase (9,10). CN in turn controls the phosphorylation of transcription factors important for the expression of immune-response genes, such as the nuclear factors of activated T cells (NFATC) [11].

Both drugs also block degranulation by mast cells, neutrophils, basophils, and cytotoxic T-lymphocytes (CTL) [12]. Further, CsA and FK block B cell division in the late activation phase (G1) of the cell cycle and treatment may occur as late as 24 hours after stimulation [13]. The principal difference between CsA and FK is the concentration or dose that is required for suppression of immune function. The immunosuppressive effect of FK is achieved at lower concentrations than CsA *in vitro*, *in vivo*, and clinically. The probable explanation for this difference lies in the higher affinity of FK for FKBP and FK:FKBP for CN.

Pharmacokinetics

CsA and FK bind erythrocytes and plasma proteins, namely lipoproteins (CsA) and albumin (FK). Whereas the absorption of FK and the microemulsion formulation of CsA are bile-independent, some CsA formulations are bile-dependent. Both CsA and FK are extensively metabolized in the liver by the cytochrome P450 3A4 (CYP3A4) system. Therefore, hepatic dysfunction alters drug clearance and half-life, increasing plasma drug concentrations and toxicity. CsA is excreted mainly by the biliary system. The half-lives for CsA and FK are 18 and 12 hours, respectively.

Drug monitoring is important for both CsA and FK because intra- and inter-subject variations make predictions of drug concentration on the basis of a given dose difficult. High performance liquid chromatography, monoclonal radioimmunoassay (RIA), and monoclonal fluorescence polarisation immunoassay (TDX) can be used to measure levels of CsA. Monoclonal RIA and TDX however give higher readings because of cross-reaction with CsA metabolites. The concentration of CsA in whole blood is approximately two-fold that in plasma. For detection of FK, enzyme-linked immunoabsorbent assay for plasma or whole blood and microparticulate enzyme immunoassay for whole blood can be used. Concentrations of FK in whole blood are approximately 10 to 20 times higher than in plasma.

Recovery of cells from CN inhibition

Inhibition of CN activity increases and falls with CsA blood levels. The inhibition of CN activity of transplant patients on CsA therapy is rapidly reversible. The recovery of CN activity *in vitro* does not require protein synthesis, is temperature-dependent, and is correlated with the efflux of CsA. There are at least two mechanisms by which CsA leaves the cell. One mechanism involves a rapid, P-glycoprotein (Pgp)-dependent efflux that is only observed in cell lines expressing high levels of Pgp and that can be blocked by competitive Pgp substrates. There is also a slower, Pgp-independent transport mechanism that requires the addition of extracellular CsA binding sites, such as erythrocytes. CsA may also leave the cells by simple diffusion, not requiring active transport. Peripheral blood leukocytes (PBL) express relatively low levels of Pgp and the Pgp-independent mechanism likely predominates. *In vitro* the recovery of CN activity is slow, likely because of the aqueous environment and the lack of extracellular binding sites [14].

Pgp functions as an adenosine triphosphate (ATP)-dependent pump for the efflux of anti-cancer drugs from multi-drug resistant tumor cell lines and its overproduction is associated with multi-drug resistance. CsA reverses multi-drug resistance by directly binding to and inhibiting Pgp. This activity is not dependent on its ability to induce immunosuppression [15]. Non-immunosuppressive CsA analogs have subsequently been proposed to increase the effectiveness of anti-cancer drugs by blocking Pgp-dependent movement of the drugs out of the cells.

Toxicity

The toxicity of immunosuppressive drugs should be considered as the general effects of interfering with the immune system (selected infections and malignancies) and the non-immune toxicities of the specific agent or class of agent. The immunodeficient states induced by FK and CsA are probably similar. Moreover the toxicology performed in experimental animals and *in vitro* with cellular systems has an unknown relevance because concentrations may not simulate clinical use.

CsA and FK share numerous non-immune adverse effects, including neph-rotoxicity, uric acid increase, and the increased incidence of infections and malignant lymphomas. Neurotoxicity, diabetes, and alopecia are more prevalent during FK therapy, and hypertension, gum hyperplasia, lipid abnormalities, hirsutism, and skin changes are more prevalent with CsA therapy. Hypertrophic cardiomyopathy has also been reported with the use of FK in pediatric transplant patients [16]. The cardiomyopathy could be reversed with lower doses of FK or conversion to CsA. Interestingly, CsA but not FK can induce smooth muscle contraction of bovine renal and coronary arteries in muscle baths *in vitro*. The effects were seen only with CsA and not FK despite the greater molar potency of FK. However, the concentrations used in this and similar *in vitro* studies are many-fold higher than those used to completely suppress immune function, and the significance is dubious. Both CN and immunophilins are ubiquitous and the drugs enter all cells. An important question that remains to be answered is why CsA and FK are not more toxic. That is, why do they not have effects on all cell types? One possibility will be discussed in a later section.

Molecular Mechanism of Action

Both CsA and FK bind to families of abundant intracellular proteins - immu-nophilins. Those that bind to CsA are termed CyP while those that bind FK are termed FKBP. Immunophilins have peptidyl-prolyl cis-trans isomerase or rotamase activity that is inhibited by the binding of CsA or FK [6,7]. It was initially believed that inhibition of the isomerase activity of immunophilin was the basis for the immunosuppressive properties of these two drugs. Subsequent experiments showed that complete inhibition of isomerase activity was not necessary for complete inhibition of the immune response and that some cyclosporine analogs could bind and inhibit isomerase activity without inhibiting the immune response [17,18]. The immunosuppressive activity of CsA and FK was then found to correlate with the inhibition of the enzymatic activity of CN by the drug: immunophilin complex [9,19,20]. Crystallization of the FK:FKBP:CN ternary complex revealed that as the drug:immunophilin complex binds more than 10 Å away from the active site of CN [21,22]. Thus FK:FKBP non-competitively inhibits CN phosphatase activity by sterically hindering the dephosphorylation of substrate. Although mutational studies have shown distinct binding interactions for CsA:CyP and FK:FKBP [23], the binding regions overlap (9) and CsA is thus assumed to have a similar mechanism of action (Figure 3).

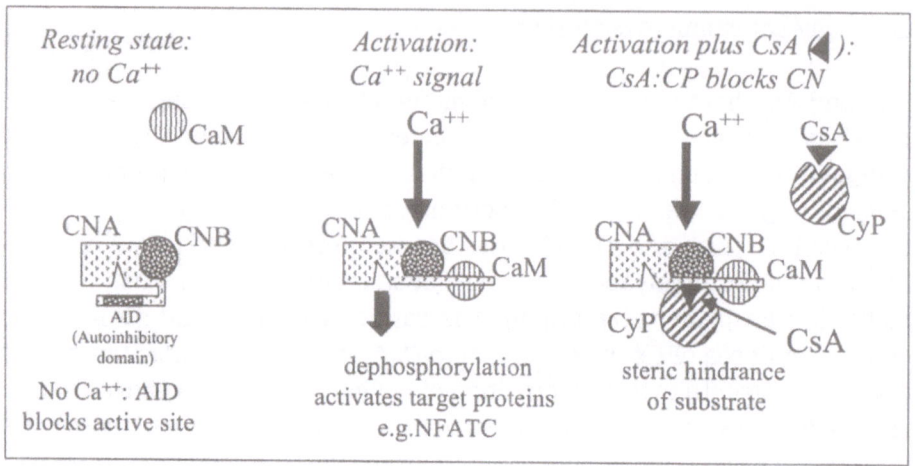

Figure 3
The mechanism of CN inhibition by CsA

Although all immunophilins can bind their respective drug, not all drug:immunophilin complexes can inhibit CN. CyPA, CyPB, FKBP12, FKBP12.6, and FKBP51 are the only ones that form active drug:immunophilin complexes which inhibit CN in the cell [24-26]. Some immunophilins such as FKBP13 and FKBP25 form inactive drug:immunophilin complexes which cannot bind CN [27]. Other immunophilins such as CyPC form active drug:immunophilin complexes but are inactive because they are sequestered away from CN by their sub-cellular localization [24]. The significance of these inactive immunophilins in relation to the action of FK and CsA is not clear. They may reduce the amount of drug available for the active immunophilins or act as reservoirs.

CALCINEURIN (CN)

Expression, Structure, and Regulation

To understand the effects of CN inhibition by CsA and FK, an understanding of the structure and functions of CN is necessary. First detected in skeletal muscle [28] and brain [29], CN is a calcium (Ca^{++})- and calmodulin (CaM)- dependent serine/threonine protein phosphatase that is ubiquitously expressed in mammalian tissues and highly conserved from yeast to humans [30,31]. Although characterized as a serine/threonine phosphatase, tyrosine dephosphorylation has also been demonstrated for CN [32]. CN is also

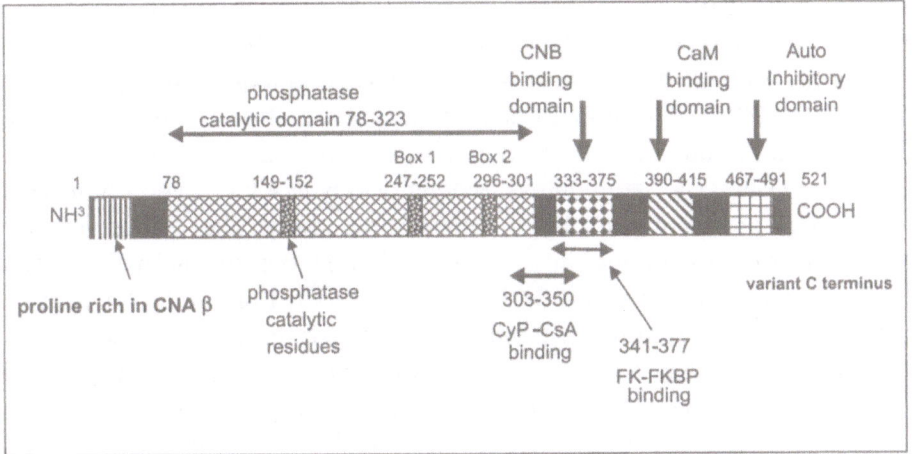

Figure 4
Human CNA alpha

known as protein phosphatase 2B and is a heterodimer of two subunits: cal-cineurin A (CNA) and calcineurin B (CNB). CNA and CNB are found tightly bound together and can only be dissociated under denaturing conditions [33]. CNA is the catalytic and CaM-binding subunit while CNB is the Ca^{++}-binding regulatory subunit [30].

Human, mouse, rat, Drosophila, and yeast sequences for CNA have been reported. Three separate genes encode CNA (58-64 kD): Aα, Aβ, and Aγ. CNAα and CNAβ are widely distributed, whereas CNAγ is testis-specific [34]. Functional differences between isoforms are not well-characterized. Except for the N- and C-terminal tails, the three isoforms exhibit 83-89% identity over 90% of their sequence [35]. As shown in Figure 4, CNA has four domains, one catalytic and three regulatory domains. The catalytic domain of CNA shows 40-50% similarity to protein phosphatase 1 and 2A. The regu-latory domains of CNA consist of a CaM-binding domain [36], a CNB-binding domain [37], and an autoinhibitory domain (AID) [38]. The AID is near the C-terminus and identified by limited proteolysis [39]. This inhibitory domain folds over and covers up the catalytic site of CNA, acting like a pseudosub-strate [38]. The Ca^{++} dependence of CN phosphatase activity is controlled by both CaM and CNB, two structurally similar but functionally different Ca^{++}-binding proteins. Binding of CaM is believed to displace the AID while the binding of Ca^{++} to CNB is thought to induce an allosteric change which alters the active site to augment its catalytic activity [40].

CNB has high affinity for Ca^{++}, but like other Ca^{++}-regulated proteins, is also regulated by Mg^{++} [30]. Two isoforms of this 19 kD protein have been demonstrated: CNB1, which associates with CNAα and CNAβ, and CNB2, which associates with CNAγ in the testes [41,42]. CNB is most homologous with CaM in the four Ca^{++}-binding domains, which are often referred to as the "EF-hand" structure and are found in most Ca^{++}-binding proteins [37]. In the absence of CaM, Ca^{++} stimulates CN activity only at a low level. Addition of CaM with Ca^{++} produces a large increase in activity. The binding of Ca^{++} to CNB modulates the interaction with and activation of CN by CaM. The V_{max} is increased by Ca^{++} and CaM without any effect on the K_m for the substrate [40]. In addition to Ca^{++}, various other metal ions also directly regulate CN phosphatase activity, such as Mg^{++} and Ni^{++}. The ability of these other metal ions to stimulate CN activity depends on the concentration, pH, and substrates used [30,43]. Further, Zn^{++} and $Fe^{++/3+}$ in the active site are thought to serve for the catalytic reaction [44].

CN is sensitive to oxidative inactivation through its Fe-Zn active centre and this can be prevented by the enzyme superoxide dismutase [45]. This may be another mechanism by which CN is regulated *in vivo* and is important to consider when assaying enzyme activity *in vitro*.

Calcium Activation

Sustained, elevated levels of intracellular Ca^{++} are required to activate CN. The mechanism by which this is achieved during T cell activation is intricate. Activation of PLC-γ1 results in the formation of two important second messenger molecules, inositol triphosphate (IP_3) and diacylglycerol (DAG). IP_3 diffuses through the cytosol and activates its receptor on the membrane of the endoplasmic reticulum (ER). Binding opens the Ca^{++} channels and releases a small burst of Ca^{++} from ER storage sites. This initial rise in intracellular Ca^{++} is insufficient to induce gene expression, cell proliferation or differentiation and is limited by inactivation of IP_3 by dephosphorylation and cytosolic extraction of Ca^{++} by the membrane Ca^{++} ATPase pump. A larger, sustained increase resulting from entry of Ca^{++} into the cell is required. The transient burst in intracellular Ca^{++} activates the intracellular Ca^{++} release activated Ca^{++} (ICRAC) channel, which is inwardly rectifying [46]. The increased entry of Ca^{++} is balanced by the increased outflux of K^+ through type *n* voltage-gated K^+ channels [47,48]. This large, sustained increase in intracellular Ca^{++} that is required to activate CN is sustained by electrochemical changes in the membrane for several hours (Figure 5).

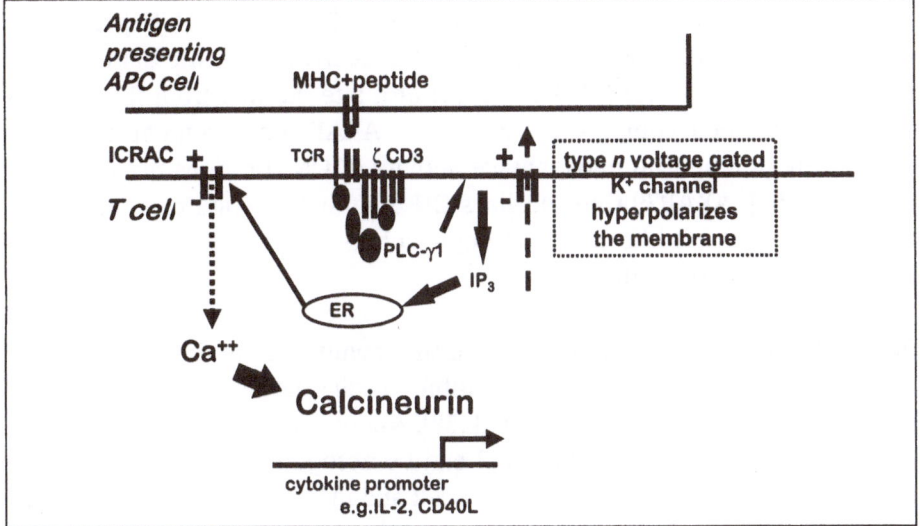

Figure 5
High cytosolic Ca^{++} activates calcineurin

Protein-protein interactions

CN is a ubiquitous enzyme that plays a role in a number of cellular processes. Cell signaling through phosphatase and kinase cascades is given structure by protein:protein interactions via scaffolding, anchoring, and adapter proteins [49]. These proteins contribute to the signal specificity by their recruitment of enzymes into signaling networks or by placing enzymes close to their substrates, regulating when and where protein kinases and phosphatases are activated in the cell. For example, receptors for activated C kinase (RACKs) tether protein kinase C (PKC) to the cytoskeleton or at submembrane sites through protein-phospholipid interactions [50]. CN also participates in a number of protein-protein interactions with various membrane bound proteins such as A-kinase anchoring protein (AKAP) [51], Bcl-2 [52], and the IP$_3$ receptor (IP$_3$R) via FKBP12 [53] (Table 1). Interaction with the IP$_3$R will be discussed later in this chapter.

AKAP79 is an anchoring protein that is enriched in neurons and present in T cells. Able to bind the membrane via its amino terminal basic region [54],

Table 1
CN scaffolding proteins

	Location
AKAP79	Plasma, cytosolic membranes
Bcl-2	Mitochondria, endoplasmic reticulum
IP$_3$R	Endoplasmic reticulum

AKAP79 is believed to anchor protein kinase A (PKA) [55], CN [51], and PKC [56] to specific microenvironments. CN binds AKAP79 at a site distinct from that for PKC or PKA. AKAP79 binds CN at a site distinct from that for the drug:immunophilin complex [57]. Binding of AKAP79 non-competitively and specifically inhibits the phosphatase activity of CN; FK does not alter this inhibition [51]. AKAP79 thus localizes CN in an inactive state. Over-expression of AKAP79 inhibits NFATC2 dephosphorylation and PMA/ionomycin-induced NFAT activity [57].

Bcl-2 is a cytoplasmic protein found on the membranes of the mitochondria and endoplasmic reticulum [58] and inhibits cell death induced by Ca^{++} signaling and growth factor withdrawal [59]. Apoptosis induced by expression of a constitutively active form of CN can be abrogated by bcl-2 expression [60]. In BHK cells co-transfected with bcl-2 and in T- and B-cell lines expressing high levels of bcl-2, a physical interaction between bcl-2 and CN can be detected [52]. CN interacts with the BH4 domain, the α-helical domain present in the anti-apoptotic members and absent in the pro-apoptotic members of the bcl-2 family. Bcl-2 does not inhibit CN phosphatase activity; instead, it anchors CN to cytoplasmic membranes and prevents an active CN from escorting NFATC into the nucleus [52]. CN is necessary to protect NFATC from rephosphorylation [61]. CsA is able to bind and inhibit the phosphatase activity of CN bound to bcl-2, indicating that the site of bcl-2 interaction on CN is distinct from that for the drug: immunophilin complex. The pro-apoptotic members of the bcl-2 family can also regulate the interaction between bcl-2 and CN [52]. Notably, an interaction between bcl-2 and CN was not detected in the cell line expressing low levels of bcl-2 and thus it is not known whether this interaction occurs in normal cells.

THE TARGET PROTEINS (SUBSTRATES) OF CN

The function of CN and the consequences of CN inhibition can be better understood by examining the actions of its substrates. CN has been shown to directly modulate the activity of a number of intracellular proteins. Some are transcription factors, such as NFATC, while others are enzymes, such as nitric oxide synthase (NOS). Substrates for CN are too numerous to discuss in any great detail. Subsequently, we will focus on NFATC, elk-1, IP_3R, NOS, and a few neuroproteins (Table 2). The indirect regulation of nuclear factor kappa in B cells (NFκB) and Jun amino-terminal kinase (JNK) by CN will also be discussed.

Table 2
Direct targets of CN

	Function
NFATC	Transcription factor
Elk-1	Transcription factor
IP$_3$R	Regulation of Ca^{++} flux
NOS	NO synthesis
MAP-2	Microtubule assembly
Tau	Microtubule assembly
Dynamin	Neurotransmitter release
Synapsin	Neurotransmitter release

NFATC

The members of the NFATC family of transcription factors are the most well-characterized substrate of CN. NFATC is found in its phosphorylated state in the cytosol in resting cells. Upon activation by an increase in intracellular Ca^{++}, CN binds to and dephosphorylates NFATC [62]. Dephosphorylation of NFATC is hypothesized to unmask a nuclear localization sequence (NLS), resulting in the nuclear translocation of the NFATC-CN complex (Figure 6) [63]. CN is required to escort and to protect NFATC from constitutively active kinases such as glycogen synthase kinase-3 [61], casein kinase 1 [64], JNK [65], and MEKK1 [64]. Once in the nucleus, NFATC forms cooperative

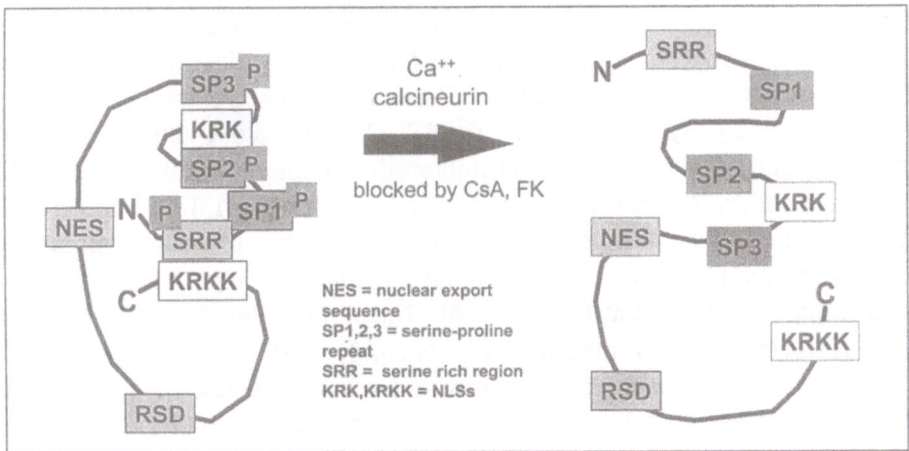

Figure 6
Phosphorylation of NFATC affects nuclear localization

Table 3 NFATC Family		
Agreed Upon	**Also Known As**	**Immune Function**
NFATC1	NFAT2, NFATc	Th2 activator
NFATC2	NFAT1, NFATp	Th2 repressor
NFATC3	NFAT4, NFATx	T cell generation and survival
NFATC4	NFAT3	Th2 repressor

complexes with Fos and Jun on DNA to induce the transcription of such genes such as IL-2 and IFN-γ. The crystal structure of the DNA-binding domains of NFATC, Fos, and Jun showed a tight association of the three transcription factors resulting in cooperative binding to DNA [66]. When Ca^{++} signaling ends, CN dissociates from NFATC and NFATC kinases rephosphorylate the NLS sequence [61,64,65]. The nuclear export of NFATC is mediated by nucleocytoplasmic shuttling factors such as Ran and crm1 [67]. Crm1 is unable to bind until CN dissociates from NFATC.

Rao *et al* have recently reviewed the first four members of the NFATC family identified [68]. The nomenclature for this area is somewhat confusing, with more than one name for each member (Table 3). Whereas NFATC1 and NFATC3 are tightly restricted to the lymphoid system in the adult system, the expression of NFATC2 and NFATC4 is fairly ubiquitous. In addition to their role in the immune system, NFATC family members have also been implicated in many other processes, such as adipogenesis [69] and cardiac morphogenesis [70,71]. NFATC knockouts have provided valuable information about the role of the various NFATC members in the immune response. The NFATC1 knockout showed hypoproliferation of peripheral T- and B-cells in response to mitogens, impaired T-cell development, and a selective decrease in IL-4 [72]. In contrast, the NFATC2 knockout showed modest splenomegaly, T- and B-cell hyperproliferation, impaired induction of FasL, and a moderate increase in Th2-type cytokines (IL-4, 5,13) [73]. Mice deficient in NFATC3 have a defect in T cell development, increased apoptosis of double-positive thymocytes, increased activation of peripheral T cells, and impaired expression of bcl-2 [74]. The double knockout of NFATC3 and NFATC2 showed massive splenomegaly and lymphadenopathy, a marked increase in mast cells and eosinophils, hyperactivated T- and B-cells, impaired expression of FasL, and a dramatic increase in Th2-type cytokines and IgG1 and IgE [75].

A recently cloned NFAT-related protein, NFAT5, differs from NFATC1-4 in its structure, DNA binding, and regulation. NFAT5 is similar in its Rel-like DNA-binding domain. However, it differs in that it does not cooperate with Fos/Jun at NFAT:AP-1 composite sites and is constitutively nuclear regardless of CN activation [76].

Elk-1

Elk-1, a member of the ternary complex factor (TCF) family of transcription factors, is also dephosphorylated by CN [77]. Unlike NFATC, elk-1 dephosphorylation results in its inactivation rather than activation. TCFs are phosphorylated and activated by members of the mitogen-activated protein (MAP) kinases family, including extracellular signal-regulated kinase (ERK) and p38, and cooperate with the serum response factor to regulate the transcriptional activity of promoters containing the serum response element (SRE), such as c-fos [78]. Both the Ras-MAP kinase pathway and Ca^{++} pathway are activated by growth factors. Thus activation of CN and its dephosphorylation of elk-1 may act as a mechanism to down-regulate elk-1 following its activation by MAP kinases. CN may also mediate cross talk between two different signaling pathways. For example, activation of TCFs by one pathway may be prevented by activation of CN by another pathway. Furthermore, inhibition of CN by CsA and FK would thus result in disregulated activation of TCF and may be the responsible for some of the toxicity and possibly the immunosuppressive effects of drugs.

IP_3R

CN regulates the intracellular Ca^{++} flux via the IP_3R. Influx of Ca^{++} across the plasma membrane may be mediated by voltage-dependent Ca^{++} channels or by release of Ca^{++} from intracellular Ca^{++} stores via intracellular Ca^{++}-release channels. The IP_3R and the ryanodine receptor (RyR) are two ligand-gated, tetrameric Ca^{++}-release channels on intracellular Ca^{++} storage sites such as the ER. While RyR is important for Ca^{++}-induced release of Ca^{++}, IP_3R is important for IP_3-induced release of Ca^{++} [79]. IP_3R is phosphorylated at three distinct sites by PKC, Ca^{++}/CaM-dependent protein kinase (CaMKII), and PKA [80]. CN appears to mainly target the PKC site of phosphorylation and regulate the activity of the channel. Ca^{++} oscillations may be mediated by the following mechanism. Ca^{++} is released from the endoplasmic reticulum through the IP_3R following activation by IP_3 and activates PKC, which then phosphorylates IP_3R and further increases the Ca^{++} flux. Elevated intracellular Ca^{++} also activates CaM and CN, which then dephosphorylates the PKC site of phosphorylation and decreases the Ca^{++}-flux [53]. FKBP12 also regulates the IP_3R and displacement of FKBP12 and CN from the receptor by FK results in leaky Ca^{++} channels [81].

NOS

CN dephosphorylates and activates NOS, which synthesizes nitric oxide (NO) from L-arginine and molecular oxygen. NO has a number of important roles in the body. For example, it functions as a neurotransmitter in the central nervous system and an endothelial-derived vasodilator. NO release is also a method by which macrophages kill tumor cells and bacteria. On the negative side, NO is also a potential mediator for glutamate neurotoxicity and hypoxic neuronal death. There are three isoforms of NOS: neuronal (nNOS), immunologic or inducible (iNOS), and endothelial (eNOS). While iNOS expression is induced by injury and its activation is Ca^{++}-independent, nNOS and eNOS are constitutively expressed and activated by Ca^{++}/CaM [82]. NOS is phosphorylated by PKA, CaM kinase II, G-kinase, and PKC. Phosphorylation of NOS by PKC inhibits its enzymatic activity; dephosphorylation of NOS by CN reverses this inhibition [83]. The unphosphorylated forms of neurogranin and neuromodulin, which can also be phosphorylated by PKC and dephosphorylated by CN, also inhibit NOS activity. CN activates NOS and increases the production of NO by at least two distinct mechanisms. FK and CsA increase the phosphorylation of NOS, inhibiting NOS activity and blocking NO production [83].

Neuroproteins

Many CN substrates have important roles in the neurosystem. The neuronal cytoskeleton is composed of microtubule polymers that are composed of tubulin. Microtubule-associated protein 2 (MAP-2) and tau (τ) are microtubule-associated proteins that promote microtubule assembly. Dephosphorylation of MAP-2 and τ by CN increases their affinity for the microtubules and stabilize microtubule length [84]; the assembly of microtubules by tubulin increases with CN-mediated dephosphorylation [85]. Whether inhibition of CN activity against these neuroproteins underlies some of the neurotoxicity of CsA and FK is unclear. However, the importance of CN, particularly CNAα, in this system is highlighted by the phenotype of the CNAα-deficient mouse, which will be discussed in more detail later.

CN has also been shown to directly regulate neurotransmitter release via the dephosphorylation of neural proteins. Synapsin is localized in the cytoplasmic surface of synaptic vesicles [86] and is involved in the regulation of translocation of synaptic vesicles to plasma membranes (87). PKA and CaM kinase II phosphorylate synapsin [88,89], reducing its binding to actin, tubulin, neurofilaments, and synaptic vesicles. Dephosphorylation of synapsin by CN increases the binding activities of synapsin to inhibit neurotransmitter release. Dynamin I, a GTPase, also plays an important role in neurotransmitter release. Dephosphorylation of dynamin I by CN decreases its GTPase activity, decreases synaptic vesicle recycling, and inhibits neurotransmitter release [90, 91]. CsA and FK treatment substantially increase glutamate release evoked by physiologic stimuli [92]. Glutamate is an excitotoxin and its enhanced release by FK and CsA treatment may underlie the drug neurotoxicity.

NFκB

NFκB is not a substrate of CN but CN has a variable and indirect effect on NFκB activation. NFκB is a ubiquitous transcription factor involved in immune reactions. First identified in B cells, NFκB was found to induce the transcription of Igκ in mature B and plasma cells. NFκB binding sites have since been demonstrated in the promoter or enhancer region of many genes, such as those encoding cytokines, chemokines, and adhesion molecules. In resting cells, NFκB can be found in an inactive complex with its inhibitor, IκB. Activation results first in the phosphorylation of IκB by IκB kinase. Phosphorylated IκB is then tagged by ubiquitin for subsequent degradation by proteosomal proteolysis. NFκB is thus released and translocates to the nucleus to induce the transcription of target genes. In some experimental systems CN plays a role in NFκB activation, and CsA inhibits NFκB activation. CN has been hypothesized to indirectly regulate NFκB by activating IκB kinase and subsequently the proteolysis of IκB [93]. CsA only partially inhibits NFκB activation and the effect is late, suggesting that the effect of CsA is indirect. Most NFκB release in most cell types may be resistant to CN inhibitors.

JNK

Another key pathway which is indirectly activated by CN is the JNK pathway. JNK or stress-activated protein kinase (SAPK) is a subgroup of MAP kinases that serine phosphorylates and increases the transcriptional activity of c-Jun. c-Jun can homo- or heterodimerize with other leucine zipper proteins such as Fos to form AP-1 complexes. JNK has also been shown to phosphorylate JunD, another possible component of AP-1. In T cells, JNK activation correlates with increased AP-1 transcriptional activity and induction of c-Jun and IL-2 gene expression. Ligation of both TCR and CD28 is required to fully activate JNK. CN significantly enhances the activation of JNK and c-Jun by PKC-θ but does not directly affect PKC-θ kinase activity [94]. Integration of the PKC-θ and CN signaling pathways likely occurs upstream.

CNAα-DEFICIENT MICE

Immunology

The immune systems of mice lacking CNAα were characterized by the Seidman group in early 1996. There was >65% reduction of CN activity in T cells from CNAα-/- mice [95]. Similarly, we found a 82-88% reduction of CN activity in the heart, brain, kidney, and spleen of CNAa-/- mice (unpublished observations). The composition and distribution of T- and B-cells were normal in thymus, spleen, lymph nodes, and bone marrow, suggesting that CNAa is not required for normal development of T and B cells. CNAα-/- mice responded normally to challenge with TNP-OVA; however, when restimulated with OVA *in vitro*, T cells harvested from lymph nodes of CNAα-/- mice proliferated less and secreted less IL-2, IL-4, and IFN-γ than T cells from wild-type mice. This defect could not be corrected by addition of normal APCs or IL-2 to the *in vitro* culture. However, stimulation with polyclonal mitogens, such as PMA plus ionomycin, ConA, or anti-CD3ε antibody showed no functional differences between CNAα-/- and wild-type T cells *in vitro*. Furthermore, T cells from CNAα-/- mice were more sensitive to inhibition by CN inhibitors CsA and FK [95]. More studies of the CNAα-deficient mouse are required to understand the discrepancy between the *in vitro* and *in vivo* findings.

Neurology

The neurological characterization of the CNAα mouse agreed with the hypothesized role of CN in the brain. Hallmark lesions of Alzheimer's disease include neurofibrillary tangles that are composed of paired helical filaments and amyloid plaques composed primarily of β-amyloid protein Aβ. The major component of the paired helical filaments, hyperphosphorylated τ, was found to accumulate in CNAa-deficient mice. As discussed previously, τ is a protein associated with the microtubule and functions to stabilize microtubules, promoting their assembly by forming cross-bridges between microtubules and between microtubules and neurofilaments. Hyperphosphorylation of τ changes its physical and functional properties, decreasing its activity. These cytoskeletal changes may explain the deficits in learning and memory observed in CNAα-deficient mice [96].

Other systems

We have examined the basic morphology of brain, thymus, liver, heart, kidney, and spleen of 4-5 month-old CNAα-deficient mice by hematoxylin and eosin (H & E) staining and Periodic Acid-Schiff (PAS) staining. No abnormalities were observed in any of the organs except for the liver and spleen. We found slightly more mitotic bodies in the liver and more prominent germinal centers in the spleen.

CN OUTSIDE THE IMMUNE SYSTEM

Cardiac System

Cardiac hypertrophy is a compensatory mechanism to maintain cardiac output in response to conditions such as hypertension and myocardial infarction. However, sustained, it can lead to heart failure and death. CN was implicated in cardiac hypertrophy when transgenic mice expressing active forms of CN developed cardiac hypertrophy and heart failure. Mice transgenic for an active form of NFATC4 also develop cardiac hypertrophy, suggesting that CN acts through activation of NFATC4. Activated NFATC4 interacts with GATA4 to induce genes leading to the hypertrophic response. CN may also act via activation of myocyte enhancer factor (MEF)-2, a myogenic transcription factor which upregulates many of the genes during hypertrophy [97,98]. CN has also been shown to play a role in cardiomyopathy resulting from defects in contractility caused by sarcomeric dysfunction [99]. CsA and FK were shown to inhibit the hypertrophic response induced by angiotensin II and phenylephrine *in vitro* through activation of NFAT [100]. Neither CsA nor FK however could prevent left ventricular hypertrophy induced by aortic banding [101,102], suggesting that CN is not the sole pathway for the hypertrophic response.

Nervous System

To summarize the previous sections with regard to the roles of CN in the nervous system, CN regulates Ca^{++} flux (IP_3-R), decreases glutamate release (synapsin, dynamin), increases stability of microtubules (τ, MAP-2, tubulin) and increases NO (NOS, neurogranin, neuromodulin). Thus, CN is necessary for normal neural functions and may also function in pathological states such as ischemic or traumatic neuronal injury. Both ischemia and trauma result in glutamate release and increases in intracellular Ca^{++}. Inhibition of NO production through inhibition of CN has been suggested to underlie the neuroprotective effects of CsA and FK in ischemic injury.

Long-term depression (LTD) is an activity-dependent decrease in synaptic efficacy that permits neural networks to store information more effectively. CN is thought to potentiate LTD by dephosphorylating and inactivating inhibitor-1, an inhibitor of protein phosphatase 1 (PP1) [103]. PP1 is then activated and dephosphorylates target proteins such a cAMP-responsive element binding protein (CREB) [104]. Phosphorylated CREB promotes the activation of genes for long-term memory. CREB may also be a direct substrate of CN [105]. Liver transplant patients on CsA have been shown to have difficulties with learning and memory.

Skeletal Muscle

Muscle growth and regeneration are important adaptive responses in health and disease states. There are three major types of muscle fibers: slow-oxidative (type 1), fast oxidative (type IIa), and fast-glycolytic (type IIb). The two main differences between them are their speed of contraction (slow/fast) and the enzymatic machinery used for ATP formation (oxidative/glycolytic). Size, strength, and speed are determined mainly by the amount and type of contractile protein incorporated [106]. Adaptation occurs over time in response to workload and pathological stimuli. Increased motor nerve activity from electrical pacing or exercise training induce fast-to-slow fiber transformation while decreased motor nerve activity from certain disease states, hypogravity, or physical inactivity induces slow-to-fast fiber transformation. CN and NFATC are abundant in skeletal muscle and have been implicated in myofiber specialization [107]. CN transcriptionally activates promoters for myoglobin (Mb) and troponin I slow (TnIs), which are expressed selectively in slow oxidative skeletal muscle fibers, but not muscle creatinine kinase, which is expressed mainly in fast, glycolytic myofibers. Transactivation of these slow-fiber-specific promoters requires collaboration among multiple transcription factors, including NFATC and MEF-2 [108]. Recently, CN has also been implicated in skeletal muscle growth [109]. Activation of GATA-2 and NFATC1 is thought to underlie the CN-mediated hypertrophy induced by insulin-like growth factor-1 (IGF-1) [109]. CsA and FK treatment has been shown to prevent muscle hypertrophy and fast-to-slow fiber transformation during functional overload, and may underlie muscle weakness in post-transplant patients [110].

TRANSFORMING GROWTH FACTOR-β (TGF-β), CSA, AND FK

TGF-β1 has recently been proposed to be a key mediator of the immunosuppressive and fibrogenic effects of CsA and FK. A multifunctional and ubiquitous cytokine, TGF-β1 is produced by many cell types including T cells. TGF-β1 inhibits T- and B cell proliferation, prevents cytotoxic T cell generation, inhibits Ig secretion, and is fibrogenic [111]. TGF-β1 transgenic mice show evidence of nephrotoxicity, glomerulosclerosis, and fibrosis of kidney while mice deficient in TGF-β1 die at 3-4 weeks of multifocal inflammatory disease [112].

CsA in mice increases progression of transplanted cancer cell lines that are regulated by TGF-β1. Human lung adenocarcinoma cells that are non-invasive *in vitro* can be induced to an invasive phenotype with CsA treatment. The phenotypic changes are reversible and can be inhibited using anti-TGF-β antibodies. Metastatic growth of tumor cells can also be induced *in vivo* in SCID-beige mice, which also suggests that the tumor-progressive effect of CsA is on the cancer cells directly and not attributable to suppression of the host immune system [113]. It is important to note that this effect of CsA has only been demonstrated in this artificial cancer model. No similar effect of CsA has been shown on pre-cancerous cells and CsA has not been implicated in the conversion of benign tumors to cancerous tumors. CsA in human populations has not been shown to affect the incidence or progression of tumors any more than any other immunosuppressive. Thus there is no evidence to date that the CN inhibitors alter cancer risks by TGF-β mechanisms or any other mechanism other than by immunosuppression.

Expression of TGF-β1 in mice and patients is increased following administration of oral CsA [114,115]. Elevated TGF-β1 has been correlated with hypertension [116] and fibrosis [117,118] associated with FK and CsA treatment. FK has been demonstrated to induce TGF-β1 expression in human peripheral blood leukocytes *in vitro*, although at concentrations that are 100-fold higher than the *in vitro* IC50 for inhibition of CN or cytokine expression (119).

IMMUNOPHILINS MAY LIMIT CN INHIBITION BY CSA AND FK AT HIGH DRUG CONCENTRATIONS

We recently explored whether differential inhibition of CN explained the differences in molar potency of FK versus CsA. We compared their effects on NFATC2 dephosphorylation using Western analysis, IFN-γ production using enzyme linked immunosorbent assay (ELISA), and CN phosphatase activity using the CN assay in human PBL and mouse spleen cell suspension. Whereas inhibition of IFN-γ secretion and NFATC2 dephosphorylation was complete, inhibition of CN phosphatase activity was incomplete with both drugs at saturation, particularly with FK. Inhibition of CN phosphatase activity was incomplete whether FK treatment was *in vivo* (in the mouse) or *in vitro* (various human and mouse tissues, especially brain). Exogenous FKBP12 or CyPA increased CN phosphatase inhibition, suggesting that incomplete inhibition of CN phosphatase activity reflected limiting amounts of active immunophilin [120]. These data contradict the prevailing assumption that active immunophilins are abundant and not limiting for inhibition of CN by CsA or FK. Further, the observation that FK and CsA completely inhibit immune function without completely inhibiting CN suggests that the inhibition of immune function is not mediated by general CN inhibition but by inhibition of a subset of CN which is critical for lymphocyte activation.

Specificity of Immunosuppressive Action

The ubiquity of CN and immunophilins raises the question of why the effects of CsA and FK inhibition of CN activity are targeted more towards the immune system versus other systems in which CN also functions. The effect that CsA and FK have on a particular tissue may be determined primarily by the amount of drug that is accumulated and the degree of CN inhibition in that tissue. Following oral administration, CsA distributes to both lymphoid and non-lymphoid tissues. We have found that CsA inhibits CN activity in most tissues comparably, with similar *in vitro* and *in vivo* IC50's. However, tissues differ in their maximal CN inhibition, probably because active immunophilins are limiting.

How then are we able to interfere with the immune response without interfering with cardiac or brain function? Limiting concentrations of active immu-nophilins suggest that some signaling pathways may be sensitive and some may be resistant to inhibition. CN is probably not a homogenous population and specific protein-protein interactions may differentially regulate the dif-ferent subsets of CN. Differing availability of immunophilins among the com-partments may then result in the selective inhibition of one CN-mediated downstream event over another. Differential expression of immunophilins among tissues may also explain the differences between CsA and FK. For example, CsA but not FK causes gum hyperplasia. Such differences may reflect more active cyclophilin than FKBP in the target tissue, and thus CsA has more effect. Sensitivity of CN to inhibition by CsA and FK varies among tissues, with the brain being most resistant *in vivo* and *in vitro*. Thus two key aspects probably determine effects on particular pathways in specific tissues: the total ratio of immunophilin to CN and the assembly of immu-nophilin and CN in a specific pathway or compartment.

NFAT peptides

Because of the ubiquitous expression and multiple substrates of CN, more specific targetting of CN activity is required. NFAT peptides (SPRIEIT or VIVIT) have been shown to be more pharmacologically specific in inhibiting the phosphatase activity of CN. The amino acid sequences of NFAT peptides correspond to one region on NFATC where CN binds. NFAT peptides are thought to disrupt the interaction between NFATC proteins and CN by bind-ing to CN at the region where NFATC needs to dock and subsequently inhib-its CN dephosphorylation of NFATC. The peptides did not interfere with CN phosphatase activity against other substrates, such as the PKA-phosphory-lated RIIα and Erk-2-phosphorylated τ [121], and selectively inhibited expres-sion of NFAT-dependent cytokine genes without affecting the expression of CN-dependent but NFAT-independent cytokine genes [122].

PUTTING IT TOGETHER: HOW DO THE DRUGS WORK IN IMMUNOSUPPRESSION?

Both CsA and FK directly bind to the isomerase site of their intracellular binding proteins CyP and FKBP. Active drug:immunophilin complexes then inhibit the phosphatase activity of CN and the activation of transcription fac-tors necessary for expression of cytokine genes and other factors needed to activate the immune response. Roles for NFATC, elk-1, JNK, and NFκB in the immune response have been demonstrated and their activities are directly or indirectly regulated by CN. Although NFATC is often considered as the principal immunological substrate for CN, mice deficient in any of the NFATC members are not immunodeficient. Dephosphorylation of elk-1 by CN results in its activation rather than inhibition, making it an unlikely downstream target for CsA or FK immunosuppression. Further, CsA only partially inhibits the activation of JNK by anti-CD3 and anti-CD28 and the activation of NFκB. Thus the crucial immunological target for CN and subsequently CsA and FK is yet to be identified. Further, although T cells are considered the principal target, the inhibition of other immune cells by CsA and FK may be as large a contributor to the immunosuppressive effect of these drugs. For example, we have shown that CsA has potent effects on IFN-γ production by non-T cells *in vivo* [123]. The role of other changes during treatment with CN inhibitors such as small increases in TGF-β is unclear.

PUTTING IT TOGETHER: THE MOLECULAR BASIS OF CN TOXICITY

Because it has been difficult to separate the nephrotoxic and neurotoxic effects of CsA and FK from their immunosuppressive effects, the mechanism of toxicity is often considered to be the same as the mechanism of immunosuppression, namely via CN. The vasoconstrictive effects of CsA and FK on endothelial cells may explain the nephrotoxic effects of these two drugs, but whether these effects are mediated by CN has not been demonstrated. It has become clear that the effects of these drugs can also be explained by non-CN mechanisms. For example, the large majority of the CN phosphatase activity in the brain is resistant to inhibition by CsA and FK. This would suggest that the neurotoxic mechanism is not simply the inhibition of CN phosphatase activity. CsA analogues that inhibit CyP isomerase activity but not CN activity have also been shown to disrupt the formation of long-term memory [124]. Thus inhibition of CyP isomerase activity but not CN activity in the brain by CsA is another possible basis for the neurotoxicity.

The observation that FK and CsA completely inhibit immune function without completely inhibiting CN suggests that the inhibition of immune function is not mediated by general CN inhibition but by inhibition of a subset of CN in a structural compartment which is critical for lymphocyte activation. New drugs could be developed which target CN relevant for immune function while leaving general CN activity intact. Possible therapies include interference with CN assemblies. Analogs of CsA or FK may also be designed to preferentially target the relevant subset of CN and spare CN pathways which if inhibited would lead to toxicity. These therapies could achieve greater specificity, less toxicity, and thus greater drug efficacy.

FUTURE PERSPECTIVES

The inhibition of CN activity against a broad range of substrates by the drug:immunophilin complexes is a possible biochemical basis for the therapeutic and adverse effects of CsA and FK. Thus as with the NFAT peptides, more selective inhibition of CN activity may be a means of lowering toxicity. A better understanding of CN the role and regulation of CN in different signaling pathways and cell types is required. Fine dissection of how established and novel CN inhibitors are similar and distinct may provide clues to more selective inhibition of CN activity. Like CsA and FK at the beginning of the decade, new CN inhibitors could be molecular probes to understanding cell signaling and lead the way to better CN-targeted inhibition of immune reactivity.

REFERENCES

1. Borel JF, Feurer C, Gubler HJ, Stahelin H . Biological effects of cyclosporin A: a new antilymphocytic agent. Agents and Actions 1976;6:468-75.
2. Kino T, Hatanaka H, Hashimoto M, Nishiyama M, Goto T, Okuhara M, Kohsaka M, Aoki H, Imanaka H. FK-506, a novel immunosuppressant isolated from a *streptomyces*. I. Fermentation, isolation, and physico-chemical and biological characteristics. J Antibiot 1987;40:1249-55.
3. Tocci MJ, Matkovich DA, Collier KA, Kwok P, Dumont F, Lin S, Degudicibus S, Siekierka JJ, Chin J, Hutchinson NI. The immunosuppressant FK506 selectively inhibits expression of early T cell activation genes. J Immunol 1989;143:718-26.
4. Elliot JF, Lin Y, Mizel SB, Bleackley RC, Harnish DG, Paetkau V. Induction of interleukin 2 messenger RNA inhibited by cyclosporine A. Science 1984;226:1439-41.
5. Kronke M, Leonard WJ, Depper JM, Arya SK, Wong-Staal F, Gallo RC, Waldman TA, Green WC. Cyclosporine A inhibits T cell growth factor gene expression at the level of mRNA transcription. Proc Natl Acad Sci USA 1984;81:5214-8.
6. Handschumacher RE, Harding MW, Rice J, Drugge RJ, Speicher DW. Cyclophilin: a specific cytosolic binding protein for cyclosporin A. Science 1984;226:544-7.
7. Harding MW, Galat A, Uehling DE, Schreiber SL. A receptor for the immunosuppressant FK506 is a cis-trans peptidyl-prolyl isomerase. Nature 1989;341:758-60.
8. Fischer G, Wittmann-Liebold K, Lang T, Kiefhaber T, Schmid FX. Cyclophilin and peptidyl-prolyl *cis-trans* isomerase are probably identical proteins. Nature 1989;337:476-8.

9. Liu J, Farmer JDJr, Lane WS, Friedman J, Weissman I, Schreiber SL. Calcineurin is a common target of cyclophilin-cyclosporin A and FKBP-FK506 complexes. Cell 1991;66:807-15.
10. Clipstone NA, Crabtree GR. Identification of calcineurin as a key signalling enzyme in T-lymphocyte activation. Nature 1992;357:695-7.
11. Emmel EA, Verweij CL, Durand DB, Higgins KM, Lacy E, Crabtree GR. Cyclosporine A specifically inhibits function of nuclear proteins involved in T cell activation. Science 1989;246:1617
12. Hultsch T, Albers MW, Schreiber SL, Hohman RJ. Immunophilin ligands demonstrate common features of signal transduction leading to exocytosis or transcription. Proc Natl Acad Sci USA 1991;88:6229-33.
13. Wicker LS, Boltz RC, Matt V. Suppression of B-cell activation by cyclosporin-A, FK506, and rapamycin. Eur J Immunol 1990;20(2277):2283
14. Batiuk TD, Pazderka F, Enns J, DeCastro L, Halloran PF. Cyclosporine inhibition of calcineurin activity in human leukocytes *in vivo* is rapidly reversible. J Clin Invest 1995;96:1254-60.
15. Foxwell BMJ, Mackie A, Ling V, Ryffel B. Identification of the multi-drug resistance-related P-glycoprotein as a cyclosporine binding protein. Mol Pharmacol 1989;36:543-6.
16. Atkison P, Joubert G, Barron A, Grant D, Paradis K, Seidman E, Wall W, Rosenberg H, Howard J, Williams S, *et al.* Hypertrophic cardiomyopathy associated with tacrolimus in paediatric transplant patients. Lancet 1995;345:894-6.
17. Sigal NH, Dumont F, Durette P, Siekierka JJ, Peterson L, Rich DH, Dunlap BE, Staruch MJ, Melino MR, Koprak SL, *et al.* Is cyclophilin involved in the immunosuppressive and nephrotoxic mechanism of action of cyclosporin A? J Exp Med 1991;173:619-28.
18. Arello F, Krupp P. Muscular disorders associated with cyclosporin. Lancet 1991;337:915
19. Liu J, Albers MW, Wandless TJ, Luan S, Alberg DG, Belshaw PJ, Cohen P, MacKintosh C, Kless CB, Schreiber SL. Inhibition of T cell signaling by immunophilin-ligand complexes correlates with loss of calcineurin phosphatase activity. Biochemistry 1992;31:3896-901.
20. Fruman DA, Klee CB, Bierer BE, Burakoff SJ. Calcineurin phosphatase activity in T lymphocytes is inhibited by FK506 and cyclosporin A. Proc Natl Acad Sci USA 1992;89:3686-90.
21. Griffith JP, Kim JL, Kim EE, Sintchak MD, Thomson JA, Fitzgibbon MJ, Fleming MA, Caron PR, Hsiao K, Navia MA. X-ray structure of calcineurin inhibited by the immunophilin-immunosuppressant FKBP12-FK506 complex. Cell 1995;82:507-22.
22. Kissinger CR, Parge HE, Knighton DR, Lewis CT, Pelletier LA, Tempczyk A, Kalish VJ, Tucker KD, Showalter RE, Moomaw EW, *et al.* Crystal structure of human calcineurin and the human FKBP12-FK506-calcineurin complex. Nature 1995;378:641-4.
23. Cardenas ME, Muir RS, Breuder T, Heitman J. Targets of immunophilin-immunosuppressant complexes are distinct highly conserved regions of calcineurin A. EMBO J 1995;14(12):2772-83.
24. Bram RJ, Hung DT, Martin PK, Schreiber SL, Crabtree GR. Identification of the immunophilins capable of mediating inhibition of signal transduction by cyclosporin A and FK506: roles of calcineurin binding and cellular location. Mol Cell Biol 1993;13(8):4760-9.
25. Sewell TJ, Lam E, Martin MM, Seszyk J, Weidner J, Calaycay J, Griffin P, Williams H, Hung S, Cryan J, *et al.* Inhibition of calcineurin by a novel FK-506-binding protein. J Biol Chem 1994;269(33):21094-102.
26. Baughman G, Wiederrecht GJ, Chang F, Martin MM, Bourgeois S. Tissue distribu-

tion and abundance of human FKBP51, an FK506-binding protein that can mediate calcineurin inhibition. Biochem Biophys Res Commun 1997;232:437-43.

27. Nigam SK, Jin Y-J, Jin M-J, Bush KT, Bierer BE, Burakoff SJ. Localization of the FK506-binding protein, FKBP 13, to the lumen of the endoplasmic reticulum. Biochem J 1993;294:511-5.

28. Stewart AA, Ingebritsen TS, Cohen P. The protein phosphatases involved in cellular regulation. 5. Purification and proterties of a Ca²⁺/calmodulin-dependent protein phosphatase (2B) from rabbit skeletal muscle. Eur J Biochem 1983;132:289-95.

29. Stewart AA, Ingebritsen TS, Manalan A, Klee CB, Cohen P. Discovery of Ca²⁺- and calmodulin-dependent protein phosphatase. Probable identity with calcineurin (CaM-BP$_{80}$). FEBS Lett 1982;137(1):80-4.

30. Klee CB, Draetta GF, Hubbard MJ. Calcineurin [review]. Advances Enzymology & Related Areas of Molecular Biology 1988;61:149-200.

31. Kincaid RL. Shenolikar S, Nairn AC, editors.Advances in Second Messenger and Phosphoprotein Research. New York, NY: Raven Press; 1993; 1, Calmodulin-dependent protein phosphatases from microorganisms to man. A study in structural conservatism and biological diversity. p. 1-23.

32. Chernoff J, Sells MA, Li HC. Characterization of phosphotyrosyl-protein phosphatase activity associated with calcineurin. Biochem Biophys Res Commun 1984;121:141-8.

33. Klee CB, Krinks MH. Purification of cyclic 3', 5'-nucleotide phosphodiesterase inhibitory protein by affinity chromatography on activator protein coupled to Sepharose. Biochemistry 1979; 17:120-6.

34. Muramatsu T, Kincaid RL. Molecular cloning and chromosomal mapping of the human gene for the testis-specific catalytic subunit of calmodulin-dependent protein phosphatase (calcineurin A). Biochem Biophys Res Commun 1992;188(1):265-71.

35. Klee CB, Ren H, Wang X. Regulation of the calmodulin-stimulated protein phosphatase, calcineurin. J Biol Chem 1998;273(22):13367-70.

36. Kincaid RL, Nightingale MS, Martin BM. Characterization of a cDNA clone encoding the calmodulin-binding domain of mouse brain calcineurin. Proc Natl Acad Sci USA 1988;85:8983-7.

37. Kakalis LT, Kennedy M, Sikkink R, Rusnak F. Characterization of the calcium-binding site of calcineurin B. FEBS Lett 1995;362:55-8.

38. Hashimoto Y, Perrino BA, Soderling TR. Identification of an autoinhibitory domain in calcineurin. J Biol Chem 1990;265:1924-7.

39. Hubbard MJ, Klee CB. Functional domain structure of calcineurin A: mapping by limited proteolysis. Biochemistry 1989;28:1868-74.

40. Perrino BA, Ng LY, Soderling TR. Calcium regulation of calcineurin phosphatase activity by its B subunit and calmodulin. J Biol Chem 1995;270(1):340-6.

41. Ueki K, Muramatsu T, Kincaid RL. Structure and expression of two isoforms of the murine calmodulin-dependent protein phosphatase regulatory subunit (calcineurin B). Biochem Biophys Res Commun 1992;187(1):537-43.

42. Mukai H, Chang C-D, Tanaka H, Ito A, Kuno T, Tanaka C. cDNA cloning of a novel testis-specific calcineurin B-like protein. Biochem Biophys Res Commun 1991;179(3):1325-30.

43. King MM, Huang CY. Activation of calcineurin by nickel ions. Biochem Biophys Res Commun 1983;114:955-61.

44. King MM, Huang CY. The calmodulin-dependent activation and deactivation of the phosphoprotein phosphatase, calcineurin, and the effect of nucleotides, pyrophosphate, and divalent metal ions. J Biol Chem 1984;259:8847-56.

45. Wang X, Culotta VC, Klee CB. Superoxide dismutase protects calcineurin from inactivation. Nature 1996;383:434-7.

46. Fanger CM, Hoth M, Crabtree GR, Lewis RS . Characterization of T cell mutants with defects in capacitative calcium entry: genetic evidence for the physiological roles of CRAC channels. J Cell Biol 1995;131(3):655-67.

47. Berridge MJ. Calcium signalling and cell proliferation [review]. BioEssays 1995; 17(6):491-500.

48. Cardenas ME, Heitman J. Means AP, editors.Advances in Second Messenger and Phosphoprotein Research. New York, NY: Raven Press, Ltd.; 1995; 9, Role of calcium in T-lymphocyte activation. p. 281-98.

49. Pawson T, Scott JD. Signaling through scaffold, anchoring, and adaptor proteins. Science 1997;278:2075-80.

50. Mochly-Rosen D. Localization of protein kinases by anchoring proteins: a theme in signal transduction. Science 1995;268:247-51.

51. Coghlan VM, Perrino BA, Howard M, Langeberg LK, Hicks JB, Gallatin WM , Scott JD. Association of protein kinase A and protein phosphatase 2B with a common anchoring protein. Science 1995;267:108-11.

52. Shibasaki F, Kondo E, Akagi T, McKeon F. Suppression of signalling through transcription factor NF-AT by interactions between calcineurin and Bcl-2. Nature 1997;386:728-31.

53. Cameron AM, Steiner JP, Roskams AJ, Ali SM, Ronnett GV, Snyder SH. Calcineurin associated with the inositol 1,4,5-triphosphate receptor-FKBP12 complex modulates Ca^{2+} flux. Cell 1995;83:463-72.

54. Dell'Acqua ML, Faux MC, Thorburn J, Thorburn A, Scott JD. Membrane-targeting sequences on AKAP79 bind phosphatidylinositol-4, 5-biphosphate. EMBO J 1998;17:2246-60.

55. Carr DW, Hausken ZE, Fraser ID, Stofko-Hahn RE, Scott JD. Association of the type II cAMP-dependent protein kinase with a human thyroid RII-anchoring protein. J Biol Chem 1992;267:13376-82.

56. Faux MC, Scott JD. Molecular glue: kinase anchoring and scaffold proteins [review]. Cell 1996;85(9):12

57. Kashishian A, Howard M, Loh C, Gallatin WM, Hoekstra MF, Lai Y. AKAP79 inhibits calcineurin through a site distinct from the immunophilin-binding region. J Biol Chem 1998;273(42):27412-9.

58. Krajewski S, Tanaka S, Takayama S, Schibler MJ, Fenton W, Reed JC. Investigation of the subcellular distribution of the bcl-2 oncoprotein: residence in the nuclear envelope, endoplasmic reticulum, and outer mitochondrial membranes. Cancer Res 1993;53(19):4701-14.

59. Linette GP, Li Y, Roth K, Korsmeyer SJ. Cross talk between cell death and cell cycle progression: Bcl-2 regulates NFAT-mediated rejection. Proc Natl Acad Sci USA 1996;93:9545-52.

60. Shibasaki F, McKeon F. Calcineurin functions in Ca^{2+}-activated cell death in mammalian cells. J Cell Biol 1995;131(3):735-43.

61. Beals CR, Sheridan CM, Turck CW, Gardner P, Crabtree GR. Nuclear export of NF-ATc enhanced by glycogen synthase kinase-3. Science 1997;275:1930-3.

62. Shaw KTY, Ho AM, Raghavan A, Kim J, Jain J, Park J, Sharma S, Rao A, Hogan PG. Immunosuppressive drugs prevent a rapid dephosphorylation of transcription factor NFAT1 in stimulated immune cells. Proc Natl Acad Sci USA 1995;92: 11205-9.

63. Beals CR, Clipstone NA, Ho SN, Crabtree GR. Nuclear localization of NF-ATc by a calcineurin-dependent, cyclosporin-sensitive intramolecular interaction. Genes Dev 1997;11:824-34.

64. Zhu J, Shibasaki F, Price R, Guillemot J-C, Yano T, Dotsch V, Wagner G, Ferrara P, McKeon F. Intramolecular masking of nuclear import signal on NF-AT4 by casein kinase I and MEKK-1. Cell 1998;93:851-61.

65. Chow C-W, Rincón M, Cavanagh J, Dickens M, Davis RJ. Nuclear accumulation

of NFAT4 opposed by the JNK signal transduction pathway. Science 1997;278: 1638-41.

66. Chen L, Glover JNM, Hogan PG, Rao A, Harrison SC. Structure of the DNA-binding domains from NFAT, Fos and Jun bound specifically to DNA. Nature 1998; 392:42-8.

67. Kehlenbach RH, Dickmanns A, Gerace L. Nucleocytoplasmic shuttling factors including Ran and crm1 mediate nuclear export of NFAT *in vivo*. J Cell Biol 1998; 141(4):863-74.

68. Rao A, Luo C, Hogan PG. Transcription factors of the NFAT family: regulation and function. Ann Rev Immunol 1997;15:707-47.

69. Ho I-C, Kim JHJ, Rooney JW, Spiegelman BM, Glimcher LH. A potential role for the nuclear factor of activated T cells family of transcriptional regulatory proteins in adipogensis. Proc Natl Acad Sci USA 1998;95(26):15537-41.

70. Ranger AM, Grusby MJ, Hodge MR, Gravallese EM, de la Brousse FC, Hoey T, Mickanin C, Baldwin HS, Glimcher LH. The transcription factor NF-ATc is essential for cardiac valve formation. Nature 1998;392:186-90.

71. de la Pompa JL, Timmerman LA, Takimoto H, Yoshida H, Elia AJ, Samper E, Potter J, Wakeham A, Marengere L, Langille BL, *et al.* Role of the NF-ATc transcription factor in morphogenesis of cardiac valves and septum. Nature 1998; 392:182-6.

72. Yoshida H, Nisina H, Takimoto H, Marengere LEM, Wakeham AC, Bouchard D, Kong Y-Y, Ohteki T, Shahinian A, Bachmann M, *et al.* The transcription factor NF-ATc1 regulates lymphocyte proliferation and Th2 cytokine production. Immunity 1998;8:115-24.

73. Viola JPB, Kiani A, Bozza PT, Rao A. Regulation of allergic inflammation and eosinophil recruitment in mice lacking the transcription factor NFAT1: role of interleukin-4 (IL-4) and IL-5. Blood 1998;91(7):2223-30.

74. Ranger AM, Hodge MR, Gravallese EM, Oukka M, Davidson L, Alt FW, de la Brousse FC, Hoey T, Grusby M, Glimcher LH. Delayed lymphoid repopulation with effects in IL-4 driven responses produced by inactivation of NF-ATc. Immunity 1998;8:125-34.

75. Ranger AM, Oukka M, Rengarajan J, Glimcher LH. Inhibitory function of two NFAT family members in lymphoid homeostasis and Th2 development. Immunity 1998;9:627-35.

76. Lopez-Rodriguez C, Aramburu J, Rakeman AA, Rao A. NFAT5, a constitutively nuclear NFAT protein that does not cooperate with Fos and Jun. Proc Natl Acad Sci USA 1999;96:7214-9.

77. Sugimoto T, Stewart S, Guan KL. The calcium/calmodulin-dependent protein phosphatase calcineurin is the major Elk-1 phosphatase. J Biol Chem 1997;272(47): 29415-8.

78. Hill CS, Treisman R. Transcriptional regulation by extracellular signals: mechanisms and specificity. Cell 1995;80:199-211.

79. Lino M. Dynamic regulation of intracellular calcium signals through calcium release channels [review]. Mol Cell Biochem 1999;190(1-2):185-90.

80. Ferris CD, Huganir RL, Bredt DS, Cameron AM, Snyder SH. Inositol triphosphate receptor: phosphorylation by protein kinase C and calcium calmodulin-dependent protein kinases in reconstituted lipid vesicles. Proc Natl Acad Sci USA 1991; 88:2232-5.

81. Cameron AM, Steiner JP, Sabatini DM, Kaplin AI, Walensky LD, Snyder SH. Immunophilin FK506 binding protein associated with inositol 1,4,5-triphosphate receptor modulates calcium flux. Proc Natl Acad Sci USA 1995;92:1784-8.

82. Marietta MA. Nitric oxide synthase: aspects concerning structure and catalysis. Cell 1994;78:927-30.

83. Dawson TM, Steiner JP, Dawson VL, Dinerman JL, Uhl GR, Snyder SH. Immunosup-

pressant FK506 enhances phosphorylation of nitric oxide synthase and protects against glutamate neurotoxicity. Proc Natl Acad Sci USA 1993;90(21):9808-12.

84. Yamamoto H, Fukunaga K, Tanaka E, Miyamoto E. Ca2+- and calmodulin-dependent phosphorylation of microtubule-associated protein 2 and τ factor, and inhibition of microtubule assembly. J Neurochemistry 1983;41:1119-25.

85. Goto S, Yamamoto H, Fukunaga K, Iwasa T, Matsukado Y, Miyamoto E. Dephosphorylation of microtubule-associated protein 2, τ factor, and tubulin by calcineurin. J Neurochemistry 1985;45:276-83.

86. De Camilli P, Harris JM, Jr., Huttner WB, Greegard P. Synapsin (protein I), a nerve terminal-specific phosphoprotein. II. Its specific association with synaptic vesicles demonstrated by immunocytochemistry in agarose-embedded synaptosomes. J Cell Biol 1983;96:1355-73.

87. Llinas R, McGuiness TL, Leonard CS, Sugimori M, Greengard P. Intraterminal injection of synapsin I or calcium/calmodulin-dependent protein kinase II alters neurotransmitter release at the squid giant synapse. Proc Natl Acad Sci USA 1985;82:3035-9.

88. Huttner WB, Greengard P. Multiple phosphorylation site in protein I and their differential regulation by cyclic AMP and calcium. Proc Natl Acad Sci USA 1979; 76:5402-6.

89. Kennedy MB, Greengard P. Two calcium/calmodulin-dependent protein kinases, which are highly concentrated in brain, phosphorylate protein I at distinct sites. Proc Natl Acad Sci USA 1981; 78:1293-7.

90. De Camilli P, Takei K. Molecular mechanisms in synaptic vesicle endocytosis and recycling. Neuron 1996;16:481-6.

91. Liu J, Sim ATR, Robinson PJ. Calcineurin inhibition of dynamin I GTPase activity coupled to nerve terminal depolarization. Science 1994;265:970-3.

92. Nichols RA, Suplick GR, Brown JM. Calcineurin-mediated protein dephosphorylation in brain nerve terminals regulates the release of glutamate. J Biol Chem 1994;269(38):23817-23.

93. Frantz B, Nordby EC, Bren G, Steffan N, Paya CV, Kincaid RL, Tocci MJ, O'Keefe SJ, O'Neill EA. Calcineurin acts in synergy with PMA to inactivate IkB/MAD3, an inhibitor of NF-kB. EMBO J 1994;13:861-70.

94. Werlen G, Jacinto E, Xia Y, Karin M. Calcineurin preferentially synergizes with PKC-theta to activate JNK and IL-2 promoter in T lymphocytes. EMBO J 1998; 17(11):3101-11.

95. Zhang W, Zimmer G, Chen J, Ladd D, Li E, Alt FW, Wiederrecht G, Cryan J, O'Neill EA, Seidman CE, et al. T cell responses in calcineurin A α -deficient mice. J Exp Med 1996;183:413-20.

96. Zhu J, McKeon F. NF-AT activation requires suppressin of crm1-dependent export by calcineurin. Nature 1999;398:256-60.

97. Liu S, Liu P, Borras A, Chatila T, Speck SH. Cyclosporin A-sensitive induction of the Epstein-Barr virus lytic switch is mediated via a novel pathway involving a MEF2 family member. EMBO J 1997;16:143-53.

98. Black BL, Olson EN. Transcriptional control of muscle development by myocyte enhancer factor-2 (MEF2) proteins. Ann Rev Cell Dev Biol 1998;14:167-96.

99. Sussman MA, Lim HW, Gude N, Taigen T, Olson EN, Robbins J, Colbert MC, Gualberto A, Wieczorek DF, Molkentin JD. Prevention of cardiac hypertrophy in mice by calcineurin inhibition. Science 1998;281:1690-3.

100. Mokentin JD, Lu J-R, Antos CL, Markham B, Richardson J, Robbins J, Grant SR, Olson EN. A calcineurin-dependent transcriptional pathway for cardiac hypertrophy. Cell 1998;93:215-28.

101. Zhang W, Kowal RC, Rusnak F, Sikkink RA , Olson EN, Victor RG. Failure of calcineurin inhibitors to prevent pressure-overload left ventribular hypertrophy in rats. Circ Res 1999;84:722-8.

102. Meguro T, Hong C, Asai K, Takagi G, McKinsey TA, Olson EN, Vatner SF. Cyclosporine attenuates pressure-overload hypertrophy in mice while enhancing susceptibility to decompensation and heart failure. Circ Res 1999;84:735-40.

103. Mulkey RM, Endo S, Shenolikar S, Malenka RC. Involvement of a calcineurin/ inhibitor-1 phosphatase cascade in hippocampal long-term depression. Nature 1994;369:486-8.

104. Bito H, Deisseroth K, Tsien RW. CREB phosphorylation and dephosphorylation: a Ca2+ and stimulus duration-dependent switch for hippocampal gene expression. Cell 1996;87:1203-14.

105. Enslen H, Sun P, Brickey D, Soderling SH, Klamo E, Soderling TR. Characterisation of Ca2+/calmodulin-dependent protein kinase IV: role of transcriptional regulation. J Biol Chem 1994;269:15520-7.

106. Schiaffino S, Riggiani C. Molecular diversity of myofibrillar proteins: gene regulation and functional significance [review]. Physiol Rev 1996;76:371-423.

107. Hoey T, Sun Y-L, Williamson K, Xu X. Isolation of two new members of the NF-AT gene family and functional characterization of the NF-AT proteins. Immunity 1995;2:461-72.

108. Chin ER, Olson EN, Richardson JA, Yang Q, Humphries C, Shelton JM, Wu H, Zhu W, Bassel-Duby R, Williams RS. A calcineurin-dependent transcriptional pathway controls skeletal muscle fiber type. Genes Dev 1998;12:2499-509.

109. Musarò A, McCullagh KJA, Naya FJ, Olson EN, Rosenthal N. IGF-1 induces skeletal myocyte hypertrophy through calcineurin in association with GATA-2 and NF-ATc1. Nature 1999;400 :581

110. Dunn SE, Burns JL, Michel RN. Calcineurin is required for skeletal muscle hypertrophy. J Biol Chem 1999;274:21908-12.

111. Letterio JJ, Roberts AB. Regulation of immune responses by TGF-b. Ann Rev Immunol 1998;16:136-61.

112. Bottinger EP, Letterio JJ, Roberts AB. Biology of TGF-β in knockout and transgenic mouse models . Kidney Int 1997;51:1355-60.

113. Hojo M, Morimoto T, Maluccio M, Asano T , Morimoto K, Lagman M, Shimbo T, Suthanthiran M. Cyclosporine induces cancer progression by a cell-autonomous mechanism. Nature 1999;397:530-4.

114. Khanna A, Kapur S, Sharma V, Li B, Suthanthiran M. *In vivo* hyperexpression of transforming growth factor-β1 in mice: stimulation by cyclosporine. Transplantation 1997;63(7):1037-9.

115. Shin G-T, Khanna A, Ding R, Sharma VK, Lagman M, Li B, Suthanthiran M. *In vivo* expression of transforming growth factor-b1 in humans. Transplantation 1998;65(3):313-8.

116. Kirk AD, Jacobson LM, Heisey DM, Fass NA, Sollinger HW, Pirsch JD. Posttransplant diastolic hypertension. Transplantation 1997;64(12):1716-20.

117. Shihab FS, Andoh TF, Tanner AM, Noble NA, Border WA, Franceschini N , Bennett WM. Role of transforming growth factor-β1 in experimental chronic cyclosporine nephropathy. Kidney Int 1996;49:1141-51.

118. Shihab FS, Bennett WM, Tanner AM, Andoh TF. Mechanism of fibrosis in experimental tacrolimus nephrotoxicity. Transplantation 1997;64(12):1829-37.

119. Khanna A, Cairns V, Hosenpud JD. Tacrolimus induces increased expression of transforming growth factor-β1 in mammalian lymphoid as well as nonlymphoid cells. Transplantation 1999;67:614-9.

120. Kung L, Halloran PF. Immunophilins may limit calcineurin inhibition by cyclosporine and tacrolimus at high drug concentrations. Transplantation 2000;70(2): 327-35.

121. Aramburu J, Garcia-Cozar F, Raghavan A, Okamura H, Rao A, Hogan PG. Selective inhibition of NFAT activation by a peptide spanning the calcineurin targeting site of NFAT. Molecular Cell 1998;1:627-37.

122. Aramburu J, Yaffe MB, López-Rodriguez C, Cantley LC, Hogan PG, Rao A . Affinity-driven peptide selection of an NFAT inhibitor more selective than cyclosporin A. Science 1999;285:2129-33.
123. Jephthah-Ochola J, Urmson J, Farkas S, Halloran PF. Regulation of MHC *in vivo*. Bacterial lipopolysaccharide induces class I and II MHC products in mouse tissues by a T cell independent, cyclosporine sensitive mechanism. J Immunol 1988;141:792-800.
124. Bennett PC, Singaretnam LG, Zhao W-Q, Lawen A, Ng KT. Peptidyl-prolyl-*cis/trans*-isomerase activity may be necessary for memory formation. FEBS Lett 1998;431:386-90.

EXPERIMENTAL

2 IMMUNOSUPPRESSIVE AGENTS

Jochen Klupp and Randall E. Morris
Department of Cardiothoracic Surgery
Stanford University
Stanford, California, USA

INTRODUCTION

Today, many new small and large molecular weight molecules are being developed for use as immunosuppressive agents. As the understanding of mechanisms of immune function improves, immunosuppressive drug discovery and development is able to more specifically target activation pathways that predominate in immune rather than nonimmune cells, thus decreasing nonspecific toxicity.

Advances in structure-based drug design enables newer versions of current drugs to show improved absorption, distribution and metabolism and is a technology that is being exploited to design entirely new molecules for several molecular targets that are important for the rejection response. For many years the primary objective in the development of immunosuppressants has been to separate the suppression of rejection from the toxic side effects of these drugs. For example, it might be possible to avoid nephrotoxic and neurotoxic side effects of calcineurin inhibitors by targeting enzymes distal to calcineurin in the activation cascade.

Since there are so many new drugs currently in development and it is impossible to predict which of them will be of clinical use (either new primary or adjuctive therapy), we have organized this chapter based on the known mechanisms of action of these new non biologic immunosuppressants.

A. W. Thomson (ed.), Therapeutic Immunosuppression, 31–54.

NEW INHIBITORS OF SIGNAL I PATHWAY

Potassium channel blockers

During T–cell activation, sustained elevated Ca^{2+} levels are needed to activate gene expression. After T cell receptor complex stimulation, IP_3 formation causes Ca^{2+} release from intracellular calcium stores. Emptying of the stores triggers Ca^{2+} influx through Ca^{2+}-release activated Ca^{2+}-channels [1], which is maintained by potassium efflux channels keeping T cell membrane polarized.

Blocking potassium channels in T lymphocytes in vitro has effects similar to calcineurin inhibitors. Ionomycin + PMA, CD2 or CD3 stimulated T cells can be inhibited as measured by ^{3}H-thymidine proliferation and IL-2 production [2]. This effect can be reversed by addition of exogenous IL-2 [1]. Nonselective potassium channel blockers like tetraethylammonium (TEA) and 4-aminopyridine (4-AP) show these effects in a very high, millimolar range [2].

Nonspecific inhibition of potassium channels, however would cause severe toxicity in clinical application. Further investigations showed that there are different subsets of potassium channels. For example, Kv1.3 a voltage-gated channel, is of special interest because it is expressed abundantly in lymphocytes, compared to lower levels in fibroblasts, brain and kidney cells [3] and dominates the membrane potential only in T lymphocytes [4].

Polypeptides isolated from scorpion venoms are able to block potassium channels in the pico-molar range. Charybdotoxin inhibits Ca^{2+} activated and voltage gated potassium channels and is able to inhibit T cell activation dose dependently [2]. Margatoxin is more specific than charybdotoxin, since margatoxin only inhibits voltage gated channels [5]. However, margatoxin is not specific for lymphocytes since it also inhibits Kv1.1 and Kv1.2 channels, which are expressed in brain, peripheral nerves and the heart [4]. In vivo studies of these toxins are complicated by the fact that, Kv1.3 is not expressed by rat cells nor cells in many other experimental animals. One study in minipigs showed that margatoxin after i.v. administration of 8µg/kg/day inhibits delayed-type hypersensitivity to tuberculin, as well as an antibody response to alloantigen as effectively as 1 mg/kg/day of tacrolimus [5]. As expected, higher doses showed neurological side effects. CP-339,818, a 1,4-dihydroquinoline compound blocks both Kv1.3 and Kv1.4, so it is not being developed for clinical use [6].

Structural changes of the sea anemone toxin, ShK, generated ShK-Dap[22] which is a highly selective and potent blocker of Kv1.3 (IC_{50} of 102 pmol) [4]. ShK-Dap[22] inhibits ^{3}H-thymidine incorporation in peripheral human T cells after mitogen stimulation, with an IC_{50} below 500 pmol. When injected into mice, ShK-Dap[22] showed only minimal toxicity: paralytic doses were reached at 200mg/kg body weight.

Although further studies are required on potassium channel blockers, this group of substances have the potential to inhibit signal 1 pathway specifically and may have the potential to suppress graft rejection. Promising substances like ShK-Dap[22] need still more development to increase its oral bioavailability and its reduce toxicity before it can be used in large animal studies or human phase I trials.

SP100030

SP100030, 2-Chloro-4-(trifluoromethyl)-5-N-phenyl-pyrimidine-carboxamide, is an agent which is able to inhibit NF-κB and AP-1 [7], both known to be crucial for Signal – 1 transduction to induce IL-1, IL-2, IL-6, IL-8, TNF-α and cell adhesion molecule transcription. SP100030 was identified by its ability to block cytokine promoter activity in cells transfected with cytokine promoter-luciferase gene constructs. SP100030 concentration – dependently inhibits immune cell proliferation with IC_{50} values of 30 nmol/l. Also, in Jurkat T cells it blocks induced production of IL-2 and IL-8 at the same IC_{50}. This effect is observed in all (including human) T cells, but not in non–T cell lines (monocytes, epithelial cells, fibroblasts, synoviocytes, osteoblasts and endothelial cells) [8, 9].

In a popliteal lymph node study (BALB/c - C3H mice) SP100030 dose-dependently suppresses the alloantigen-induced PLN weight: 10 mg/kg caused 52% inhibition, compared to 12 mg/kg cyclosporine which caused only 35% inhibition. In a murine ear – heart transplant model, 15 to 20 mg/kg SP100030 administered intraperitoneally prolongs graft survival significantly for more than 30 days. Also adjuvant arthritis is reduced effectively in Lewis rats (20 – 30 mg/kg i.p.). No body weight changes or other toxicological side effects have been observed in these studies.

Although the experience with SP100030 is limited to rodent models, the results obtained show that, focusing on key enzymes of Signal 1 pathway should be able to produce significant immunosuppression with a good safety profile.

Tepoxalin

Another potent inhibitor of NF-κB activation is Tepoxalin (5-[4-chlorophenyl]-N-hydroxy-[4-methoxyphenyl]-N-methyl-1-H-pyrazole-3-propanamide; molecular weight:385). It was first discovered as a dual inhibitor of 5-lipoxygenase (LO) and cyclooxygenase (CO) and is effective in preventing inflammation and synovitis in several animal models [10]. Due to its inability to inhibit gastric prostaglandin synthesis, Tepoxalin does not cause gastric mucosa damage at anti-inflammatory doses [11]. Further investigations showed that naproxen and other CO inhibitors, as well as zileuton (a LO inhibitor), do not show the same antiproliferative effects as tepoxalin [10, 12].

Later it was shown that tepoxalin inhibits NF-κB activation in a dose related manor [13]. Tepoxalin inhibits OKT3 (IC_{50}: 5.9), PMA + ionomycin (IC_{50}: 1.6) and IL-2 induced (IC_{50}: 2.75) T cell stimulation. The antiproliferative effect is more pronounced on activated PBLs than on spontaneous proliferating cell lines [14]. It also blocks PMA + ionomycin induced IL-2R production and IL-2 induced cell proliferation and signal transduction [14]. Together with cyclosporine in suboptimal concentrations, tepoxalin suppresses T cell proliferation synergistically. Furthermore it was shown that tepoxalin suppresses IL-6, IL-8 and IFN-γ production [15, 16].

By its inhibition of NF-κB tepoxalin also suppresses expression of the cell adhesion molecules CD62E (E-selectin), CD11b/CD18 (Mac-1) and CD106 (VCAM-1), but not CD11a/CD18 (LFA-1) and CD54 (ICAM – 1) [16]. Since CD11b/CD18 and CD106 are effective in monocyte adhesion processes, tepoxalin is expected to modulate atherosclerosis and inflammation [16] as well as neutrophil migration [15]. MLR was suppressed with an IC_{50} of 1.3 μMol.

In vivo, tepoxalin suppresses local graft-versus-host responses by about 40% in mice. In skin transplantation (BALB/cByJ ($H-2^d$) to C3H/HeJ ($H-2^k$) mice), tepoxalin prolongs median survival time to 15 days with a 50 mg/kg dose, compared to 8 days in the control group [12]. Coadministration of suboptimal doses of tepoxalin (12.5 mg/kg) and cyclosporine (50 mg/kg) prolongs skin graft survival for more than 40 days [12], suggesting synergism between both drugs.

The toxicological and pharmacological profiles of tepoxalin are showing promising results. In mice and rats LD_{50} is more than 10-fold higher than immunosuppressive doses (>400 mg/kg) [12]. In healthy human volunteers [17], oral doses from 35 to 300 mg were absorbed rapidly and reached t_{max}

after 2 to 3 hours of administration. Except at the 300 mg dose, tepoxalin was not detected 24 hours after dosing ($t_{1/2}$ 1.3 to 8 hours). Tepoxalin is converted to RWJ20142, an active metabolite ($t_{1/2}$ 7 to 24 hours), which also blocks cyclooxygenase and lipooxygenase. Inhibition of NF-κB was not determined in this study. No major adverse events have been recorded. Five out of 20 healthy participants reported abdominal discomfort, diarrhea or lightheadness.

In summary, by blocking NF-κB, tepoxalin is mechanistically different from cyclosporine and tacrolimus and acts synergistically with cyclosporine. With only minor toxicity and a good pharmacological profile, transplantation studies in larger animals could be promising.

Dithiocarbamates

Dithiocarbamates are defined by possession of a $(R_1)(R_2)N-C(S)-S-R_3$ functional group [18]. They are known as anti-oxidants and they have agricultural (fungicides and insecticides, Tetramethylthiuram disulphide) and clinical (alcohol aversion therapy, Disulphiran DSF) applications. Especially Diethyldithiocarbamate (DDTC) and Pyrrolidine Dithiocarbamate (PDTC) are used for cell biology investigations. Like other antioxidants used as anti-inflammatory agents or radical scavengers (Acetylsalicylate ASS, Sulfasalazine 5-ASA, N-Acetylcystein NAC), PDTC and DDTC are able to inhibit activation of the NF-κB transcription factor [18-22] by preventing IκBα phosphorylation [23]

Similar to NAC, PDTC not only inhibits NF-κB, but also activates AP-1 [19]. Furthermore DTCs strongly inhibit NFAT and are able to inhibit T cell activation, CD25 expression in response to costimulation with CD28 and CD2 antibodies, as well as IL-2 secretion by costimulation with antibodies against CD3 and CD28 [19]. Due to the AP-1 stimulation, CD69 expression is not completely blocked by DTCs after PMA and ionophore activation in T cells and ICAM-1 expression is activated in endothelial cells by PDTC. However, DTCs lead to blockade of IL-2 and thereby to inhibition of T cell activation.

Since NF-κB also promotes HIV-1 replication, all the drugs mentioned above have been investigated for antiviral therapy [20, 21]. The role of DTCs in preventing apoptotic cell death is still controversial: in doses which are able to block NF-κB (50 – 500 μM) PDTC is able to prevent apoptosis in human promyelocytic leukemia (HL-60) cells [24] but stimulates apoptosis of rabbit osteoclasts [25]. When thymocytes are incubated with PDTC or DDTC for incubation periods longer than six hours, cells show typical signs of apoptosis [18]. It is suggested that toxicity of PDTC is related to its ability to chelate metal in a lipophilic membrane-permeable complex [18]. PDTC has also been reported to induce apoptosis in vascular smooth muscle cells [26]. Another member of this family of metal chelators, DSF, enhances in vivo accumulation of copper in the cerebellum and hippocampus of treated rats [18].

Due to this potentially toxic profile, it is doubtful if PDTC or DDTC will ever enter larger animal trials. However, these substances will remain excellent instruments to investigate gene transcription in activated T cells furthermore.

Protein Tyrosine Kinase inhibitors

Genistein (5,7,4'-trihydroxyflavone), an isoflavanoid compound, has been shown to specifically inhibit protein tyrosine kinases (PTK) [27]. Genistein is able to reduce activated killer T lymphocyte mediated lysis of tumor cells by 50% in a 100 micromolar solution [28]. Other PTK inhibitors like herbimycin A showed a higher potency in the same experimental setting (93% inhibition by 2 µMol). Genistein (180 µMol) ininhibits the induction of Fas-based cytotoxicity [29] and is also able to inhibit PMA or PHA / anti-CD28 stimulated T cell proliferation in a 40 µMol solution [30]. Also IL2-R and IL2 production are inhibited by genistein at the same concentrations needed for inhibition of proliferation [30].

PT I, a synthetic derivative of genistein was further evaluated in an in vivo

Table 1 Anecdotally cited signal 1 inhibitors under development		
Hydroquinone	Inhibits NFκB reversibly. Possible cause of toxicity of cigarettes	[97]
Momordins	Reduces Jan/Fos binding to Ap-1	[98]
Ro 09-2210	Small molecule isolated from fungus FC2506. Able to block CD3 and CD25 induced T cell proliferation; inhibits AP-1 and selectively MEK1	[99]
YM-53792	Inhibitor of NF-AT activation but not of AP-1 or NFκB. Inhibits IL-2, IL-4, IL-5 in peripheral blood	[100]
Lymphostatin	Inhibits protein-tyrosine kinase p56lck dose dependently. Suppresses IL-2 production in vitro and MLR	[101, 102]

study with pancreatic islet allograft transplantation: Lewis rats treated with 3 mg/kg *PT I* for 15 days accepted Wistar-Furth islet allografts for almost 100 days. [31]

Others

Other signal 1 inhibitors are listed in Table 1. Reports of these drugs are only anecdotal and their future importance remains to be seen.

NEW INHIBITORS OF SIGNAL II PATHWAY

Methylxanthine derivatives

Methylxanthine derivatives are known to have some immunomodulatory effects. However, the IC_{50}'s of theophylline (>400 µmol) and pentoxifylline (113 µmol) are higher than plasma levels which can be achieved in clinical settings [32]. By inhibition of cAMP phosphodiesterase activity methylxanthine derivatives are able to suppress T cell proliferation to alloantigens and mitogens, inhibit generation of cytotoxic T lymphocytes and natural killer cell-mediated cytolysis [33]. These effects are mainly due to suppression of TH_1 function by reducing production of inflammatory cytokines, including TNF-α, IFN-γ and IL-2 [34]. Due to high plasma levels required, pentoxifylline showed no effect on the incidence of rejection episodes in renal transplant patients [35].

A802715, 7-propyl-1-(5-hydroxy-5 methylhexyl)-3 methylxanthin, was further developed due to its lower IC_{50} (41 µmol) in suppressing TNF-α and IFN-γ production after LPS stimulation [32]. Additionally A802715 enhances TH_2 driven cytokines like IL-6 and IL-10. [36]. In contrast to other methylxanthine derivatives, A802715 is able to suppress not only CD3 stimulated human T cells, but also CD28 stimulated human T cells [37]. In vitro, a synergistic effect between A802715 and cyclosporine was shown with a high combination index (1/CI=9, where 1/CI > 1 is synergistic) in MLR and cell-mediated lympholysis assays [37]. Whereas signal 1 inhibition can be ascribed to cAMP elevation, the mechanism of additional signal 2 inhibition of A802715 is not known.

In vivo, this effect could also be proven [38]: Minimally effective oral doses of A802715 (100mg/kg/day) in combination with cyclosporine (7.5 mg/kg/day) for 30 days led to long term survival of cardiac allografts in rats. In an MHC compatible model (Wag/Rij – R/A), this combination results in donor specific tolerance by suppressing cytotoxic T cells and persisting TH$_2$ cells. Tolerance could not be achieved in a MHC incompatible model (WKAH – PVG).

Methylxanthines may also be beneficial by decreasing cyclosporine side effects: cyclosporine induced nephrotoxicity may be caused by decreased cAMP levels [39] and pentoxifylline was effective in decreasing cyclosporine induced toxicity, probably related to an effect on endothelin release and vasoconstriction [40].

The combination of methylxanthine derivatives with an additional inhibitory effect on signal 2, like A802715, with cyclosporine is promising not only because of its synergistic effect in immunosuppression, but also by its potential reversal of cyclosporine nephropathy.

NEW INHIBITORS OF NUCLEOTIDE SYNTHESIS

VX-497

Based on the three dimensional crystal structure of IMPDH, VX-497 was rationally designed. VX-497 belongs to a new class of phenyl oxazole inhibi-

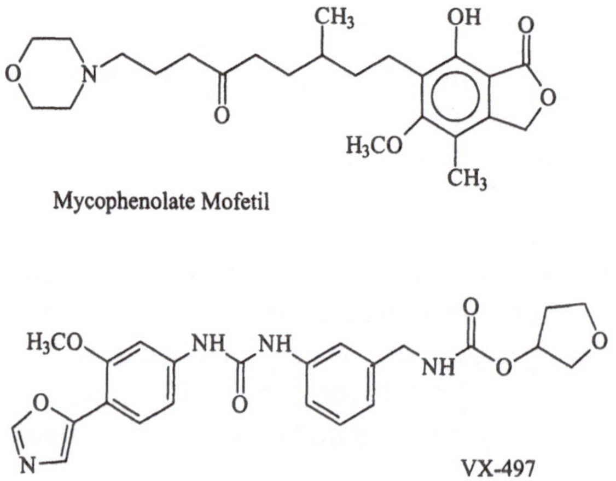

Mycophenolate Mofetil

VX-497

Figure 1
Comparison of the chemical structures of the IMPDH inhibitors MMF and VX-497

tors of IMPDH [41] and is structurally unrelated to other IMPDH inhibitors (Figure 1) like MPA or ribavirin. In vitro this uncompetitive and reversible inhibitor of IMPDH down regulates proliferation of human lymphocytes dose dependently. In vivo VX-497 prolongs skin graft survival in mice and prolongs heterotopic heart graft survival in a Brown Norway to Lewis heart transplant model [41]. In this study, graft survival was prolonged to 28 days with 75 mg/kg BID dosing.

The main difference between VX497 and MPA is the absence of enterohepatic circulation for VX-497. Since this enterohepatic recirculation is thought to be the main reason for gastrointestinal toxicity from treatment with mycophenolate mofetil, this aspect of VX-497 may lead to an improved tolerability. In effective doses (75 mg/kg BID) VX-497 caused no enteritis in histopathological studies.

Although only limited data are available for VX-497, this drug offers a new perspective in drug development: using structure based drug design to create a new molecule that inhibits a validated target (IMPDH) while simultaneous increasing safety by altering its route of excretion [42]. Future work will be needed to determine whether VX-497 is as effective as mycophenolate mofetil and to determine whether this new chemical entity can be used safely.

Malononitrilamides

Leflunomide (HWA 486) was first reported as a new chemical entity in 1976, but its ability to suppress immune function was not reported till 1985 [43]. Since then, the clinical, pharmacological and pharmacokinetic profiles of the drug itself and the active metabolite A77 1726 have become better understood [44]. The active metabolite of leflunomide (A77 1726) has a long plasma half life of 11 to 16 days [45]. Therefore, changes in dose are not rapidly translated into changes in levels. This is not a problem in the treatment of rheumatoid arthritis since patients are on a fixed dose, but if leflunomide were to be used in transplant patients and if it were to require constant dose adjustment to maintain a narrow range of plasma levels, its long half life would be a liability. There are no plans to develop leflunomide for transplantation since it is at the end of its patent life. Since nothing is known about the doses and levels needed to suppress rejection in man and since drug-drug interactions between leflunomide and other medications used in transplant patients have not be investigated, use of leflunomide off label does incur a risk.

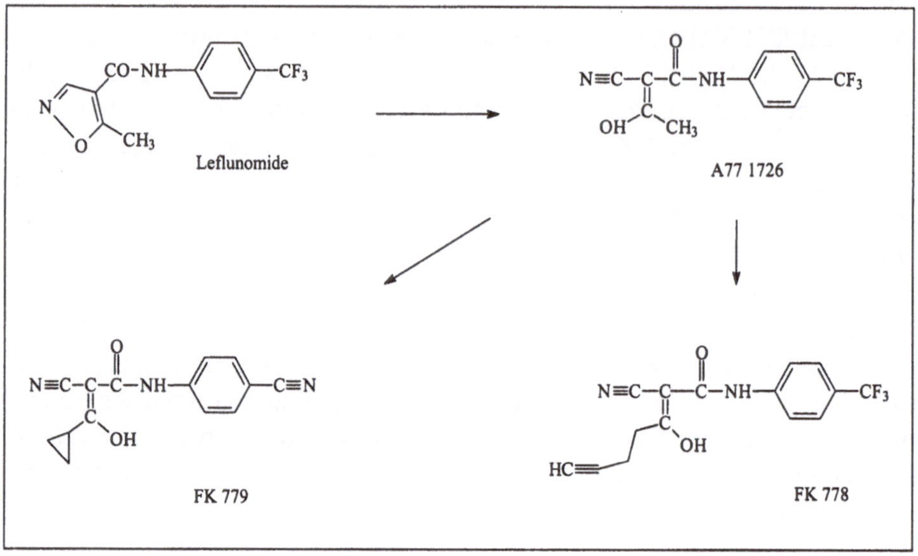

Figure 2
The MNA's Leflunomide, A77 1726, FK778 and FK779

In the last decade more than 80 derivatives of the MNA, A77 1726 have been created, by systematically exchanging molecular side groups [46]. Two compounds, MNA279 and MNA715, have been selected for further development. These are now known as FK779 and FK778. FK779 is 2-cyano-N-(4-cynaophenyl)-3-cyclopropyl-3-hydroxy-propenoic acid amid ($C_{14}H_{11}N_3O_2$) and has a molecular weight of 253,26 Da; FK778 is chemically named 2-cyano-3-hydroxy-N-[4-(trifluoromethyl)-phenyl]-2-hepten-6-ynoic acid ($C_{15}H_{11}F_3N_2O_2$) and has a molecular weight of 308,26 Da (Figure 2). In contrast to leflunomide, FK778 and especially FK779 have a shorter half life in rodents. Both have a very good oral bioavailability [47]. Like A77 1726 [48, 49], both are able to bind specifically to dihydro-orotate-dehydrogenase (DHODH) and inhibit dose dependently de novo pyrimidine biosynthesis [44, 47, 50]. DHODH is the fourth enzyme in the de novo pathway for pyrimidine biosynthesis (Figure 3) and is located on the inner membrane of the mitochondria [51]. Pyrimidine nucleotides are essential for RNA and DNA synthesis and for membrane lipid biosynthesis and protein glycosylation. Activated T and B cells rely primarily on the de novo pathway for both purine and pyrimidine biosynthesis, whereas other cell types and resting T and B cells are able to synthesize purines and pyrimidines using the salvage pathway [52].

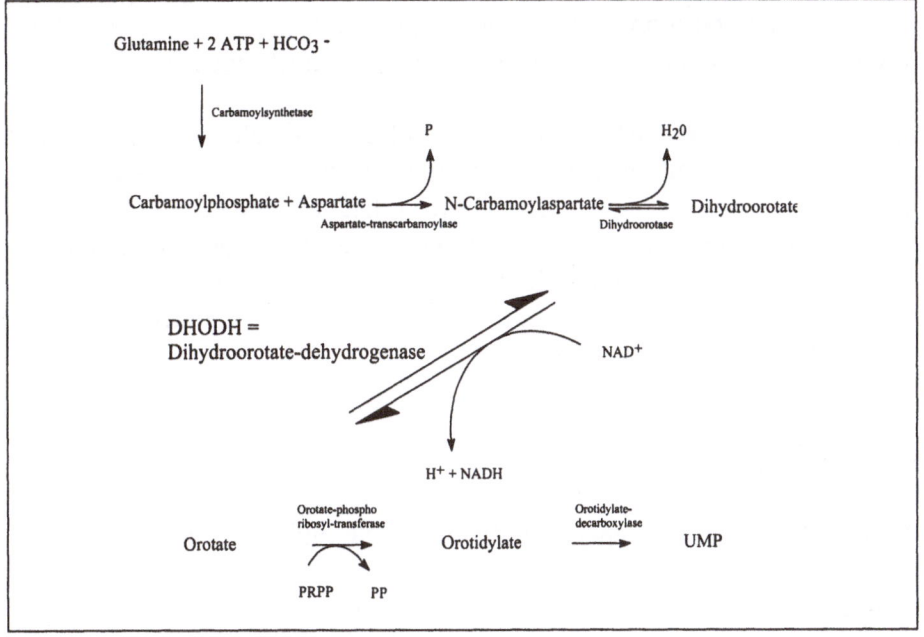

Figure 3
De novo pyrimidine synthesis. DHODH is the fourth enzyme in the synthesis, which is inhibited by the MNA's.

Mechanism of action

Leflunomide and its active metabolite A77 1726 are able to inhibit T cell activation directly, T cell independent B cell activation, IgG and IgM antibody production, and smooth muscle cell proliferation in vitro [44, 53]. Thus it was expected that the MNA's would have the same mechanism of action. Data showed that FK 778 inhibited human T cell activation (IC_{50} < 10 umol/L), with a potency that is independent of the type of the mode of stimulation of T cells by mitogen or of a combination of TCR signal and CD28-mediated activation [54]. In a culture of purified human B cells, activated by the presence of BHK_{CD40L} cells, FK 778 effectively inhibit the proliferative response and also IgG and IgM synthesis [54]. FK 779 and 778 show also an effect on monocyte function and are able to reduce oxygen radical formation [55].

Comparing different MNA's with A77 1726 in different species, it was shown, that the antiproliferative potency of FK778 is equal to the active metabolite and more potent than FK779 in cultures of human and baboon immune cells and less potent then FK779 in cultures of rat and pig immune cells [56]. In whole blood lymphocyte stimulation FK778 was more effective than FK779 in rhesus monkeys, dogs and cats and the rat T-cells were highly resistant to the effect of both analogues when compared with A77 1726 [57]. Both MNA's also inhibit growth-factor stimulated rat smooth muscle cells [58].

The primary mechanism by which MNA's inhibit cell proliferation is believed by some to be inhibition of membrane receptor-associated protein tyrosine kinase [59]. However, later studies showed that concentrations required for inhibiting tyrosine kinase far exceed the concentration [60] required for anti-proliferative effects. It is possible that concentrations of MNA's in vivo could be high enough that inhibition of tyrosine kinase activity contributes to the antiproliferative effect of these drugs.

Preclinical animal studies

So far, all published in vivo studies for FK778 and 779 have been in the rodent. After single and multiple oral dose studies in the rat, the AUC increases dose-dependently [44]. In contrast to A77 1726, FK778 and 779 show a decreased clearance after multiple dosing compared to single dosing. For a given dose of MNA or leflunomide, the exposure (AUC) differs (FK778 > FK779 > A77 1726). The pharmacokinetics show high interindividual variability at a given dose.

Prompted by their ability to suppress T and B cell proliferation, including IgG and IgM response, FK778 and 779 were examined for treatment of graft-versus-host-disease (GvHD) [47]. In an acute life-threatening GvHD model involving injection of $1x10^8$ parenteral C57BL/6 splenocytes into B6C3F1 hybrid recipient mice, both MNA's were able to prolong survival in a dose dependent manner (2.5 to 20 mg/kg). With high concentrations mortality was prevented completely [61-64].

In different rodent models (Lewis to Fisher (F344), Dark Agouti to Lewis) FK778 and 779 were able to prolong skin allograft survival in a dose dependent manner after oral gavage. The minimum effective dose (2.5mg/kg) prolonged graft survival for 5 to 10 days. Both MNA's showed similar dose response curves and an efficacy equal to cyclosporine in preventing acute skin graft rejection [65]. For reversal of acute rejection, again both MNA's were effective at a dose of 10 mg/kg, whereas a delayed treatment with cyclosporine (20mg/kg) failed to rescue the skin grafts [65]. Potentiation of efficacy was also shown between tacrolimus and MNAs for prevention and treatment of skin allograft rejection. Using a combination of ineffective doses of tacrolimus dose (0.2 mg/kg) and FK778 or FK779 (20mg/kg), tolerance induction (survival > 75 days) was achieved after withdrawal of immunosuppression at day 20.

After heterotopic heart transplantation between different strains of rats, oral treatment of 10mg/kg FK778 resulted in indefinite graft survival. Even after stopping immunosuppression more than half of the grafts survived more than 3 months [66]. Delayed treatment from postoperative day 4 on, pro-longed graft survival from 38 to more than 100 days [67]. Furthermore, the MNA's potentiated the immunosuppressive effect of cyclosporine in the rat heart model [47, 50]

In a life dependent kidney transplantation trial (DA to PVG), 10 days of FK779 treatment (10 mg/kg) prolongs animal survival to 36.5 ± 34.0 days versus 9 days in the control group [47]. In a dose evaluation study 50% of the treated rats died after dosing with 15 mg/kg FK779 due to gastrointestinal side effects. At 7.5mg/kg, no toxicity was observed and kidney allograft sur-vival was prolonged for up to 34 days, with only slight increases in urea and creatinine [47].

The ability of the MNA's to prevent smooth muscle cell proliferation led to studies preventing and treating graft vascular disease and chronic rejection. It could be demonstrated that in BN femoral allograft segments transplanted orthotopically into LEW rats, intimal thickening was reduced by MNA's at a dose of 10/mg/kg [68].

Blocking T cell independent B cell activation and antibody formation is a promising mode of action for suppressing responses to xenografts. In the mouse to rat skin xenograft model, FK778 and 779 prolong skin graft survival dose dependently (10 – 20 mg/kg). Also, delayed therapy increases graft survival significantly. Xenoantibody formation was reduced at a dose of 20 mg/kg [47, 69]. Both cyclosporine and tacrolimus, potentiate the efficacy of the MNAs, whereas single therapy with an ineffective dose of cyclosporine (10 mg/kg) or tacrolimus (0.2 mg/kg) is not able to prolong xenograft survival [70, 71].

In the hamster to rat cardiac xenotransplantation model, a combination of cyclosporine and MNA's results in a long-term xenograft survival [66]. After administration of 10 mg/kg cyclosporine and 10 mg/kg of FK778 graft sur-vival is prolonged for over 30 days.

In summary these studies demonstrate that the MNA's are promising new immunosuppressive agents. Blocking T- and B-cell proliferation and poten-tiation of the efficacy of cyclosporine or tacrolimus support ongoing development of these MNAs and other members of this class for suppression of allo- and xenograft rejection. Ongoing preclinical efficacy studies in nonhuman primates and human Phase I trials will provide the pharmacokinetic, efficacy, and safety data that will determine which of the MNA's enters Phase II trials.

Deazaguanine analogues

Purine nucleoside phosphorylase (PNP) is an essential enzyme of the purine salvage pathway. It has been shown that humans with an inherited deficiency of PNP have a relatively selective depletion of T cells, while B-cell immunity remains intact [72]. Most likely, this selective inhibition of T cells is secondary to an accumulation of deoxyguanosine-triphosphate (dGTP), which apparently suppresses ribonucleotide reductase activity and hence, DNA synthesis [73].

8-amino-guanosine and 8-amino-9-benzyl-guanine derivatives have been developed to inhibit PNP. However, they showed high toxicity in doses required for T cell suppression [72]. Applying crystallographic methods and structure-based design, new PNP-inhibitors (9-deazaguanine derivatives) were developed for treatment of T cell-mediated inflammatory response, T cell-leukemia and prevention of organ rejection [74]. BCX-34 (2-amino-1,5-dihydro-7-(3-pyridinylmethyl)-4H-pyrrolo[3,2-d]pyrimidin-4-one) (Figure 4) is a potent 9-deazaguanine derivative, which is not only able to increase intracellular dGTP in human cells, but also to decrease intracellular guanosine-triphosphate (GTP) [73]. Decreased pools of GTP caused by mycophenolic acid are, known to suppress T cell proliferation [75].

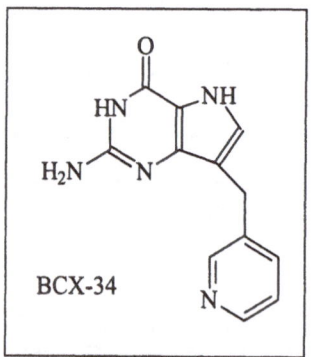

BCX-34

Figure 4
BCX-34 (2-amino-1,5-dihy-dro-7- (3-pyridinylmethyl)-4H-pyrrolo [3,2-d] pyrimidin-4-one) is a potent 9-deazaguanine derivative.

In vitro BCX-34 inhibits human, mouse and rat red blood cell PNP with IC_{50}'s of 36, 32 and 5 nMol, respectively. In a T cell culture of human leukemia cells (CCRF-CEM) BCX-34 inhibits cell proliferation in the presence, but not in the absence of deoxyguanine (dGuo). Deoxycytidine reverses the inhibition caused by BCX-34 and dGuo [73]. The maximum inhibitory effect on human PNP and T cell proliferation is about 80%, whereas BCX-34 is not able to inhibit rat or mouse T cell proliferation. Since PNP in rodent

T cells is inhibited, the reason for its lack of efficacy is explained by the fact that rodent T cells do not accumulate dGTP, but the mechanism responsible for the failure of rodent cells to accumulate dGTP is not understood. Additional in vitro studies [76] showed that BCX-34 is not only acting in malignant human T cell-lines, but also in peripheral blood mononuclear cells. After OKT3, tetanus toxoid and IL-2 induced proliferation, BCX-34 showed IC_{50}'s of 4 µMol, 0.7 µMol and 14.6 µMol. BCX-34 does not inhibit tetanus toxoid induced IL-2 release, which confirms the hypothesis that this drug arrests cells late in their cell cycle. The human mixed lymphocyte reaction is also inhibited by BCX-34 dose dependently [77].

The pharmacokinetics of BCX-34 showed a rapid disappearance after iv injection (within 3 hours; 1mg/kg in rats) and a good oral bioavailability of 76%. Half-lives were not calculated in these studies, but detectable plasma levels were observed 12 hours after a 10 mg/kg oral dose of BCX-34 [73]. Toxicological data have not been published and only neurological disorders of PNP deficient patients suggest what the adverse effects of this drug may be.

Since BCX-34 is not able to inhibit rodent T cell proliferation, no in vivo efficacy data are available yet. Clinical trials are testing BCX-34 in dermal applications for psoriasis and T cell lymphoma [73]. Based on its mechanism of action, its high bioavailability, and its capability to potentiate the efficacies of cyclosporine and tacriolimus, BCX-34 may be used in transplantation. Further toxicological trials and efficacy studies in non-human primates would have to be done to better predict its future for use in transplant patients.

OTHERS

FTY720

Myriocin (ISP-1) was isolated from the ascomycete Isaria sinclairii, which is parasitic in insects and plants. Extracts from this fungi imperfecti, have been used widely in traditional Chinese medicine. However ISP-1 produced fatal side effects in experimental animals during drug evaluation and further development was stopped. FTY720, 2-amino-2-(2-[4-octylphenyl]ethyl)-1,3-propanediol hydrochloride ($C_{19}H_{33}NO_2$–HCL, Figure 1) with a molecular weight of 343.94 Da is a synthetic structural analog of ISP-1. [78, 79]

FTY720 has a completely new mechanism of action, which is not related to

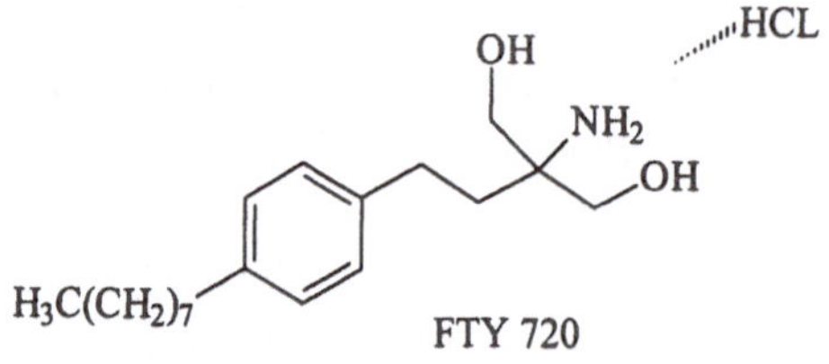

Figure 5
FTY 720 acts by promoting homing of lymphocytes into Payer's Plaques and lymph nodes.

any other mechanism of action of any known immunosuppressive agents. It inhibits T cell dependent and independent immunity and suppresses T cell infiltration into grafted organs by depletion of peripheral lymphocytes to 3% of the original cell count within 3 hours after oral application [80]. FTY 720 does not effect T or B cell function in vitro in concentrations which are able to modulate immune response in vivo. Although the mechanism of action is not yet fully understood, it is likely that FTY720 acts by a combination of altered T cell traffic but probably not by inducing apoptosis as originally thought [81, 82].

Mechanism of action
ISP-1 and related compounds inhibit allogenic mixed lymphocyte reactions (MLR) and interleukin-2 dependent proliferation in a mouse cell line [80]. However, FTY720 in doses up to 1000 nmol/l does not inhibit MLR, IL-2 production, mRNA expression by antigen- or mitogen-stimulated T cells [83], cytokine-driven cell proliferation, or cytotoxic T cell generation or action [84]. High concentrations (4×10^{-6} M) added in vitro to rat lymphocytes induce chromatin condensation, formation of apoptotic bodies and DNA fragmentation [82, 84, 85]. Two lines of evidence led to the hypothesis that FTY720 leads to apoptotic cell death: First, FTY720 (10mg/kg) induces a marked reduction of peripheral lymphocytes in rats, and second, dead cells increased with time in spleen cells cultured with FTY720 [85].

More recent reports however indicate, that FTY720 acts by selectively depleting T and B cells from blood and sequesters lymphocytes into lymph nodes and Peyer's plaques [86-88]. The initial explanations for this mechanism of action were, that FTY720 increases adhesion of lymphocytes to high endothelial venules in the lymphoid tissues by up-regulating LFA-1, ICAM-1 and L-selectin [87, 89]. Later analysis showed that FTY720 does not modulate selectins and adhesion molecule expression in lymphocytes and high endothelial venules. Since the effect of FTY720 is blocked by pertussis toxin, it has been suggested that FTY720 functions through G-protein coupled receptors and that an increased response of the lymphocytes to chemokines may cause the homing into lymph nodes and Peyer's plaques (Brinkmann V. et al.; unpublished data). Supporting the hypothesis that FTY720 is acting by increasing the homing of lymphocytes rather than by inducing T cell death is that FTY720 does not alter the function of the resting memory T cell pool. For example, mice immune to Lymphocytic Choriomeningitis Virus efficiently eliminate the virus from lung, kidney, liver spleen and blood after ending FTY720 treatment.

Toxicity and Pharmacokinetics

While ISP-1 induces severe digestive disorders at a dose of 1 mg/kg, resulting in death of the animals, the toxicologic profile of FTY720 is completely different: It was observed to have no toxic effects in rats (3 mg/kg) and monkeys (0.3 mg/kg) at doses that are immunosuppressive [80, 85]. LD_{50} in rats is 300 to 600 mg/kg and no deaths were reported in dogs that received a single dose of less than 200 mg/kg [80]. Rats gained weight during 5 mg/kg treatment and showed only slightly increased levels of BUN , creatinine, and transaminase [90]. In other toxicologic studies (Brinkmann et al., not published) no renal, pancreatic or bone marrow toxicity was observed. At high concentrations adverse effects on the lungs have been recorded.

Oral bioavailability in rats (80%), dogs (60%), and monkeys (40%) is good , with a half life of 12 to 29 hours in a dose range between 0.1 and 3 mg/kg [80]. None of the identified metabolites is immunosuppressive. The metabolites are excreted in urine and feces at ratios between 20 to 50% in different species.

Preclinical animal studies

In autoimmune and anti-inflammatory models FTY720 inhibited hypersensitivity responses in mice (0.03 mg/kg), joint destruction in an arthritis model in rats (0.1 mg/kg) and allergic encephalomyelitis [80]. In dose response studies, 0.1 to 10 mg/kg FTY720 prolongs skin, heart, liver and small bowel survival in rats [80, 84, 91]. Also in graft-versus-host disease in rats, FTY720 causes unresponsiveness (0.1 – 0.3 mg/kg) [92]. In canine kidney transplantation FTY720 given twice (5 mg/kg) at before and on the day of operation day results in a median graft survival of 21 days versus 9 days in the control group [85]. Posttransplant daily dosing (5 mg/kg) is not effective. However FTY 720 when combined with a subtherapeutic dose of cyclosporine (10 mg/kg) prolongs graft survival significantly [85]. Synergistic interaction with cyclosporine (CI = 0.15 – 0.37) or sirolimus (CI = 0.22 – 0.53) was also reported in heart, liver and small bowel transplantation in rats [84, 93] and with tacrolimus in heart transplantation [94]. In a nonhuman primate kidney model, FTY720 and subtherapeutic cyclosporine prolongs graft survival in a supra-additive effect [80]. Furthermore, FTY720 (5 mg/kg) is able to reverse ongoing rejections after heterotopic heart [94] and orthotopic liver transplants [85] in rats and after kidney transplantation in dogs [95]. Together with allochimeric class I MHC antigen FTY720 induces tolerance in a Wistar Furth to ACI rat heart transplant model [96].

In summary, FTY720 shows promising results in different animal studies. Its different mode of action and acceptable safety profile in animals suggests this drug will have a role in clinical transplantation in combination with other drugs or as rescue therapy for ongoing rejections.

REFERENCES

1. Garcia ML, Hanner M, Kaczorowski GJ. Scorpion toxins: tools for studying K+ channels. Toxicon 1998;36(11):1641-50.
2. Lin CS, Boltz RC, Blake JT, et al. Voltage-gated potassium channels regulate calcium-dependent pathways involved in human T lymphocyte activation. Journal of Experimental Medicine 1993;177(3):637-45.
3. Lewis RS, Cahalan MD. Potassium and calcium channels in lymphocytes. Annual Review of Immunology 1995;13:623-53.
4. Kalman K, Pennington MW, Lanigan MD, et al. ShK-Dap22, a potent Kv1.3-specific immunosuppressive polypeptide. Journal of Biological Chemistry 1998;273(49): 32697-707.
5. Koo GC, Blake JT, Talento A, et al. Blockade of the voltage-gated potassium channel Kv1.3 inhibits immune responses in vivo. Journal of Immunology 1997; 158(11):5120-8.
6. Nguyen A, Kath JC, Hanson DC, et al. Novel nonpeptide agents potently block the C-type inactivated conformation of Kv1.3 and suppress T cell activation. Molecular Pharmacology 1996;50(6):1672-9.
7. Sullivan RW, Bigam CG, Erdman PE, et al. 2-Chloro-4-(trifluoromethyl)pyrimidine-5-N-(3',5'- bis(trifluoromethyl)phenyl)-carboxamide: a potent inhibitor of NF-kappa B- and AP-1-mediated gene expression identified using solution-phase combinatorial chemistry. Journal of Medicinal Chemistry 1998;41(4):413-9.
8. Morikawa M, Shorthouse RA, Suto MJ, Goldman ME, Morris RE. A novel inhibitor of nuclear factor-kappa B and activator protein-1 transcription factors in T cells suppresses host-versus-graft alloreactivity in vivo. Transplantation Proceedings 1997;29(1-2):1269-70.
9. Goldman ME, Ransone LJ, Anderson DW, et al. SP100030 is a novel T-cell-specific transcription factor inhibitor that possesses immunosuppressive activity in vivo. Transplantation Proceedings 1996;28(6):3106-9.
10. Ritchie DM, Argentieri DC, Aparicio BL, Plante RK, Lau CY, Barbone AG. Cytokine-modulating activity of tepoxalin, a new potential antirheumatic. International Journal of Immunopharmacology 1995;17(10):805-12.

11. Wallace JL, Cirino G, Cicala C, Anderson DW, Argentieri D, Capetola RJ. Comparison of the ulcerogenic properties of tepoxalin with those of non-steroidal anti-inflammatory drugs (NSAIDs). Agents & Actions 1991;34(1-2):247-50.

12. Fung-Leung WP, Pope BL, Chourmouzis E, Panakos JA, Lau CY. Tepoxalin, a novel immunomodulatory compound, synergizes with CsA in suppression of graft-versus-host reaction and allogeneic skin graft rejection. Transplantation 1995;60(4):362-8.

13. Kazmi SM, Plante RK, Visconti V, Taylor GR, Zhou L, Lau CY. Suppression of NF kappa B activation and NF kappa B-dependent gene expression by tepoxalin, a dual inhibitor of cyclooxygenase and 5-lipoxygenase. Journal of Cellular Biochemistry 1995;57(2):299-310.

14. Zhou L, Ritchie D, Wang EY, Barbone AG, Argentieri D, Lau CY. Tepoxalin, a novel immunosuppressive agent with a different mechanism of action from cyclosporin A. Journal of Immunology 1994;153(11):5026-37.

15. Zhou L, Pope BL, Chourmouzis E, Fung-Leung WP, Lau CY. Tepoxalin blocks neutrophil migration into cutaneous inflammatory sites by inhibiting Mac-1 and E-selectin expression. European Journal of Immunology 1996;26(1):120-9.

16. Lee DH, Tam SS, Wang E, Taylor GR, Plante RK, Lau CY. The NF-kappa B inhibitor, tepoxalin, suppresses surface expression of the cell adhesion molecules CD62E, CD11b/CD18 and CD106. Immunology Letters 1996;53(2-3):109-13.

17. Waldman SA, Vitow C, Osborne B, et al. Pharmacokinetics and pharmacodynamics of tepoxalin after single oral dose administration to healthy volunteers. Journal of Clinical Pharmacology 1996;36(5):462-8.

18. Orrenius S, Nobel CS, van den Dobbelsteen DJ, Burkitt MJ, Slater AF. Dithiocarbamates and the redox regulation of cell death. Biochemical Society Transactions 1996;24(4):1032-8.

19. Martinez-Martinez S, Gomez del Arco P, Armesilla AL, et al. Blockade of T-cell activation by dithiocarbamates involves novel mechanisms of inhibition of nuclear factor of activated T cells. Molecular & Cellular Biology 1997;17(11):6437-47.

20. Wahl C, Liptay S, Adler G, Schmid RM. Sulfasalazine: a potent and specific inhibitor of nuclear factor kappa B. Journal of Clinical Investigation 1998;101(5):1163-74.

21. Kopp E, Ghosh S. Inhibition of NF-kappa B by sodium salicylate and aspirin [see comments]. Science 1994;265(5174):956-9.

22. Lin KI, Lee SH, Narayanan R, Baraban JM, Hardwick JM, Ratan RR. Thiol agents and Bcl-2 identify an alphavirus-induced apoptotic pathway that requires activation of the transcription factor NF-kappa B. Journal of Cell Biology 1995; 131(5):1149-61.

23. Beauparlant P, Hiscott J. Biological and biochemical inhibitors of the NF-kappa B/Rel proteins and cytokine synthesis. Cytokine & Growth Factor Reviews 1996; 7(2):175-90.

24. Bessho R, Matsubara K, Kubota M, et al. Pyrrolidine dithiocarbamate, a potent inhibitor of nuclear factor kappa B (NF-kappa B) activation, prevents apoptosis in human promyelocytic leukemia HL-60 cells and thymocytes. Biochemical Pharmacology 1994;48(10):1883-9.

25. Ozaki K, Takeda H, Iwahashi H, Kitano S, Hanazawa S. NF-kappa B inhibitors stimulate apoptosis of rabbit mature osteoclasts and inhibit bone resorption by these cells. FEBS Letters 1997;410(2-3):297-300.

26. Henkel T, Machleidt T, Alkalay I, Kronke M, Ben-Neriah Y, Baeuerle PA. Rapid proteolysis of I kappa B-alpha is necessary for activation of transcription factor NF-kappa B. Nature 1993;365(6442):182-5.

27. Akiyama T, Ishida J, Nakagawa S, et al. Genistein, a specific inhibitor of tyrosine-specific protein kinases. Journal of Biological Chemistry 1987;262(12):5592-5.

28. Stewart BH, Hoskin DW. Inhibition of protein tyrosine kinases or protein kinase C prevents nonspecific killer T lymphocyte-mediated tumoricidal activity. Biochi-

mica et Biophysica Acta 1997;1356(3):333-42.

29. Anel A, Buferne M, Boyer C, Schmitt-Verhulst AM, Golstein P. T cell receptor-induced Fas ligand expression in cytotoxic T lymphocyte clones is blocked by protein tyrosine kinase inhibitors and cyclosporin A. European Journal of Immunology 1994;24(10):2469-76.

30. Atluru S, Atluru D. Evidence that genistein, a protein-tyrosine kinase inhibitor, inhibits CD28 monoclonal-antibody-stimulated human T cell proliferation. Transplantation 1991;51(2):448-50.

31. Fiedor P, Kozerski L, Dobrowolski JC, et al. Immunosuppressive effects of synthetic derivative of genistein on the survival of pancreatic islet allografts. Transplantation Proceedings 1998;30(2):537.

32. Semmler J, Gebert U, Eisenhut T, et al. Xanthine derivatives: comparison between suppression of tumour necrosis factor-alpha production and inhibition of cAMP phosphodiesterase activity. Immunology 1993;78:520-5.

33. Tilg H, Eibl B, Pichl M, et al. Immune response modulation by pentoxifylline in vitro. Transplantation 1993;56(1):196-201.

34. Jewett A, Bonavida B. Pentoxifylline suppresses interleukin-2-mediated activation of immature human natural killer cells by inhibiting endogenous tumor necrosis factor-alpha secretion. J Clin Immunol 1994;14(1):31-8.

35. Koenigsrainer A, Aichberger C, Riedmann B, Steurer W, Oefner D, Margreiter R. Pentoxifylline as an adjunct to cyclosporine -based immunosuppression does not improve the outcome of renal transplantation. Transpl Proc 1995;27(1):1062-3.

36. Jilg S, Barsig J, Leist M, Kusters S, Volk HD, Wendel A. Enhanced release of interleukin-10 and soluble tumor necrosis factor receptors as novel principles of methylxanthine action in murine models of endotoxic shock. Journal of Pharmacology & Experimental Therapeutics 1996;278(1):421-31.

37. Lin Y, Goebels J, Rutgeerts O, et al. Use of the methylxanthine derivative A802715 in transplantation immunology: I. Strong in vitro inhibitory effects on CD28-costimulated T cell activities. Transplantation 1997;63(12):1813-8.

38. Lin Y, Segers C, Mikhalsky D, Tjandra-Maga TB, Schonharting M, Waer M. Use of the methylxanthine derivative A802715 in transplantation immunology: II. In vivo experiments. Transplantation 1997;63(12):1734-8.

39. Schwaninger M, Blume R, Oetjen E, Knepel W. The immunosuppressive drugs cyclosporin A and FK506 inhibit calcineurin phosphatase activity and gene transcription mediated through the cAMP-responsive element in a nonimmune cell line. Naunyn-Schmiedebergs Archives of Pharmacology 1993;348(5):541-5.

40. Bennett WM, Elzinga LW, Porter GA, Rosen S. The effects of pentoxifylline on experimental chronic cyclosporine nephrotoxicity. Transplantation 1992;54(6):1118-20.

41. Gummert JF, Barten MJ, Boeke K, et al. Structure-based immunosuppressive drug design: Efficacy and pharmacokinetics of VX-497, a novel inhibitor of inosine monophosphate dehydrogenase, in rat heart allograft recipients. (submitted for publication) 1999.

42. Navia MA. Rational design of new immunosuppressive drugs. Transpl Proc 1999; 31(1-2):1097-8.

43. Bartlett RR, Schleyerbach R. Immunopharmacological profile of a novel isoxazol derivative, HWA 486, with potential antirheumatic activity--I. Disease modifying action on adjuvant arthritis of the rat. International Journal of Immunopharmacology 1985;7(1):7-18.

44. Silva Junior HT, Morris RE. Leflunomide and malononitrilamides. American Journal of the Medical Sciences 1997;313(5):289-301.

45. Mladenovic V, Domljan Z, Rozman B, et al. Safety and effectiveness of leflunomide in the treatment of patients with active rheumatoid arthritis. Results of a randomized, placebo-controlled, phase II study. Arthritis & Rheumatism 1995;

38(11):1595-603.

46. Kuo EA, Hambleton PT, Kay DP, et al. Synthesis, structure-activity relationships, and pharmacokinetic properties of dihydroorotate dehydrogenase inhibitors: 2-cyano-3-cyclopropyl-3-hydroxy-N-[3'-methyl-4'-(trifluoromethyl)phenyl] propenamide and related compounds. Journal of Medicinal Chemistry 1996;39(23): 4608-21.

47. Schorlemmer H, Bartlett R, Kurrle R. Malononitrilamides: a new strategy of immunosuppression for allo- and xenotransplantation. Transplantation Proceedings 1998;30(3):884-90.

48. Bruneau JM, Yea CM, Spinella-Jaegle S, et al. Purification of human dihydro-orotate dehydrogenase and its inhibition by A77 1726, the active metabolite of leflunomide. Biochemical Journal 1998;336(Pt 2):299-303.

49. Williamson RA, Yea CM, Robson PA, et al. Dihydroorotate dehydrogenase is a high affinity binding protein for A77 1726 and mediator of a range of biological effects of the immunomodulatory compound. Journal of Biological Chemistry 1995;270(38):22467-72.

50. Qi Z, Ekberg H. Malononitrilamides 715 and 279 prolong rat cardiac allograft survival, reverse ongoing rejection, inhibit allospecific antibody production and interact positively with cyclosporin. Scandinavian Journal of Immunology 1998;48(4): 379-88.

51. Angermuller S, Loffler M. Localization of dihydroorotate oxidase in myocardium and kidney cortex of the rat. An electron microscopic study using the cerium technique. Histochemistry & Cell Biology 1995;103(4):287-92.

52. Simmonds HA. Diagnosis and treatment of inborn errors of purine and pyrimidine metabolism: an overview. Advances in Experimental Medicine & Biology 1994;370:1-6.

53. Gummert JF, Ikonen T, Morris RE. New Immunosuppressive Agents. J Am Soc Nephrol 1999;in press.

54. Kurrle R, Bartlett R, Ruuth E, Lauffer L, Schorlemmer HU. Malononitrilamides inhibit T- and B-cell responsiveness. Transplantation Proceedings 1996;28(6): 3053-6.

55. Schorlemmer HU, Bartlett RR, Kurrle R. Malononitrilamides prevent the generation of oxygen radicals in mononuclear phagocytes and graft rejection in a rat model. Transplantation Proceedings 1999;31(1-2):851-3.

56. Kurrle R, Ruuth E, Bartlett R, Lauffer L, Schorlemmer HU. Malononitrilamides inhibit T- and B-cell responsiveness in different species. Transplantation Proceedings 1997;29(1-2):1302-3.

57. Gregory CR, Silva HT, Patz JD, Morris RE. Comparative effects of malononitriloamide analogs of leflunomide on whole blood lymphocyte stimulation in humans, rhesus macaques, cats, dogs, and rats. Transplantation Proceedings 1998;30(4):1047-8.

58. Nair RV, Cao W, Morris RE. Inhibition of smooth muscle cell proliferation in vitro by leflunomide, a new immunosuppressant, is antagonized by uridine. Immunology Letters 1995;47(3):171-4.

59. Xu X, Williams JW, Bremer EG, Finnegan A, Chong AS. Inhibition of protein tyrosine phosphorylation in T cells by a novel immunosuppressive agent, leflunomide. Journal of Biological Chemistry 1995;270(21):12398-403.

60. Cao WW, Kao PN, Chao AC, Gardner P, Ng J, Morris RE. Mechanism of the antiproliferative action of leflunomide. A77 1726, the active metabolite of leflunomide, does not block T-cell receptor-mediated signal transduction but its antiproliferative effects are antagonized by pyrimidine nucleosides. Journal of Heart & Lung Transplantation 1995;14(6 Pt 1):1016-30.

61. Schorlemmer HU, Kurrle R, Bartlett RR. Malononitrilamides inhibit the development of various murine graft-vs-host diseases. Transplantation Proceedings

1996;28(6):3043-7.

62. Schorlemmer HU, Ruuth E, Kurrle R. The alloreactivity in the popliteal lymph node (PLN) assay is regulated by malononitrilamides (MNAs). International Journal of Tissue Reactions 1997;19(3-4):157-61.

63. Schorlemmer HU, Kurrle R, Bartlett RR. The new immunosuppressants, the malononitrilamides MNA 279 and MNA 715, inhibit various graft-vs.-host diseases (GvHD) in rodents. Drugs Under Experimental & Clinical Research 1997; 23(5-6):167-73.

64. Schorlemmer HU, Kurrle R, Bartlett RR. Various graft vs. host diseases (GvHD) in rodents can be prevented and treated by malononitrilamides (MNAs). Inflammation Research 1997;46(Suppl 2):S165-6.

65. Schorlemmer HU, Schwab W, Ruuth E, Kurrle R. Acute skin graft rejection can be prevented and treated in rat models by malononitrilamides. Transplantation Proceedings 1996;28(6):3048-50.

66. Lin Y, Segers C, Waer M. Efficacy of the malononitrilamide X 920715 as compared with leflunomide in cardiac allo- and xenotransplantation in rats. Transplantation Proceedings 1996;28(6):3036.

67. Morris RE, Huang X, Cao W, Zheng B, Shorthouse RA. Leflunomide (HWA 486) and its analog suppress T- and B-cell proliferation in vitro, acute rejection, ongoing rejection, and antidonor antibody synthesis in mouse, rat, and cynomolgus monkey transplant recipients as well as arterial intimal thickening after balloon catheter injury. Transplantation Proceedings 1995;27(1):445-7.

68. Morris RE, Huang X, Gregory CR, et al. Studies in experimental models of chronic rejection: use of rapamycin (sirolimus) and isoxazole derivatives (leflunomide and its analogue) for the suppression of graft vascular disease and obliterative bronchiolitis. Transplantation Proceedings 1995;27(3):2068-9.

69. Schorlemmer HU, Kurrle R. Malononitrilamides reduce IgM and IgG xenoantibodies and prolong skin xenograft survival in a mouse-to rat model. Transplantation Proceedings 1998;30(4):976-9.

70. Schorlemmer HU, Kurrle R. Control of mouse-to-rat skin xenograft rejection by malononitrilamides. Transplantation Proceedings 1996;28(6):3037-9.

71. Schorlemmer HU, Kurrle R. Combination therapy of malononitrilamides and tacrolimus (FK 506) induced long-term xenograft survival. Transplantation Proceedings 1998;30(8):4170-3.

72. St Georgiev V. Enzymes of the purine metabolism: inhibition and therapeutic potential. Annals of the New York Academy of Sciences 1993;685:207-16.

73. Bantia S, Montgomery JA, Johnson HG, Walsh GM. In vivo and in vitro pharmacologic activity of the purine nucleoside phosphorylase inhibitor BCX-34: the role of GTP and dGTP. Immunopharmacology 1996;35(1):53-63.

74. Montgomery JA, Niwas S, Dose JR, et al. Structure-based design of inhibitors of purine nucleoside phosphorylase: 9-(arylmethyl) derivatives of 9-deazaguanine. J Med Chem 1993;36:55-69.

75. Allison AC, Eugui EM. Immunosuppressive and other Effects of Mycophenolic Acid and an Ester Prodrug, Mycophenolate Mofetil. Immunol Rev 1993;136:5-28.

76. Conry RM, Bantia S, Turner HS, et al. Effects of a novel purine nucleoside phosphorylase inhibitor, BCX-34, on activation and proliferation of normal human lymphoid cells. Immunopharmacology 1998;40(1):1-9.

77. Iwata H, Wada Y, Walsh M, et al. In vitro study of BCX-34: a new human T-lymphocyte-specific purine phosphorylase inhibitor. Transplantation Proceedings 1998;30(4):983-6.

78. Fujita T, Inoue K, Yamamoto S, et al. Fungal metabolites. Part 11. A potent immunosuppressive activity found in Isaria sinclairii metabolite. Journal of Antibiotics 1994;47(2):208-15.

79. Fujita T, Hirose R, Yoneta M, et al. Potent immunosuppressants, 2-alkyl-2-amino-

propane-1,3-diols. Journal of Medicinal Chemistry 1996;39(22):4451-9.

80. Kahan BD. FTY720: a new immunosuppressive agent with novel mechanism(s) of action. Transplantation Proceedings 1998;30(5):2210-3.

81. Suzuki S, Li XK, Shinomiya T, et al. The in vivo induction of lymphocyte apoptosis in MRL-lpr/lpr mice treated with FTY720. Clinical & Experimental Immunology 1997;107(1):103-11.

82. Li XK, Shinomiya T, Enosawa S, Kakefuda T, Amemiya H, Suzuki S. Induction of lymphocyte apoptosis by a novel immunosuppressant FTY720: relation with Fas, Bcl-2 and Bax expression. Transplantation Proceedings 1997;29(1-2):1267-8.

83. Chiba K, Hoshino Y, Suzuki C, et al. FTY720, a novel immunosuppressant possessing unique mechanisms. I. Prolongation of skin allograft survival and synergistic effect in combination with cyclosporine in rats. Transplantation Proceedings 1996;28(2):1056-9.

84. Wang ME, Tejpal N, Qu X, et al. Immunosuppressive effects of FTY720 alone or in combination with cyclosporine and/or sirolimus. Transplantation 1998;65(7): 899-905.

85. Suzuki S, Enosawa S, Kakefuda T, et al. A novel immunosuppressant, FTY720, with a unique mechanism of action, induces long-term graft acceptance in rat and dog allotransplantation. Transplantation 1996;61(2):200-5.

86. Yanagawa Y, Sugahara K, Kataoka H, Kawaguchi T, Masubuchi Y, Chiba K. FTY720, a novel immunosuppressant, induces sequestration of circulating mature lymphocytes by acceleration of lymphocyte homing in rats. II. FTY720 prolongs skin allograft survival by decreasing T cell infiltration into grafts but not cytokine production in vivo. Journal of Immunology 1998;160(11):5493-9.

87. Chiba K, Yanagawa Y, Masubuchi Y, et al. FTY720, a novel immunosuppressant, induces sequestration of circulating mature lymphocytes by acceleration of lymphocyte homing in rats. I. FTY720 selectively decreases the number of circulating mature lymphocytes by acceleration of lymphocyte homing. Journal of Immunology 1998;160(10):5037-44.

88. Chiba K, Yanagawa Y, Kataoka H, Kawaguchi T, Ohtsuki M, Hoshino Y. FTY720, a novel immunosuppressant, induces sequestration of circulating lymphocytes by acceleration of lymphocyte homing. Transplantation Proceedings 1999;31(1-2):1230-3.

89. Li XK, Enosawa S, Kakefuda T, Amemiya H, Suzuki S. FTY720, a novel immunosuppressive agent, enhances upregulation of the cell adhesion molecular ICAM-1 in TNF-alpha treated human umbilical vein endothelial cells. Transplantation Proceedings 1997;29(1-2):1265-6.

90. Xu M, Antoniou EA, Afford SC, et al. Effect of peritransplant FTY720 alone or in combination with posttransplant FK 506 in a rat model of cardiac allotransplantation. Transplantation Proceedings 1997;29(7):2964-6.

91. Hoshino Y, Suzuki C, Ohtsuki M, Masubuchi Y, Amano Y, Chiba K. FTY720, a novel immunosuppressant possessing unique mechanisms. II. Long-term graft survival induction in rat heterotopic cardiac allografts and synergistic effect in combination with cyclosporine A. Transplantation Proceedings 1996;28(2):1060-1.

92. Masubuchi Y, Kawaguchi T, Ohtsuki M, et al. FTY720, a novel immunosuppressant, possessing unique mechanisms. IV. Prevention of graft versus host reactions in rats. Transplantation Proceedings 1996;28(2):1064-5.

93. Stepkowski SM, Wang M, Qu X, et al. Synergistic interaction of FTY720 with cyclosporine or sirolimus to prolong heart allograft survival. Transplantation Proceedings 1998;30(5):2214-6.

94. Xu M, Pirenne J, Antoniou EA, Afford SC, D'Silva M, McMaster P. Effect of peritransplant FTY720 alone or in combination with post-transplant tacrolimus in a rat model of cardiac allotransplantation. Transplant International 1998;11(4): 288-94.

95. Yuzawa K, Otsuka M, Taniguchi H, et al. Rescue effect of FTY720 on acute renal rejection in dogs. Transplantation Proceedings 1999;31(1-2):872.
96. Chueh SC, Tian L, Wang M, Wang ME, Stepkowski SM, Kahan BD. Induction of tolerance toward rat cardiac allografts by treatment with allochimeric class I MHC antigen and FTY720. Transplantation 1997;64(10):1407-14.
97. Pyatt DW, Stillman WS, Irons RD. Hydroquinone, a reactive metabolite of benzene, inhibits NF-kappa B in primary human CD4+ T lymphocytes. Toxicology & Applied Pharmacology 1998;149(2):178-84.
98. Lee DK, Kim B, Lee SG, et al. Momordins inhibit both AP-1 function and cell proliferation. Anticancer Research 1998;18(1A):119-24.
99. Williams DH, Wilkinson SE, Purton T, Lamont A, Flotow H, Murray EJ. Ro 09-2210 exhibits potent anti-proliferative effects on activated T cells by selectively blocking MKK activity. Biochemistry 1998;37(26):9579-85.
100. Kuromitsu S, Fukunaga M, Lennard AC, Masuho Y, Nakada S. 3-(13-Hydroxytridecyl)-1-[13-(3-pyridyl)tridecyl]pyridinium chloride (YM-53792), a novel inhibitor of NF-AT activation. Biochemical Pharmacology 1997;54(9): 999-1005.
101. Nagata H, Ochiai K, Aotani Y, et al. Lymphostin (LK6-A), a novel immunosuppressant from Streptomyces sp. KY11783: taxonomy of the producing organism, fermentation, isolation and biological activities. Journal of Antibiotics 1997;50(7): 537-42.
102. Aotani Y, Nagata H, Yoshida M. Lymphostin (LK6-A), a novel immunosuppressant from Streptomyces sp. KY11783: structural elucidation. Journal of Antibiotics 1997;50(7):543-5.

3 POLYCLONAL AND MONOCLONAL ANTIBODIES

Lucienne Chatenoud
Immunologie Clinique
INSERM U25, Hôpital Necker
Paris, France

The introduction, more than thirty years ago, of polyclonal anti-lymphocyte antibodies in clinical kidney transplantation was a major step in the history of therapeutic immunosuppression [1]. Not only were these biological agents very efficient in prolonging allograft survival but they represented the first immunosuppressants having a selective action on immune cells, in great distinction with the chemical agents available at that time namely, cortico-steroids and azathioprine. In parallel, the experimental work conducted in rodents by the group of A. Monaco disclosed the unique tolerogenic proper-ties of polyclonal antilymphocyte sera (ALS). Tolerance to skin allografts was obtained combining ALS treatment and post-transplant donor bone marrow infusion [2, 3]. The effect was antigen specific since third party grafts were rapidly rejected; lymphohemopoietic microchimerism was observed in toler-ant animals [2, 3]. These were the first results suggesting that an adequate alloantigen delivery under the cover of a treatment using a biological anti-lymphocyte agent could recreate, in such transiently immunosuppressed adult hosts, the same "permissive" environment for the establishment of transplantation tolerance initially reported in the neonate by Billingham, Brent and Medawar [4].

Therapeutic monoclonal antibodies to T cell surface receptors, produced by hybridomas, started to be developed in the early 1980s as an appealing alter-native to ALS [5, 6]. They were in fact much easier to produce and stan-dardize. They included homogeneous sets of antibodies with predefined specificity for a single antigenic determinant or epitope and they could be administered at smaller doses as compared to those used for polyclonal prep-arations. Importantly, it rapidly appeared that, just as ALS, some monoclonal

A. W. Thomson (ed.), Therapeutic Immunosuppression, 55–80.

antibodies exhibited tolerogenic properties in various transplantation and autoimmunity models, not only in rodents but also in non human primates [7-11, 11-21]

The clinical use of first generation rodent monoclonal antibodies was mostly restricted to the field of transplantation essentially due to their side effects linked to their immunogenicity and, for some particular specificities such as CD3, their mitogenicity and cytokine releasing potential. However, the situation is now evolving due to the ever growing panel made available of "humanized" monoclonal antibodies, that are much better tolerated, and represent promising therapeutic tools not only in transplantation but also in autoimmunity.

Our aim will be to review the data that highlight the importance of polyclonal and monoclonal antibodies as therapeutic tools to control aberrant immune responses and to discuss their potential as part of novel immunointervention strategies aimed at promoting immune tolerance to both alloantigens and autoantigens.

I. MAIN THERAPEUTIC TARGETS OF POLYCLONAL AND MONOCLONAL ANTIBODIES

Depending on their fine specificity, therapeutic antibodies impact at distinct levels of the immune response through two non mutually exclusive biological effects that are the physical destruction of the target cells and/ or their functional inactivation. This inactivation may be secondary to antibody-mediated cytokine or cytokine receptor neutralization or to the direct interaction with specialized membrane receptors involved in the transduction of still ill defined "immunoregulatory" signals. Receptors involved in the delivery of costimulatory signals (CD28/ CTLA4, CD40/ CD40Ligand) appear very important in this context [11, 22].

Polyclonal antilymphocyte preparations for clinical use (antilymphocyte globulins (ALG) or antithymocyte preparations (ATG)) are serum IgG fractions recovered from rabbits or horses upon immunization with human immune cells [23]. The source of antigen is variable depending on the preparation and includes thymocytes, thoracic duct cells, cultured lymphoblasts or continuous T cell lines such as CD3+ Jurkat cells. Serum IgG fractions are purified and adsorbed to eliminate contaminating antibody specificities (to platelets, red cells and some serum proteins). Despite these purification steps only a minor fraction of the immunoglobulins thus obtained react to human T lymphocytes (estimated to 1-2% depending on the preparation). This explains both the difficulties in standardizing the preparations and the quite variable and sometimes very high dosages of xenogeneic IgGs that need to be administered to achieve the desired therapeutic effect (up to 10-20 mg/kg/day with some preparations). In terms of their fine specificity, anti-T lymphocyte antibodies contained in ALG or ATG preparations are mixtures including, in variable proportions, antibodies to CD2, CD3, the T cell receptor (TCR), CD4, CD8, CD11a, CD25, CD40 and CD54 [24-26]. Differences in the concentration and the affinity of each of these antibody specificities do explain the variable therapeutic potency of ALG and ATG preparations [27].

Monoclonal antibodies are homogeneous sets of immunoglobulins, produced in vitro, sharing identical physicochemical characteristics and specific for single epitopes expressed by cell receptors or soluble mediators. Among the vast panel of monoclonal antibodies interfering with immune cells cooperation pathways some are of particular interest for therapeutic purposes.

These include monoclonal antibodies directed at receptors involved in antigen recognition such as CD3 and CD4. CD3 is a set of five to six invariant polypeptide chains termed γ, δ, ε, ζ, η and, in some cases, it also includes the γ chain of the FcεRI and FcγRIII (CD16) [28]. CD3 is associated with the TCR$\alpha\beta$ and TCR $\gamma\delta$ at the T cell surface. Stoichiometry data suggest that the CD3/ TCR cluster expresses as follows : $(\alpha\beta)_2$ $(\gamma\delta\varepsilon)_2$ $(\zeta\zeta)_4$ [29]. CD3 plays a fundamental role in transducing TCR-mediated activation signals. The CD3 antibodies used in vivo for clinical or experimental studies are specific for the ε chain [6, 30, 31].

CD4 defines one of the two major subsets of mature T lymphocytes. In humans, at variance with rodents, CD4 is also expressed on monocytes, macrophages, Langerhans' cells, eosinophils, endothelial cells of hepatic sinusoids, sperm and brain cells [32]. Only in lymphocytes the intracytoplasmic carboxyterminal domain of CD4 is non-covalently linked to the protein-tyrosine kinase p56^{lck}. Upon antigen binding CD4 forms a cluster with the TCR/CD3 complexes and, through its intracytoplasmic domain associated kinase p56^{lck}, it interacts with the "activated" (i.e. phosphorylated) CD3 $\zeta\zeta$-ZAP-70 complexes and plays a major role in stabilizing the TCR/CD3-peptide/MHC interaction and amplifying the signal transduction through TCR [33-36]. Given this contribution of CD4 to TCR/CD3-mediated signalling it has been proposed that CD4 antibody-mediated coating not only interferes with lymphocyte binding to MHC class II bearing cells but also triggers therapeutically relevant negative "signals" that, interestingly enough, seem to differentially affect naive versus memory T cells [37-42] .

As we already mentioned, of great interest are also the antibodies or fusion proteins interacting with surface molecules delivering costimulatory signals (CD28, CTLA4/ B7 and CD40/ CD40Ligand) or those specific for soluble cytokines or particular cytokine receptors selectively expressed on the surface of activated T cells (the IL-2 receptor α chain or CD25) [11, 22, 43-45]. These major topics are the subject of two independent contributions of this book.

The case of antibodies to CD52, a small glycosylphosphatidylinositol (GPI)-anchored protein expressed at the surface of human B cells, T cells as well as monocyte/ macrophages which function is presently unknown, is also interesting to discuss since they have been extremely potent at promoting long term acceptance of organ allografts as well as prolonged remission of established, and otherwise intractable, autoimmune diseases (multiple sclerosis, vasculitis, rheumatoid arthritis) [46-48].

II. BIOLOGICAL EFFECTS OF POLYCLONAL OR MONOCLONAL ANTIBODIES

Antilymphocyte sera are cell-depleting agents. Target cell lysis usually occurs upon complement binding or following opsonisation and subsequent trapping and destruction by reticuloendothelial cells especially in the spleen, liver and lungs [23, 49, 50]. More recent in vitro data have also shown that, at submitogenic concentrations, ALG may trigger apoptosis of activated T cells, an effect that is tightly dependent on the presence of antibodies to CD2 and CD3 in the preparation [51]. However, cell depletion is not the only mode of action of ALS since T cells that reappear in the periphery after cessation of treatment (usually within 2 to 3 weeks depending on the dose administered) are functionally impaired. This cell inactivation may be secondary to coating of surface receptors and/or antigenic modulation as first suggested by Levey and Medawar in their "blindfolding" hypothesis [52]. Moreover, some data, from both mouse and monkey models, have also suggested that treatment with ALS promoted the generation of non specific suppressor T cells that could mediate the prolonged therapeutic effects observed [53, 54].

Some T cell directed monoclonal antibodies also express very efficient lytic capacities but, at variance with polyclonal antibodies, the mechanisms mediating the target destruction in vivo are more complex and cannot be predicted, as initially expected, from the antibody isotype [55, 56]. In fact, there is now compelling evidence to show that the monoclonal antibody fine specificity will also influence its lytic capacity.

This is well illustrated by the case of CD52 antibodies (Campath-1). The first Campath-1 antibody was a rat IgM characterized in 1983 and a CDR-grafted humanized version, Campath-1H, was produced by genetic engineering [57]. Both the rat and the humanized antibody expressed a highly depleting capacity. This explains that rat IgM and IgG2b Campath-1 antibodies have been extensively used, in vitro and in vivo, to purge T cells from allogeneic bone marrow prior to transplant for prevention graft versus host disease [58, 59]. Interestingly, various isotype variants of the CDR-grafted Campath-1H antibody were produced including an IgG4, normally considered as a non-depleting human isotype. Although, in vitro, this antibody did not exhibit major Fc related effector functions, when administered in vivo it produced a significant cell depletion [60].

The density and the distribution of the antigen on the target cell surface will also greatly influence the monoclonal antibody lytic capacity. Thus antigens that easily undergo antigenic modulation (i.e. the disappearance of a receptor from the cell membrane upon binding to the specific monoclonal antibody [61, 62]) may be a poor target for lysis. This is in fact the case for T cell antigen receptors (CD3-TCR) and, indeed, monovalent antibodies, that avoid antigenic modulation, display a significantly increased lytic potential [63-65].

Concerning the mechanisms mediating the monoclonal antibody mediated cell lysis, direct complement dependent depletion may occur with humanized monoclonals but not with mouse and rat antibodies that express a rather poor lytic capacity in presence of human complement. Other mechanisms are the opsonization and trapping by reticuloendothelial cells, redirected T cell lysis upon bridging cytotoxic T cells to the target [66] and, as shown antibodies to CD3, CD4 and MHC class I, the induction of apoptosis or programmed cell death [67-70].

Depending on the fine specificity of the antibody used, depletion may globally affect leucocytes (CD52 antibodies) or T cells (polyclonal ALG or ATG, CD3 antibodies) or T cell subsets (CD4 antibodies). Short lived T cells will rapidly reappear after short term depletion. Conversely, recirculating long lived T cells will take several weeks in the mouse and several months in man to replenish initial cell pools. The case of depleting monoclonal antibodies to CD4 deserves a special word of caution since peripheral CD4+ T cell counts may remain very low for several consecutive months after the end of treatment. This was for instance the experience with the chimeric CD4 antibody MT-512 (human IgG1) that has been administered to both organ allograft recipients and patients presenting with rheumatoid arthritis. Some of the patients who received the antibody at high doses (700mg of cumulated dosage) maintained low circulating CD4 (up to 60% from baseline) for over 18-30 months [71].

As already discussed for ALS, some monoclonal antibodies will inhibit or down modulate the functional capacity of immune cells. This may be accomplished through antibody-mediated cell coating, as observed for non depleting antibodies to CD4 or through antigenic modulation of the target cell receptor, as typically seen with CD3 antibodies.

Very rapidly after their first administration, CD3 antibodies promote the redistribution of the CD3/ TRC complex that ultimately caps at a pole of the cell and disappears upon internalization or shedding [61, 62]. This is why in both humans and mice, at the doses usually administered (5mg/ day in patients and 5-20µg/ day in mice) depletion is partial and only affects 30 to 40% of CD3+ cells. Residual CD3+ lymphocytes, both in the periphery and within target organ infiltrates, undergo antigenic modulation and thus express a particular phenotype : CD3⁻TCR⁻CD4+ or CD3⁻TCR⁻CD8+ [61, 62, 72]. This phenomenon, reverses within 8 to 12hours once the antibody is cleared [61]. Importantly, CD3-modulated cells are fully unresponsive to antigen-specific or mitogen stimulation [61, 62], thus suggesting that this mechanism is probably central to the mode of action of CD3 antibodies and the in vivo immunosuppression/ unresponsiveness they induce [73-76].

Finally, although less well defined in cellular and molecular terms, another crucial in vivo effect of ALS and some anti-T cell antibodies, we already alluded to, is the triggering of "immunoregulatory" pathways which translate, especially over long-term, in the establishment of an "operational" immune tolerance with evidence, depending on the models, for cell anergy, immune deviation and/ or dominant or infectious tolerance. These latter phenomena have been documented especially upon use of antibodies to CD4, associations of CD4 and CD8 and CD3 [7, 9, 12, 13, 18, 20, 21, 75, 77].

III. THE BENEFITS OF HUMANIZED MONOCLONAL ANTIBODIES

It was the general experience that xenogeneic monoclonal antibodies generated a strong humoral immune response [78-83]. This occurred in the clinical setting in spite of the relatively low doses administered (5 mg/ day in the case of OKT3) when compared to those used for polyclonal antibodies. This anti-globulin response is deleterious due to its ability to rapidly and completely neutralize the therapeutic effect of the monoclonal antibody [78, 80, 82, 84]. Independently from the fine specificity of the injected antibody the humoral response presented some interesting peculiarities. First, anti-monoclonal globulins are highly restricted in their specificity and only include anti-isotypic and anti-idiotypic antibodies [78, 79, 85, 86]. Anti-idiotypic antibodies represent the majority if not the totality of the neutralizing component due to their capacity to compete with the target in binding the monoclonal antibody [78, 84]. Anti-isotypic antibodies appear for most of them to be essentially non-neutralizing [86]. Secondly, studies performed on affinity purified anti-idiotypic antibodies showed that the response was oligoclonal [87]. The fact that only a few specific B cell clones are recruited in the response suggest that quantitatively the overall amount of anti-monoclonal immunoglobulins produced is not massive. This is in keeping with the clinical observation that, at variance with what is observed with polyclonal antibodies, serum sickness is not a side effect of monoclonal antibody administration (the amount of immune complexes formed is probably insufficient to elicit a generalized reaction). Anaphylaxis is another potential risk that in practice has been extremely rare [88].

In the first few years following the introduction of OKT3 in transplantation the sensitization appeared as a clinically relevant problem [76, 78, 80-82, 84]. In fact, patients presenting with circulating neutralizing anti-OKT3 immunoglobulins could not be retreated with the monoclonal. The problem was mostly circumvented by adapting the associated immunosuppressive treatment. Thus, in the case of OKT3, the association with corticosteroids, azathioprine and cyclosporin at adequate doses decreased the frequency of sensitization from 90-95% to 15-25% [89]. Although effective, this strategy was, for obvious reasons, only a partial solution to the problem. In particular, it was not applicable to clinical situations such as autoimmunity where heavy drug associations are, as compared to transplantation, not frequently applied. A more radical approach was the possibility of generating "humanized" antibodies through molecular engineering.

Two sorts of humanized antibodies have been derived that are chimeric antibodies, presenting intact variable regions, from the parental rodent antibody, combined to a human immunoglobulin constant portion and complementarity determining region (CDR)-grafted antibodies, expressing the rodent hypervariable regions, that specifically interact with the antigen, inserted into human immunoglobulin frameworks [57, 90, 91]. Both of these approaches allow to produce "à la carte" monoclonal antibodies combining a given specificity with a selected human Fc fragment that may impact on the final antibody effector capacities (complement fixation, opsonisation and antibody-dependent cell cytotoxicity (ADCC) and their potential mitogenic and cytokine releasing capacity).

Despite the fact rodent hypervariable regions, carrying the idiotypic determinants, are still present in humanized antibodies the data recovered from trials, both in transplantation and autoimmunity, using chimeric or CDR-grafted monoclonal antibodies, fully confirmed their hypothesized low immunogenicity [44, 45, 92, 93]. Only in cases where the humanized antibodies were administered alone (in the absence of associated immunosuppressants) and for more than 2 consecutive treatment courses there were reports of an anti-idiotypic response arising [94]. One may hope that in the not too distant future the problem will be completely solved by using fully human monoclonal antibodies. Three different methods have been described that allow the production of human therapeutic monoclonal antibodies.

One method uses mice in which endogenous immunoglobulin genes have been knocked out and that, in addition, have been made transgenic for human constant and variable immunoglobulin encoding genes. Thus, upon immunization, B lymphocytes in these animals only produce high affinity human antibodies expressing a significant diversity [95, 96].

Phage display is another possibility. cDNA libraries from human B cells are expressed in filamentous phages that allow a rapid in vitro selection of antibodies with the desired specificity [97].

The third approach has been described by Lubin et al. and consists of the establishment of human-mouse chimeras. Irradiated mice are reconstituted with bone marrow cells from scid mice. Human lymphocytes from presensitized donors are then injected into the reconstituted mice that are boosted with defined antigens and used for fusion with myeloma cells [98].

In the particular case of CD3 antibodies, the humanization is a unique way to abrogate not only their immunogenicity but also their deleterious mitogenic potential. In fact, one major side effect linked to the administration of

OKT3 was the acute "flu-like" syndrome that invariably followed the first injections of the monoclonal antibody [80-82, 99-103]. The symptoms mainly included high fever, chills and headache, repeated episodes of vomiting, diarrhea and severe prostration. Although fully reversible within 48 to 72 hours this syndrome was a real limitation to the more extensive use of OKT3 in clinical transplantation and has totally prevented its application to other clinical contexts such as autoimmunity [104]. The reaction is linked to the massive though transient systemic release of several cytokines (TNF, IFNγ, IL-2 , IL-3, IL-4, IL-6, IL-10, GM-CSF) [99-103, 105-107]. Importantly, the mitogenic capacity of CD3 antibodies is monocyte dependent, due to the ability of the Fc portion of the monoclonal to interact with monocyte/ macrophages Fc receptors [75, 108, 109, 109-111]. Thus, engineered humanized non mitogenic CD3 antibodies have been produced by introducing modifications (mutations and aglycosylations) within the constant Fc portion to inhibit their interactions with monocyte/ macrophage Fc receptors [112, 113].

At present two humanized non-mitogenic CD3 antibodies have been reported and are under study in pilot clinical trials.

One has been characterized by the group of H. Waldmann. It is derived from the rat YTH 12.5 [113, 114] and is a humanised CDR-grafted IgG1 antibody which γ1 constant region lacks the CH2 domain glycosylation site. As other aglycosylated antibodies this CD3 monoclonal is unable to bind to Fc receptors or activate complement. Results of preclinical studies showed that aglycosyl IgG1 YTH 12.5 does not induce T cell proliferation in the presence of human serum, it possesses a significantly reduced ability to redirect T cell lysis, and, as the parental YTH 12.5 antibody, it does suppress proliferation mixed lymphocyte reactions [113]. Moreover, when injected into mice expressing a human CD3-ε transgene the aglycosyl IgG1 YTH 12.5 antibody, at variance with the parental mitogenic monoclonal, did not induce a significant cytokine release [113].

The second non-mitogenic humanized CD3 antibody was produced by the group of J. Bluestone and was derived from OKT3. This humanized γOKT3-5 antibody has been mutated in the Fc region and expresses a 100-fold decrease in its affinity for human Fc receptors as compared to the parental monoclonal. The γOKT3-5 antibody is not mitogenic in vitro and it did not show a significant in vivo cytokine releasing capacity in an experimental model in which human splenocytes from cadaveric organ donors were inoculated into severe combined immunodeficient mice (hu-SPL-SCID mice) [112].

Results from pilot trials are very encouraging since they seem to fully confirm both the good tolerance as well as the capacity of these humanized CD3 antibodies to reverse ongoing kidney allograft rejection [115, 116].

IV. CLINICAL USE OF MONOCLONAL ANTIBODIES

Transplantation

Initially the clinical use of monoclonal antibodies was mostly confined to transplantation. Probably the best example to quote is that of the mouse IgG2a monoclonal OKT3, specific for the ε chain of the human CD3 complex that was introduced for the treatment and the prevention of renal allograft rejection in the early 1980s [61, 73, 76, 78, 117-119]. The dose administered was 5mg/day, for 10 to 15 consecutive days in association to corticosteroids and azathioprine and, in most cases, cyclosporin was applied by the end of OKT3 therapy. Based on the therapeutic effectiveness observed in these first trials large randomized studies were undertaken that fully confirmed the initial findings and supported the commercial distribution of the antibody [81]. Subsequently, the use of OKT3 was extended to the treatment of renal allograft rejection resistant to other therapies ("rescue") and to liver and heart allograft recipients [120-130].

Despite its evident therapeutic effectiveness the risk of sensitization and the occurrence of the "flu-like" syndrome represented a major limitation explaining that various centers did not adopt OKT3 as a routine treatment especially as an induction therapy for the prevention of allograft rejection.

The situation may rapidly evolve if the preliminary data reported with humanized non mitogenic CD3 antibodies can be confirmed on a large scale basis [115, 116].

As compared to OKT3 the clinical experience with other murine monoclonal antibodies was limited and never reached the point of a large scale distribution although encouraging results were reported. This was the case for antibodies such as CD25 or LFA-1 [131-135].

Here again the panorama may now rapidly evolve with the advent of humanized antibodies. Very recently two humanized CD25 antibodies (one chimeric and one CDR-grafted), that are very well tolerated and are effective as induction therapy, have been launched in the market [43-45].

Of particular interest are also the recent data reported by the group of R. Calne with the CD52 antibody Campath-1H [46]. Campath 1H was administered to 31 renal allograft recipients at a dose of 20 mg (i.v.) on days 0 and 1 after transplant. The patients were maintained on low-dose monotherapy with cyclosporine initiated 72hrs after transplant. At 15-28 months of follow-up 29 patients present with functioning grafts. Six rejection episodes were scored that were responsive to conventional steroid therapy.

Autoimmunity

Contrasting with their extensive use in transplantation the application of first generation murine monoclonal antibodies for the treatment of autoimmune diseases has been more problematic essentially because of their side effects, the more so since in such clinical context monoclonal antibodies were mostly applied alone in the absence of other immunosuppressants. Despite its potential effectiveness OKT3 was not applicable because of the very serious consequences of the cytokine release syndrome as shown by the data from the few patients presenting a multiple sclerosis and treated with this monoclonal [104]. Mouse antibodies to human CD4 were also applied based on the large evidence showing the effectiveness of CD4 antibodies in the prevention and the treatment of experimental autoimmune diseases. The first pilot trials enrolled patients presenting with long-standing rheumatoid arthritis, psoriasis, inflammatory bowel disease or uveitis [32, 136-141]. The treatment was well tolerated, only rare cases of mild side effects after the first injection (linked to minor cytokine release) have been reported [32]. The antibodies used essentially induced partial and transient disappearance of circulating CD4+ cells; coating of CD4+ cells was also observed, with dose-dependent saturation of CD4 binding sites. When present, antigenic modulation only affected a minor proportion of CD4 receptors. One major drawback in all these trials was the sensitizing effect of the murine monoclonals. The antiglobulin response frequently observed associated with the relatively short half life of murine monoclonals probably explains that most of these pilot studies showed no major long lasting clinical effects [32, 71, 136-140, 142].

Humanized antibodies represented a radical solution to this problem. One very good example is that of humanized antibodies to TNF which use has completely revolutionized the treatment of rheumatoid arthritis as a consequence of the pioneer experimental and clinical work conducted by the groups of M. Feldmann and T. Maini. The first crucial in vitro finding was that neutralizing antibodies to TNF significantly decreased the production of most of the pro-inflammatory cytokines (i.e. IL-1, IL-6, IL-8, GM-CSF) normally found in vitro cultures of cells infiltrating synovial membranes from rheumatoid arthritis patients [143]. Moreover, in vivo, mice expressing a human TNF transgene develop a chronic arthritis that was fully prevented by treatment with antibodies to TNF [143]. In another model of experimental collagen type II-induced arthritis, neutralizing antibodies to TNF did also exhibit a significant therapeutic effect [143].

The results of the first randomized placebo-controlled double-blind study showing the effectiveness of the chimeric neutralising antibody to TNF cA2 (human IgG1) for the treatment of long-standing rheumatoid arthritis were reported in 1994 [144]. They fully confirmed the data from the initial phase I/II open trial showing no acute toxicity and significant therapeutic benefit, as assessed by the clinical and laboratory parameters, lasting for several weeks after the end of treatment. Some of the patients having disease relapse underwent 2 or more cycles of retreatment; disease flares were sensitive to retreatment but the mean duration of the induced remissions progressively diminished probably due to the appearance of an antiglobulin response [94]. Subsequent studies fully supported the effectiveness of this TNF neutralizing strategy using as tools both antibodies to TNF or soluble TNF receptor fusion proteins [145]. Presently, trials are being conducted that associate these molecules to methotrexate in the attempt to obtain longer lasting clinical remissions [146].

Another condition where antibodies to TNF were used with success was the treatment of severe ulcerative colitis [147]. Although the pathophysiology of this disease remains unclear there is evidence for a significant role played by inflammatory cytokines [148]. The therapeutic benefit obtained upon TNF antibody treatment correlated with a decrease in IFNγ production by mononuclear cells infiltrating the lamina propria [149].

Concerning humanized CD4 antibodies several of the published studies focussed on the use of the chimeric cM-T412 antibody (human IgG1) that is depleting. In rheumatoid arthritis results from open studies seemed encouraging especially when cumulated doses raging 350-700mg were used [150]. Only minor adverse events were reported such as fever associated with myalgia, malaise and asymptomatic hypotension that were correlated to transient elevations of circulating IL-6 [151]; mild sensitization was reported in a majority of the patients [150, 151]. One major problem was, however, that the therapeutic effect could not be confirmed in the context of a large randomized, double-blind placebo controlled study including patients with early rheumatoid arthritis [152]. One may recall at this point the very interesting data showing that in a model of collagen type II-induced arthritis in which the animals develop a chronic arthritis, CD4 antibodies alone could not reverse established disease (swollen joints, bone erosions). However, combining the CD4 therapy with sub-optimal doses of the TNF antibody, which per se were of no benefit, a significant improvement was observed [153]. This synergistic effect of TNF and CD4 antibodies may be explained by the need to neutralize the "inflammation" vicious circle, that is a hallmark of self-perpetuating ongoing autoimmunity, to "sensitise" the system to the effect of T-cell directed immunointervention.

A last point concerning the cM-T412 antibody was, as previously mentioned, the very long-lasting CD4+ cell depletion observed that was not noted with the parental mouse M-T151 anti-CD4 antibody [71, 142].

Results from an open pilot study suggested that humanized non depleting antibodies to CD4 could be very effective for the treatment of severe forms of psoriasis [154]. Patients with recalcitrant plaque psoriasis (PASI>12) received the humanized non-depleting monoclonal antibody to CD4 OKTcdr4a. The antibody was well tolerated. Four weeks from treatment, the mean decrease in PASI score was 46% and in half of the patients disease remission was prolonged for up to 6 months. These results pointed to the relevance of CD4+ lymphocytes in psoriasis at the time they showed that depletion of CD4+ cells was not mandatory to achieve therapeutic effectiveness [154].

Campath-1H has been administered in patients presenting with declared autoimmunity. This CD52 antibody has been applied in patients with rheumatoid arthritis. At 3 and 6 months of treatment an improvement in the Paulus score was observed in about half of the patients [155, 156].

Severe systemic vasculitis was another situation in which Campath-1H proved to be particularly effective [47, 48]. The antibody was initially applied to rare vasculitis which pathogenesis is thought to involve mainly T cell-mediated mechanisms; subsequently, patients with Wegener's granulomatosis were also treated with success. Particularly impressive in this clinical context were the long-term remissions that could be obtained when combining antibodies to CD52 and to CD4 [47, 48].

Very promising are also the results that have been obtained in multiple sclerosis [157-159]. In a vast majority of the patients a stabilisation of the clinical symptoms has been observed and over 6-12 months follow-up the long lasting lymphocyte depletion seemed to correlate with a marked decrease in the appearance of new lesions in the central nervous system as assessed by NMR scanning.

V. ANTIBODIES TO T CELL RECEPTORS AS UNIQUE TOLERANCE-PROMOTING TOOLS

The experiments of R. Billingham, L. Brent and P. Medawar were the first to establish that immunological tolerance was an acquired state [4]. The authors showed that mouse neonates injected with allogeneic cells, as adults, indefinitely accepted skin grafts sharing the same haplotype as the cells injected at birth. Importantly, this tolerant state was specific since the animals could reject third party allogeneic skin [4]. At variance with what was initially thought, central deletion of alloreactive T cells is not the only mechanism explaining neonatal tolerance. Peripheral tolerance mechanisms also operate to sustain the unresponsiveness. Thus, lymphoid cells from treated animals can transfer tolerance to adult syngeneic recipients [160]. A Th2 type immune deviation has also been evidenced in tolerant animals since upon specific activation, alloreactive T cells produce low IFNγ but high IL-4 levels [161]. Moreover, neonatal tolerance is abrogated when IL-4 neutralizing antibodies or IL-12 are administered in combination with the allogeneic cells at birth [161].

Among the strategies attempted to recreate in adult hosts an immune environment "permissive" to tolerance induction those using polyclonal or monoclonal antibodies seem to held great promise for the foreseeable future clinical applications. The ground breaking experiments performed by Monaco and Wood in the 1960's settled the conceptual basis for this strategy by showing that a combination of ALS treatment and post-transplantation donor bone marrow infusion could induce specific unresponsiveness to skin allografts [2, 3]. In their model, skin graft survival was significantly prolonged; by thymectomising adult mice prior to ALS treatment 90% of the grafts survived over 100 days and 40% permanently. Recent data suggest that rapamycin, used at dosages that are ineffective on their own in promoting skin graft survival, can successfully replace adult thymectomy [162].

Since then, various groups have reproduced and extended these findings showing that:

1. tolerance to vascularized and non-vascularized allografts was not only

induced by ALS but also by different monoclonal antibodies or fusion proteins interfering with T cell surface receptors or their ligands i.e. CD3, CD4 and CD8, costimulation receptors such as CD28, CTLA4 and CD40Ligand [7-13]

2. several of these biological immunosuppressants [i.e. ALS, CD3-immuno-toxin, CD4 antibodies, CD40Ligand antibodies together with CTLA4 Ig] reproduced the same result in larger animals such as monkeys, that are valuable preclinical models [11, 14-21]

3. donor bone marrow was not indispensable in both the rodent and monkey models [18-21, 163] and,

4. some anti-T cell monoclonal antibodies also represent invaluable tools to restore self-tolerance in established autoimmunity.

In this context one may quote the quite impressive therapeutic effectiveness of CD3 antibodies in the non obese diabetic [NOD] mouse. NOD mice develop a spontaneous T cell mediated, autoimmune, insulin-dependent diabetes mellitus that closely resembles the human disease [164, 165]. Diabetogenic T cells, that transfer acute diabetes into immunoincompetent syngeneic recipients, are present in high frequency in the spleen of diabetic NOD mice and include both CD4+ (essentially IFNγ producing Th1 cells) and CD8+ lymphocytes [166-172]. In parallel to these effector cells, co-transfer experiments have identified a subset of CD4+CD62L+ T cells in the spleen and the thymus of prediabetic animals mediating "active tolerance" namely, exerting an active control or a down-regulatory effect on diabetogenic lymphocytes or their precursors. These cells fully prevent the transfer of disease by diabetogenic cells [173, 174].

A low-dose CD3 treatment (5 to 20μg for 5 consecutive days) administered to overtly diabetic NOD mice (presence of glycosuria and glycemia $\geq$ 4g/l) induced permanent disease remission in 60-80% of mice [75, 111]. The remission was durable and the effect was not related to generalized long standing immunosuppression since 8 to 10 weeks after treatment all mice responded normally to exogenous antigens. The long term effect was specific for ß-cell-associated antigens since mice showing remission after CD3 antibody treatment did not destroy syngeneic islet grafts as untreated diabetic NOD females normally do [75]. Non mitogenic F(ab')2 fragments of 145 2C11 were as effective as the whole mitogenic antibody in promoting permanent remission of overt diabetes [111]. These results suggest that already available non-mitogenic engineered antibodies to human CD3 [113, 175] could represent interesting therapeutic tools in patients presenting with recent onset diabetes. They also open the prospect of using this same therapeutic strategy in other T-cell dependent autoimmune diseases.

At present, the precise cellular and molecular mechanisms underlying this immune tolerance are still ill defined. This explains that "operational tolerance", meaning an in vivo status of antigen specific unresponsiveness in the absence of generalized immunosuppression, is the general term frequently used to define this situation.

What is known, however, is that in nearly all the models we mentioned the tolerance is not deletional, i.e. not based on the physical elimination of the alloreactive or autoreactive effector T cells. Instead, the tolerant hosts frequently show potent T cell-mediated regulatory mechanisms that effectively control, down modulate or suppress pathogenic effectors. Of particular interest is the fact that tolerance, once induced, is frequently dominant or "infectious" according to the term initially coined by Gershon [176] and can be acquired by non-tolerant T cells in the absence of further immunosuppression [21]. In some transplantation models it was also shown that the tolerance can also spread to additional antigenic determinants provided that all determinants are presented together on the same antigen presenting cell, a phenomenon termed "linked suppression" [177]. The underlying principle is that tolerance to one antigen in one tissue allograft will facilitate tolerance to other alloantigens on other transplants, provided that the determinants are presented by the same antigen presenting cell, in other words that there is, at least partly, an alloantigen sharing between the different grafts [21, 177].

One interesting hypothesis put forward some years ago suggested that, based on the Th1/ Th2 paradigm [178], most of these phenomena were explained by an exclusive immune deviation from a Th1 allo or autodestructive response to a Th2 non destructive or even protective response. The data from some models of CD4 antibody induced tolerance to cardiac and renal allografts were in support of this assumption [179]. However, no firm evidence could confirm that T cells mediating transferable or infectious tolerance expressed a Th2 cytokine producing pattern [9]. One possible explanation for these results is that there may be other significant routes for T cell immune deviation than Th1 and Th2. The case of Th3 or Tr1 regulatory cells that mediated their effect through TGFβ and IL-10 production respectively, is interesting to mention [180, 181]. Another possibility is that cytokines are not the exclusive effectors of the immunoregulation.

It was also proposed that tolerant cells would be to some extent anergic i.e. providing no help, and compete for antigen presenting cell binding with potentially reactive effectors. There is interesting in vitro evidence to sustain this hypothesis. Thus, anergic human T cell clones could suppress the proliferation of potentially reactive non anergic cells provided the same antigen presenting cell was presenting the peptides specific for both partners [182]. Competition for the antigen presenting cell surface and locally produced IL-2 has been proposed as the mechanism for this effect while excluding a role for "inhibitory" cytokines [i.e. IL-4, IL-10] secreted by the anergic cells [182]. This type of effect is an interesting explanation for the in vivo linked suppression phenomenon [9, 177].

VI. CONCLUSIONS

The future for humanized monoclonal antibodies is promising and exiting. They have already significantly improved our therapeutic approach to transplantation and autoimmunity. The recent data in relevant preclinical models fully confirmed the expectations from rodent work in that anti-T cell monoclonals express therapeutic activities that are unique and not shared by most conventional chemical immunosuppressants.

The better understanding of the immune mechanisms that induce and/ or maintain "operational" tolerance will set the basis for devising suitable in vitro tests to monitor for antigen specific unresponsiveness. This will be a major step supporting the establishment of clinical protocols that will aim at tolerance and will dispense from the need for long term treatments with non specific immunosuppressants and all inherent major risks.

REFERENCES

1. Starzl TE. Heterologous antilymphocyte globulin. New Engl J Med 1968;279: 700-705.
2. Monaco AP, Wood ML, Russell PS. Studies on heterologous antilymphocyte serum in mice. III. Immunological tolerance and chimerism produced across the H2-locus with adult thymectomy and antilymphocyte serum. Ann N Y Acad Sci 1966;129:190-209.
3. Wood ML, Monaco AP, Gozzo JJ, Liegeois A. Use of homozygous allogeneic bone marrow for induction of tolerance with antilymphocyte serum: dose and timing. Transplant Proc 1971;3:676-679.
4. Billingham RE, Brent L, Medawar PB. Actively acquired tolerance to foreign cells. Nature 1953;172:603-606.
5. Kohler G, Milstein C. Continuous cultures of fused cells secreting antibody of predefined specificity. Nature 1975;256:495-497.
6. Kung P, Goldstein G, Reinherz EL, Schlossman SF. Monoclonal antibodies defining distinctive human T cell surface antigens. Science 1979;206:347-349.
7. Nicolls MR, Aversa GG, Pearce NW, et al. Induction of long-term specific tolerance to allografts in rats by therapy with an anti-CD3-like monoclonal antibody.

Transplantation 1993;55:459-468.

8. Qin S, Cobbold SP, Pope H, et al. "Infectious" transplantation tolerance. Science 1993;259:974-977.

9. Cobbold SP, Adams E, Marshall SE, Davies JD, Waldmann H. Mechanisms of peripheral tolerance and suppression induced by monoclonal antibodies to CD4 and CD8. Immunol Rev 1996;149:5-33.

10. Larsen CP, Elwood ET, Alexander DZ, et al. Long-term acceptance of skin and cardiac allografts after blocking CD40 and CD28 pathways. Nature 1996;381: 434-438.

11. Kirk AD, Burkly LC, Batty DS, et al. Treatment with humanized monoclonal antibody against CD154 prevents acute renal allograft rejection in nonhuman primates [see comments. Nat Med 1999;5:686-693.

12. Bushell A, Niimi M, Morris PJ, Wood KJ. Evidence for immune regulation in the induction of transplantation tolerance: a conditional but limited role for IL-4. J Immunol 1999;162:1359-1366.

13. Niimi M, Pearson TC, Larsen CP, et al. The role of the CD40 pathway in alloantigen-induced hyporesponsiveness in vivo. J Immunol 1998;161:5331-5337.

14. Thomas JM, Carver FM, Foil MB, Hall WR, Adams C, Fahrenbruch GB. Renal allograft tolerance induced with ATG and donor bone marrow in outbred rhesus monkeys. Transplantation 1983;36:104-106.

15. Thomas J, Carver M, Cunningham P, Park K, Gonder J, Thomas F. Promotion of incompatible allograft acceptance in rhesus monkeys given posttransplant antithymocyte globulin and donor bone marrow. I. In vivo parameters and immunohistologic evidence suggesting microchimerism. Transplantation 1987;43:332-338.

16. Thomas JM, Carver FM, Cunningham PR, Olson LC, Thomas FT. Kidney allograft tolerance in primates without chronic immunosuppression--the role of veto cells. Transplantation 1991;51:198-207.

17. Thomas J, Alqaisi M, Cunningham P, et al. The development of a posttransplant TLI treatment strategy that promotes organ allograft acceptance without chronic immunosuppression. Transplantation 1992;53:247-258.

18. Thomas FT, Ricordi C, Contreras JL, et al. Reversal of naturally occuring diabetes in primates by unmodified islet xenografts without chronic immunosuppression. Tansplantation 1999;67:846-854.

19. Hamawy MM, Knechtle SJ. trategies for tolerance induction in nonhuman primates. Curr Opin Immunol 1998;10:513-517.

20. Thomas JM, Neville DM, Contreras JL, et al. Preclinical studies of allograft tolerance in rhesus monkeys: a novel anti-CD3-immunotoxin given peritransplant with donor bone marrow induces operational tolerance to kidney allografts. Tansplantation 1997;64:124-135.

21. Cobbold S, Waldmann H. Infectious tolerance. Curr Opin Immunol 1998;10: 518-524.

22. Larsen CP, Pearson TC. The CD40 pathway in allograft rejection, acceptance, and tolerance. Current Opinion In Immunology 1997;9:641-647.

23. Bach JF, Strom TB. Antilymphocyte antibodies. In: Bach JF, Strom TB, editors. The Mode of Action of Immunosuppressive Agents. Amsterdam: Elsevier, 1985: 271-391.

24. Bonnefoy-Berard N, Vincent C, Revillard JP. Antibodies against functional leukocyte surface molecules in polyclonal antilymphocyte and antithymocyte globulins. Tansplantation 1991;51:669-673.

25. Rebellato LM, Gross U, Verbanac KM, Thomas JM. A comprehensive definition of the major antibody specificities in polyclonal rabbit antithymocyte globulin. Tansplantation 1994;57:685-694.

26. Bourdage JS, Hamlin DM. Comparative polyclonal antithymocyte globulin and antilymphocyte/antilymphoblast globulin anti-CD antigen analysis by flow cytom-

etry. Tansplantation 1995;59:1194-1200.

27. Balner H, Eysvoogel VP, Cleton FJ. Testing of anti-human lymphocyte sera in chimpanzees and lower primates. Lancet 1968;1:19-22.

28. Clevers H, Alarcon B, Wileman T, Terhorst C. The T cell receptor/CD3 complex: a dynamic protein ensemble. Annu Rev Immunol 1988;6 :629-662.

29. Davis MM, Chien YH. T cell antigen receptors. In: Paul WE, editors. Fundamental Immunology. New York: Raven Press, 1999:341-366.

30. Leo O, Foo M, Sachs DH, Samelson LE, Bluestone JA. Identification of a monoclonal antibody specific for a murine T3 polypeptide. Proc Natl Acad Sci USA 1987;84:1374-1378.

31. Nooij FJ, Jonker M, Balner H. Differentiation antigens on rhesus monkey lymphocytes. II. Characterization of RhT3, a CD3-like antigen on T cells. Eur J Immunol 1986;16:981-984.

32. Emmrich F, Bach JF. Therapeutic anti-CD4 antibodies. In: Bach JF, editors. T-Cell-Directed Immunointervention. Oxford: Blackwell, 1993:176-200.

33. Emmrich F, Rieber P, Kurrle R, Eichmann K. Selective stimulation of human T lymphocyte subsets by heteroconjugates of antibodies to the T cell receptor and to subset-specific differentiation antigens. Eur J Immunol 1988;18:645-648.

34. Julius M, Maroun CR, Haughn L. Distinct roles for CD4 and CD8 as co-receptors in antigen receptor signalling. Immunol Today 1993;14:177-183.

35. Rudd CE. CD4, CD8 and the TCR-CD3 complex: a novel class of protein-tyrosine kinase receptor. Immunol Today 1990;11:400-406.

36. Thome M, Duplay P, Guttinger M, Acuto O. Syk and ZAP-70 mediate recruitment of p56lck/CD4 to the activated T cell receptor/CD3/zeta complex. J Exp Med 1995;181:1997-2006.

37. Bank I, Chess L. Perturbation of the T4 molecule transmits a negative signal to T cells. J Exp Med 1985;162:1294-1303.

38. Emmrich F, Kanz L, Eichmann K. Cross-linking of the T cell receptor complex with the subset-specific differentiation antigen stimulates interleukin 2 receptor expression in human CD4 and CD8 T cells. Eur J Immunol 1987;17:529-534.

39. Jabado N, Le Deist F, Fisher A, Hivroz C. Interaction of HIV gp120 and anti-CD4 antibodies with the CD4 molecule on human CD4+ T cells inhibits the binding activity of NF-AT, NF-kappa B and AP-1, three nuclear factors regulating interleukin-2 gene enhancer activity. Eur J Immunol 1994;24:2646-2652.

40. Jabado N, Pallier A, Jauliac S, Fischer A, Hivroz C. gp160 of HIV or anti-CD4 monoclonal antibody ligation of CD4 induces inhibition of JNK and ERK-2 activities in human peripheral CD4+ T lymphocytes. Eur J Immunol 1997;27:397-404.

41. Jabado N, Pallier A, Le Deist F, Bernard F, Fischer A, Hivroz C. CD4 ligands inhibit the formation of multifunctional transduction complexes involved in T cell activation. J Immunol 1997;158:94-103.

42. Jauliac S, Mazerolles F, Jabado N, et al. Ligands of CD4 inhibit the association of phospholipase Cgamma1 with phosphoinositide 3 kinase in T cells: regulation of this association by the phosphoinositide 3 kinase activity. Eur J Immunol 1998;28:3183-3191.

43. Waldmann TA, O'Shea J. The use of antibodies against the IL-2 receptor in transplantation. Current Opinion In Immunology 1998;10:507-512.

44. Nashan B, Moore R, Amlot P, Schmidt AG, Abeywickrama K, Soulillou JP. Randomised trial of basiliximab versus placebo for control of acute cellular rejection in renal allograft recipients. CHIB 201 International Study Group [published erratum appears in Lancet 1997 Nov 15;350[9089]:1484. Lancet 1997;350: 1193-1198.

45. Vincenti F, Kirkman R, Light S, et al. Interleukin-2-receptor blockade with daclizumab to prevent acute rejection in renal transplantation. New England Journal of Medicine 1998;338:161-165.

46. Calne R, Moffatt SD, Friend PJ, et al. Campath IH allows low-dose cyclosporine monotherapy in 31 cadaveric renal allograft recipients. Transplantation 1999;68: 1613-1616.

47. Lockwood CM, Thiru S, Isaacs JD, Hale G, Waldmann H. Long-term remission of intractable systemic vasculitis with monoclonal antibody therapy. Lancet 1993; 341:1620-1622.

48. Lockwood CM, Thiru S, Stewart S, et al. Treatment of refractory Wegener's granulomatosis with humanized monoclonal antibodies Qjm 1996;89:903-912.

49. Martin WJ, Miller JF. Cell to cell interaction in the immune response. IV. Site of action of antilymphocyte globulin. J Exp Med 1968;128:855-874

50. Greaves MF, Tursi A, Playfair JH, Torrigiani G, Zamir R, Roitt IM. Immunosuppressive potency and in vitro activity of antilymphocyte globulin. Lancet 1969;1: 68-72

51. Genestier L, Fournel S, Flacher M, Assossou O, Revillard JP, Bonnefoy-Berard N. Induction of Fas [Apo-1, CD95]-mediated apoptosis of activated lymphocytes by polyclonal antithymocyte globulins. Blood 1998;91:2360-2368.

52. Levey RH, Medawar PB. Some experiments on the action of antilymphoid antisera. Ann N Y Acad Sci 1966;129:164.

53. Maki T, Simpson M, Monaco AP. Development of suppressor T cells by antilymphocyte serum treatment in mice. Transplantation 1982;34:376-381.

54. Thomas FT, Carver FM, Foil MB, et al. Long-term incompatible kidney survival in outbred higher primates without chronic immunosuppression. Ann Surg 1983; 198:370-378.

55. Bindon CI, Hale G, Waldmann H. Importance of antigen specificity for complement-mediated lysis by monoclonal antibodies. Eur J Immunol 1988;18:1507-1514.

56. Isaacs JD, Clark MR, Greenwood J, Waldmann H. Therapy with monoclonal antibodies. An in vivo model for the assessment of therapeutic potential. J Immunol 1992;148:3062-3071.

57. Riechmann L, Clark M, Waldmann H, Winter G. Reshaping human antibodies for therapy. Nature 1988;332:323-327.

58. Hale G, Waldmann H. Control of graft-versus-host disease and graft rejection by T cell depletion of donor and recipient with Campath-1 antibodies. Results of matched sibling transplants for malignant diseases Bone Marrow Transplantation 1994;13:597-611.

59. Hale G, Zhang MJ, Bunjes D, et al. Improving the outcome of bone marrow transplantation by using CD52 monoclonal antibodies to prevent graft-versus-host disease and graft rejection. Blood 1998;92:4581-4590.

60. Isaacs JD, Wing MG, Greenwood JD, Hazleman BL, Hale G, Waldmann H. A therapeutic human IgG4 monoclonal antibody that depletes target cells in humans. Clinical & Experimental Immunology 1996;106:427-433.

61. Chatenoud L, Baudrihaye MF, Kreis H, Goldstein G, Schindler J, Bach JF. Human in vivo antigenic modulation induced by the anti-T cell OKT3 monoclonal antibody. Eur J Immunol 1982;12:979-982.

62. Chatenoud L, Bach JF. Antigenic modulation: a major mechanism of antibody action. Immunol Today 1984;5:20-25.

63. Abbs IC, Clark M, Waldmann H, Chatenoud L, Koffman CG, Sacks SH. Sparing of first dose effect of monovalent anti-CD3 antibody used in allograft rejection is associated with diminished release of pro-inflammatory cytokines. Therapeutic Immunology 1994;1:325-331.

64. Routledge EG, Lloyd I, Gorman SD, Clark M, Waldmann H. A humanized monovalent CD3 antibody which can activate homologous complement. Eur J Immunol 1991;21:2717-2725.

65. Clark M, Bindon C, Dyer M, et al. The improved lytic function and in vivo efficacy of monovalent monoclonal CD3 antibodies. Eur J Immunol 1989;19:381-388.

66. Wong JT, Colvin RB. Selective reduction and proliferation of the CD4+ and CD8+ T cell subsets with bispecific monoclonal antibodies: evidence for inter-T cell-mediated cytolysis. Clin Immunol Immunopathol 1991;58:236-250.

67. Smith CA, Williams GT, Kingston R, Jenkinson EJ, Owen JJ. Antibodies to CD3/T-cell receptor complex induce death by apoptosis in immature T cells in thymic cultures. Nature 1989;337:181-184.

68. Wesselborg S, Janssen O, Kabelitz D. Induction of activation-driven death [apoptosis] in activated but not resting peripheral blood T cells. J Immunol 1993;150: 4338-4345.

69. Choy EH, Adjaye J, Forrest L, Kingsley GH, Panayi GS. Chimaeric anti-CD4 monoclonal antibody cross-linked by monocyte Fc gamma receptor mediates apoptosis of human CD4 lymphocytes. Eur J Immunol 1993;23:2676-2681.

70. Genestier L, Paillot R, Bonnefoy-Berard N, et al. Fas-independent apoptosis of activated T cells induced by antibodies to the HLA class I alpha1 domain. Blood 1997;90:3629-3639.

71. Moreland LW, Pratt PW, Bucy RP, Jackson BS, Feldman JW, Koopman WJ. Treatment of refractory rheumatoid arthritis with a chimeric anti-CD4 monoclonal antibody. Long-term followup of CD4+ T cell counts. Arthritis Rheum 1994;37: 834-838.

72. Caillat-Zucman S, Blumenfeld N, Legendre C, et al. The OKT3 immunosuppressive effect. In situ antigenic modulation of human graft-infiltrating T cells. Transplantation 1990;49:156-160.

73. Cosimi AB, Colvin RB, Burton RC, et al. Use of monoclonal antibodies to T-cell subsets for immunologic monitoring and treatment in recipients of renal allografts. N Engl J Med 1981;305:308-314.

74. Vigeral P, Chkoff N, Chatenoud L, et al. Prophylactic use of OKT3 monoclonal antibody in cadaver kidney recipients. Utilization of OKT3 as the sole immunosuppressive agent. Transplantation 1986;41:730-733.

75. Chatenoud L, Thervet E, Primo J, Bach JF. Anti-CD3 antibody induces long-term remission of overt autoimmunity in nonobese diabetic mice. Proc Natl Acad Sci USA 1994;91:123-127.

76. Debure A, Chkoff N, Chatenoud L, et al. One-month prophylactic use of OKT3 in cadaver kidney transplant recipients. Transplantation 1988;45:546-553.

77. Pearson TC, Madsen JC, Larsen CP, Morris PJ, Wood KJ. Induction of transplantation tolerance in adults using donor antigen and anti-CD4 monoclonal antibody. Transplantation 1992;54:475-483.

78. Chatenoud L, Baudrihaye MF, Chkoff N, Kreis H, Goldstein G, Bach JF. Restriction of the human in vivo immune response against the mouse monoclonal antibody OKT3. J Immunol 1986;137:830-838.

79. Benjamin RJ, Cobbold SP, Clark MR, Waldmann H. Tolerance to rat monoclonal antibodies. Implications for serotherapy. J Exp Med 1986;163:1539-1552.

80. Cosimi AB, Burton RC, Kung PC, et al. Evaluation in primate renal allograft recipients of monoclonal antibody to human T-cell subclasses. Transplant Proc 1981;13:499-503.

81. Ortho X. A randomized clinical trial of OKT3 monoclonal antibody for acute rejection of cadaveric renal transplants. Ortho Multicenter Transplant Study Group. N Engl J Med 1985;313:337-342.

82. Goldstein G, Fuccello AJ, Norman DJ, Shield Cf 3D, Colvin RB, Cosimi AB. OKT3 monoclonal antibody plasma levels during therapy and the subsequent development of host antibodies to OKT3. Transplantation 1986;42:507-511.

83. Norman DJ, Shield Cf 3D, Henell KR, et al. Effectiveness of a second course of OKT3 monoclonal anti-T cell antibody for treatment of renal allograft rejection. Transplantation 1988;46:523-529.

84. Legendre C, Kreis H, Bach JF, Chatenoud L. Prediction of successful allograft

rejection retreatment with OKT3. Transplantation 1992;53:87-90.

85. Villemain F, Jonker M, Bach JF, Chatenoud L. Fine specificity of antibodies produced in rhesus monkeys following in vivo treatment with anti-T cell murine monoclonal antibodies. Eur J Immunol 1986;16:945-949.

86. Baudrihaye MF, Chatenoud L, Kreis H, Goldstein G, Bach JF. Unusually restricted anti-isotype human immune response to OKT3 monoclonal antibody. Eur J Immunol 1984;14:686-691.

87. Chatenoud L, Jonker M, Villemain F, Goldstein G, Bach JF. The human immune response to the OKT3 monoclonal antibody is oligoclonal. Science 1986;232:1406-1408.

88. Abramowicz D, Crusiaux A, Goldman M. Anaphylactic shock after retreatment with OKT3 monoclonal antibody. N Engl J Med 1992;327:736.

89. Hricik DE, Mayes JT, Schulak JA. Inhibition of anti-OKT3 antibody generation by cyclosporine--results of a prospective randomized trial. Transplantation 1990; 50:237-240.

90. Morrison SL, Johnson MJ, Herzenberg LA, Oi VT. Chimeric human antibody molecules: mouse antigen-binding domains with human constant region domains. Proc Natl Acad Sci USA 1984;81:6851-6855.

91. Winter G, Milstein C. Man-made antibodies. Nature 1991;349:293-299.

92. Lazarovits AI, Rochon J, Banks L, et al. Human mouse chimeric CD7 monoclonal antibody [SDZCHH380] for the prophylaxis of kidney transplant rejection. J Immunol 1993;150:5163-5174.

93. Rebello PR, Hale G, Friend PJ, Cobbold P, Waldmann H. Anti-globulin responses to rat and humanized CAMPATH-1 monoclonal antibody used to treat transplant rejection. Transplantation 1999;68:1417-1420.

94. Elliott MJ, Maini RN, Feldmann M, et al. Repeated therapy with monoclonal antibody to tumour necrosis factor alpha [cA2] in patients with rheumatoid arthritis. Lancet 1994;344:1125-1127.

95. Bruggemann M, Taussig MJ. Production of human antibody repertoires in transgenic mice. Current Opinion In Biotechnology 1997;8:455-458.

96. Bruggemann M, Neuberger MS. Strategies for expressing human antibody repertoires in transgenic mice. Immunology Today 1996;17:391-397.

97. Marks JD, Hoogenboom HR, Bonnert TP, McCafferty J, Griffiths AD, Winter G. By-passing immunization. Human antibodies from V-gene libraries displayed on phage. J Mol Biol 1991;222:581-597.

98. Lubin I, Segall H, Marcus H, et al. Engraftment of human peripheral blood lymphocytes in normal strains of mice. Blood 1994;83:2368-2381.

99. Abramowicz D, Schandene L, Goldman M, et al. Release of tumor necrosis factor, interleukin-2, and gamma-interferon in serum after injection of OKT3 monoclonal antibody in kidney transplant recipients. Transplantation 1989;47:606-608.

100. Chatenoud L, Ferran C, Legendre C, et al. In vivo cell activation following OKT3 administration. Systemic cytokine release and modulation by corticosteroids. Transplantation 1990;49:697-702.

101. Chatenoud L, Ferran C, Reuter A, et al. Systemic reaction to the anti-T-cell monoclonal antibody OKT3 in relation to serum levels of tumor necrosis factor and interferon-gamma. N Engl J Med 1989;320:1420-1421.

102. Ferran C, Sheehan K, Dy M, et al. Cytokine-related syndrome following injection of anti-CD3 monoclonal antibody: further evidence for transient in vivo T cell activation. Eur J Immunol 1990;20:509-515.

103. Hirsch R, Gress RE, Pluznik DH, Eckhaus M, Bluestone JA. Effects of in vivo administration of anti-CD3 monoclonal antibody on T cell function in mice. II. In vivo activation of T cells. J Immunol 1989;142:737-743.

104. Weinshenker BG, Bass B, Karlik S, Ebers GC, Rice GP. An open trial of OKT3 in patients with multiple sclerosis. Neurology 1991;41:1047-1052.

105. Durez P, Abramowicz D, Gerard C, et al. In vivo induction of interleukin 10 by anti-CD3 monoclonal antibody or bacterial lipopolysaccharide: differential modulation by cyclosporin A. J Exp Med 1993;177:551-555.
106. Yoshimoto T, Paul WE. CD4pos, NK1.1pos T cells promptly produce interleukin 4 in response to in vivo challenge with anti-CD3. J Exp Med 1994;179:1285-1295.
107. Flamand V, Abramowicz D, Goldman M, et al. Anti-CD3 antibodies induce T cells from unprimed animals to secrete IL-4 both in vitro and in vivo. J Immunol 1990;144:2875-2882.
108. Van Lier RA, Boot JH, de Groot ER, Aarden LA. Induction of T cell proliferation with anti-CD3 switch-variant monoclonal antibodies: effects of heavy chain isotype in monocyte-dependent systems. Eur J Immunol 1987;17:1599-1604.
109. Hirsch R, Bluestone JA, de Nenno L, Gress RE. Anti-CD3 F[ab']2 fragments are immunosuppressive in vivo without evoking either the strong humoral response or morbidity associated with whole mAb. Transplantation 1990;49:1117-1123.
110. Parlevliet KJ, Ten Berge IJ, Yong SL, Surachno J, Wilmink JM, Schellekens PT. In vivo effects of IgA and IgG2a anti-CD3 isotype switch variants. J Clin Invest 1994;93:2519-2525.
111. Chatenoud L, Primo J, Bach JF. CD3 antibody-induced dominant self tolerance in overtly diabetic NOD mice. J Immunol 1997;158:2947-2954.
112. Alegre ML, Peterson LJ, Xu D, et al. A non-activating "humanized" anti-CD3 monoclonal antibody retains immunosuppressive properties in vivo. Tansplantation 1994;57:1537-1543.
113. Bolt S, Routledge E, Lloyd I, et al. The generation of a humanized, non-mitogenic CD3 monoclonal antibody which retains in vitro immunosuppressive properties. Eur J Immunol 1993;23:403-411.
114. Routledge EG, Falconer ME, Pope H, Lloyd IS, Waldmann H. The effect of aglycosylation on the immunogenicity of a humanized therapeutic CD3 monoclonal antibody. Tansplantation 1995;60:847-853.
115. Woodle ES, Xu D, Zivin RA, et al. Phase I trial of a humanized, Fc receptor non-binding OKT3 antibody, huOKT3gamma1[Ala-Ala] in the treatment of acute renal allograft rejection. Tansplantation 1999;68:608-616.
116. Friend PJ, Hale G, Chatenoud L, et al. Phase I study of an engineered aglycosylated humanized CD3 antibody in renal transplant rejection. Transplantation 1999;68:1632-1637.
117. Cosimi AB, Burton RC, Colvin RB, et al. Treatment of acute renal allograft rejection with OKT3 monoclonal antibody. Transplantation 1981;32:535-539.
118. Frey DJ, Matas AJ, Gillingham KJ, et al. Sequential therapy--a prospective randomized trial of MALG versus OKT3 for prophylactic immunosuppression in cadaver renal allograft recipients. Transplantation 1992;54:50-56.
119. Abramowicz D, Goldman M, de Pauw L, Vanherweghem JL, Kinnaert P, Vereerstraeten P. The long-term effects of prophylactic OKT3 monoclonal antibody in cadaver kidney transplantation--a single-center, prospective, randomized study. Transplantation 1992;54:433-437.
120. Goldstein G. Overview of the development of Orthoclone OKT3: monoclonal antibody for therapeutic use in transplantation. Transplant Proc 1987;19:1-6.
121. Hricik DE, Zarconi J, Schulak JA. Influence of low-dose cyclosporine on the outcome of treatment with OKT3 for acute renal allograft rejection. Transplantation 1989;47:272-277.
122. Norman DJ, Barry JM, Bennett WM, et al. The use of OKT3 in cadaveric renal transplantation for rejection that is unresponsive to conventional anti-rejection therapy. Am J Kidney Dis 1988;11:90-93.
123. Colonna Jo 2D, Goldstein LI, Brems JJ, et al. A prospective study on the use of monoclonal anti-T3-cell antibody [OKT3] to treat steroid-resistant liver transplant rejection. Arch Surg 1987;122:1120-1123.

124. Woodle ES, Thistlethwaite Jr JR, Emond JC, et al. OKT3 therapy for hepatic allograft rejection. Differential response in adults and children. Transplantation 1991;51:1207-1212.

125. Goldstein G, Kremer AB, Barnes L, Hirsch RL. OKT3 monoclonal antibody reversal of renal and hepatic rejection in pediatric patients. J Pediatr 1987;111:1046-1050.

126. Farges O, Samuel D, Bismuth H. Orthoclone OKT3 in liver transplantation. Transplant Sci 1992;2:16-21.

127. Farges O, Ericzon BG, Bresson-Hadni S, et al. A randomized trial of OKT3-based versus cyclosporine-based immunoprophylaxis after liver transplantation. Long-term results of a European and Australian multicenter study. Tansplantation 1994;58:891-898.

128. Millis JM, McDiarmid SV, Hiatt JR, et al. Randomized prospective trial of OKT3 for early prophylaxis of rejection after liver transplantation. Transplantation 1989;47:82-88.

129. Eason JD, Cosimi AB. Biologic immunosuppressive agents. In: Ginns LC, Cosimi AB, Morris PJ, editors. Transplantation. Malden, USA: Blackwell Science, 1999:196-224.

130. Robbins RC, Oyer PE, Stinson EB, Starnes VA. The use of monoclonal antibodies after heart transplantation. Transplantation Science 1992;2:22-27.

131. Le Mauff B, Hourmant M, Rougier JP, et al. Effect of anti-LFA1 [CD11a] monoclonal antibodies in acute rejection in human kidney transplantation. Transplantation 1991;52:291-296.

132. Maraninchi D, Mawas C, Stoppa AM, et al. Anti LFA1 monoclonal antibody for the prevention of graft rejection after T cell-depleted HLA-matched bone marrow transplantation for leukemia in adults. Bone Marrow Transplantation 1989;4:147-150.

133. Soulillou JP, Cantarovich D, Le Mauff B, et al. Randomized controlled trial of a monoclonal antibody against the interleukin-2 receptor [33B3.1] as compared with rabbit antithymocyte globulin for prophylaxis against rejection of renal allografts. N Engl J Med 1990;322:1175-1182.

134. Kriaa F, Hiesse C, Alard P, et al. Prophylactic use of the anti-IL-2 receptor monoclonal antibody LO-Tact-1 in cadaveric renal transplantation: results of a randomized study. Transplantation Proceedings 1993;25:817-819.

135. Kirkman RL, Shapiro ME, Carpenter CB, et al. A randomized prospective trial of anti-Tac monoclonal antibody in human renal transplantation. Transplantation 1991;51:107-113.

136. Herzog C, Walker C, Muller W, et al. Anti-CD4 antibody treatment of patients with rheumatoid arthritis: I. Effect on clinical course and circulating T cells. J Autoimmun 1989;2:627-642.

137. Horneff G, Burmester GR, Emmrich F, Kalden JR. Treatment of rheumatoid arthritis with an anti-CD4 monoclonal antibody. Arthritis Rheum 1991;34:129-140.

138. Wendling D, Wijdenes J, Racadot E, Morel-Fourrier B. Therapeutic use of monoclonal anti-CD4 antibody in rheumatoid arthritis. J Rheumatol 1991;18:325-327.

139. Nicolas JF, Chamchick N, Thivolet J, Wijdenes J, Morel P, Revillard JP. CD4 antibody treatment of severe psoriasis. Lancet 1991;338:321.

140. Emmrich J, Seyfarth M, Fleig WE, Emmrich F. Treatment of inflammatory bowel disease with anti-CD4 monoclonal antibody. Lancet 1991;338:570-571.

141. Goldberg D, Morel P, Chatenoud L, et al. Immunological effects of high dose administration of anti-CD4 antibody in rheumatoid arthritis patients. J Autoimmun 1991;4:617-630.

142. Reiter C, Kakavand B, Rieber EP, Schattenkirchner M, Riethmuller G, Kruger K. Treatment of rheumatoid arthritis with monoclonal CD4 antibody M-T151. Clinical results and immunopharmacologic effects in an open study, including

repeated administration. Arthritis Rheum 1991;34:525-536.

143. Brennan FM, Feldmann M. Cytokines in autoimmunity. Curr Opin Immunol 1992;4:754-759.

144. Elliott MJ, Maini RN, Feldmann M, et al. Randomised double-blind comparison of chimeric monoclonal antibody to tumour necrosis factor alpha [cA2] versus placebo in rheumatoid arthritis. Lancet 1994;344:1105-1110.

145. Moreland LW, Baumgartner SW, Schiff MH, et al. Treatment of rheumatoid arthritis with a recombinant human tumor necrosis factor receptor [p75]-Fc fusion protein [see comments. N Engl J Med 1997;337:141-147.

146. Maini RN, Breedveld FC, Kalden JR, et al. Therapeutic efficacy of multiple intravenous infusions of anti-tumor necrosis factor alpha monoclonal antibody combined with low-dose weekly methotrexate in rheumatoid arthritis [see comments. Arthritis & Rheumatism 1998;41:1552-1563.

147. Van Dullemen HM, Van Deventer SJ, Hommes DW, et al. Treatment of Crohn's disease with anti-tumor necrosis factor chimeric monoclonal antibody [cA2]. Gastroenterology 1995;109:129-135.

148. Van Deventer SJ. Tumour necrosis factor and Crohn's disease [see comments]. [Review] [76 refs. Gut 1997;40:443-448.

149. Plevy SE, Landers CJ, Prehn J, et al. A role for TNF-alpha and mucosal T helper-1 cytokines in the pathogenesis of Crohn's disease. J Immunol 1997;159:6276-6282.

150. Van Der Lubbe PA, Reiter C, Breedveld FC, et al. Chimeric CD4 monoclonal antibody cM-T412 as a therapeutic approach to rheumatoid arthritis. Arthritis & Rheumatism 1993;36:1375-1379.

151. Van Der Lubbe PA, Reiter C, Miltenburg AM, et al. Treatment of rheumatoid arthritis with a chimeric CD4 monoclonal antibody [cM-T412]: immunopharmacological aspects and mechanisms of action. Scand J Immunol 1994;39:286-294.

152. Van Der Lubbe PA, Dijkmans BA, Markusse HM, Nassander U, Breedveld FC. A randomized, double-blind, placebo-controlled study of CD4 monoclonal antibody therapy in early rheumatoid arthritis. Arthritis & Rheumatism 1995;38:1097-1106.

153. Williams RO, Mason LJ, Feldmann M, Maini RN. Synergy between anti-CD4 and anti-tumor necrosis factor in the amelioration of established collagen-induced arthritis. Proc Natl Acad Sci USA 1994;91:2762-2766.

154. Bachelez H, Flageul B, Dubertret L, et al. Treatment of recalcitrant plaque psoriasis with a humanized non-depleting antibody to CD4. J Autoimmun 1998;11:53-62.

155. Watts RA, Isaacs JD, Hale G, Hazleman BL, Waldmann H. CAMPATH-1H in inflammatory arthritis. Clinical & Experimental Rheumatology 1993;11 Suppl 8:S165-S167.

156. Isaacs JD, Watts RA, Hazleman BL, et al. Humanised monoclonal antibody therapy for rheumatoid arthritis. Lancet 1992;340:748-752.

157. Moreau T, Thorpe J, Miller D, et al. Preliminary evidence from magnetic resonance imaging for reduction in disease activity after lymphocyte depletion in multiple sclerosis Lancet 1994;344:298-301.

158. Coles AJ, Wing MG, Smith S, et al. Pulsed monoclonal antibody treatment and autoimmune thyroid disease in multiple sclerosis. Lancet 1999;354:1691-1695.

159. Coles AJ, Wing MG, Molyneux P, et al. Monoclonal antibody treatment exposes three mechanisms underlying the clinical course of multiple sclerosis. Ann Neurol 1999;46:296-304.

160. Roser BJ. Cellular mechanisms in neonatal and adult tolerance. Immunol Rev 1989;107:179-202.

161. Donckier V, Flamand V, Desalle F, et al. IL-12 prevents neonatal induction of transplantation tolerance in mice. Eur J Immunol 1998;28:1426-1430.

162. Bobbio SA, Wood ML, Monaco AP. Significant augmentation of specific unresponsiveness by rapamycin in ALS-treated, bone marrow injected mice. Transplant Sci 1993;3:51-55.

163. Qin SX, Wise M, Cobbold SP, et al. Induction of tolerance in peripheral T cells with monoclonal antibodies. Eur J Immunol 1990;20:2737-2745.

164. Castano L, Eisenbarth GS. Type-I diabetes: a chronic autoimmune disease of human, mouse, and rat. Annu Rev Immunol 1990;8:647-679.

165. Bach JF. Insulin-dependent diabetes mellitus as an autoimmune disease. Endocrine Rev 1994;15:516-542.

166. Bendelac A, Carnaud C, Boitard C, Bach JF. Syngeneic transfer of autoimmune diabetes from diabetic NOD mice to healthy neonates. Requirement for both L3T4+ and Lyt-2+ T cells. J Exp Med 1987;166:823-832.

167. Wicker LS, Miller BJ, Mullen Y. Transfer of autoimmune diabetes mellitus with splenocytes from nonobese diabetic [NOD] mice. Diabetes 1986;35:855-860.

168. Miller BJ, Appel MC, O'Neil JJ, Wicker LS. Both the Lyt-2+ and L3T4+ T cell subsets are required for the transfer of diabetes in nonobese diabetic mice. J Immunol 1988;140:52-58.

169. Yagi H, Matsumoto M, Kunimoto K, Kawaguchi J, Makino S, Harada M. Analysis of the roles of CD4+ and CD8+ T cells in autoimmune diabetes of NOD mice using transfer to NOD athymic nude mice. Eur J Immunol 1992;22:2387-2393.

170. Haskins K, Portas M, Bergman B, Lafferty K, Bradley B. Pancreatic islet-specific T-cell clones from nonobese diabetic mice. Proc Natl Acad Sci USA 1989;86:8000-8004.

171. Katz JD, Benoist C, Mathis D. T helper cell subsets in insulin-dependent diabetes. Science 1995;268:1185-1188.

172. Healey D, Ozegbe P, Arden S, Chandler P, Hutton J, Cooke A. In vivo activity and in vitro specificity of CD4+ Th1 and Th2 cells derived from the spleens of diabetic NOD mice. J Clin Invest 1995;95:2979-2985.

173. Boitard C, Yasunami R, Dardenne M, Bach JF. T cell-mediated inhibition of the transfer of autoimmune diabetes in NOD mice. J Exp Med 1989;169:1669-1680.

174. Hutchings PR, Cooke A. The transfer of autoimmune diabetes in NOD mice can be inhibited or accelerated by distinct cell populations present in normal splenocytes taken from young males. J Autoimmun 1990;3:175-185.

175. Alegre ML, Collins AM, Pulito VL, et al. Effect of a single amino acid mutation on the activating and immunosuppressive properties of a "humanized" OKT3 monoclonal antibody. J Immunol 1992;148:3461-3468.

176. Gershon RK, Kondo K. Infectious immunological tolerance. Immunology 1971;21:903-914.

177. Davies JD, Leong LY, Mellor A, Cobbold SP, Waldmann H. T cell suppression in transplantation tolerance through linked recognition. J Immunol 1996;156:3602-3607.

178. Mosmann TR, Coffman RL. TH1 and TH2 cells: different patterns of lymphokine secretion lead to different functional properties. Annu Rev Immunol 1989;7:145-173.

179. Nickerson P, Steurer W, Steiger J, Zheng X, Steele AW, Strom TB. Cytokines and the Th1/Th2 paradigm in transplantation. Curr Opin Immunol 1994;6:757-764.

180. Weiner HL, Friedman A, Miller A, et al. Oral tolerance: immunologic mechanisms and treatment of animal and human organ-specific autoimmune diseases by oral administration of autoantigens. Annu Rev Immunol 1994;12:809-837.

181. Groux H, O'Garra A, Bigler M, et al. A CD4+ T-cell subset inhibits antigen-specific T-cell responses and prevents colitis. Nature 1997;389:737-742.

182. Lombardi G, Sidhu S, Batchelor R, Lechler R. Anergic T cells as suppressor cells in vitro. Science 1994;264:1587-1589.

CYTOKINES AND THEIR RECEPTORS AS THERAPEUTIC TARGETS

4

Peter Nickerson
Depts of Internal Medicine and Immunology
University of Manitoba
Winnipeg, Manitoba, Canada

INTRODUCTION

A major advance in our understanding of the development effector T cells programs came in 1986 when Mosmann and Coffman observed that individual CD4$^+$ T helper (Th) cell clones express phenotypically distinct cytokine profiles [1]. Since then numerous investigators have explored the regulation of these polarized Th cytokine programs, which has given rise to a unifying concept - 'the Th1/Th2 paradigm' (Fig. 1). Central to this paradigm is the role of certain cytokines that act as cross regulators of Th1/Th2 cell function. IFNγ, a Th1 product, inhibits expression of the Th2 program while IL-4 and IL-10, Th2 products, can act to block the Th1 program. In appreciation of these facts, an intensive effort has been launched to reach an understanding of the CD4$^+$ T-cell programs associated with allograft rejection and tolerance. Indeed, therapeutic strategies based on the concept of manipulating cytokine networks have been put forward as a possible means to control the allograft response. These strategies include: (i) inhibition of production/effects of Th1 cytokines, (ii) enhancing systemic or local levels of Th2 cytokines, and (iii) targeting key cytokine receptors.

Recently it has become apparent that the Th1/Th2 model, while providing a valuable framework for probing various models, has undoubtedly oversimplified the complexity of cytokine responses by individual T-cells in vivo [2, 3]. Indeed, as suggested by Mossman and Kelso, these two patterns of cytokine expression likely represent extremes of many possible outcomes. The aim of this chapter then is to review the experimental data that supports or refutes the validity of the Th1/Th2 model in the context of allograft rejection and tol-

81

A. W. Thomson (ed.), Therapeutic Immunosuppression, 81–99.
© 2001 *Kluwer Academic Publishers.*

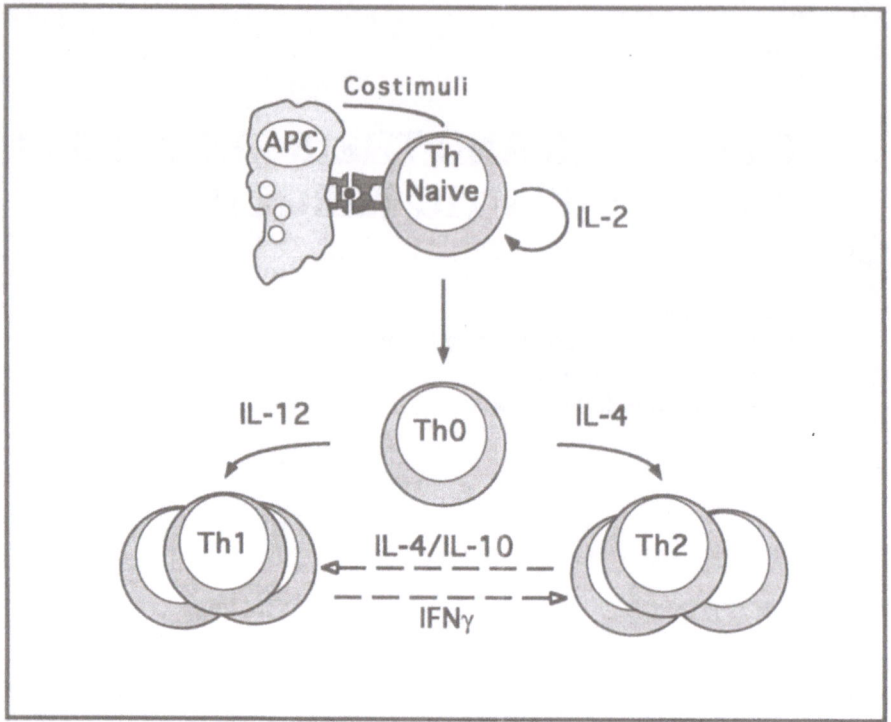

Figure 1
CD4⁺ T-cell activation programs (solid arrows indicate positive effect, hatched arrows indicate inhibitory effect).

erance and ask whether the manipulation of cytokine networks will provide a robust opportunity for inducing transplantation tolerance in the clinic.

T-CELL ACTIVATION AND THE TH1/TH2 PARADIGM

The current understanding of naive T-cell activation and the development of cytokine effector programs has evolved rapidly in the last 5 years (reviewed in [4-6]). T-cell activation is a two-step process in which occupancy of the T-cell receptor (TCR) by processed antigen/major histocompatibility complex (Ag/MHC) provides the first signal for full activation. Signal two ('costimulation') is derived from cognate ligand-ligand interactions between proteins expressed upon the surfaces of antigen-presenting cells (APCs) and T-cells. Dendritic cells (DC) are the most potent APCs in providing these costimulation signals to naive T-cells, whereas all APCs (i.e. DC, activated macrophages or B-cells) are able to stimulate primed T-cells [7, 8].

In studies that utilize α/β-TCR transgenic animals, primary in vitro stimulation with antigen pulsed APCs initially results in low level IL-2, but not IL-4 or IFNγ, production by naive CD4$^+$ T-cells [9, 10] (Fig. 1). Continued stimulation evokes IL-2, IL-4, IL-5, IL-6, and IFNγ production (Th0). With chronic stimulation, naive Th cells mature to a Th1 or Th2 phenotype, which is thought to be via passage through this common precursor (Th0) stage. This concept is indirectly supported by data showing that naive T-cells which become IL-4 producers (i.e. Th2 cells) require exposure to IL-2 as well as IL-4 to acquire this phenotype [11, 12]. To directly test this hypothesis a transgenic mouse was created in which the IL-4 promoter was placed upstream of the gene for herpes simplex virus (HSV) thymidine kinase (TK) [13]. Upon activation of naive T-cells exposed to ganciclovir, which kills cells expressing the IL-4 gene, production of both IFNγ and IL-4 was eliminated. Thus, effector cells producing IL-4 (Th2) or IFNγ (Th1) appear to differentiate from a common precursor expressing IL-4 (i.e. the Th0 cell).

To date studies suggest that the decision to commit to a Th1 vs. Th2 response is primarily dependent upon the cytokine microenvironment present at the time of naive T-cell activation (i.e. the presence of IL-12, IFNγ, or IL-4) (reviewed in [5, 6]). IL-12, a 75kDa heterodimer derived from DC or macrophages, favors the expression of a Th1 cell program (e.g. augments IFNγ production) [14-17]. Functional receptors for IL-12 are restricted to activated uncommitted T-cells and to Th1 cells, and are lost on Th2 cells [18]. Anti-IL-12 antiserum blocks expression of the Th1 phenotype and IL-12 knockout mice have a greatly diminished Th1 response [19]. IFNγ, derived from NK and T-cells, promotes Th1 development, in part, via enhancing IL-12 production by macrophages and maintaining IL-12 receptor β2 chain expression on CD4$^+$ cells [20-22]. Conversely, in vitro, if primary stimulation is accompanied by IL-4, CD4$^+$ T-cells commit to a Th2 cytokine profile (i.e. IL-4, IL-5, IL-13) while provision of an αIL-4 mAb in the primary culture promotes expression of a Th1 phenotype (i.e. IFNγ, lymphotoxin). The mechanism of action of IL-4 is not entirely clear, but IL-4 has been found to inhibit IL-12 production by DC and macrophages, as well as to downregulate the expression of IL-12Rβ2 chain on Th2 cells [14, 16, 21-24]. Moreover, IL-4 is dominant over IL-12 when both are present at the time of naive T-cell activation [14, 25]. The source of IL-4 at the time of naive T-cell activation remains a matter of debate, potential sources include memory CD4$^+$ cells, CD4$^+$ NK1.1$^+$ cells, mast cells, basophils and eosinophils [5]. Taken together these studies support the concept that naive T-cells are not precommitted to a Th1 or Th2 phenotype but rather the cytokine environment at the time of activation determines the subsequent program.

Recently, two groups have challenged the central role of cytokines in determining naive T-cell commitment to a Th1 vs. Th2 effector population. First, in a rather elegant study, Bird et al demonstrated that the number of cell cycles controlled the ability of naive T-cells to express specific cytokines [26]. Specifically, IL-2 was shown to be expressed with stimulation of naive T-cells independent of cell cycle progression. IFNγ expression increased progressively with cell division but required entry into the S phase of the cell cycle. Expression of IL-4, however, did not occur until at least 3 cell divisions had taken place. Interestingly, the addition of IL-12 or IL-4 at the time of naive T-cell stimulation, while leading to an enhanced Th1 or Th2 program respectively, did not change the dependence on cell cycle requirements for the expression of IFNγ or IL-4. This suggests that IL-12 and IL-4 can direct more polarized states only by increasing or limiting the initial number of effector cytokine-expressing cells. Indeed, the absolute requirement for IL-12 or IL-4 in the instruction of a Th1 or Th2 effector program has been called into question (reviewed in [4]). Other factors, have also been implicated in determining the naive T-cell commitment to a Th1 vs. Th2 program. For example the dose and nature of the antigen, the type of the APC costimulators involved (B7-1 vs. B7-2), and the strength of the antigen/MHC-TCR interaction have all been shown to play a potential role [27-29]. Moreover, in a recent study, Rissoan et al suggest that the origin of the dendritic cell itself may control naive T cell differentiation into Th1 vs. Th2 effector responses [30]. In this study, monocyte derived DC (DC1) produce IL-12 and induce Th1 differentiation, while plasmacytoid derived DC (DC2), though not producing IL-4, induce Th2 differentiation by a mechanism that was independent of IL-12 or IL-4. This suggests that DC2 elicit a Th2 response from naive T-cells by a unique pathway. What is not clear is the nature of the signals that elicit a DC1 vs. a DC2 response upon antigen exposure. Thus, there is accumulating evidence that the commitment of naive T-cells to Th1 or Th2 effector programs is more complex than originally envisioned based on cytokine regulation alone.

Once Th1 and Th2 cell programs are activated they further intensify the committed response via the cross-regulation of one another in vivo through the release of IFNγ or IL-4 and IL-10, respectively, into the microenvironment (Fig. 1). One could envision then therapeutic strategies that attempt to use cytokines to deviate a mature Th1 program to a Th2 program and visa versa. Indeed, Perez et al found that naive CD4+ T-cells which initially express a Th1 phenotype after the addition of exogenous IL-12 during Ag-APC induced activation, could be deviated to a Th2 phenotype by exposing these T-cells to IL-4 during subsequent Ag challenge [31]. The corollary was not true, naive T-cells which expressed a Th2 phenotype via exposure to exogenous

IL-4 during initial Ag challenge did not deviate to a Th1 phenotype upon subsequent Ag challenge in the presence of IL-12. Unfortunately, to date more mature Th1 and Th2 phenotypes appear to be terminally differentiated programs [4, 6].

From the aforementioned, it is clear that Th1 and Th2 programs are polar extremes and indeed appear to act as negative regulators of each other. What is not clear, and will be developed below in the context of the alloimmune response, is whether one Th program is protective over the other (i.e. is a Th2 response anti-inflammatory when it is present and excluding a Th1 response?). It should also be emphasized that other CD4$^+$ T-cell programs are known to exist that are distinct from Th1 or Th2 effector cells (reviewed in [32]). Indeed, a number of groups have demonstrated that CD4$^+$ T-cells that express IL-10 or TGFβ are capable of immunoregulation of both Th1 and Th2 mediated inflammatory responses [33-36]. It is with this background in mind that we turn to the validity of the Th1/Th2 paradigm in the context of the immune response to alloantigens.

CYTOKINE PROGRAMS AND ALLOGRAFT REJECTION

Intragraft IL-2, IFNγ, and the CTL specific marker granzyme B, proteins and/or transcripts have been detected in rejecting allografts while IL-4 expression has not been as consistently detected [37-40]. Moreover, the sequential analysis of either rejecting experimental allografts [37-39] or human renal allografts biopsies [41], usually detects IL-2 and IFNγ gene expression preceding graft dysfunction. The precise roles of IFNγ and IL-2 in graft rejection are uncertain. However, several CD4$^+$ T-cell dependent effector mechanisms (i.e. delayed type hypersensitivity (DTH), complement and antibody dependent cellular cytotoxicity (i.e. CDC and ADCC), and cytotoxic T-lymphocyte (CTL) activity) participate in acute allograft rejection (Fig. 2). In this context, IL-2 is believed to stimulate both the proliferation of T-cells and activation of cytotoxic function of CTLs. IFNγ is thought to recruit macrophages into the graft, cause macrophage activation, enhance CTL activation, upregulate MHC expression by the graft and induce IgG isotype switching to IgG1 and IgG3 that can bind high affinity Fcγ receptors and complement.

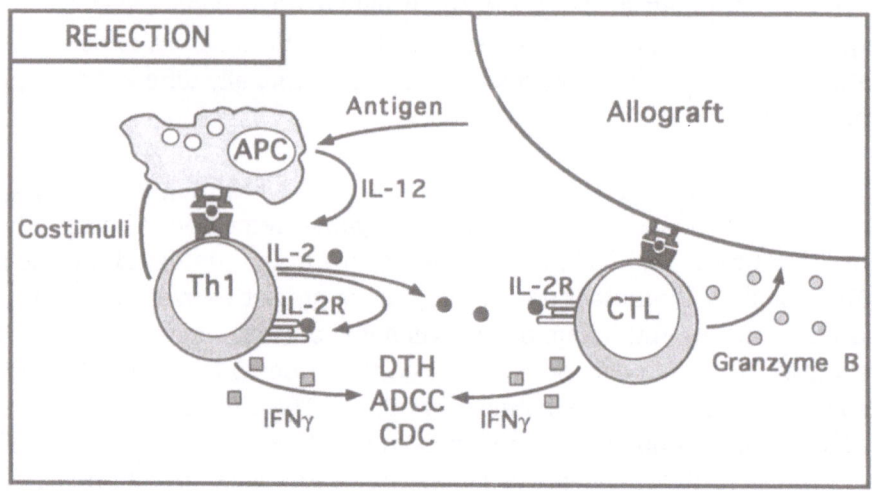

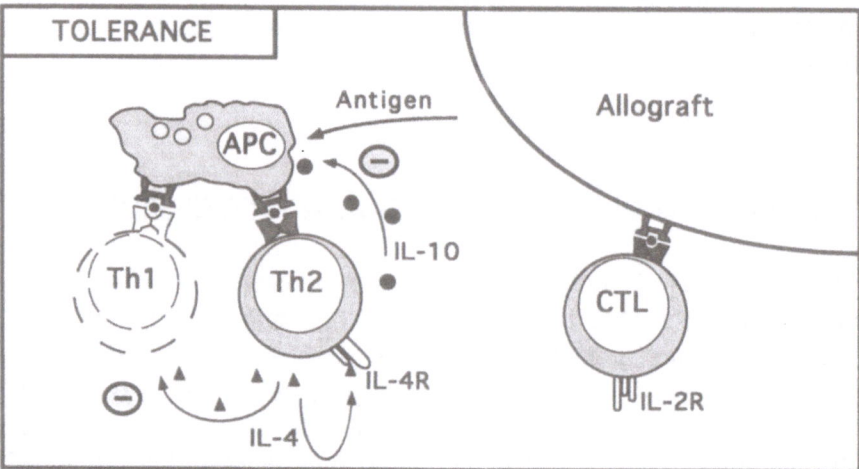

Figure 2
A model of T-cell cytokine programs associated with allograft rejection (upper panel) and a model of T-cell cytokine programs associated with tolerance (lower panel).

Targeting cytokine growth factors to abrogate the alloimmune response

Clearly IL-2 expression is strongly associated with the rejection process [37-39, 41] and IL-2, when administered as an adjunct to various tolerizing regimens, precludes long-term engraftment [42-44]. Does this mean that the absence of IL-2 gene expression will lead to tolerance? Several studies have demonstrated that application of tolerance inducing therapies often skews the allograft response from a Th1 pattern usually noted during unmodified rejection to a Th2 pattern [38, 44-46]. The possibility exists that tolerance might directly result from an allograft response conducted in the absence of IL-2 expression and in the presence of IL-4 expression [44, 46-48]. To test this hypothesis Steiger et al transplanted allogeneic islets into mice whose IL-2 gene had been functionally silenced by targeted gene disruption (IL-2 knockout mice, [49]). Interestingly, all IL-2 knockout mice rejected their allografts at a tempo that was only modestly delayed in comparison to mice with two copies of the intact IL-2 gene. Immunohistologic analysis of the allograft response in IL-2 knockout graft recipients reveals CD4$^+$ and CD8$^+$ T-cells infiltrates in rejecting grafts [50]. Indeed, the intragraft pattern of gene expression in IL-2 knockout recipient mice demonstrated the presence of transcripts for IL-4, IFNγ, and the CTL specific marker granzyme B, but not IL-2. These findings have been confirmed by Dai et al, in a murine cardiac allograft model [51]. Moreover, IL-2 knockout recipients were able to generate alloantigen specific CTL responses [50, 51]. Thus, the absence of IL-2 gene expression, even in the presence of IL-4 gene expression does not inevitably lead to graft tolerance.

Which growth factors might support IL-2 independent T-cell proliferation? IL-4, IL-7, IL-9 and IL-15 are potent T-cell growth factors [52, 53]. IL-7 triggered signals, not blocked by cyclosporine, are important for lymphocyte differentiation and stimulation of CTL proliferation [54]. IL-15 is produced by a wide variety of cell types with the notable exception of mature T-cells [53]. Interestingly, IL-15 binds to a trimolecular receptor complex which includes two members of the IL-2 receptor complex (i.e. the IL-2-Rβ, and common gamma (γc), chain as well as the IL-15 selective IL-15Rα chain. IL-15 supports the proliferation of CD4$^+$ and CD8$^+$ T-cells; IL-15 driven proliferation is blocked by anti-IL-2Rβ, but not anti-IL-2Rα mAb. Further, IL-15 supports CTL activity, albiet suboptimal in the absence of IL-2 (reviewed in [53]). Interestingly, the allograft response elicited in IL-2 and IL-4 double knockout mice, and studies of human renal transplant biopsies, amplified IL-7 and IL-15 gene expression in tissues undergoing rejection [55, 56]. Clearly, allograft rejection elicits the expression of multiple T-cell growth factor programs: there is a complex cytokine network that is able to supports T-cell proliferation in response to alloantigen.

Targeting proinflammatory cytokines to abrogate the alloimmune response

An alternative to targeting cytokines that support T-cell proliferation would be to neutralize or prevent the expression of proinflammatory cytokine programs, which are expressed during allograft rejection. In theory, this approach could be effected through blockade of gene expression with anti-sense oligonucleotides, neutralization with antibodies or soluble cytokine receptor fusion proteins (reviewed in [57]). While appealing one must ask, as in the case of T-cell growth factors, whether the plethora of proinflammatory cytokines exerting overlapping function will nullify this approach. Indeed, as reviewed below preclinical studies utilizing this approach highlight inherent difficulties and complexities.

As previously discussed, IL-12 is a key regulatory cytokine that is able to promote the development of a Th1 effector program (i.e. IFNγ) while inhibiting Th2 effector programs. In order to determine the relative requirement for IL-12 in the allograft response, Piccotti et al treated cardiac allograft recipients with a neutralizing anti-IL-12 mAb or with the IL-12 receptor antagonist IL-12 p40 homodimer [58]. Interestingly, while both forms of IL-12 antagonism induced intra-graft Th2 cytokine expression, the time to graft rejection was accelerated rather that prolonged. Moreover, IL-12 blockade failed to prevent IFNγ gene expression in the grafts. Subsequently it was shown that while the IL-12 p40 homodimer was able to preclude alloreactive Th1 development, it induced IFNγ expression in alloreactive CD8$^+$ T-cells [59]. In order to confirm the lack of a requirement for IL-12 during an allograft response the same group transplanted allogeneic hearts into IL-12 p40 knockout recipients [60]. As before, the allografts were rejected in an accelerated fashion. While IFNγ expression was diminished, as compared to wild type hosts, it was readily detectable in p40 knockout allograft recipients and the source appeared to be a CD8$^+$ T-cell population. Thus, these studies demonstrate that targeting IL-12, while able to enhance a Th2 cytokine program in the graft, is unable to preclude a Th1 like program (i.e. IFNγ) from arising. This calls into question the relative importance of enhancing a Th2 immune response in the context of allograft rejection.

Given the central role of IFNγ in mediating proinflammatory immune responses (vida supra) it has been hypothesized that targeting this Th1 cytokine may be beneficial in the context of allograft rejection. However, IFNγ knockout hosts reject heterotopic heart transplants with a time course and histologic pattern similar to that of the wild type host and the expression of other proinflammatory cytokines noted during the allograft response in IFNγ knockout mice is unchanged (i.e. TNFα) [61]. Similarly, islet allograft rejection in IFNγ receptor knockout hosts is brisk and remains T-cell dependent [62]. Moreover, studies that have employed IFNγ neutralizing antibodies have failed to prolong allograft survival [60, 63].

To date it would appear that individual proinflammatory cytokines are not indispensable in eliciting an allograft response. Thus, it is unlikely that targeting any one T-cell cytokine pathway will prevent clinical graft rejection. Moreover, given the complex nature of cytokine networks, it may prove difficult to block the production or neutralization of the myriad of cytokines that are apparently involved in supporting alloantigen specific T-cell activation, proliferation and effector functions.

Targeting cytokine receptors to preclude the allograft response

Members of a given cytokine family often utilize common receptor subunits (reviewed in [64]). Therefore, it may prove feasible to inhibit intracellular signaling pathways that are activated by several cytokine receptors. For example, the IL-2 receptor complex is comprised of a $\alpha,\beta,\gamma c$ heterotrimer. IL-15 and IL-2, both bind to the IL-2Rβ and γc chains and utilize these chains for signal transduction [65]. Moreover, other cytokines, which act as T-cell growth factors (i.e. IL-4, IL-7, IL-9), also utilize the γc of the IL-2R, in addition to their own, cytokine specific α receptor chains, as receptor components [66-68]. The discovery that X-linked severe combined immunodeficiency (XSCID) is caused by a defect in the γc chain proves that the lack of signaling through this pathway affects multiple cytokines and leads to far more profound immunodeficiency than noted in IL-2 knockout mice [49, 69]. Thus, γc chains are critical for signal transduction for a number of cytokine T-cell growth factors.

It has been hypothesized that the selective destruction of T cell activation induced growth factor receptor, i.e. IL-2Rα bearing T cells with cytolytic anti-IL-2Rα mAb, or blocking their ability to bind growth factors with anti-γc mAb, or blocking the common pathway of intracellular growth factor signaling with drugs such as rapamycin, may well lead to graft prolongation in the clinic [70, 71]. Indeed, Li et al demonstrated in an islet allograft model that blockade of the γc chain with a non-cytolytic mAb at the time of transplantation resulted in allograft tolerance [72]. In vitro blockade of the γc chain with this mAb inhibits allospecific proliferation while enhancing activation induced cell death (ACID) in allospecific T-cell populations [72, 73]. Thus, targeting common cytokine receptor proteins would appear to be a successful strategy and the use of these agents in large animal preclinical transplant models will be awaited with great interest.

IMMUNOREGULATORY CYTOKINES AND ALLOGRAFT TOLERANCE

Active immunoregulatory phenomena are central to the creation and/or maintenance of peripheral allograft tolerance. Many laboratories, perhaps most elegantly in the demonstration of infectious tolerance by Qin et al [74], have shown the presence of donor specific regulatory cells through the use of passive transfer systems. One hypothesis suggests that tolerance is due to the ability of Ag-specific, T-cell clones to migrate to the target tissue and release immunoregulatory cytokines into the local microenvironment. Indeed, as stated previously, a number of groups have demonstrated that $CD4^+$ T-cells that express IL-10 or TGFβ are capable of immunoregulation of both Th1 and Th2 mediated inflammatory responses [33-36]. Thus, the data would support the existence of cytokine driven immunoregulatory networks in vivo.

What evidence exists for a role of immunoregulatory cytokines in either the induction or the maintenance of allograft tolerance? In animal models, tolerizing therapies appear to inhibit the magnitude and/or alter the quality of $CD4^+$ T-cell activation during the induction of tolerance. A switch from the expression of IL-2 and IFNγ, detected in the grafts of acutely rejecting hosts, to the expression of IL-4 in the grafts of hosts being treated with tolerizing therapies is often manifest [38, 44, 45, 74]. In an extension of the "Th1/Th2 paradigm" it has been suggested that induction of tolerance to an allograft is dependent upon immune deviation of the $CD4^+$ T-cell program to a Th2 phenotype (i.e. IL-4, IL-10) and away from the Th1 (i.e. IFNγ) profile associated with rejection [75, 76] (Fig. 2). Interestingly, there is a suspicion that immune deviation to a Th2 like pattern, while permissive for long term engraftment may paradoxically support chronic rejection [77]. Moreover, a recent study by Larson's group has raised the possibility that chronic vascular rejection in a heterotopic cardiac allograft model is associated with an ongoing immune response characterized by prolonged cytokine expression. In this model, long term acceptance and avoidance of chronic rejection requires a silencing of both Th1 and Th2 cytokine programs [78].

Immunoregulation of the allograft response and the role of Th2 cytokines

What role might IL-10 have in abrogating allograft rejection? In vitro studies have determined that rIL-10 exerts inhibitory effects upon: IFNγ release, proliferation of Th1 cells stimulated by Mø, MHC class II expression on monocytes, IL-12 release from Mø, and the expression of B7 costimulatory ligands on the surface of Mø [79-82]. Thus, IL-10 appears to be a potent blocker of Th1 responses. However, the effects of IL-10 are not uniformly immunosuppressive or anti-inflammatory, IL-10 augments IL-2 supported proliferation of CD8[+] T-cells and enhances IL-2 induced cytotoxicity by these cells [83]. Finally, IL-10 stimulates monocyte FcγRI surface expression and ADCC [84]. Thus, depending on the nature of the local microenvironment IL-10 may exert anti- or pro- inflammatory effects.

Initial studies suggest that mammalian IL-10 may not readily block allograft rejection. In a transgenic mouse model in which the murine IL-10 gene was constitutively expressed by the pancreatic β cells, islets from these transgenic mice were transplanted into MHC incompatible recipients. Despite documented IL-10 expression within the microenvironment of the graft, allograft rejection was not delayed [85]. Zheng et al demonstrated that systemic administration of a long acting IL-10-Ig fusion protein did not delay the onset of allograft rejection [86]. Indeed, IL-10-Ig treatment resulted in an augmented CTL response to the graft. Moreover, Li et al found that anti-IL-10 mAb prolonged organ allograft survival rather than accelerating rejection [87]. Interestingly, Qin et al have found that retroviral transfection of cardiac grafts with viral (v)IL-10, not murine (m)IL-10, leads to prolonged but not indefinite cardiac allograft survival [88] suggesting that the structural differences of vIL-10 and mIL-10 may determine whether the immunosuppressive vs. immunostimulatory effects of IL-10 are exerted during the allograft response. Together these studies highlight the inherent difficulty of extrapolating the reductionist approach of in vitro studies (i.e. the immunoregulation by IL-10 on T-cell activation) to the complex dynamics of in vivo biology.

Does IL-4 inhibit graft rejection and directly promote allograft tolerance? In vitro high levels of IL-4 skew Th0 cells toward a Th2 response and away from a Th1 response (Fig 1). As previously stated, the expression of IL-4 during the period of administration of tolerizing therapies and the concomitant silencing of IL-2 gene expression are frequent markers for tolerance induction [38, 44, 45]. Nevertheless, there is mounting evidence against a key role for IL-4 in supporting tolerance induction. First, the expression of IL-4 in the absence of IL-2 is not sufficient for the induction of tolerance [50, 51]. Indeed, the induction of IL-4 by IL-12 blockade was unable to abrogate a Th1 response (IFNγ) [58]. Second, the administration of a soluble IL-4 receptor to allograft recipients leads to graft prolongation not hastened rejection [89]. Third, overexpression of IL-4 in an islet allograft is unable to significantly prolong allograft survival [90]. Fourth, long-term allograft acceptance can occur in IL-4 knockout recipients [43, 91]. These studies suggest that

IL-4 by itself is insufficient and/or the importance of the detection of IL-4 during tolerance induction lies not in the expression of IL-4 but rather the absence of IL-2 and IFNγ expression.

The aforementioned does not allow one to conclude that IL-4 plays no role in allograft tolerance. Notably, the capacity of donor specific transfusion (DST) to create a state of tolerance may be IL-4 dependent [92]. Moreover, the adoptive transfer of tolerance, initially induced by non-depleting anti-CD4 and anti-CD8 monoclonal antibodies, in a minor histocompatibility skin allograft model was shown to be partially dependent on IL-4 [93]. Thus, in some circumstances IL-4 can aid tolerance induction; however, IL-4 is not a universal requirement for the induction of peripheral tolerance (vida supra). There is no evidence that IL-4 is primarily responsible for the maintenance of tolerance, although expression of IL-4 may aid in the induction of tolerance through the capacity of IL-4/IL-10 to shut down the Th1 program.

Immunoregulation of the allograft response and the role of Th1 cytokines

Recent seminal studies have suggested that, while IL-2 and IFNγ have pro-inflammatory effects, they may also be essential to limit an alloimmune response in vivo. Dia et al found that cardiac allografts in wild-type mice would survive indefinitely after tolerance induction with CTLA4Ig treatment, while engraftment could not be achieved in wild-type mice treated with anti-IL-2 mAb or in IL-2 knockout mice [51]. Similarly, Konieczny et al were unable to induce long-term engraftment in cardiac allograft recipients with costimulation blockade when they were concomitantly treated with an anti-IFNγ mAb [94]. These studies clearly support the concept that IL-2 and IFNγ have immunoregulatory functions in vivo.

The mechanisms by which IL-2 and IFNγ mediate a regulatory influence are becoming clearer. IFNγ knockout mice are characterized by an increase in the proliferative response to antigenic challenge [95]. Hassan et al, found that endogenous IFNγ facilitates cardiac allograft tolerance induction by its ability to limit the proliferation of alloantigen specific T-cells [96]. IL-2, IL-2Rα and β chain knockout mice are characterized by marked hyperplasia of the lymphocyte compartments and the development of autoimmune disease [97-99]. Moreover, it has been shown that IL-2 plays a role in potentiating Fas-mediated apoptosis as activated IL-2Rα -/- T cells are resistant to Fas-mediated activation-induced cell death (AICD) [100]. This potentiation appears to be due to the ability of IL-2 to induce Fas ligand expression on T-cells, while suppressing the expression of FLIP, an inhibitor of apoptosis [101]. Taken together, these studies suggest that IL-2 and IFNγ have both pro- and anti-inflammatory roles in the context of an immune response. Thus, strategies that specifically aim to block these cytokines in order to prevent allograft rejection may at the same time preclude the development of allograft tolerance.

CONCLUSION

With the recent insights into the role of cytokines during naive T-cell activation and the development of CD4$^+$ T effector programs, numerous strategies have been devised to target specific cytokine pathways. To date however, the results of these strategies have been disappointing. This is largely due to the complexity that exists in cytokine networks. As was seen in the case of IL-10, IL-2 and IFNγ, cytokines are pleiotropic; they may have both immunoregulatory and proinflammatory properties. Even in the case of TGFβ there is debate as to whether it can be considered solely anti-inflammatory (reviewed in [102]). Moreover, as was the case for T-cell growth factors, cytokine networks have a degree of redundancy.

It is notable that in no circumstances to date has allograft tolerance been achieved via specifically blocking the production/effects of a proinflammatory cytokine (e.g. IL-2, IFNγ, IL-12), and/or enhancing the endogenous production, or local/systemic administration of a cytokine with immunoregulatory properties (e.g. IL-4, IL-10, TGFβ). At the very least, multiple cytokine pathways need to be blocked, as was the case when targeting the common γc receptor. More commonly, models of allograft tolerance apply therapies, which prevent optimal T-cell activation during alloantigen recognition by naive T-cells (i.e. a phase which is cytokine independent). Furthermore, it has been suggested that peripheral tolerance exists at multiple levels (i.e. immune deviation, anergy, apotosis) [103]. Thus cytokine therapy in isolation is unlikely to be sufficient to induce or maintain the complex series of events that are crucial to the generation and maintenance of "tolerance".

REFERENCES

1.   Mossmann TR, Cherwinski H, Bond MW, Giedlin MA, Coffman RL. Two types of murine helper T cell clone. I. Definition according to profiles of lymphokine activities and secreted proteins. J Immunol 1986;136:2348-2357.

2. Kelso A. Th1 and Th2 subsets: paradigms lost? Immunology Today 1995;16: 374-379.
3. Mosmann TR, Sad S. The expanding universe of T-cell subsets: Th1, Th2 and more. Immunology Today 1996;17:138-146.
4. Reiner S, Seder R. Dealing from the evolutionary pawnshop: How lymphocytes make decisions. Immunity 1999;11:1-10.
5. O'Garra A. Cytokines induce the development of functionally heterogeneous T helper cell subsets. Immunity 1998;8:275-283.
6. Abbas A, Murphy K, Sher A. Functional diversity of helper T lymphocytes. Nature 1996;383:787-793.
7. Macatonia SE, Hsieh C-Y, Murphy KM, O'Garra A. Dendritic cells and macrophages are required for Th1 development of CD4+ T cells from $\alpha\beta$ TCR transgenic mice: IL-12 substitution from macrophages to stimulate IFN-γ production is IFN-γ-dependent. International Immunology 1993;5:1119-1128.
8. Steinman RM. The dendritic cell system and its role in immunogenicty. Annu Rev Immunol 1991;9:271-296.
9. Hsieh C-S, Heimberger AB, Gold JS, O'Garra A, Murphy KM. Differential regulation of T helper phenotype development by interleukins 4 and 10 in an $\alpha\beta$ T-cell-receptor transgenic system. Proc Natl Acad Sci USA 1992;89:6065-6069.
10. Seder RA, Paul WE, Davis MM, Fazekas de St. Groth B. The presence of interleukin 4 during in vitro priming determines the lymphokine-producing potential of CD4+ T cells from T cell receptor transgenic mice. J Exp Med 1992;176: 1091-1098.
11. LeGros G, Ben-Sasson SZ, Seder R, Finkelman FD, Paul WE. Generation of interleukin 4 [IL-4] -producing cells in vivo and in vitro: IL-2 and IL-4 are required for in vitro generation of IL-4 -producing cells. J Exp Med 1990;179:921-929.
12. Seder RA, Germain RN, Linsley PS, Paul WE. CD28-Mediated costimulation of Interleukin 2(IL-2) production plays a critical role in T cell priming for IL-4 and Interferon γ production. J Exp Med 1994;179:299-304.
13. Kamogawa Y, Minasi L, Carding SR, Bottomly K, Flavell RA. The relationship of IL-4 and IFNγ -producing T cells studied by lineage ablation of IL-4-producing cells. Cell 1993;75:985-995.
14. Hsieh C-S, Macatonia SE, Tripp CS, Wolf SF, O'Garra A, Murphy KM. Development of Th1 CD4+ T cells through IL-12 produced by Listeria-induced macrophages. Science 1993;260:547-549.
15. Manetti R, Parronchi P, Giudizi MG, et al. Natural Killer cell stimulatory factor (interleukin 12 [IL-12]) induces T helper type 1 (Th1)-specific immune responses and inhibits the development of IL-4 producing Th cells. J Exp Med 1993;177:1199-1204.
16. Macatonia S, Hosken N, Litton M, et al. Dendritic cells produce IL-12 and direct the development of Th1 cells from naive CD4+ T cells. J Immunol 1995;154: 5071-5079.
17. Scheicher C, Mehlig M, Dienes H-P, Reske K. Uptake of microparticle-adsorbed protein antigen by bone marrow-derived dendritic cells results in up-regulation of interleukin-1a and interleukin-12 p40/p35 and triggers prolonged, efficient antigen presentation. Eur J Immunol 1995;25:1566-1572.
18. Szabo SJ, Jacobson NG, Dighe AS, Gubler U, Murphy KM. Developmental commitment to the Th2 lineage by exinction of IL-12 signalling. Immunity 1995;2: 665-675.
19. Magram J, Connaughton SE, Warrier RR, et al. IL-12-deficient mice are defective in IFN-g production and type 1 cytokine responses. Immunity 1996;4:471-481.
20. Trinchieri G. Interleukin-12: a proinflammatory cytokine with immunoregulatory functions that bridge innate resistance and antigen-specific adaptive immunity. Annu Rev Immunol 1995;13:251-276.

21. Szabo S, Dighe AS, Gubler U, Murphy KM. Regulation of the interleukin (IL)-12B2subunit expression in developing T helper 1 (Th1) and Th2 cells. J Exp Med 1997;185:817-824.
22. Rogge L, Barberis-Maino L, Biffi M, et al. Selective expression of an interleukin-12 receptor component by human T helper 1 cells. J Exp Med 1997;185:825-831.
23. Koch F, Stanzl U, Jennewein P, et al. High level IL-12 production by murine dendritic cells: upregulation via MHC class II and CD40 molecules and downregulation by IL-4 and IL-10. J Exp Med 1996;184:741-746.
24. Murphy EE, Terres G, Macatonia SE, et al. B7 and interleukin 12 cooperate for proliferation and interferon γ production by mouse T helper clones that are unresponsive to B7 costimulation. J Exp Med 1994;180:223-231.
25. Seder RA, Paul WE. Acquisition of lymphokine-producing phenotype by CD4+ T cells. Annu Rev Immunol 1994;12:635-673.
26. Bird JJ, Brown DR, Mullen AC, et al. Helper T cell differentiation is controlled by the cell cycle. Immunity 1998;9:229-237.
27. Hosken NA, Shibuya K, Heath AW, Murphy KM, O'Garra A. The effect of antigen dose on CD4+ T cell phenotype development in an αβ-TCR-transgeneic mouse model. J Exp Med 1995;182:1579-1584.
28. Constant S, Pfeiffer C, Woodard A, Pasqualini T, Bottomly K. Extent of T cell receptor ligation can determine the functional differentiation of naive CD4+ T cells. J Exp Med 1995;182:1591-1596.
29. Kuchroo VJ, Prabhu Das M, Brown JA, et al. B7-1 and B7-2 costimulatory molecules activate differentially the Th1/Th2 developmental pathways: application to autoimmune disease therapy. Cell 1995;80:707-718.
30. Rissoan M-C, Soumelis V, Kadowaki N, et al. Reciprocal Control of T helper cell and dendritic cell differentiation. Science 1999;283:1183-1186.
31. Perez VL, Lederer JA, Lichtman AH, Abbas AK. Stability of Th1 and Th2 populations. Int Immunol 1995;7:869-875.
32. Mason D, Powrie F. Control of immune pathology by regulatory T cells. Curr Opin Immunol 1998;10:649-655.
33. Chen Y, Kuchroo VK, Inobe J-I, Hafler DA, Weiner HL. Regulatory T cell clones induced by oral tolerance: suppression of autoimmune encephalomyelitis. Science 1994;265:1237-1240.
34. Groux H, O'Garra A, Bigler M, et al. A CD4+ T-cell subset inhibits antigen-specific T-cell responses and prevents colitis. Nature 1997;389:737-742.
35. Powrie F, Carlino J, Leach MW, Mauze S, Coffman RL. A critical role for transforming growth factor-beta but not interleukin 4 in the suppression of T helper type 1-mediated colitis by CD45RB(low) CD4+ T cells. J Exp Med 1996;183:2669-2674.
36. Bridoux F, Badou A, Saoudi A, et al. Transforming growth factor β (TGF-β)-dependent inhibition of T helper 2 (Th2)-induced autoimmunity by self-major histocompatibility complex (MHC) class II-specific, regulatory CD4+ T cell lines. J Exp Med 1997;186:1769-1775.
37. O'Connell PJ, Pacheco-Silva A, Nickerson PW, et al. Unmodified pancreatic islet allograft rejection results in the preferential expression of certain T cell activation transcripts. J Immunol 1993;150:1093-1104.
38. Takeuchi T, Lowry RP, Konieczny B. Heart allografts in murine systems: the differential activation of Th2-like effector cells in peripheral tolerance. Transplantation 1992;53:1281-1294.
39. Dallman MJ, Larsen CP, Morris PJ. Cytokine gene transcription in vascularised organ grafts: Analysis using semiquantitative polymerase chain reaction. J Exp Med 1991;174:493-496.
40. Lipman ML, Stevens AC, Strom TB. Heightened intragraft cytotoxic T lymphocyte gene expression in acutely rejecting renal allografts. J Immunol 1994;152:

5120-5127.

41. McLean AG, Hughes D, Welsh KI, et al. Patterns of graft infiltration and cytokine gene expression during the first 10 days of kidney transplantation. Transplantation 1997;3:374-380.

42. Dallman MJ, Shiho O, Page TH, Wood KJ, Morris PJ. Peripheral tolerance to alloantigen results from altered regulation of the interleukin 2 pathway. J Exp Med 1991;173:79-87.

43. Nickerson P, Zheng X, Steiger J, et al. Prolonged islet allograft acceptance in the absence of interleukin 4 expression. Transplant Immunology 1996;4:81-85.

44. Sayegh MH, Akalin E, Hancock WW, et al. CD28-B7 blockade after alloantigenic challenge in vivo inhibits Th1 cytokines but spares Th2. J Exp Med 1995;181: 1869-1874.

45. Nickerson PW, Pacheco-Silva A, O'Connell PJ, Steurer W, Rubin Kelley V, Strom TB. Analysis of cytokine transcripts in pancreatic islet cell allografts during rejection and tolerance induction. Transplant Proc 1993;25:984-985.

46. Bugeon L, Cuturi M-C, Hallet M-M, Paineau J, Chabannes D, Soulillou J-P. Peripheral tolerance of an allograft in adult rats- characterization by low interleukin-2 and interferon-γ mRNA levels and by strong accumulation of major histocompatibility complex transcripts in the graft. Transplantation 1992;54:219-225.

47. Hancock WW, Sayegh MH, Kwok CA, Weiner HL, Carpenter CB. Oral, but not intravenous, alloantigen prevents accelerated allograft rejection by selective intragraft Th2 cell activation. Transplantation 1993;55:219-225.

48. Kupiec-Weglinski JW, Wasowska B, Papp I, et al. CD4 mAb therapy modulates alloantibody production and intracardiac graft deposition in association with selective inhibition of Th1 lymphokines. J Immunol 1993;151:5053-5061.

49. Schorle H, Holtschke T, Hünig T, Schimpl A, Horak I. Development and function of T cells in mice rendered interleukin-2 deficient by gene targeting. Nature 1991;352:621-623.

50. Steiger J, Nickerson PW, Steurer W, Moscovitch-Lopatin M, Strom TB. IL-2 Knockout recipient mice reject islet cell allografts. J Immunol 1995;155:489-498.

51. Dai Z, Konieczny BT, Baddoura FK, Lakkis FG. Impaired alloantigen-mediated T cell apoptosis and failure to induce long-term allograft survival in IL-2-deficient mice. J Immunol 1998;161:1659-1663.

52. Chazen GD, Pereira GMB, LeGros G, Gillis S, Shevach EM. Interleukin 7 is a T cell growth factor. Proc Natl. Acad Sci USA 1989;86:5923-5927.

53. Tagaya Y, Bamford RN, DeFilippis AP, Waldman TA. IL-15: A pleiotropic cytokine with diverse receptor/signaling pathways whose expression is controlled at multiple levels. Immunity 1996;4:329-336.

54. Alderson MR, Sassenfeld HM, Widmer MB. IL-7 enhances cytolytic T lymphocyte generation and induces lymphokine activated killer cells from human peripheral blood. J. Exp. Med. 1990;172:577-587.

55. Li XC, Roy-Chaudhury P, Hancock WW, et al. IL-2 and IL-4 double knockout mice reject islet allografts: a role for novel T cell growth factors in allograft rejection. J Immunol 1998;161:890-896.

56. Strehlau J, Pavlakis M, Lipman M, et al. Quantitative detection of immune activation transcripts as a diagnostic tool in kidney transplantation. Proc Natl Acad Sci USA 1997;94:695-700.

57. Debets R, Savelkoul HFJ. Cytokine antagonists and their potential therapeutic use. Immunology Today 1994;15:455-458.

58. Piccotti JR, Chan SY, Goodman RE, Magram J, Eichwald EJ, Bishop DK. IL-12 antagonism induces T helper 2 responses, yet exacerbates cardiac allograft rejection. Evidence against a dominant protective role for T helper cytokines in alloimmunity. J Immunol 1996;157:1951-1957.

59. Piccotti JR, Chan SY, Li K, Eichwald EJ, Bishop DK. Differential effects of IL-12

receptor blockade with IL-12 p40 homodimer on the induction of CD4+ and CD8+ IFN-gamma-producing cells. J Immunol 1997;158:643-648.

60. Piccotti JR, Li K, Chan SY, et al. Alloantigen-reactive Th1 development in IL-12 deficient mice. J Immunol 1998;160:1132-1138.

61. Konieczny BT, Saleem SS, Lowry RP, Lakkis FG. Vigorous cardiac and skin allograft rejection in the absence of IFNγ. JASN 1996;7:1887.

62. Steiger J, Nickerson P, Ryffel B, Thiel G, Strom TB, Heim M. Islet cell transplantation in IFNγ receptor deficient mice. Are Th2 cells upregulated? JASN 1996; 7:1896.

63. Stevens HP, van der Kwast TH, van der Meide PH, Vuzevski VD, Buurman WA, Jonker M. Synergistic immunosuppression effects of monoclonal antibodies specific for interferon-gamma and tumor necrosis factor alpha. A skin transplantation study in the rhesus monkey. Transplantation 1990;50:856-861.

64. Kishimoto T, Taga T, Akira S. Cytokine signal transduction. Cell 1994;76: 253-262.

65. Takeshita T, Asao H, Ohtani K, et al. Cloning of the γ chain of the human IL-2 receptor. Science 1992;257:379-382.

66. Kondo M, Takeshita T, Ishii N, et al. Sharing of the interleukin-2 (IL-2) receptor γ chain between receptors for IL-2 and IL-4. Science 1993;262:1874-1877.

67. Noguchi M, Nakamura Y, Russell SM, et al. Interleukin-2 receptor γ chain: A functional compontent of the interleukin-7 receptor. Science 1993;262:1877-1880.

68. Russell SM, Keegan AD, Harada N, et al. Interleukin-2 receptor γ chain: A functional component of the interleukin-4 receptor. Science 1993;262:1880-1883.

69. Noguchi M, Yi H, Rosenblatt H, et al. Interleukin-2 receptor γ chain mutation results in X-linked severe combined immunodificiency in humans. Cell 1993;73: 147-157.

70. Strom TB, Kelley VR, Murphy JR, Nichols J, Woodworth TG. Interleukin-2 receptor-directed therapies:Antibody- or cytokine-based targeting molecules. Annu Rev Med 1993;44:343-353.

71. Waldmann TA. The IL-2/IL-2 receptor system: A target for rational immune intervention. Immunol Today 1993;14:264-270.

72. Li XC, Li Y, Dodge I, Zheng XX, Malek TR, Strom TB. Block the common γ chain of cytokine receptors induces permanent allograft tolerance. Transplantation 1999; 67:S21.

73. Dai Z, Arakelov A, Wagener M, Konieczny BT, Lakkis FG. Antibodies which target the common cytokine receptor gamma (γc) chain enhance activation-induced apoptosis of allospecific CD8+ T-cells. Transplantation 1999;67:S21.

74. Qin S, Cobbold SP, Pope H, et al. "Infectious" transplantation tolerance. Science 1993;259:974-977.

75. Lowry RP. The relationship of IL-4, IL-10, and other cytokines to transplantation tolerance. Transplant Sci 1993;3:104-112.

76. Paul WE, Seder RA. Lymphocyte responses and cytokines. Cell 1994;76(2): 241-251.

77. Hancock W, Shi C, Picard M, Bianchi C, Russell M. LEW-to-F344 carotid artery allografts: analysis of a rat model of posttransplant vascular injury involving cell-mediated and humoral responses. Transplantation 1995;60:1565-1572.

78. Larsen CP, Elwood ET, Alexander DZ, et al. Long-term acceptance of skin and cardiac allografts after blocking CD40 and CD28 pathways. Nature 1996;381: 434-438.

79. Macatonia SE, Doherty TM, Knight SC, O'Garra A. Differential effect of IL-10 on dendritic cell-induced T cell proliferation and IFNγ production. J Immunol 1993; 150:3755-3765.

80. de Waal Malefyt R, Haanen J, Spits H, et al. Interleukin 10 (IL-10) and viral IL-10 strongly reduce antigen-specific human T cell proliferation by diminishing the

antigen-presenting capacity of monocytes via downregulation of class II major histocompatibilty complex expression. J Exp Med 1991;174:915-924.

81. D'Andrea A, Aste-Amezaga, Valiante NM, Ma X, Kubin M, Trinchieri G. Interleukin 10 (IL-10) inhibits human lymphocyte interferony production by suppressing natural killer cell stimulatory factor/IL-12 synthesis in accessory cells. J Exp Med 1993;178:1042-1048.

82. Ding L, Linsley PS, Huang L-Y, Germain RN, E.M. S. IL-10 inhibits macrophage costimulatory activity by selectively inhibiting the up-regulation of B7 expression. J Immunol 1993;151:1224-1234.

83. Chen WF, Zlotnik A. IL-10: A novel cytotoxic T cell differentiation factor. J Immunol 1991;147:528-534.

84. te Velde AA, Malefijt RdW, Huijbens RJF, de Vries JE, Figdor CG. IL-10 stimulates monocyte FcγR surface expression and cytotoxic activity. J Immunol 1992;149:4048-4052.

85. Lee M-S, Wogensen L, Shizuru J, Oldstone MBA, Sarventnick N. Pancreatic islet production of murine interleukin10 does not inhibit immune-mediated tissue destruction. J Clin Invest 1994;93:1332-1338.

86. Zheng XX, Steele AW, Nickerson PW, Steurer W, Steiger J, Strom TB. Administration of non-cytolytic IL-10/Fc in murine models of LPS-induced septic shock and allogeneic islet transplantation. J Immunol 1995;154:5590-5600.

87. Li W, Fu F, Lu L, et al. Systemic administration of anti-interleukin-10 antibody prolongs organ allograft survival in normal and presensitized recipients. Transplantation 1998;66:1587-1596.

88. Qin L, Chavin KD, Ding Y, et al. Multiple vectors effectively achieve gene transfer in a murine cardiac transplantation model. Transplantation 1995;59:809-816.

89. Fanslow WC, Clifford KN, Park LS, et al. Regulation of alloreactivity in vivo by IL-4 and the soluble IL-4 receptor. 1991 1991;147:535-540.

90. Mueller R, Davies JD, Krahl T, Sarvetnick N. IL-4 expression by grafts from transgenic mice fail to prevent rejection. J Immunol 1997;159:1599-1603.

91. Lakkis FG, Konieczny BT, Saleem S, et al. Blocking the CD28-B7 T cell costimulation pathway induces long term cardiac allograft acceptance in the absence of IL-4. J Immunol 1997;158:2443-2448.

92. Bushell A, Niimi M, Morris PJ, Wood KJ. Evidence for immune regulation in the induction of transplantation tolerance: a conditional but limited role for IL-4. J Immunol 1999;162:1359-1366.

93. Davies JD, Martin G, Phillips J, Marshall SE, Cobbold SP, Waldman H. T cell regulation in adult transplantation tolerance. J Immunol 1996;157:529-533.

94. Konieczny BT, Dai Z, Elwood ET, et al. IFN-gamma is critical for long-term allograft survival induced by blocking the CD28 and CD40 ligand T cell costimulation pathways. J Immunol 1998;160:2059-2064.

95. Dalton DK, Pitts-Meek S, Keshav S, Figari IS, Bradley A, Stewart TA. Multiple defects of immune cell function in mice with disrupted interferon-gamma genes. Science 1993;259:1739-1742.

96. Hassan AT, Dai Z, Konieczny BT, et al. Regulation of alloantigen-mediated T-cell proliferation by endogenous interferon-gamma: Implications for long-term allograft acceptance. Transplantation 1999;68:124-129.

97. Sadlack B, Lohler J, Schorle H, et al. Generalized autoimmune disease in interleukin-2-deficient mice is triggered by an uncontrolled activation and proliferation of CD4+ Tcells. Eur J Immunol 1995;25:3053-3059.

98. Willerford DM, Chen J, Ferry JA, Davidson L, Ma A, Alt FW. Interleukin-2 receptor alpha chain regulates the size and content of the peripheral lymphoid compartment. Immunity 1995;3:521-530.

99. Suzuki H, Kunkig TM, Furlonger C, et al. Deregulated T cell activation and autoimmunity in mice lacking interleukin-2 receptor β. Science 1995;268:1472-1476.

100. Van Parijs L, Biuckians A, Ibragimov A, Alt FW, Willerford DM, Abbas AK. Functional responses and apoptosis of CD25 (IL-2R alpha)-deficient T cells expressing a transgenic antigen receptor. J Immunol 1997;158:3738-3745.
101. Refaeli Y, Van Parijs L, London CA, Tschopp J, Abbas AK. Biochemical mechanisms of IL-2-regulated Fas-mediated T cell apoptosis. Immunity 1998;8: 615-623.
102. Wahl SM. Transforming growth factor β: The good, the bad, and the ugly. J Exp Med 1994;180:1587-1590.
103. Arnold B, Schonrich G, Hammerling GJ. Multiple levels of peripheral tolerance. Immunology Today 1993;14:12-14.

NOVEL STRATEGIES USING
MHC PEPTIDES

5

Colm C. Magee and Mohamed H. Sayegh
Department of Medicine
Brigham & Women's Hospital and Harvard University
Boston, Massachusetts, USA

INTRODUCTION

Advances in our understanding of the structure and function of MHC molecules, the mechanisms of antigen processing and the molecular interactions occurring between the T cell receptor (TCR) complex and the major histocompatibility complex (MHC)-peptide complex have stimulated research into MHC-peptide based strategies of immunosuppression. We now know that MHC bound peptides play an important role in the T cell selection processes within the thymus, and in regulating the immune response to antigen in the periphery. Many of these bound peptides are derived from MHC molecules themselves. The appreciation of the role that the indirect allorecognition pathway plays in both acute and chronic rejection (see below) has further emphasised the pathological importance of these peptides. Investigation of the immunomodulatory effects of MHC peptides or their derivatives is therefore a logical strategy. This investigation has been greatly assisted by our ability to now efficiently synthesise peptides corresponding to sequences of specific regions of mammalian MHC molecules.

The goal of researching such compounds is their ultimate use in human patients undergoing transplantation or with autoimmune disease. Studies of MHC derived peptides in experimental transplantation and autoimmune disease already suggest several advantages of peptide immunotherapy: (i) specific rather than generalized immunosuppression (ii) the ability to induce tolerance in some models and (iii) the relative non-immunogenicity of certain peptides compared to monoclonal antibodies.

A. W. Thomson (ed.), Therapeutic Immunosuppression, 101–126.
© 2001 *Kluwer Academic Publishers.*

This chapter will briefly review current knowledge regarding the structure and function of the MHC-peptide complex and the pivotal role it plays in allograft rejection and autoimmune disease. MHC peptides are then divided into broad groups for discussion: (i) those derived from conserved (non-poly-morphic) regions of the MHC, (ii) those derived from variable (polymorphic) regions of the MHC and (iii) those which disrupt CD4/8 – MHC interactions (some of these also belong to the first group).

THE MAJOR HISTOCOMPATIBILITY COMPLEX

The major histocompatibility complex (MHC) is located on the short arm of chromosome 6 and includes at least 200 genes. The complex is divided into 3 parts: class I (HLA-A, -B, -C), class II (HLA-DR, -DP, -DQ) and class III (genes encoding TNF and complement factors). The products of the class I and II MHC genes are co-dominantly expressed and these class I and II MHC molecules, along with their bound peptides, are the focus of this article.

Class I MHC

Class I MHC molecules are expressed on the surface of virtually all nucleated cells. A schematic diagram of a class I MHC molecule is shown in figure 1. These molecules primarily display peptides derived from nuclear and cyto-solic proteins. Loading of newly synthesised class I MHC molecules with peptide fragments requires transport of peptides into the endoplasmic retic-ulum by transporter associated with antigen presentation (TAP). Peptides bound within the cleft region of class I MHC are typically 9-11 amino acids in length. This cleft is formed by 2 parallel strands of α-helix and 8 strands of β-pleated sheet, all derived from the $\alpha 1$ and $\alpha 2$ domains. Binding of the CD8 molecule occurs mainly via the non-polymorphic $\alpha 3$ domain.

Class II MHC

In contrast to class I MHC molecules, the expression of class II MHC mol-ecules is normally restricted to the surface of mononuclear phagocytes, B lymphocytes and endothelial cells. A schematic diagram of a class II MHC molecule is shown in figure 2. Peptides presented by class II MHC are usu-ally derived from the extracellular milieu. Loading of class II MHC with peptide requires the co-ordinate action of the invariant chain (Ii) polypep-

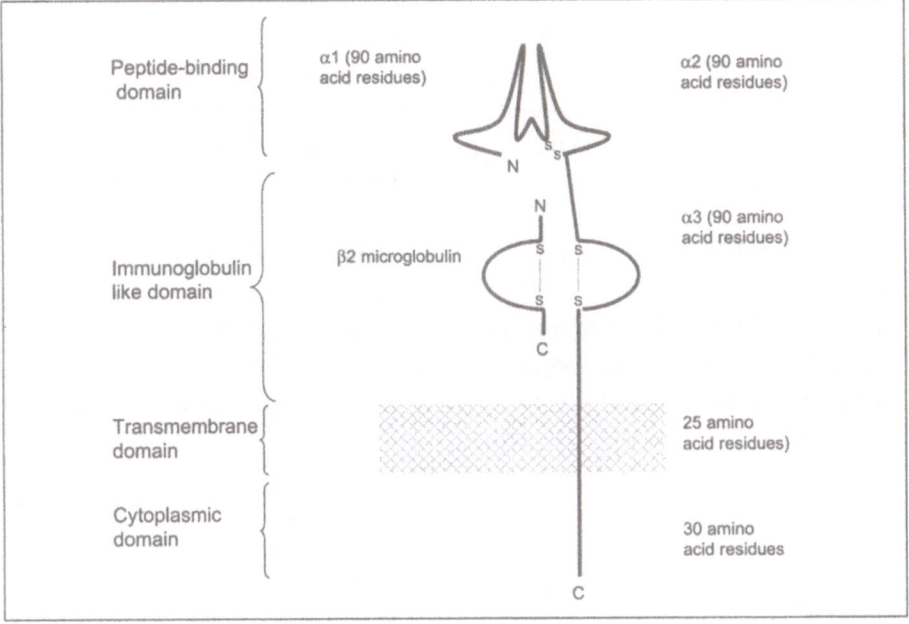

Figure 1
Schematic diagram of a human class I MHC molecule.

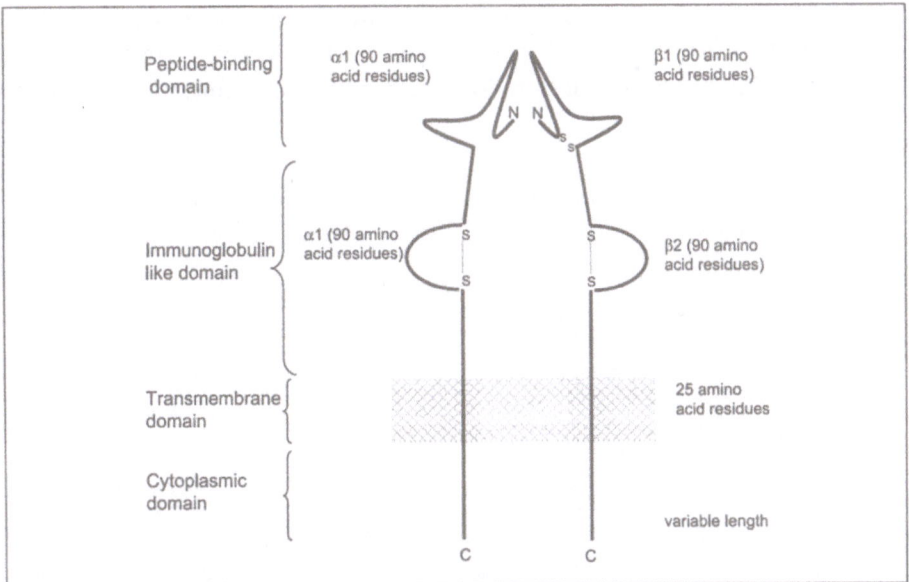

Figure 2
Schematic diagram of a human class II MHC molecule.

tide, its derivative the class II associated invariant chain peptide (CLIP) and HLA-DM. The peptide binding cleft of class II MHC molecules is also formed by an α-helical, β-pleated sheet structure. In contrast to class I MHC, the cleft is formed by the α1 and β1 domains. Another difference is that the cleft structure allows binding of longer peptides: typically 10-30 amino acids in length. Binding of CD4 occurs mainly via the non-polymorphic β2 domain.

Note that both antigen presentation pathways allow display of self and foreign peptides on the surface of the antigen presenting / target cell for "sampling" by CD4 or CD8 lymphocytes. Of course, self-tolerance requires that immune responses to self peptide-MHC complexes are controlled. Autoimmune disease is thought to result in some cases from breakdown of this form of tolerance.

ALLORECOGNITION: THE ROLE OF PEPTIDES

Activation of antigen specific CD4+ T cells plays a pivotal role in initiation of the alloimmune response. This activation can occur through two distinct but not mutually exclusive allorecognition pathways (Figure 3) [1,2]. In the direct pathway, recipient T cells recognize allo-MHC molecules + peptide on the surface of donor cells. In the indirect pathway, recipient T cells recognize self MHC + processed allopeptide on the surface of recipient antigen presenting cells (APCs). Indirect is a somewhat misleading description because in the normal immune response to foreign microbes etc., antigen recognition

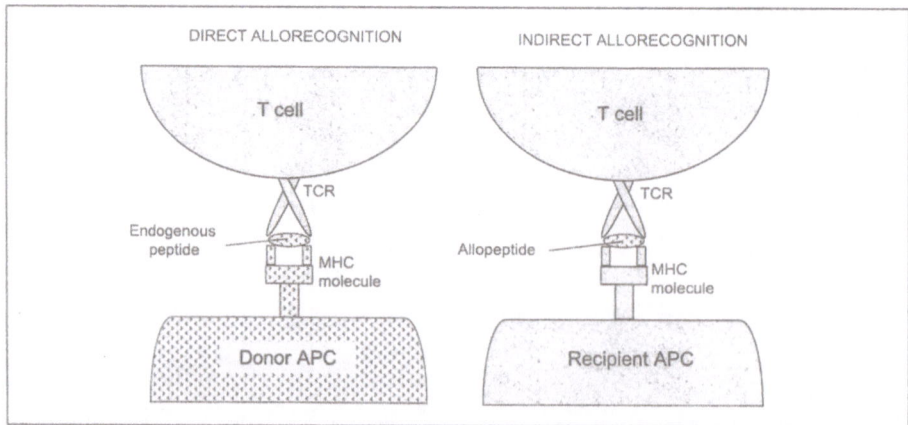

Figure 3
Pathways of allorecognition.

occurs through this pathway. The relative importance of these pathways in rejection of allografts is debated. Traditionally, the direct pathway has been considered the primary mechanism by which allorecognition occurs. There is increasing evidence from animal and human studies that indirect allorecognition plays an important role in both acute and chronic rejection [1,3-7]. Furthermore, recent registry data suggest that poorer long-term renal allograft survival is associated with greater mismatching of those class I MHC peptides which would be preferentially expressed on recipient HLA molecules [8]. The principal difference to be considered here is that in the direct pathway, allo-MHC *molecules* activate CD4 lymphocytes; in the indirect method, allo-MHC *peptides* or other (non-MHC derived) incompatible peptides activate CD4 lymphocytes. Thus, administration of synthetic peptides might modulate the indirect pathway through mechanisms such as competitive binding etc.

An important feature of the indirect pathway of allorecognition is that T cell responses to alloantigen may be limited to only a few dominant (immunodominant) antigenic determinants. Tolerising to, or blocking, these peptide determinants may then successfully inhibit indirect T cell alloresponses. Of course, the clinical usefulness of such a strategy is dependent on the relative contribution of the indirect (as opposed to the direct) allorecognition pathway to rejection.

NON-POLYMORPHIC CLASS I MHC DERIVED PEPTIDES

Peptides derived from the non-polymorphic α helical regions of human class I MHC have been extensively investigated. The α-helical regions of the class I MHC molecule not only define the site for binding of antigenic peptide but also provide potential sites for interaction of the MHC molecule with the T-cell receptor (see above). Initial studies of a panel of peptides corresponding to residues 60-84 of the $\alpha 1$ domain of five human MHC class I alleles showed that some blocked CTL maturation and mature CTL function, some blocked maturation alone while others had no such effects [9]. The carboxy 10 (75-84) amino acids were responsible for these immunomodulatory effects.

Subsequent work has focused mainly on 2 peptides (or their dimeric forms): HLA-B7 (75-84) and HLA-B2702 (75-84) (later licensed as Allotrap[R] peptides by Sangstat). In the original report by Nisco *et al.*, co-administration of a subtherapeutic dose of cyclosporin A (CsA) and the HLA-B7.75-84 peptide resulted in long-term cardiac allograft survival in the majority of rodent recipients [10]. Furthermore, these animals were rendered specifically tolerant: second allografts from the same donor strain were accepted whereas third-party grafts were rejected. The peptide was effective when administered by the intravenous or oral route. Mechanistic studies suggested that the immunosuppressive effects were mediated via induction of anergy. Cuturi *et al.*[11] and Hanaway *et al.* [12] evaluated the same peptide in lower responder-stimulator combinations where CsA could be withheld, allowing study of the peptide's effect alone. Both groups found prolonged survival in the peptide treated animals. Analysis of graft infiltrating leukocytes from 07.75-84 peptide treated animals in the former study showed marked decreases in allospecific and spontaneous (NK cell) cytotoxic activity. Hanaway's group also demonstrated a donor specific decrease in CTL function and, in addition, evidence of decreased T helper cell activation. In a stringent mouse skin transplant model, the 2702.75-84 but not the 07.75-84 peptide prolonged graft survival as monotherapy or with CsA [13]. Gao *et al.* also found prolongation of mouse cardiac allograft survival in 2702.75-84 treated recipients; the combination of peptide with low dose CsA was again much more effective [14]. Interestingly, the L-isomer form of 2702.75-84 which is more resistant to proteolytic breakdown had a longer serum half-life (30 to 60 minutes) and enhanced *in vivo* immunosuppressive activity compared to the conventional D-isomer form. More recent studies have

Table 1
Animal studies of HLA-B7.75-84 and HLA-B27.75-84 peptides (ALS=anti-lymphocyte serum)

Refs	
B7.75-84	
10	Peptide + low dose CsA: prolonged cardiac allograft survival; induced donor specific tolerance
11,12	Peptide prolonged cardiac allograft survival; decreased NK & CTL function
15	Peptide + low dose CsA: prolonged small bowel allograft survival
17	In a chronic rejection model, peptide + low dose CsA: prolonged cardiac allograft survival; prevented graft arteriosclerosis
B27.75-84	
13	Peptide prolonged skin allograft survival, alone or with CsA
14	Peptide + low dose CsA prolonged cardiac allograft survival; L-isomer more effective than D- isomer
16	Peptide prolonged pancreatic islet xenograft survival, alone or with ALS

shown prolongation of graft survival with these peptides in rat small bowel allotransplant [15] and in pig-to-mouse pancreatic xenotransplant models [16]. Prevention of chronic rejection in one of the standard animal models has also been reported [17].The *in vivo* studies of these Allotrap[R] peptides are summarised in Table 1. Note that the 07.75-84 peptide is effective in rat transplant models whereas the 2702.75-84 peptide is effective in mouse models.

Recently, a new 'in silico screening' approach was used to develop potentially more effective derivatives of the 2702.75-84 peptide [18]. Importantly, this approach did not require knowledge of the peptides' site(s) of action - a requirement for standard structure-based design techniques. Immunosuppressive activities, physico-chemical properties and molecular dynamic studies of substituted forms of the 2702.75-84 peptide were computer analyzed to construct new more potent derivatives. One derivative, RDP 1258 peptide, although possessing an amino acid sequence quite distinct from the parent compound, was significantly more potent at inhibiting human and mouse T lymphocyte cytotoxicity. Studies of this peptide in our laboratory demonstrated inhibition of the rat, mouse and human MLR; experimental renal allograft survival was prolonged when the peptide was combined with low dose CsA [19].

The above results in animal models have been sufficiently impressive to stimulate interest in human studies. A small randomized, double blind (phase II) trial to assess the safety and pharmacokinetics of the 07.75-84 peptide in recipients of a first cadaveric renal allograft was recently completed [20]. Patients received standard CsA + steroid + azathioprine therapy and variable doses of peptide or placebo. Those patients treated with the highest dose of peptide developed significantly reduced peripheral blood natural killer (NK) cell cytotoxicity to K562 targets (a commonly used human tumour cell line) several days after completing the ten day treatment course and this effect persisted for as long as two months. Although the biological significance of this finding is uncertain, the study does demonstrate that MHC peptides can exert immunomodulatory effects in humans. Acute rejection still occurred in peptide treated patients; in fact there was a trend towards more acute rejection episodes and herpetic infections with peptide treatment. No patient became immunized to the peptide and the plasma half-life of the peptide was shown to be extremely short (minutes).

Although these class I MHC peptides function, at least in part, by inhibiting NK cell and specific CTL mediated lysis of foreign cells, their *in vivo* mechanism of action is incompletely understood. The allele non-specific effects of the 07.75-84 and 2702.75-84 peptides and the fact that both L- and D-iso-mers of peptide 2702.75-84 prolong graft survival suggest that the peptides' immunomodulatory activity is not based on direct interaction with the T-cell receptor or on presentation by MHC molecules. Using biotinylated forms of various class I MHC peptides and their inverted dimers, Nossner *et al.* found that the 2702.75-84 peptide and its inverted dimer bound to the heat shock proteins (HSPs), HSP70 and HSC702 from human T cell lysates and that binding affinity correlated highly with inhibition of human CTL activity [21]. They postulated that the immunomodulatory peptides mediated their effects via binding to these HSPs which possibly had an immunophilin type role within the T cell. A subsequent study has found poor correlation between peptide immunomodulating activity and binding to HSPs [22]. For example, the D-isomer of HLA-B27.75-84 was more potent than its L- coun-terpart, but did not bind to HSC70. The binding of peptides by HSPs reported by Nossner may be non-specific. There is now strong evidence that these peptides function, at least in part, by upregulation of haem oxygenase-1 (HO-1) activity. Affinity chromatography with one of these immunomodula-tory peptides identified HO-1 as a potential receptor [23]. All of the biolog-ically active peptides derived from 2702.75-84 were shown to inhibit HO activity *in vitro*. Similar to that observed with other inhibitors of HO, *in vivo* administration of the peptides to mice resulted in rapid *upregulation* of HO-1 protein expression.

Haem oxygenase is one of a number of protective genes whose expression is upregulated by stresses such as ischaemia, acute inflammation [24] and experimental allograft rejection [25]. Administration of protoporphyrin com-pounds which upregulate HO activity can attenuate the acute inflammatory response [24] and prevent the development of chronic rejection in allograft models [26]. The mechanisms by which upregulation of HO exerts these effects are not fully understood but are postulated to involve the increased synthesis of the products of heme catabolism: biliverdin, bilirubin and carbon monoxide [27]. Bile pigments (biliverdin and bilirubin) show anti-oxi-dant and anti-complement effects *in vitro* [28,29], inhibit lymphocyte prolif-erative responses to mitogen [30] and impair NK-cell mediated cytotoxicity [31]. Carbon monoxide may function as a gaseous messenger to modulate the activity of cGMP, nitric oxide synthase [32] and enzymes involved in ara-chidonaté metabolism [33]. In addition, due to the haem protein nature of nitric oxide synthase, induction of HO may modulate the production of nitric oxide, an important effector molecule in immune and inflammatory reactions [34].

NON-POLYMORPHIC CLASS II MHC DERIVED PEPTIDES

Boytim *et al.* studied a peptide derived from a conserved region of the $\alpha 1$ domain α helix of class II MHC molecules (specifically residues 65-79 of the HLA-DQA1*03011 allele) [35]. This region forms part of the peptide binding cleft, as discussed above. This DQ peptide inhibited human lymphocyte proliferation *in vitro* to both mitogenic and antigenic stimuli. Inhibition of proliferation was not allele specific, suggesting that its receptor is broadly expressed. Early events in T cell activation were not affected: rather the peptide functioned by inhibiting cyclin-dependent kinases and thus arresting cell cycle progression. This effect on cell cycle progression was analogous to that of rapamycin. The receptors of these two compounds are distinct, however, because the DQA1*03011 peptide did not compete with rapamycin for binding to FKBP. Recent work by the same group has identified proliferating cell nuclear antigen (PCNA) as the probable binding protein [36].

Research in our own laboratory has focused on peptides derived from non-polymorphic regions of the α chain of certain rat and human class II MHC molecules. Initial *in vitro* studies showed that a peptide derived from rat RT1.D[u] (51-75) inhibited the MLR and generation of CTL [37]. The active component of this peptide was composed of amino acid residues 61-75. Peptides derived from corresponding regions of rat RT1.B[a] and the human alleles HLA-DQA1*0101 and DQB1*0501 (residues 62-77 in the case of human MHC) were then tested [38]. All α chain peptides but not the β chain derived peptide exhibited immunosuppressive effects *in vitro* with the HLA-DQA1*0101 peptide being the most potent. This peptide inhibited the rat, human and mouse MLR, irrespective of donor or stimulator MHC type. IL-2 and INF-γ production in the MLR was also inhibited. The HLA-DQA1*0101 peptide also inhibited CTL generation in the MLR but had no effect on the cytolytic activity of preformed CTLs. Thus, the peptide inhibited mainly CD4 lymphocyte function. The immunomodulatory effects of this peptide appear to be mediated, at least in part, by apoptosis of antigen activated cells [38]. The binding sites of the DQA1*0101 peptide have not yet been characterised.

It is interesting to note that although the HLA-DQA1*03011 and the HLA-DQA1*0101 peptides are derived from similar regions of different MHC alleles, have significant overlap in amino acid sequence (Table 2) and are allele non-specific immunosuppressants *in vitro*, their mechanisms of action are very different. Further comparison of these immunomodulatory peptides *in vivo* is planned.

Table 2
Amino acid sequences of HLA-DQA1*0101(62-77) and HLA-DQA1*03011(65-79)

	62	63	64	65	66	67	68	69	70	71	72	73	74	75	76	77	78	79
DQA1*0101	A	L	R	N	M	A	V	A	K	H	N	L	N	I	M	I		
DQA1*03011				N	I	A	V	L	K	H	N	L	N	I	V	I	K	R

POLYMORPHIC MHC DERIVED PEPTIDES

In rodent models, peptides derived from polymorphic regions of MHC molecules can induce alloantigen specific tolerance when administered by certain routes. Systemic administration of anti-lymphocyte serum is usually required at the time of intrathymic innoculation with allopeptides for this strategy to be successful. In such cases, the peptides presumably exert their immunosuppressive effects by modulating the indirect pathway of allorecognition. Intrathymic innoculation of recipient animals with class I allopeptides or antigens was shown to prolong cardiac allograft and pancreatic islet survival [39,40]. In a donor-recipient combination mismatched for one class I MHC molecule, Shirwan et al. found long-term cardiac allograft survival after intrathymic injection of a mixture of three MHC class I allopeptides [41,42]. These peptides had previously been shown to be immunodominant in the same rat allograft rejection model [43]. Long-term engraftment was associated with production of certain IgG subtypes [41]. Despite evidence of high levels of donor microchimerism in recipients with long-term surviving grafts, graft histology showed chronic rejection [42]. This study illustrates the importance of correlating "tolerance" with graft histological findings: in much of the literature concerning MHC derived peptides, graft histology is *not* reported.

Intrathymic injection of polymorphic class II MHC allopeptides has also yielded encouraging results in experimental organ transplant models. In a rat renal allograft model, intrathymic injection of polymorphic class II MHC allopeptides (from RT1.B^u and RT1.D^u of the WF rat) was shown to induce antigen specific unresponsiveness [44] - important evidence for the role of T cell recognition of class II peptides in vascularized allograft rejection. In this model, the immunogenic but not the non-immunogenic allopeptides were effective tolerogens [45,46]. The induction phase of this acquired thymic tolerance required an intact thymus and was mediated by peripheral T cell anergy. The maintenance phase was thymus-independent and possibly mediated by deletion of specific alloreactive T cell clones [45,46]. A separate study showed that intrathymic injection of the above WF peptides with systemic administration of anti-CD3 monoclonal antibody prolonged the survival of pancreatic islet xenografts in a WF rat into C57BL/6J mouse model [47]. Donor-specific unresponsiveness did not last indefinitely and all xenografts were eventually rejected. Nevertheless, the study results suggest that useful manipulation of the indirect pathway in xenotransplantation is achievable. It is noteworthy that intrathymic administration of the immunodominant class I *or* II MHC alloantigens – rather than both classes of antigens – is sufficient to induce long-term allograft acceptance in rodents. This strategy must now be assessed in higher mammals.

Oral administration of class II MHC polymorphic peptides has been shown to downregulate alloimmune responses such as specific delayed type hypersensitivity (DTH) reactions to the same allopeptides or to analogous allogeneic cells. LEW rats fed the above RT1.B^u and RT1.D^u allopeptide mixture for five days developed antigen specific reduction of DTH responses to both the allopeptide mixture and to RT1^u expressing WF splenocytes [48]. Only the immunogenic peptides were tolerogenic [49,50]. Histology of the DTH lesions showed a switch in production from Th1 to Th2 cytokines [49]. Lymphocytes derived from peptide fed LEW animals exhibited specific reduction in proliferation and CTL generation against allogeneic WF cells in the MLR [50].

The use of allochimeric proteins (in which polymorphic regions/epitopes of donor MHC are incorporated into a backbone of recipient MHC) has been pioneered by Kahan's group [51]. Using a modified polymerase chain reaction and gene splicing technique, nucleotides encoding polymorphic amino acids of the α helical region of RT1.A^u were superimposed onto the analogous RT1.A^a coding region [51]. Three allochimeric or hybrid proteins were then produced *in vitro*. A single perioperative injection of one such protein into the portal vein of the ACI (RT1.A^a) recipient of a WF (RT1.A^u) heart induced donor specific tolerance; another peptide was equally effective when combined with a short course of CsA. This approach allowed identification of tolerogenic epitopes in class I alloantigens; in this case, located in the polymorphic α1 helical region of RT1.A^u. The mechanism of action of these hybrid proteins is not fully understood. One hypothesis is that peptides generated by recipient processing of the allo-chimeric protein deliver anergic signals to the T lymphocytes specific for the 'wild type' alloantigen [51].

Finally, there is evidence to suggest that manipulation of the indirect pathway of allorecognition in human transplant recipients may be clinically advantageous. Suciu-Foca and colleagues have demonstrated that, in the early post-transplant period, recipients of a two HLA-DR mismatched cardiac allograft may exhibit indirect alloreactivity against donor HLA-DR antigens which is limited to a single peptide determinant of an allogeneic HLA-DR molecule and restricted by one self HLA-DR molecule [7]. In addition, *in vitro* immunization studies have shown that T cell lines responding to an HLA-DR derived allopeptide express a limited number of TCR variable genes [52]. Together these findings suggest that targeting the relevant limited number of dominant allopeptides or their binding sites might suffice in blocking indirect alloresponses. One caveat is the occurrence of intramolecular and intermolecular spreading of epitopes recognized through the indirect allorecognition pathway in patients with recurrent and / or chronic rejection [53,54]. In such cases, effective downregulation of the indirect pathway might require targeting a large number of potential epitopes (including cryptic epitopes). Another issue is that indirect alloresponses to class I MHC peptides in human transplantation have not been assessed to the same extent as those to class II MHC peptides. Class I MHC will be quantitatively more expressed than class II molecules in graft tissue and are likely to form a large source of alloantigens for uptake by recipient APCs.

OTHER STRATEGIES FOR TARGETING THE INDIRECT PATHWAY OF ALLORECOGNITION

Possible strategies for modulating the indirect pathway in humans include (i) *intrathymic or oral administration* of immunodominant peptides (as discussed above) (ii) *peptide blockade* of the recipient's MHC molecule(s), (iii) *high zone tolerance* in which high concentrations of antigen stimulate initial T cell activation followed by death and (iv) *TCR antagonism.* The applicability of thymus based strategies of immunomodulation in humans, particularly adults is questionable. With regard to oral tolerising regimens, studies to date in the autoimmune disease, multiple sclerosis (using myelin antigen) have proved disappointing.

Peptide induced MHC blockade

A given MHC molecule can bind a large number of peptide antigens in its cleft region [55]. Peptides binding to the same MHC molecule can compete with each other for presentation to T lymphocytes *in vitro* [56]. Thus, a molar excess of competitor peptide would inhibit adequate interaction of TCRs with wild type peptide-MHC complexes. Co-administration of antigen and a competitor peptide (which binds to the same class II MHC molecule) can inhibit lymphocyte activation and antibody responses *in vivo* [57,58]. This strategy has been successfully used to prevent experimental autoimmune diabetes [59] and experimental allergic encephalomyelitis (EAE) [60,61]. A peptide named S9M with high binding affinities for H-2D^b (class I MHC) prevented H-2D^b restricted, CTL mediated destruction of virally infected pancreatic cells in a virus-induced autoimmune diabetes model [62]. This blocking peptide was designed to bind with high affinity to the class I MHC D^b allele but to lack the crucial TCR interactive residues. Clearance of the virus was not affected because of H-2K^b restricted CTL lysis of virally infected cells. Mechanistic studies showed that expansion of H-2D^b restricted, anti-viral CTL was inhibited by the blocking peptide and that adoptive transfer of S9M specific CTLs did not prevent diabetes mellitus (strongly suggesting that induction of regulatory cells did not occur).

There is at least one report of peptide blockade prolonging experimental allograft survival. However, in this study, the inhibitory peptide was derived from the TCR Vβ8 variable region [63]. In the mouse strain combinations used, allogeneic responses to the class I MHC, L^d molecule were mainly restricted to TCR Vβ8 lymphocytes. Administration of the TCR Vβ8 peptide specifically prolonged L^d disparate skin allografts. Binding assays showed that the peptide did not compete for binding to the L^d antigen binding groove. The authors speculated that the synthetic TCR Vβ8 peptide bound the L^d molecule in a manner similar to the intact TCR, thus competing with the TCR for interaction with the L^d molecule.

There are a number of difficulties with peptide induced MHC blockade *in vivo*: the epitope(s) to be blocked must be clearly defined, the binding affinity of the blocking agent must be equal or greater than that of the targeted epitope; efficacy is limited by the short half-life of these peptides and they work best when given at the time of initial exposure to antigen. Furthermore, their effect is likely to be short-lived [60,62,64]. Lack of specificity due to binding of non-targeted MHC molecules could also occur.

High zone tolerance

High doses of antigen can paradoxically suppress immune responses by extrathymic mechanisms in adult animals. Exposure of the T lymphocyte to large doses of antigen can induce initial cell activation but then anergy or death. Activation induced cell death is thought to be an important mechanism of maintaining peripheral tolerance. This is mediated in lymphocytes by signalling through Fas or TNF receptors and is facilitated by the presence of IL-2 [65]. This area is further reviewed in [66]. Repetitive administration of myelin basic protein attenuated the severity of EAE in a mouse model [65]. Use of this intervention in experimental transplantation has not been reported. However, Liu *et al.* found that high doses of an HLA-DR4 derived allopeptide suppressed the blastogenic response of a T lymphocyte line reactive to this peptide [67]. Production of IL-4 but not IL-2 was inhibited.

Altered peptide ligands / TCR antagonists

Recent studies have shown that T cell "stimulation" using synthetic peptides with substituted amino acids (particularly those amino acids which interact with the TCR) can have varying effects on subsequent T cell responses [68-71]. Co-presentation of an altered peptide ligand (APL) with wild type antigen may inhibit T lymphocyte proliferation to antigen: this phenomenon is called TCR antagonism. When the APL delivers a partial signal to the T cell, the term partial antagonism is used; delivery of no signal is termed full antagonism. In some cases, presentation of APLs renders the T cell anergic to subsequent challenge with wild type antigen [71].

TCR antagonism has been described with both CD4 and CD8 lymphocytes. The exact mechanisms by which such antagonism occurs are unclear. Simple competitive inhibition of binding of the wild type antigen is one possibility but this idea has been criticised on the basis that the antagonist would need to engage nearly all TCRs [72]. It is postulated by others that TCR antagonists disrupt oligomerization of the TCR or its interaction with co-receptors [72,73]. Readers are referred to reference [74] for more discussion of the hypothetical models of TCR signalling and its disruption by APLs. With regard to effects downstream of the TCR complex, there is now strong evidence that at least some APLs induce a limited and atypical form of intracellular signal transduction [74,75]. Compared to typical agonist ligands, APLs induced an "abnormal" pattern of TCRζ and CD3ϵ tyrosine phosphorylation, which resulted in inactivation of ZAP-70, a critical tyrosine kinase in T cell activation [76,77]. Such downstream effects may result in global T cell anergy (dominant negative signal hypothesis). This hypothesis has been challenged, however by a recent report. Daniels et al. generated T cells bearing two TCRs of known, non-overlapping specificity [78]. Antagonism of one TCR by an altered ligand did not impair the ability of the other TCR to transmit an activational signal.

An important advantage of TCR antagonists is their greater potency (more than ten-fold) than MHC blockers [79,80]. Interestingly, APLs are proving to be useful tools for studying the TCR mediated signalling cascade and T cell selection processes within the thymus [72]. Moreover, the existence of endogenous APLs has recently been appreciated [81,82]. In certain situations, antigen processing may generate both stimulatory and inhibitory peptides from the same immunogenic epitope [83]. There is now fascinating evidence that viruses may display altered epitopes which act as natural TCR antagonists and thus inhibit CTL responses against these epitopes [84].

It should be emphasized that most of the above work involved T cell clones where a single TCR interacted with a single ligand - a condition unlikely to occur in vivo. However, Matsushita et al. studied a battery of synthetic peptides of random sequences and proscribed length and found that certain peptides did inhibit polyclonal responses of unseparated human PBMCs (to PPD, crude mite extract or allogeneic human cells) [85]. With regard to in vivo studies, TCR antagonists have not yet been tested in transplant models. Substituted forms of the encephalitogenic epitopes of MBP have successfully prevented EAE [79,86,87] and ameliorated early established disease [86].

There are several issues regarding the applicability of APLs/TCR antagonism to humans [72]. Firstly, in human disease, the immune response may be directed against multiple epitopes and involve multiple TCR specificities. Thus, multiple TCR antagonists - an impractical approach - would be required to treat disease. Secondly, APLs which function as effective antagonists of T cell clones in vitro may behave as agonists of other T cells in vivo, thus worsening disease [87]. Lastly, the antigen(s) targeted in autoimmune disease are frequently unknown. However, de Koster et al. recently described an efficient method for designing TCR antagonists of alloreactive T cells using peptide libraries enriched for HLA-binding motifs [88]. This method does not require knowledge of the original allostimulatory peptide.

INHIBITORS OF CD4/CD8 – MHC INTERACTIONS

Analogs of "critical" regions on CD4/CD8 molecules

The main functions of the CD4 or CD8 co-receptors are: (i) promotion of adhesion between the T cell and the APC/target cell and (ii) signal transduction. Interaction between the CD4/CD8 and class II/I MHC molecules plays a critical role in normal T cell activation. This binding occurs mainly via the two N-terminal Ig-like domains of CD4 and the non-polymorphic β2 domain of the class II MHC molecule; or via the analogous regions of CD8 and the non-polymorphic α3 domain of the class I MHC molecule. Although these co-receptors and their cognate MHC molecules are large proteins, these molecules interact via a limited number of small surface binding epitopes. Appropriately designed small molecule analogues of these epitopes may thus disrupt the normal interaction between parent macromolecules. Design of such compounds has been greatly facilitated by nuclear magnetic resonance structural analysis of molecules and computer screening of molecular data bases. This "rational design" of peptide or non-peptide blockers can potentially be applied to many macromolecular interactions important in alloimmune responses. It also allows the design of more stable derivatives, resistant to enzymatic breakdown *in vivo.*

Inhibition of CD4 - class II MHC interaction

Peptides corresponding to the CD4 binding domain of class II MHC were assessed by Clayberger *et al.* [89]. A synthetic peptide corresponding to residues 134-152 of the HLA-DR β-chain inhibited the differentiation of CTL precursors and the proliferation of an alloreactive CD4 cell clone to antigen [89]. These inhibitory effects could be overcome by the addition of exogenous IL-2. This strategy was also assessed in an analogous mouse model [90]. *In vitro,* low doses of the I-A^b(134-148) peptide stimulated and high doses inhibited the mouse MLR; antigen specific T cell responses were actually enhanced by these peptides, however.

rD-mPGPtide is a 13 amino acid peptide designed to mimic the CDR (complementarity determining region)3-domain 1 (D1) region of the murine CD4 molecule, but consisting of D- rather than L- amino acids to slow proteolytic breakdown. This region is thought to be a contact site for class II MHC [91]. *In vitro,* rD-mPGPtide inhibited the mouse MLR [92,93]; *in vivo,* it markedly attenuated the severity of EAE [92] and enhanced bone marrow engraftment in various mouse models [93,94]. Combining rD-mPGPtide with CsA in the bone marrow transplant model had an additive survival effect and allowed reduction in CsA dosage [95]. A single injection of rD-mPGPtide significantly prolonged skin allograft survival in a class II MHC disparate strain combination [96]. These *in vivo* studies of rD-mPGPtide are summarized in Table 3. The mechanism of action of this peptide analogue is incompletely understood: it may function by disruption of CD4 dimerisation which would impair the tripartite TCR-class II MHC-peptide interaction. Potential advantages

Table 3
New immunomodulatory peptides developed by structure-based design techniques to inhibit CD4 or CD8 function.

Compound	Design features	Effects	Refs
rD-mPGPtide	Mimics the CDR3-D1 region of CD4; consists of D- rather than L- amino acids to slow proteolytic breakdown	Inhibited MLR; prolonged bone marrow allograft survival (mouse models); decreased severity of EAE	91-96
hPGP(N)	Analogue of CDR3-like region of the D1 domain of human CD4	Inhibited proliferation of (CD4+) T cells in human MLR	97
Cyclic heptapeptide IV	Mimics the CD4 domain 1 CC' surface loop (may serve as a critical functional epitope for CD4-class II MHC binding)	Inhibited human MLR; prolonged bone marrow and skin allograft survival (mouse models); decreased severity of EAE	98
TJU103	Non-peptide ligand of CD4 D1 surface-binding pocket	Inhibited human MLR; prolonged skin allograft survival (mouse models); decreased severity of EAE	99
Cyclic peptide SC4	Derived from CDR2 region of mouse CD8	Inhibited generation and activation of CTLs in vitro; prolonged skin allograft survival	100
CD8 DE region peptides	Mimic DE loop region of CD8 (interacts with class I MHC)	Inhibited CD8-class I MHC adhesion and blocked CTL mediated lysis of target cells in vitro	102

over anti-CD4 antibodies are its ease of synthesis, non-immunogenicity (in the limited animal models studied to date) and its inhibition of activated antigen-specific T cells rather than all CD4 cells.

Using computer-assisted molecular modelling techniques, peptide analogues of the CDR3-like region of the D1 domain of the human CD4 molecule have been constructed. These peptides inhibited CD4+ T cell proliferation in MLR assays [97]. Similarly, a heptapeptide was designed to mimic the CD4 domain 1 CC' surface loop, involved in CD4-class II MHC interaction [98]. *In vitro*, this analogue blocked stable CD4-class II MHC interaction, as assessed by rosette formation; *in vivo*, this peptide exerted immunosuppressive effects in autoimmune and transplant models [98]. Computer assisted structural/rational design of immunomodulatory molecules is now being extended to include compounds other than peptides [99].

Inhibition of CD8 – class I MHC interaction

Peptides corresponding to the CD8 binding region of the class I MHC α chain were assessed by Clayberger *et al.* (see reference [89] above). A synthetic peptide corresponding to residues 222-235 of the class I MHC α chain blocked the differentiation of CTL precursors into activated CTLs; unlike the HLA-DR β-chain peptide, this peptide did not inhibit lymphocyte proliferation. Korngold's group are now using the structure-based design approach described above to synthesise peptide inhibitors of CD8 lymphocyte function. Cyclic peptides corresponding to sequences from the 3 CDRs of mouse CD8 were synthesised [100]. These CDR-like regions (found in most members of the Ig superfamily) are likely to be involved in CD8 interactions with other surface molecules. Four of these peptides inhibited the generation and/or activity of CTLs. Furthermore, one of these peptides prolonged the survival of class I - but not class II - MHC disparate mouse skin grafts. The crystal structure of the human CD8-class I MHC complex has recently been described [101]. This model shows that the DE loop region of CD8, in addition to the CDR-like regions, interacts with class I MHC. Small peptide mimics of this DE loop inhibited CD8-class I MHC adhesion and blocked CTL mediated lysis of target cells *in vitro*, indicating that the DE loop is a functionally important epitope [102]. Further studies of these peptides *in vivo* are underway.

Comment on structure-based design of immunomodulatory peptides

The purpose of structure-based drug design is to use structural and biological data to create synthetic compounds with biological function [103]. It is apparent from the above studies which have used peptide mimics of functionally critical regions of CD4 and CD8 molecules that this technique has much potential to inhibit specific components of the immune response. For example, structure-based peptide design is now being used to block the interaction of IgE with its high affinity Fc receptor and thus inhibit mast cell degranulation [103]. Proposed advantages of designed peptide drugs are their low cost, low immunogenicity and perhaps oral bioavailability [100].

OTHER PEPTIDES

The class II associated invariant chain peptide (CLIP) is known to play an important role in the orderly traffic of newly synthesized class II MHC molecules within APCs and in the correct "loading" of these molecules with peptide before transport of the peptide-MHC complex to the cell surface. Incubation of APCs with CLIP *in vitro* or CLIP immunization *in vivo* have been shown to decrease antigen specific T cell responses, presumably by inhibiting both the loading of antigenic peptide onto class II MHC and the subsequent expression of peptide-MHC complexes on the cell surface [104]. This technique has yet to be tested in transplantation models.

CONCLUSION

Many MHC derived or associated peptides have been shown to possess clinically relevant immunomodulatory effects. In many cases, the mechanisms of action of these compounds remain under investigation. The putative sites of action of some of these peptides are summarised in figure 4. Elucidation of these mechanisms is also providing us with important information about fundamental immune processes such as TCR-MHC interaction. In general, non-polymorphic peptides suppress immune responses in a non-allele specific manner whereas polymorphic peptides induce antigen specific unresponsiveness. The clinical applicability of strategies utilising polymorphic

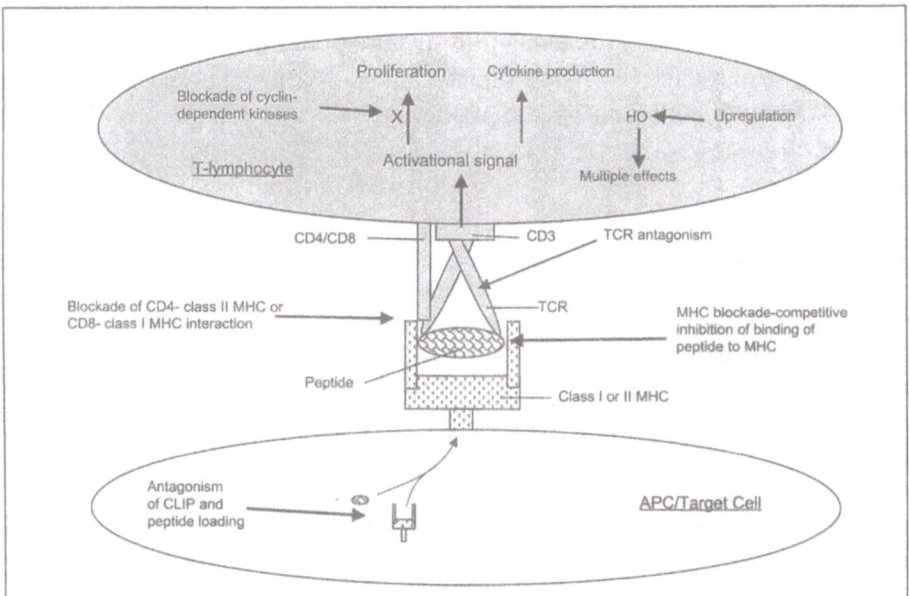

Figure 4
Possible mechanisms of peptide mediated immunomodulation.

peptides will be enhanced if the role of indirect allorecognition and the phenomenon of limited dominance of allo-MHC peptides are firmly established in human transplantation. Powerful information technology is now allowing structure-based design of immune molecule antagonists and rapid screening of peptide libraries for suitable agents [105]. Potential advantages of such designed compounds are high specificity, non-immunogenicity and slow biodegradability.

Of course, much further research is required before the use of MHC peptides can become a clinical reality in human transplantation and autoimmune disease. The success of the studies described above needs to be repeated in more genetically outbred animals and higher mammals. The feasibility of intrathymic administration of peptides to primates or humans has yet to be determined. The current low acute rejection rates achievable in human organ transplantation with standard immunosuppressive agents mean that the beneficial effects of additional agents - such as peptides - may be difficult to demonstrate, at least in the short-term. Nevertheless, protocols incorporating MHC peptides are likely to enter the clinical research arena in the near future.

Finally, since indirect allorecognition is associated with chronic allograft rejection [3-6,106,107], synthetic MHC peptides may be used to develop assays of post-transplant self-restricted CD4/CD8 T cell activity and to correlate this activity with chronic allograft dysfunction. Early downregulation of this specific alloreactivity using the strategies discussed above may attenuate the development of chronic rejection.

REFERENCES

1. Gould DS, Auchincloss H, Jr. Direct and indirect recognition: the role of MHC antigens in graft rejection. Immunol Today 1999;20(2):77-82.
2. Sayegh MH, Watschinger B, Carpenter CB. Mechanisms of T cell recognition of alloantigen. The role of peptides. Transplantation 1994;57(9):1295-302.
3. SivaSai KS, Smith MA, Poindexter NJ, et al. Indirect recognition of donor HLA class I peptides in lung transplant recipients with bronchiolitis obliterans syndrome. Transplantation 1999;67(8):1094-8.
4. Hornick PI, Mason PD, Yacoub MH, et al. Assessment of the contribution that direct allorecognition makes to the progression of chronic cardiac transplant rejection in humans. Circulation 1998;97(13):1257-63.
5. Fluck N, Witzke O, Morris PJ, Wood KJ. Indirect allorecognition is involved in both acute and chronic allograft rejection. Transplant Proc 1999;31(1-2):842-3.
6. Suciu-Foca N, Ciubotariu R, Itescu S, Rose EA, Cortesini R. Indirect allorecognition of donor HLA-DR peptides in chronic rejection of heart allografts. Transplant

Proc 1998;30(8):3999-4000.

7. Liu Z, Colovai AI, Tugulea S, et al. Indirect recognition of donor HLA-DR peptides in organ allograft rejection. J Clin Invest 1996;98:1150-7.

8. Takemoto SK, Cecka JM, Gjertson DW, Terasaki PI. Class I peptides involved in the indirect pathway of allorecognition. Transplant Proc 1999;31(1-2):781.

9. Clayberger C, Lyu SC, Pouletty P, Krensky AM. Peptides corresponding to T-cell receptor-HLA contact regions inhibit class I-restricted immune responses. Transplant Proc 1993;25(1 Pt 1):477-8.

10. Nisco S, Vriens P, Hoyt G, et al. Induction of allograft tolerance in rats by an HLA class-I-derived peptide and cyclosporine A. J Immunol 1994;152(8):3786-92.

11. Cuturi MC, Josien R, Douillard P, et al. Prolongation of allogeneic heart graft survival in rats by administration of a peptide (a.a. 75-84) from the alpha 1 helix of the first domain of HLA-B7 01. Transplantation 1995;59(5):661-9.

12. Hanaway MJ, Geissler EK, Wang J, et al. Immunosuppressive effects of an HLA class I-derived peptide in a rat cardiac allograft model. Transplantation 1996;61(8):1222-8.

13. Buelow R, Veyron P, Clayberger C, Pouletty P, Touraine JL. Prolongation of skin allograft survival in mice following administration of ALLOTRAP. Transplantation 1995;59(4):455-60.

14. Gao L, Woo J, Buelow R. Both L- and D-isomers of allotrap 2702 prolong cardiac allograft survival in mice. J Heart Lung Transplant 1996;15(1):78-87.

15. Willetts IE, Tam PK, Morris PJ, Dallman MJ. Treatment with an HLA-peptide and cyclosporine A prolongs rat small bowel allograft survival. J Pediatr Surg 1997;32(3):469-72.

16. Squiers EC, Hodell M, Tice D, Buelow R. Prolongation of porcine islet xenograft survival in mice after therapy with immunosuppressive peptides. Transplantation 1998;66(11):1558-61.

17. Murphy B, Kim KS, Buelow R, Sayegh MH, Hancock WW. Synthetic MHC class I peptide prolongs cardiac survival and attenuates transplant arteriosclerosis in the Lewis-->Fischer 344 model of chronic allograft rejection. Transplantation 1997;64(1):14-9.

18. Grassy G, Calas B, Yasri A, et al. Computer-assisted rational design of immunosuppressive compounds. Nat Biotechnol 1998;16(8):748-52.

19. Magee C, Azuma H, Knoflach A, et al. In vitro and in vivo immunomodulatory effects of RDP 1258, a novel synthetic peptide. J Am Soc Nephrol 1999;10:1997-2005.

20. Giral M, Cuturi MC, Nguyen JM, et al. Decreased cytotoxic activity of natural killer cells in kidney allograft recipients treated with human HLA-derived peptide. Transplantation 1997;63(7):1004-11.

21. Nossner E, Goldberg JE, Naftzger C, et al. HLA-derived peptides which inhibit T cell function bind to members of the heat-shock protein 70 family. J Exp Med 1996;183(2):339-48.

22. Woo J, Iyer S, Cornejo MC, et al. Immunosuppression by D-isomers of HLA class I heavy chain (amino acid 75 to 84)-derived peptides is independent of binding to HSC70. Transplantation 1997;64(10):1460-7.

23. Iyer S, Woo J, Cornejo MC, et al. Characterization and Biological Significance of Immunosuppressive Peptide D2702.75-84(E --> V) Binding Protein. Isolation of heme oxygenase-1. J Biol Chem 1998;273(5):2692-7.

24. Willis D, Moore AR, Frederick R, Willoughby DA. Heme oxygenase: a novel target for the modulation of the inflammatory response. Nat Med 1996;2(1):87-90.

25. Agarwal A, Kim Y, Matas AJ, Alam J, Nath KA. Gas-generating systems in acute renal allograft rejection in the rat. Co-induction of heme oxygenase and nitric oxide synthase. Transplantation 1996;61(1):93-8.

26. Hancock WW, Buelow R, Sayegh MH, Turka LA. Antibody-induced transplant

arteriosclerosis is prevented by graft expression of anti-oxidant and anti-apoptotic genes. Nat Med 1998;4(12):1392-6.

27. Platt JL, Nath KA. Heme oxygenase: protective gene or Trojan horse [news]. Nat Med 1998;4(12):1364-5.

28. Stocker R, Yamamoto Y, McDonagh AF, Glazer AN, Ames BN. Bilirubin is an anti-oxidant of possible physiological importance. Science 1987;235(4792):1043-6.

29. Nakagami T, Toyomura K, Kinoshita T, Morisawa S. A beneficial role of bile pigments as an endogenous tissue protector: anti-complement effects of biliverdin and conjugated bilirubin. Biochim Biophys Acta 1993;1158(2):189-93.

30. Haga Y, Tempero MA, Kay D, Zetterman RK. Intracellular accumulation of unconjugated bilirubin inhibits phytohemagglutin-induced proliferation and interleukin-2 production of human lymphocytes. Dig Dis Sci 1996;41(7):1468-74.

31. Haga Y, Tempero MA, Zetterman RK. Unconjugated bilirubin inhibits in vitro major histocompatibility complex-unrestricted cytotoxicity of human lymphocytes. Biochim Biophys Acta 1996;1316(1):29-34.

32. White KA, Marletta MA. Nitric oxide synthase is a cytochrome P-450 type hemoprotein. Biochemistry 1992;31(29):6627-31.

33. Martasek P, Schwartzman ML, Goodman AI, et al. Hemin and L-arginine regulation of blood pressure in spontaneous hypertensive rats. J Am Soc Nephrol 1991;2(6):1078-84.

34. Maines MD. The heme oxygenase system: a regulator of second messenger gases. Annu Rev Pharmacol Toxicol 1997;37(517):517-54.

35. Boytim ML, Lyu SC,Jung R, Krensky AM, Clayberger C. Inhibition of cell cycle progression by a synthetic peptide corresponding to residues 65-79 of an HLA class II sequence: functional similarities but mechanistic differences with the immunosuppressive drug rapamycin. J Immunol 1998;160(5):2215-22.

36. Murphy B, Krensky AM. HLA-derived peptides as novel immunomodulatory therapeutics. J Am Soc Nephrol 1999;10:1346-55.

37. Murphy B, Akalin E, Watschinger B, Carpenter CB, Sayegh MH. Inhibition of the alloimmune response with synthetic nonpolymorphic class II MHC peptides. Transplant Proc 1995;27(1):409-10.

38. Murphy B, Magee CC, Alexander SI, et al. Inhibition of allorecognition by a human class II MHC-derived peptide through the induction of apoptosis. J Clin Invest 1999;103(6):859-67.

39. Oluwole SF, Chowdhury NC, Jin MX, Hardy MA. Induction of transplantation tolerance to rat cardiac allografts by intrathymic inoculation of allogeneic soluble peptides. Transplantation 1993;56(6):1523-7.

40. Oluwole SF, Jin MX, Chowdhury NC, Ohajekwe OA. Effectiveness of intrathymic inoculation of soluble antigens in the induction of specific unresponsiveness to rat islet allografts without transient recipient immunosuppression. Transplantation 1994;58(10):1077-81.

41. Mhoyan A, Cramer DV, Baquerizo A, Shirwan H. Induction of allograft nonresponsiveness after intrathymic inoculation with donor class I allopeptides. I. Correlation of graft survival with antidonor IgG antibody subclasses. Transplantation 1997;64(12):1665-70.

42. Shirwan H, Wu GD, Barwari L, Liu A, Cramer DV. Induction of allograft nonresponsiveness after intrathymic inoculation with donor class I allopeptides. II. Evidence for persistent chronic rejection despite high levels of donor microchimerism. Transplantation 1997;64(12):1671-6.

43. Shirwan H, Leamer M, Wang HK, Makowka L, Cramer DV. Peptides derived from alpha-helices of allogeneic class I major histocompatibility complex antigens are potent inducers of CD4+ and CD8+ T cell and B cell responses after cardiac allograft rejection. Transplantation 1995;59(3):401-10.

44. Sayegh MH, Perico N, Imberti O, et al. Thymic recognition of class II major histo-

compatibility complex allopeptides induces donor-specific unresponsiveness to renal allografts. Transplantation 1993;56(2):461-5.

45. Sayegh MH, Perico N, Gallon L, et al. Mechanisms of acquired thymic unresponsiveness to renal allografts. Thymic recognition of immunodominant allo-MHC peptides induces peripheral T cell anergy. Transplantation 1994;58(2):125-32.

46. Remuzzi G, Perico N, Carpenter CB, Sayegh MH. The thymic way to transplantation tolerance [editorial]. J Am Soc Nephrol 1995;5(9):1639-46.

47. Zeng Y, Torres M, Wang Y, Montag A, Thistlethwaite JR, Jr. Intrathymic xenogeneic pancreatic islet transplantation--induction of donor-specific unresponsiveness by MHC class II peptides. Transplant Proc 1995;27(1):176-7.

48. Sayegh MH, Khoury SJ, Hancock WW, Weiner HL, Carpenter CB. Induction of immunity and oral tolerance with polymorphic class II major histocompatibility complex allopeptides in the rat. Proc Natl Acad Sci U S A 1992;89(16):7762-6.

49. Hancock WW, Khoury SJ, Carpenter CB, Sayegh MH. Differential effects of oral versus intrathymic administration of polymorphic major histocompatibility complex class II peptides on mononuclear and endothelial cell activation and cytokine expression during a delayed-type hypersensitivity response. Am J Pathol 1994;144(6):1149-58.

50. Sayegh MH, Khoury SJ, Hancock WW, Weiner HL, Carpenter CB. Mechanisms of oral tolerance by MHC peptides. Ann N Y Acad Sci 1996;778(338):338-45.

51. Wang M, Stepkowski SM, Yu J, Wang M, Kahan BD. Localization of cryptic tolerogenic epitopes in the alpha1-helical region of the RT1.Au alloantigen. Transplantation 1997;63(10):1373-9.

52. Liu Z, Sun YK, Xi YP, et al. Limited usage of T cell receptor V beta genes by allopeptide-specific T cells. J Immunol 1993;150(8 Pt 1):3180-6.

53. Suciu-Foca N, Harris PE, Cortesini R. Intramolecular and intermolecular spreading during the course of organ allograft rejection. Immunol Rev 1998;164:241-6.

54. Ciubotariu R, Liu Z, Colovai AI, et al. Persistent allopeptide reactivity and epitope spreading in chronic rejection of organ allografts. J Clin Invest 1998;101(2):398-405.

55. Engelhard VH. Structure of peptides associated with MHC class I molecules. Curr Opin Immunol 1994;6(1):13-23.

56. Babbitt BP, Matsueda G, Haber E, Unanue ER, Allen PM. Antigenic competition at the level of peptide-Ia binding. Proc Natl Acad Sci U S A 1986;83(12):4509-13.

57. Guery JC, Sette A, Leighton J, Dragomir A, Adorini L. Selective immunosuppression by administration of major histocompatibility complex (MHC) class II-binding peptides. I. Evidence for in vivo MHC blockade preventing T cell activation. J Exp Med 1992;175(5):1345-52.

58. Adorini L, Muller S, Cardinaux F, et al. In vivo competition between self peptides and foreign antigens in T- cell activation. Nature 1988;334(6183):623-5.

59. Hurtenbach U, Lier E, Adorini L, Nagy ZA. Prevention of autoimmune diabetes in non-obese diabetic mice by treatment with a class II major histocompatibility complex-blocking peptide. J Exp Med 1993;177(5):1499-504.

60. Lamont AG, Sette A, Fujinami R, et al. Inhibition of experimental autoimmune encephalomyelitis induction in SJL/J mice by using a peptide with high affinity for IAs molecules. J Immunol 1990;145(6):1687-93.

61. Sakai K, Zamvil SS, Mitchell DJ, et al. Prevention of experimental encephalomyelitis with peptides that block interaction of T cells with major histocompatibility complex proteins. Proc Natl Acad Sci U S A 1989;86(23):9470-4.

62. von Herrath MG, Coon B, Lewicki H, et al. In vivo treatment with a MHC class I-restricted blocking peptide can prevent virus-induced autoimmune diabetes. J Immunol 1998;161(9):5087-96.

63. Goss JA, Alexander-Miller MA, Gorka J, et al. Specific prolongation of allograft survival by a T-cell-receptor- derived peptide. Proc Natl Acad Sci U S A 1993;90(21):

9872-6.

64. Guery JC, Adorini L. Selective immunosuppression of class II-restricted T cells by MHC class II-binding peptides. Crit Rev Immunol 1993;13(3-4):195-206.

65. Critchfield JM, Racke MK, Zuniga-Pflucker JC, et al. T cell deletion in high antigen dose therapy of autoimmune encephalomyelitis. Science 1994;263(5150): 1139-43.

66. Bishop GA, Sun J, Sheil AG, McCaughan GW. High-dose/activation-associated tolerance: a mechanism for allograft tolerance. Transplantation 1997;64(10): 1377-82.

67. Liu Z, Harris PE, Colovai AI, et al. Suppression of the indirect pathway of T cell reactivity by high doses of allopeptide. Autoimmunity 1995;21(3):173-84.

68. Allen PM. Introduction: T-cell recognition of variant ligands. Semin Immunol 1996;8(2):61.

69. Evavold BD, Allen PM. Separation of IL-4 production from Th cell proliferation by an altered T cell receptor ligand. Science 1991;252(5010):1308-10.

70. Evavold BD, Sloan-Lancaster J, Hsu BL, Allen PM. Separation of T helper 1 clone cytolysis from proliferation and lymphokine production using analog peptides. J Immunol 1993;150(8 Pt 1):3131-40.

71. Sloan-Lancaster J, Evavold BD, Allen PM. Induction of T-cell anergy by altered T-cell-receptor ligand on live antigen-presenting cells. Nature 1993;363(6425): 156-9.

72. Sette A, Alexander J, Snoke K, Grey HM. Antigen analogs as tools to study T-cell activation function and activation. Semin Immunol 1996;8(2):103-8.

73. Bachmann MF, Speiser DE, Zakarian A, Ohashi PS. Inhibition of TCR triggering by a spectrum of altered peptide ligands suggests the mechanism for TCR antagonism. Eur J Immunol 1998;28(10):3110-9.

74. Madrenas J, Germain RN. Variant TCR ligands: new insights into the molecular basis of antigen- dependent signal transduction and T-cell activation. Semin Immunol 1996;8(2):83-101.

75. Ruppert J, Alexander J, Snoke K, et al. Effect of T-cell receptor antagonism on interaction between T cells and antigen-presenting cells and on T-cell signaling events. Proc Natl Acad Sci U S A 1993;90(7):2671-5.

76. Madrenas J, Wange RL, Wang JL, et al. Zeta phosphorylation without ZAP-70 activation induced by TCR antagonists or partial agonists. Science 1995;267(5197): 515-8.

77. Sloan-Lancaster J, Shaw AS, Rothbard JB, Allen PM. Partial T cell signaling: altered phospho-zeta and lack of zap70 recruitment in APL-induced T cell anergy. Cell 1994;79(5):913-22.

78. Daniels MA, Schober SL, Hogquist KA, Jameson SC. Cutting edge: a test of the dominant negative signal model for TCR antagonism. J Immunol 1999;162(7): 3761-4.

79. Franco A, Southwood S, Arrhenius T, et al. T cell receptor antagonist peptides are highly effective inhibitors of experimental allergic encephalomyelitis. Eur J Immunol 1994;24(4):940-6.

80. Serra HM, Crimi C, Sette A, Celis E. Fine restriction analysis and inhibition of antigen recognition in HLA- DQ-restricted T cells by major histocompatibility complex blockers and T cell receptor antagonists. Eur J Immunol 1993;23(11):2967-71.

81. Hsu BL, Evavold BD, Allen PM. Modulation of T cell development by an endogenous altered peptide ligand. J Exp Med 1995;181(2):805-10.

82. Vidal K, Allen PM. The effect of endogenous altered peptide ligands on peripheral T-cell responses. Semin Immunol 1996;8(2):117-22.

83. Carson RT, Desai DD, Vignali KM, Vignali DA. Immunoregulation of Th cells by naturally processed peptide antagonists. J Immunol 1999;162(1):1-4.

84. Bertoletti A, Sette A, Chisari FV, et al. Natural variants of cytotoxic epitopes are

T-cell receptor antagonists for antiviral cytotoxic T cells. Nature 1994;369(6479): 407-10.

85. Matsushita S, Matsuoka T. Peptide length-dependent TCR antagonism on class II HLA-restricted responses of peripheral blood mononuclear cells and T cell clones. Eur J Immunol 1999;29(2):431-6.

86. Kuchroo VK, Greer JM, Kaul D, et al. A single TCR antagonist peptide inhibits experimental allergic encephalomyelitis mediated by a diverse T cell repertoire. J Immunol 1994;153(7):3326-36.

87. Anderton SM, Manickasingham SP, Burkhart C, et al. Fine specificity of the myelin-reactive T cell repertoire: implications for TCR antagonism in autoimmunity. J Immunol 1998;161(7):3357-64.

88. de Koster HS, Vermeulen CJ, Hiemstra HS, et al. Definition of agonists and design of antagonists for alloreactive T cell clones using synthetic peptide libraries. Int Immunol 1999;11(4):585-91.

89. Clayberger C, Lyu SC, DeKruyff R, Parham P, Krensky AM. Peptides corresponding to the CD8 and CD4 binding domains of HLA molecules block T lymphocyte immune responses in vitro. J Immunol 1994;153(3):946-51.

90. Shen X, Hu B, McPhie P, et al. Peptides corresponding to CD4-interacting regions of murine MHC class II molecules modulate immune responses of CD4+ T lymphocytes in vitro and in vivo. J Immunol 1996;157(1):87-100.

91. Zhang X, Piatier-Tonneau D, Auffray C, et al. Synthetic CD4 exocyclic peptides antagonize CD4 holoreceptor binding and T cell activation. Nat Biotechnol 1996;14(4):472-5.

92. Jameson BA, McDonnell JM, Marini JC, Korngold R. A rationally designed CD4 analogue inhibits experimental allergic encephalomyelitis. Nature 1994;368(6473): 744-6.

93. Townsend RM, Briggs C, Marini JC, Murphy GF, Korngold R. Inhibitory effect of a CD4-CDR3 peptide analog on graft-versus-host disease across a major histocompatibility complex-haploidentical barrier. Blood 1996;88(8):3038-47.

94. Koch U, Korngold R. A synthetic CD4-CDR3 peptide analog enhances bone marrow engraftment across major histocompatibility barriers. Blood 1997;89(8):2880-90.

95. Townsend RM, Gilbert MJ, Korngold R. Combination therapy with a CD4-CDR3 peptide analog and cyclosporin A to prevent graft-vs-host disease in a MHC-haploidentical bone marrow transplantation model. Clin Immunol Immunopathol 1998;86(1):115-9.

96. Koch U, Choksi S, Marcucci L, Korngold R. A synthetic CD4-CDR3 peptide analog enhances skin allograft survival across a MHC class II barrier. J Immunol 1998; 161(1):421-9.

97. Friedman TM, Reddy AP, Wassell R, Jameson BA, Korngold R. Identification of a human CD4-CDR3-like surface involved in CD4+ T cell function. J Biol Chem 1996;271(37):22635-40.

98. Satoh T, Aramini JM, Li S, et al. Bioactive Peptide Design Based on Protein Surface Epitopes. A cyclic heptapeptide mimics CD4 domain 1 CC' loop and inhibits CD4 biological function. J Biol Chem 1997;272(18):12175-80.

99. Li S, Gao J, Satoh T, et al. A computer screening approach to immunoglobulin superfamily structures and interactions: discovery of small non-peptidic CD4 inhibitors as novel immunotherapeutics. Proc Natl Acad Sci U S A 1997;94(1):73-8.

100. Choksi S, Jameson BA, Korngold R. A structure-based approach to designing synthetic CD8alpha peptides that can inhibit cytotoxic T-lymphocyte responses. Nat Med 1998;4(3):309-14.

101. Gao GF, Tormo J, Gerth UC, et al. Crystal structure of the complex between human CD8alpha(alpha) and HLA- A2. Nature 1997;387(6633):630-4.

102. Li S, Choksi S, Shan S, et al. Identification of the CD8 DE loop as a surface functional epitope. Implications for major histocompatibility complex class I binding

and CD8 inhibitor design. J Biol Chem 1998;273(26):16442-5.

103. McDonnell JM, Beavil AJ, Mackay GA, et al. Structure based design and characterization of peptides that inhibit IgE binding to its high-affinity receptor. Nat Struct Biol 1996;3(5):419-26.

104. Zechel MA, Chaturvedi P, Lee CE, Rider BJ, Singh B. Modulation of antigen presentation and class II expression by a class II-associated invariant chain peptide. J Immunol 1996;156(11):4232-9.

105. Schneider G, Schrodl W, Wallukat G, et al. Peptide design by artificial neural networks and computer-based evolutionary search. Proc Natl Acad Sci U S A 1998;95(21):12179-84.

106. Vella JP, Spadafora FM, Murphy B, et al. Indirect allorecognition of major histocompatibility complex allopeptides in human renal transplant recipients with chronic graft dysfunction. Transplantation 1997;64(6):795-800.

107. Renna-Molajoni E, Cinti P, Evangelista B, et al. Role of the indirect recognition pathway in the development of chronic liver allograft rejection. Transplant Proc 1998;30(5):2140-1.

COSTIMULATORY BLOCKADE AS A THERAPEUTIC REGIMEN FOR PROLONGING ALLOGRAFT SURVIVAL AND INDUCING TOLERANCE: AN OVERVIEW OF RECENT RESEARCH

6

Majed M. Hamawy, Clifford S. Cho and Stuart J. Knechtle
Department of Surgery
University of Wisconsin
Madison, Wisconsin, USA

BACKGROUND

T lymphocytes are essential components of the immune response to allografts. Therefore, T lymphocytes are the target for almost all of the therapeutic regimens currently employed to prevent or control the immune response to the allograft. Indeed, monoclonal antibodies targeting the T cell antigen receptor (TCR) and the receptor for interleukin-2 (IL-2) have proved useful for controlling the acute immune response to the allograft. Furthermore, inhibitors of TCR signal transduction pathways such as cyclosporin A (CsA) and FK506, inhibitors of the serine/threonine phosphatase calcineurin, have revolutionized the short-term survival rate of allografts. However, despite the marked increase in the survival rate of allografts past one year, no significant increase in long-term allograft survival has been achieved. Furthermore, because the currently employed therapeutic regimens do not discriminate between allograft-specific T cells and allograft-nonspecific T cells, such regimens induce a general and a marked immunosuppression that may render the patient susceptible to infection and to tumor progression.

Indeed, in the past two decades there has been an explosion in research

A. W. Thomson (ed.), Therapeutic Immunosuppression, 127–158.
© 2001 *Kluwer Academic Publishers.*

involving the molecular and cellular basis of transplant immunology. In particular, there have been rapid and profound advances in elucidating the mechanisms of T cell activation and in defining membrane molecules, other than the subunits of the TCR, that are critical for regulating TCR activation and function. Accordingly, such exciting discoveries have led to the development of promising new therapeutic regimens to control the outcome of the immune response to allografts. In this chapter we will focus on describing the different costimulatory molecules in T cells and will discuss the therapeutic regimens that target such molecules.

T CELL ACTIVATION

Activation of T cells is initiated by the interactions between the TCR on T cells with peptide antigen (Ag) presented in the context of the major histocompatibilty complex (MHC) by antigen presenting cells (APC). TCR engagement initiates an array of intracellular signals, leading to the increase in the transcriptional activity of cytokine genes, cell adhesion, proliferation, and differentiation. Cytokines released from activated T cells stimulate antibody production, induce maturation of cytotoxic effector cells, and activate various accessory cells such as phagocytes. The α and β subunits, which make up the Ag-binding portion of the TCR, each possess short intracytoplasmic chains with no known roles in signal transduction [1,2]. However, each TCR associates with six transmembrane polypeptides collectively known as the CD3 complex. Each of the CD3 complex proteins possesses a relatively long cytoplasmic portion that is critical for initiating and transducing TCR signaling. Localized within these cytoplasmic sequences are immune receptor tyrosine-based activation motifs, or ITAMs [1,3-5]. The significance of these ITAMs lies in the fact that, once phosphorylated by protein tyrosine kinases (PTKs), they serve as high-affinity binding sites for multiple proteins that contain src homology-2 (SH2) domains. In this manner, cytoplasmic enzymes containing SH2 domains are effectively recruited to the TCR complex for purposes of TCR-mediated signal transduction [6].

TCR ligation has been shown to trigger an array of intracellular signals, including the stimulation of PTKs, the generation of inositol triphosphate and diacylglycerol, the activation of protein kinase C (PKC), the increase in intracellular Ca^{2+}, the activation of the Ras and Rho family of GTPases, and the activation of several mitogen-activated protein kinases (MAPKs) (Figure 1) [3,4]. Stimulated MAPKs translocate from the cytoplasm to the nucleus where they phosphorylate and in turn activate transcription factors such

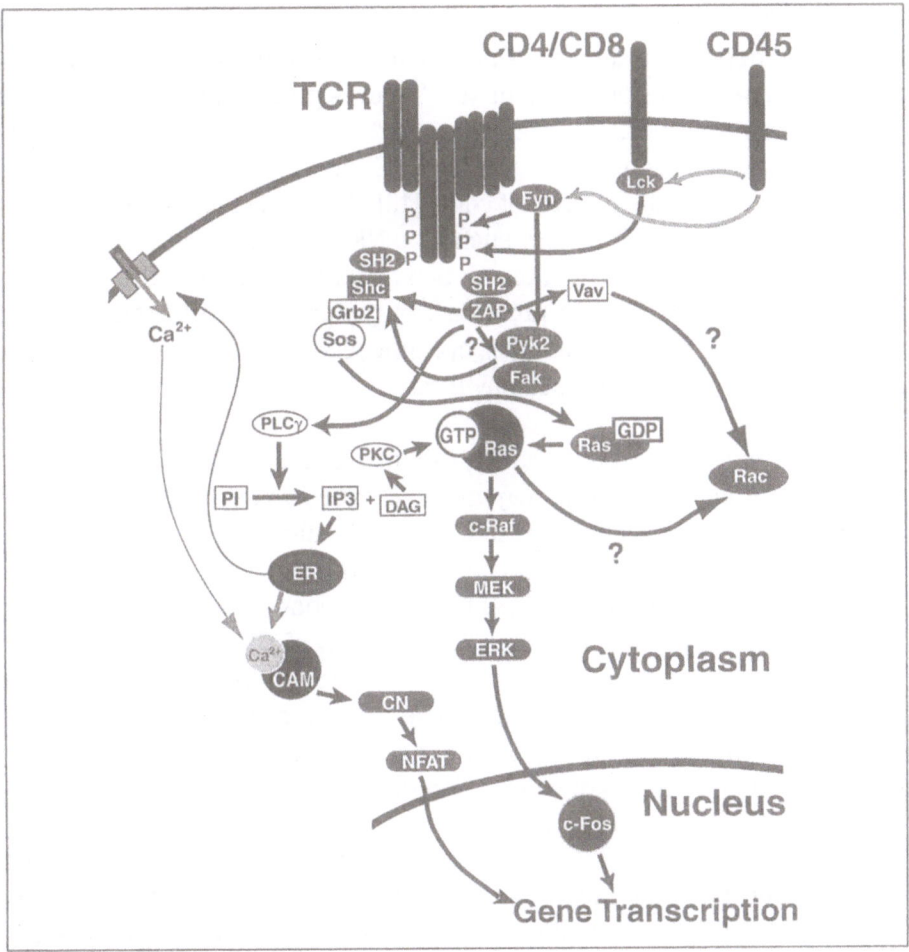

Figure 1
Scheme of some TCR-induced signals. TCR ligation activates CD45, which will dephosphorylate Fyn and Lck leading to the activation of the PTKs and to the phosphorylation of ITAMs in the TCR-subunits. ZAP-70 binds phosphorylated CD3ζ-ITAMs and is activated for the phosphorylation of downstream signals including PCLγ, Vav, and Shc. Activated PCLγ catalyses the hydrolysis of PI to PI3 and DAG, which mobilize Ca^{2+} from intracellular stores and activate PKC, respectively. Ca^{2+} binds calmodulin leading to the activation of calcineurin, which then induces the translocation of NF-AT to the nucleus. Shc binds through its SH2 to phosphorylated CD3ζ-ITAMs and becomes phosphorylated by ZAP-70. Phosphorylated Shc associates with the SH2 of Grb2-Sos complex, linking TCR to Ras signaling pathway. Pyk2 and Fak tyrosine phosphorylated after TCR may associate with the SH2 domain of Shc-Grb2-Sos complex and may link TCR to Ras pathway. Activated Ras stimulates the Raf-ERK signaling cascade leading to the activation of ERK, and in turn, to the phosphorylation and activation of the transcription factor c-Fos. Tyrosine phosphorylated Vav and activated Ras may link TCR to the Rho signaling cascade. c-Jun and c-Fos form AP-1 and together with NF-AT and other transcription factors initiate gene transcription.

as c-Fos, c-Jun, Elk-1, and c-Myc [7,8]. The increase in intracellular Ca^{2+} following TCR ligation stimulates various enzymes such as the Ca^{2+}/calmodulin-dependent kinases (CaMKs) and the serine/threonine phosphatase calcineurin, key enzymes in the T cell signal transduction cascade [9-14]. Activated CaMKs phosphorylate and upregulate the transcriptional activity of transcription factors such as CRE-binding protein (CREB), which in turn upregulates the activity of c-Fos [15]. Stimulated calcineurin dephosphorylates transcription factors such as c-NF-AT, Elk-1, Oct-1, and NF-κB, leading to modulation of the transcription factors' activity [16-18]. Activated transcription factors bind to promoters of genes, leading to the transcription of genes that encode cytokines, cytokine receptors, and protooncogenes such as c-Myc, c-Fos, and Src family PTKs.

It is now widely accepted that T cell activation is a complex process that involves not only the engagement of TCR by Ag/MHC, but also the engagement of the so-called costimulatory molecules on T cells. Interactions between costimulatory molecules on T cells with their ligands on APCs can play critical roles in determining the T cell response that occurs following TCR stimulation. For example, the engagement of CD28 has been shown to optimize TCR-mediated release of critical growth factors and cytokines from T cells. In contrast, the engagement of the costimulatory molecules cytotoxic T lymphocyte Ag-4 (CTLA-4) and CD2 has been shown to downregulate, rather than upregulate, TCR signaling.

The mechanisms by which costimulatory signals modulate TCR function are not clear, but may involve any one or more of the following: 1) they may provide additional, distinct signaling events, thereby complementing or downregulating those initiated through TCR; 2) costimulatory molecules may enhance the magnitude and/or duration of a TCR-induced signal, causing it to reach a threshold needed to activate further downstream signaling cascades; 3) costimulatory molecules may provide signals similar to the TCR complex but at different time points, which may result in repetitive stimulation required to maintain a proliferative or functional activation status.

In addition to positively or negatively regulating TCR-initiated signals, the failure to engage certain costimulatory molecules at the time of TCR:Ag/MHC interaction has been shown to lead to a state of unresponsiveness to subsequent stimulation known as anergy. This phenomenon is often observed after TCR ligation in the absence of CD28 engagement. The interaction of TCR:Ag/MHC without costimulatory molecules interaction has also been shown to result in a complete disregard of the MHC or antigen/MHC complex by the T cell (so-called ignorance) and/or apoptotic self-destruction of the T cell. The process of determining which of the three potential abortive outcomes takes place in the absence of costimulatory activity is not understood. Yet, the elicitation of these negative responses promises to be a door to inducing organ allograft tolerance.

COSTIMULATORY MOLECULES

The most widely studied costimulatory molecule/ligand pairs include CD4/MHC class II, CD8/MHC class I, CD28/B7, CTLA-4/B7, CD154/CD40, CD45/?, CD2/CD48(CD58), LFA-1/ICAM, and CD44/hyaluronic acid (Table 1). Costimulatory molecules on T cells have similar structural organization in that they all possess prominent extracellular domains, hydrophobic transmembrane regions, and a cytoplasmic tail that is often involved in cell signal transduction. Unlike TCR and MHC, they lack polymorphic regions of structural variability in their extracellular domains; therefore, they bind specific ligands that are present on the surfaces of their counterpart cells.

CD4 and CD8

The CD4 and CD8 proteins confer MHC restriction to their T cells by specifically binding to the MHC class II and I, respectively [19]. CD4, also known as Leu-3 or T4, is found (under normal circumstances) on approximately 65% of mature peripheral T cells. CD4 is ~58kDa glycoprotein characterized by 4 Ig V-like domains in its N-terminal extracellular component, a hydrophobic transmembrane region and a highly basic 40 amino acid intracytoplasmic tail. Its binding target is thought to be in an invariant region of the MHC class II (perhaps within the constant $\alpha2$ or $\beta2$ domains). Notably, CD4 has also been found to be the viral target for entry of the human immunodeficiency virus.

CD8, also named Leu-2 or T8, is typically found on roughly 35% of mature peripheral T cells. Unlike CD4, it exists either as a homodimer of two ~34kD CD8α chains, or occasionally as a heterodimer of CD8α and CD8β chains. Each chain of the dimer is an Ig superfamily derivative, characterized by an extracellular N-terminal Ig V-like domain, a hydrophobic transmembrane region, and a highly basic 25 to 27 amino acid intracytoplasmic tail. In a fashion analogous to the binding tendencies of CD4, CD8 is thought to bind specifically to a segment of the class I MHC invariant $\alpha3$ domain, thereby mediating its own MHC class-restricting function.

Table 1
Costimulatory molecules on T cells

Costimulatory molecule	Alternate names	Molecular weight	Gene superfamily	Ligands	Distribution
CD4	Leu-3 T4	55-58 kDa	Ig	MHC II	~65% mature peripheral T cells
CD8	Leu-2	30-38 kDa	Ig	MHC I	~35% mature peripheral T cells
CD28	Tp44	80-90 kDa	Ig	B7-1 B7-2	mature peripheral T cells developing thymocytes
CD152	CTLA-4 Ly56	35-75 kDa	Ig	B7-1 B7-2	activated T cells
CD80	B7-1 Ly53	55 kDa	Ig	CD28 CD152	stimulated B cells macrophages dendritic cells Langerhans'cells fibroblasts
CD86	B7-2 Ly58	80 kDa	Ig	CD28 CD152	stimulated B cells macrophages dendritic cells Langerhans'cells granulocytes
CD154	CD40 ligand Ly62 gp39	39 kDa	TNF	CD40	activated helper T cells mast cells eosinophils dendritic cells endothelial cells platelets

CD45	T200 Ly5 LCA	18-240 kDa	?	?	leukocytes
CD2	LFA-2 LFA-3 ligand Ly37	45-58 kDa	Ig	CD58 LFA-3	mature peripheral T cells immature T cells NK cells
CD11a/CD18	LFA-1	180 kDa / 95 kDa heterodimer	integrin ($\beta2$)	ICAM-1 ICAM-2	ubiquitous
CD54	ICAM-1 Ly47 MALA2	80-114 kDa	Ig	LFA-1	most hematopoietic cells fibroblasts keratinocytes endothelial cells
CD102	ICAM-2 Ly60	58-68 kDa	Ig	LFA-1	most hematopoietic cells platelets endothelial cells
CD44	Ly24 Pgp1	75-250 kDa	cartilage link	hyaluronic acid fibronectin laminin collagen	most hematopoietic cells fibroblasts

Table 1 Continued.

133

In addition to dictating MHC class restriction, CD4 and CD8 also facilitate the costimulation of T cells. This is manifested by the rapid phosphorylation of their cytoplasmic serine residues and by the physical association of their cytoplasmic regions with the critical Src family PTK Lck [20,21]. Thus, the formation of the TCR:Ag/MHC complex and the simultaneous interaction between CD4/CD8 and the MHC appear to bring the cytoplasmic tail of CD4/CD8 and the associated Lck into close proximity to CD3, leading to the rapid phosphorylation of the tyrosine residues of the ITAMs in CD3. The tyrosine phosphorylated ITAMs of CD3 act as docking sites for the SH2 domains of various enzymes and signaling molecules and therefore are essential for propagating TCR signaling. Indeed, mutations in Lck that render the enzyme inactive almost completely abort signaling through TCR.

CD28 and CTLA-4

CD28, also named Tp44, is typically found as an 80-90 kDa homodimer expressed constitutively on 80-95% of all CD4$^+$ T cells and approximately 50% of all CD8$^+$ T cells; occasionally it may exist in a monomeric form [22,23]. CD28 is expressed on both resting and activated T cells, but its expression is modestly upregulated on activated T cells.

CD28 is critical for T cell activation [24-26]. For example, mice lacking CD28 because of targeted gene disruption show significant immune system defects consistent with defective T cell function [24-28]. Furthermore, TCR-induced cytokine production and cell proliferation are markedly reduced in the absence of CD28 ligation [29-32]. Because of its role in regulating T cell activation, CD28 has been implicated in playing important roles in the immune response to tumors [33-35], in controlling TCR-induced cell death through apoptosis [36-38], and in the process of allograft rejection [39,40]. In addition to providing signals required for optimal activation of T cells, CD28-initiated signals appear to also prevent the state of unresponsiveness (anergy) that develops in T cells stimulated through TCR in the absence of CD28 ligation [41-44]. This characteristic of T cell activation is of particular interest for studies aimed at designing strategies to prolong allograft survival [40]. Interestingly, in some T cell clones, unresponsiveness or anergy can be reversed by CD28 ligation, an event of potential importance in the generation of cytolytic responses against tumors [34,35].

An analogue to CD28 is CTLA-4, also known as CD152 or Ly-56. CTLA-4 is ~70 kDa homodimer glycoprotein, which is structurally similar to CD28 and found in both homodimeric and monomeric forms. Unlike CD28, however, CTLA-4 is only expressed on activated T cells, with maximal expression found approximately 48 hours after T cell stimulation. Also in contrast to CD28, ligation of CTLA-4 on T cells has been shown to inhibit TCR function [24,26,45-47]. For example, ligation of CTLA-4 has been shown to inhibit TCR/CD28-mediated IL-2 production and to delay cell cycle progression, whereas in vivo blockade of CTLA-4 B7 interaction enhances autoreactive and tumor-specific activity [48-51]. Accordingly, the CTLA-4 knockout mouse exhibits a profound spontaneous autoimmune disease, and at 2-3 weeks of age, the CTLA-4 knockout mouse manifests a massive lymphoproliferative disorder and develops an apparent autoimmune myocarditis and pancreatitis [52]. Treating the CTLA-4 knockout mouse with CTLA-4-Ig, a fusion protein synthesized by fusing the extracellular CTLA-4 domain to the constant region of IgG, prevents the lymphoproliferation and the fatal multiorgan tissue damage.

Both CD28 and CTLA-4 specifically bind to counterparts found on APCs known as B7-1 and B7-2. Both B7 proteins are typical Ig superfamily members with extracellular Ig V- and C-like domains. B7-1, also known as CD80, is expressed on stimulated B cells, macrophages, dendritic cells, Langerhans' cells and fibroblasts. B7-2, or CD86, is expressed on stimulated B cells, macrophages, dendritic cells, Langerhans' cells, and granulocytes. B7-2 expression on activated APCs is typically induced more rapidly and to higher concentrations than is B7-1 expression. Although both CD28 and CTLA-4 bind specifically to both B7-1 and B7-2, CTLA-4 binds B7 approximately 100 times more avidly than CD28, and B7-1 binds both CD28 and CTLA-4 approximately 2 to 3 times more avidly than B7-2.

As with TCR signaling, CD28 signal transduction pathways also involve protein tyrosine phosphorylations that are critical for CD28 function (Figure 2). Thus, CD28 ligation induces the tyrosine phosphorylation of several proteins, including the cytoplasmic region of CD28 [53-64]. Although CD28 lacks a consensus binding site for the SH2 domains of Src kinases (YXX(I/L)) [65], studies have implicated the Src family PTKs Lck and Fyn in the tyrosine phosphorylation of CD28 [53,57]. Tyrosine phosphorylated CD28 associates with several SH2-containing proteins including phosphatidylinositol 3-kinase (PI 3-kinase), Itk (a member of the Tec family), and growth factor receptor-bound protein 2 (Grb2) [53,54,62,63,66-77]. CD28-Grb2 association may link CD28 signaling pathways to the small GTPase Ras [7,78]. The activation of PI 3-kinase after CD28 ligation could link CD28 signaling pathways to Akt/protein kinase B, p70 S6 kinase, Ras, PKC, and the Rho family GTPases. The involvement of Rho family GTPases in CD28 signal transduction pathways is further supported by recent studies in which CD28

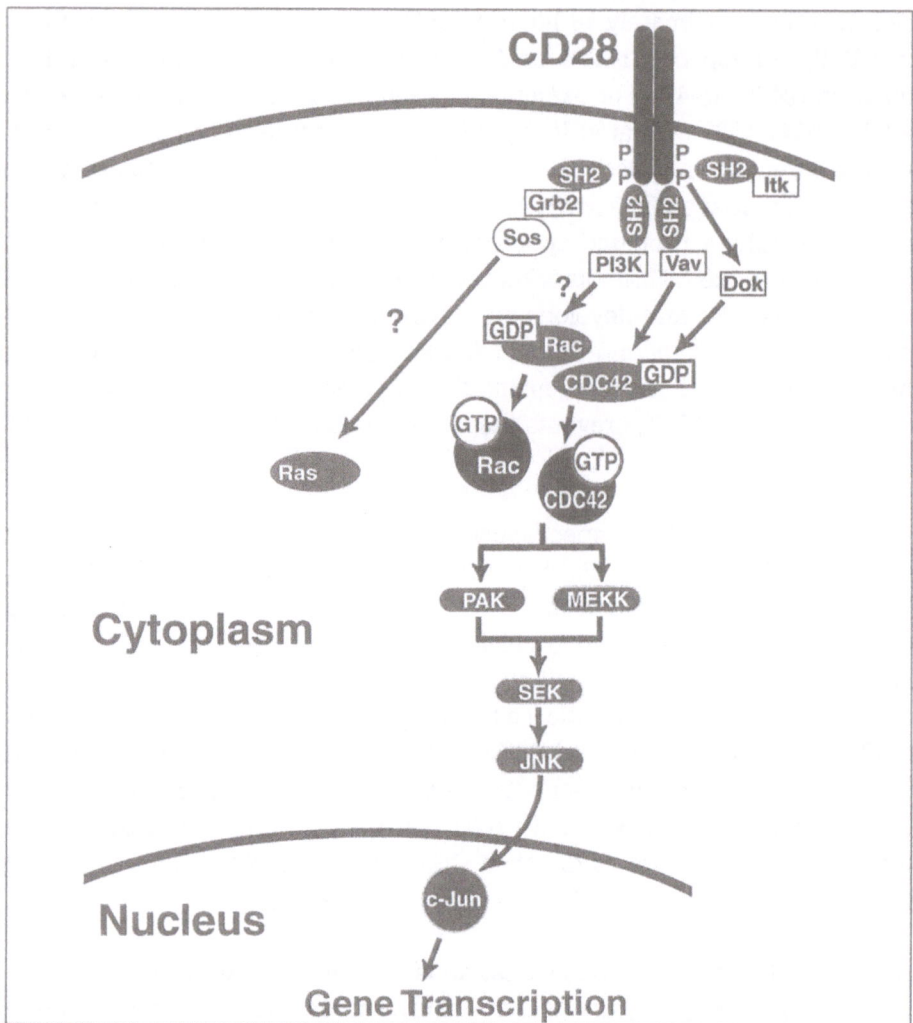

Figure 2
Scheme of some of the CD28-induced signals. CD28 ligation leads to the phosphorylation of tyrosine residues in the cytoplasmic domain of CD28, presumably by Lck and Fyn. Proteins including Grb2-Sos, PI 3-kinase, Vav, and Dok associate through their SH2 domains with tyrosine phosphorylated CD28. Itk is constitutively associated through its SH3 domain with CD28. Grb2-Sos may link CD28 to the Ras signaling cascade. Tyrosine phosphorylated Vav associated with phosphorylated CD28 may link CD28 to the Rho family GTPases Rac and Cdc42 signaling cascade. PI 3-kinase and Dok are upstream of Rho and may link CD28 to Rho pathways. Pyk2 tyrosine phosphorylation and activation after CD28 ligation could function upstream of Rho GTPases and in turn link CD28 to Rho signaling pathways. Activated Rho GTPases stimulate the JNK signaling cascade leading to the phosphorylation and activation of the transcription factor c-Jun.

ligation was shown to induce tyrosine phosphorylation and activation of Vav, a guanine nucleotide exchange factor (GNF) for Rho family GTPases [54,59,69,78], and to promote the formation of focal adhesion-like sites where these GTPases accumulate [79]. Rho family GTPases are implicated in regulating the activation of the c-Jun NH2-terminal kinase (JNK; also known as stress activated protein kinase (SAPK)) [7,80,81]. Accordingly, CD28-initiated signals have been reported to regulate JNK activation in T cells [82-84].

However, despite the apparent similarity between TCR and CD28 signaling pathways, recent studies suggest that some of CD28-triggered signaling pathways are distinct from those of TCR. For example, IL-2 production induced by the TCR in conjunction with phorbol 12-myristate 13-acetate (PMA) is almost completely inhibited by CsA and FK506, drugs that inhibit the Ca^{2+}-dependent Ser/Thr phosphatase calcineurin; yet, these drugs have no effect on the production of IL-2 by the ligation of CD28 in conjunction with PMA [85,86]. Accordingly, CsA only partially inhibits IL-2 production induced by the coligation of CD28 and TCR [85,87]. Thus, T cell activation appears to involve a bipartite signal transduction mechanism with calcineurin-dependent and calcineurin-independent components. These data, together with the fact that CD28 but not TCR induces the tyrosine phosphorylation of the adapter protein Dok [56,59,61], support the notion that some of the intracellular signals initiated after CD28 ligation are different from those triggered by TCR ligation. Yet, current models assume that CD28 and TCR signal transduction pathways are integrated on the level of the protein kinases that are involved in JNK signaling cascade, since these kinases require both TCR and CD28 signals for full activation [82-84]. Activated JNK phosphorylates c-Jun, resulting in the activation of c-Jun's transcriptional activity.

The molecular mechanisms initiated after CTLA-4 are not as clear as those initiated after TCR or CD28 ligation. Recent transfection in vitro studies have shown that CTLA-4 can become tyrosine phosphorylated by the Src family PTKs Lck and Fyn [88,89]. Notably, the cytoplasmic tail of CTLA-4 has been shown to associate in a tyrosine phosphorylation-independent manner with the clathrin-associated adaptor complex AP-2, a process that is critical for the internalization and the expression of CTLA-4 [90-93]. Importantly, CTLA-4 has been shown to associate with the CD3 complex of TCR, a process that appears to be enhanced by the activation of Lck by yet unknown mechanisms [94]. CTLA-4 also associates with the tyrosine phosphatase SHP-2, a molecule critical for the regulation of TCR signaling and T cell activation [94,95]. Thus, it is proposed that the ligation of TCR and the subsequent activation of Lck lead to association of CTLA-4 with the CD3 complex of TCR, and in turn, to the recruitment of the CTLA-4-associated SHP-2 to the TCR complex. Once in close proximity to the TCR complex, SHP-2 promotes CD3 dephosphorylation either directly or indirectly by regulating Lck activity. The dephosphorylation of CD3 and/or Lck will terminate signaling through TCR and in turn aborts T cell activation. Accordingly, CTLA-4 has been shown to attenuate the activity of ERK, JNK, AP-1, NF-AT, and NF-κB in activated T cells [96,97]. Furthermore, T cells from CTLA-4 knockout mouse exhibit hyperphosphorylation of the CD3ζ chain as well as increased activity of the TCR-associated PTKs Fyn, Lck, and ZAP-70 [95]. Notably, CTLA-4 has also been shown to block CD28-induced activation of ERK, JNK, NF-κB, and AP-1 in T cells [96,98,99].

CD154

CD154, also known as CD40 ligand, Ly-62, or gp39, was initially studied in regard to its ability to serve as a second costimulatory signal on helper T cells in B cell activation [100-102]. CD154 is a 36 kDa glycoprotein, a member of the tumor necrosis factor superfamily, and is found mainly on activated helper T cells, mast cells, eosinophils, dendritic cells, endothelial cells and platelets. A soluble variant of CD154 (thought to result from post-translational modification) has also been identified, although its role is unclear. The receptor for CD154 is CD40, which is ~50 kDa glycoprotein that is structurally analogous to tumor necrosis factor-receptor. CD40 has been localized to B cells and to other APCs like monocytes and dendritic cells, as well as on epithelial and endothelial cells.

CD154:CD40 interaction is important for the development of thymus-dependent humoral immunity, as CD154-CD40 interaction is essential for proliferation, differentiation, isotype switching and survival of B cells in germinal centers [103]. Accordingly, mutations in CD154 result in the X-linked hyper-IgM syndrome, an immunodeficiency characterized by elevated IgM levels and inefficient isotype switching due to impaired B cell stimulation [104]. Interestingly, CD154:CD40 interaction has recently been shown to be important for mediating T cell help for cytotoxic T cells. For example, blockade of CD154 inhibits cytotoxic T cell priming [105]. Moreover, the impaired cytotoxic T cell response in mice depleted of CD4+ T helper cells was restored by a single injection of an anti-CD40 activating antibody. Recent studies also suggest that CD154 engagement activates T cells [106]. For example, the defect in the maturation of germinal centers in the CD154 knockout mouse can be corrected by injection of CD40-Fc proteins. Furthermore, ligating CD154 with monoclonal antibodies (mAb) has been shown to induce the tyrosine phosphorylation of several proteins in T cells [107]. However, it is not clear whether CD154-triggered signals contribute to or modulate the signaling pathways of TCR.

Importantly, the CD154:CD40 system appears to interact closely with the CD28:B7 system to facilitate T cell activation. For example, the activation of T cells increases the expression of CD154 on T cells. As a result, the enhanced CD154-CD40 interaction increases the expression of B7 molecules on APC which in turn engage more CD28 on T cells. This positive feedback augments TCR signaling leading to enhanced proliferation and cytokine release.

CD45

CD45, also termed T-200, Ly-5, or leukocyte common antigen (LCA), is a family of cell surface tyrosine phosphatases that range in size from 180 to 240 kDa [108,109]. These membrane glycoproteins are synthesized as the variable exon splicing products of a single gene. CD45 is found on both immature and mature T cells, B cells, mononuclear phagocytes and polymorphonuclear leukocytes. Considerable experimental evidence suggests that surface expression of this molecule is critical for normal signaling events to occur in T and B cells [108,109]. For example, expression of CD45 is essential for the TCR to couple with the phosphatidylinositol second messenger pathway and for TCR-mediated proliferation of T lymphocytes [110]. Furthermore, CD45 has been shown to be capable of reversing the phosphorylation of CD3ζ [111] and of multiple tyrosine residues of Lck in vitro, a tyrosine kinase critical for initiating TCR signaling [112,113]. Moreover, CD45 appears to also modulate early signaling events in B cell receptor signal transduction pathways, including PLCγ phosphorylation, which regulates phosphoinositide hydrolysis and the calcium mobilization response [114].

CD2

CD2, also named LFA-2, LFA-3 ligand, and Ly-37, is a ~50 kDa glycoprotein found specifically on most mature and immature T cells as well as most natural killer (NK) cells [115,116]. On immature T cells, it is expressed on cell surfaces before TCR:CD3 complexes are seen. It is structurally comprised of two Ig-like extracellular domains, a transmembrane region, and a 116 amino acid intracytoplasmic tail. Its specific counterpart is CD58, or LFA-3, which is ~70 kDa glycoprotein localized to a spectrum of hematopoietic and nonhematopoietic cells as well as endothelial cells. In vitro, ligation of CD2 alone by monoclonal antibodies appears to induce T cells to synthesize and release cytokines and undergo cell proliferation [117]. For this reason, it has been hypothesized that CD2 binding may represent an alternative pathway to T cell activation independent of TCR:Ag/MHC interaction. The presence of CD2 early in the development of T cells may imply a role for CD2 in stimulating immature T cell proliferation [118]. Recently, CD2 has been shown to associate with the Src family Fyn and to induce the transcriptional activity of NF-AT [117].

LFA-1 (CD11a/CD18)

LFA-1 (lymphocyte function-associated antigen 1) is an integrin family-type membrane protein found on nearly all hematopoietic cells [119]. LFA-1 facilitates cell-cell adhesion by binding its ligand ICAM (intercellular adhesion molecule), a surface molecule found on T cell surfaces, as well as a broad array of both hematopoietic and nonhematopoietic cell types and endothelial cells [120]. LFA-1:ICAM interaction is thought to mediate lymphocyte functions that depend on intercellular adhesion, such as CTL-mediated cytolysis, helper T cell stimulation, and transendothelial migration. Activation of LFA-1 is a prerequisite for ligand binding. Circulating lymphocytes generally express an inactive (low avidity) form of LFA-1 [121]; this is crucial to maintain homeostasis, since constitutively active LFA-1 would cause instantaneous aggregation of circulating cells and clogging of the vessels. Several stimuli, including TCR, have been shown to induce intracellular signals that transiently activate and in turn increase the avidity of LFA-1:ICAM interaction [121,122]. This upregulation in avidity is thought to result from conformational changes which take place in the extracellular portion of LFA-1 as a result of the phosphorylation of intracytoplasmic amino acid residues (the so-called inside-out signaling process) by signals initiated by stimuli such as the TCR. In addition to simply enhancing cell:cell interaction, LFA-1 is capable of mediating a true costimulatory signal, as manifested by an increase in protein tyrosine phosphorylation upon LFA engagement [123,124] and by the ability of soluble ICAM to enhance T cell activation in vitro [125].

Interestingly, recent studies in LFA-1 and CD28 knockout mice suggest that LFA-1 and CD28 exhibit distinct, nonoverlaping mechanisms to modulate T cell activation [126]. Thus, CD28 ligation lowered the number of TCR that had to be aggregated to activate T cells and also permitted the activation of

T cells by low affinity ligands. LFA-1, on the other hand, facilitated TCR signaling by lowering the amount of antigen required for T cell ligation. Thus, in the absence of LFA-1, 100-fold more Ag was required for T cell-APC conjugation and for the subsequent T cell activation. Thus, CD28 appears to modulate TCR-induced T cell activation by providing additional distinct signals that modulate TCR signaling. In contrast, LFA-1 appears to facilitate the generation of TCR signaling, and in turn TCR-mediated activation by promoting T cell-APC adhesion. Notably, in these studies CD28 but not LFA-1 prevented induction of T cell anergy after TCR stimulation.

Additional evidence for distinct roles for LFA-1 and CD28 in T cell costimulation is shown by in vitro studies in which B7 and ICAM-1 differently regulated the negative selection of thymocytes [127]. Thus, negative selection was augmented by B7, but was inhibited by ICAM-1 activation.

CD44

CD44, also known as Pgp-1 or Ly-24, is a family of cell surface adhesion molecules found on the cell surfaces of a broad spectrum of hematopoietic cells. CD44 proteins demonstrate a high affinity for extracellular matrix structures, including hyaluronic acid, fibronectin, laminin, and collagen [128]. The multiple glycoprotein isoforms (75-250 kDa) are encoded by a single gene by alternative splicing and are further modified by a range of post-translational modifications. CD44 proteins are single chain molecules comprising an N-terminal extracellular domain, a membrane proximal region, a transmembrane domain, and a cytoplasmic tail. CD44 is thought to be involved in a variety of lymphocyte functions, including lymphopoiesis, lymphocyte homing and cell migration [129,130]. Interestingly, TCR ligation has been shown to increase CD44 binding to its ligand, an event that may be critical for T cell extravasation at inflammatory sites [130].

COSTIMULATORY MOLECULE BLOCKADE

Numerous studies have examined the usefulness of blocking the interactions between costimulatory molecules and their ligands on graft survival. mAb are the tool of choice to study the effect of the costimulation blockade on allograft survival. However, caution should be taken when interpreting data obtained with mAb, for in addition to blocking the interaction between the molecules, mAb also may crosslink their targets. Because most of the costimulatory molecules and their ligands associate with enzymes such as PTKs and phosphatases, crosslinking these enzymes may elicit signals that could modulate the cellular response to TCR engagement by the Ag. Furthermore, because many of the costimulatory molecules on T cells and their ligands are also present on cells other than T cells, the effect of crosslinking the molecules on other cells should also be taken into consideration when interpreting the data with mAb. As described below, soluble costimulatory molecules and their ligands have also been used to determine the effect of costimulation blockade on allograft survival.

CD4 blockade

A good deal of success has been achieved in the delaying of graft rejection in numerous animal models after administration of anti-CD4 mAb. Skin, cardiac, renal and pancreatic islet allograft models in mice, rats and nonhuman primates have all been applied to the study of anti-CD4 mAb, often with the resultant induction of what appeared to be at least transient donor graft-specific tolerance [131]. Admittedly, some of the success of anti-CD4 mAb-based therapy has been a result of significant pre-transplantation depletion of CD4+ T cells. However, it has become clear that non-depleting forms of anti-CD4 mAb are in fact capable of inducing donor-specific tolerance, supporting the role of true costimulatory signal blockade [132]. Interestingly, much of the success in CD4 blockade has required pre-transplantation administration of mAb [133]. Thus, it appears that in order to prolong allograft acceptance, CD4 blockade must take place prior to the initiation of the TCR:Ag/MHC complex. Because CD4 interaction with the antigen/MHC complex normally occurs only on T cells being actively exposed to antigen and not upon resting T cells, the resting state before exposure to alloantigen provides a window of opportunity to thoroughly prevent future interaction of CD4 to MHC. Attempts to administer anti-CD4 mAb as single agent therapy at or after the time of transplantation typically confer only marginal benefit to the recipient. The significance of CD4-directed costimulatory blockade preventing natural CD4:MHC interaction is further strengthened by the observation that allograft survival is prolonged when anti-MHC II mAb is coadministered with anti-CD4 mAb [134].

Success has also been met with the coadministration of anti-CD4 mAb with smaller amounts of donor alloantigen in the form of donor-specific transfusions in the pre-transplantation period [135]. It has been suggested that pretreatment with non-depleting anti-CD4 mAb with donor specific transfusions promotes the development and expansion of a population of regulatory cells, which may maintain donor-specific tolerance after introduction of the allograft. This hypothesis is strengthened by the observation that anti-CD4 mAb-induced tolerance may be adoptively transferred to naïve hosts by the transfer of spleen cells collected from mAb-treated animals. Specifically, mice demonstrate indefinite cardiac allograft acceptance after receiving pre-transplant donor-specific transfusion and anti-CD4 mAb. By transferring spleen cells from these tolerant recipients to naïve secondary recipients, these secondary recipients will subsequently accept the same donor car-diac allografts without any additional immunosuppressive therapy. This transfer of donor-specific graft acceptance can even be transferred from primary recipients who receive the pretreatment protocol of donor-specific transfusion and anti-CD4 mAb alone, without subsequent cardiac allotrans-plantation [136]. Also in agreement with the hypothetical presence of such regulatory cells is the observation that, within some tolerized rat cardiac allografts, an exuberant infiltration of inflammatory cells can be observed without any evidence of consequent graft injury [137]. Presumably, the recip-ient remains capable of mounting an immune response against alloanti-gens, but the potentially injurious results of this response are held in check. Attempts to characterize this presumed immunoregulatory subpopulation of cells as the IL-4 and IL-10-dependent TH2 cell have not been consistently borne out [138].

Although apparently successful in preventing acute rejection in many animal models of allotransplantation, the potential of CD4 blockade in preventing chronic rejection is not at all clear. Histologic examination of some long-term cardiac allografts in mice which have received anti-CD4 mAb therapy dem-onstrates the presence of a fairly continuous process of gradual inflamma-tory infiltration, microvascular endothelial activation and graft remodeling suggestive of both acute and chronic graft rejection [139]. Nevertheless, the success of CD4-directed costimulatory blockade has prompted the initia-tion of human clinical studies. A murine anti-human anti-CD4 mAb, OKT4A, has been employed in a clinical trial pilot study as an adjunct to a standard immunosuppressive regimen of cyclosporine, prednisone and azathioprine in cadaveric renal transplant recipients. Of note, as would be expected with the unpredictability of cadaveric renal transplantation, OKT4A could not be administered in the pretransplant setting. OKT4A has been shown to be a non-depleting mAb which appears to be well-tolerated by recipients. Although preliminary graft survival results do appear to show an improve-ment in 2 year graft survival of 95% compared to 83% in control patients, OKT4A recipients have certainly not been free of episodic acute rejection, as a three-month acute rejection rate of 37% was noted. The likely role of a gradual neutralization or enervation effect caused by the development of a human anti-mouse antibody reaction measured in 84% of patients has not been characterized [178].

CD28/B7 blockade

Perhaps the most extensive work in the field of costimulatory blockade has been applied to the CD28:B7 interaction. Much of this work has employed CTLA-4-Ig. Like native CTLA-4, CTLA-4-Ig binds B7 molecules with a much higher avidity than does CD28, thereby providing an effective mechanism of blocking the critical positive costimulatory signals induced by CD28:B7 interaction.

In numerous rat and mouse skin, cardiac, renal, hepatic and pancreatic allograft models, administration of CTLA-4-Ig to graft recipients has demonstrated impressive prolongation of graft survival, and even the occasional induction of tolerance [131]. More recently, use of CTLA-4-Ig in nonhuman primates has demonstrated significant prolongation of renal and pancreatic islet allograft survival [140-142]. Incomplete blockade of B7, as illustrated by the use of a CTLA-4-Ig mutant which binds B7-1 but not B7-2, is ineffective in mediating graft acceptance [143]. Interestingly, unlike CD4 blockade, the efficacy of CTLA-4-Ig appears to be highest when administered after transplantation [144]. It is very possible that activated T cells are simply more susceptible to the blockade of costimulation than are resting T cells. Furthermore, it is not until the T cell is activated that endogenous cell surface CTLA-4 is expressed; therefore, delayed administration of CTLA-4-Ig probably permits some endogenous CTLA-4:B7 interaction to take place first, which can then transduce its own intracellular downregulatory signals [145]. The importance of endogenous CTLA-4:B7 interaction in the induction of tolerance is further illustrated by the general inability of B7 blockade alone by anti-B7 mAb to facilitate long-term allograft acceptance [146], although this observation has recently been confused by the demonstration of some long-term allograft acceptance with anti-B7-2 mAb alone [147]. Although unilateral blockade of B7 would prevent the costimulatory signal transduced via CD28 ligation, B7 blockade would theoretically also prevent any stimulation of native CTLA-4, thus blocking its inhibitory effect of T cell activation. In fact, early administration of CTLA-4-Ig in rat pancreatic islet allograft studies appears to inhibit the efficacy of other tolerance-inducing regimens which may be in part dependent upon CTLA-4:B7-induced downregulation [146]. This concept is supported by the ability of anti-CTLA-4 mAb pre-treatment to prevent any induction of allograft tolerance by standard CD28:B7 interaction blockade [147]. These phenomena suggest that selective blockade of CD28, which would prevent the pro-stimulatory CD28:B7 interaction while permitting the pro-inhibitory CTLA-4:B7 interaction, could provide successful allograft acceptance. Indeed, rat cardiac allotransplantation using anti-CD28 mAb can significantly prolong allograft survival, although without promoting true graft tolerance [148].

As opposed to the anti-CD4 mAb data discussed earlier, appropriately administered CTLA-4-Ig has also been shown to be effective in the prevention of some models of chronic rejection. CTLA-4-Ig administered two days following cardiac allotransplantation in rats not only produces significant prolongation of graft survival, but histologic examination of explanted cardiac allografts from long-term survivors demonstrates significantly less arteriosclerosis than that seen in allografts from cyclosporine-treated recipients [149]. This possible protective effect of CTLA-4-Ig against changes suggestive of chronic rejection appears to be abrogated by the coadministration of cyclosporine; long-term cardiac rat allografts explanted from rats receiving both CTLA-4-Ig and traditional cyclosporine exhibited an accelerated coronary arteriosclerosis not seen in rats having received only CTLA-4-Ig [150]. Perhaps even more striking has been the ability of CTLA-4-Ig administered after the onset of acute graft rejection to prevent chronic rejection. Rats undergoing renal allotransplantation treated with a short course of post-transplantation cyclosporine inevitably developed changes suggestive of acute rejection; those rats who received a dose of CTLA-4-Ig 8 weeks after transplantation subsequently avoided the progressive proteinuria and histologic inflammatory infiltration, glomerulosclerosis and vascular hyperplasia which non-CTLA-4-Ig-treated subjects all developed [150].

CD154/CD40 blockade

Blockade of the CD154:CD40 interaction has received close attention in the pursuit of tolerance induction. mAb directed against CD154 has effectively prolonged cardiac and pancreatic islet allograft survival in mice [151,152]. Of note, prolongation of allograft survival was only seen when anti-CD154 therapy was initiated at the time of transplantation; therapy initiated on post-transplant day five was unable to appreciably prolong graft acceptance [151]. In large animals, anti-CD154 mAb has produced remarkable prolongation of rejection-free survival of nonhuman primate renal and cardiac allografts [153]. Just as extraordinary has been the ability of anti-CD154 mAb "rescue therapy" retreatment to reverse episodes of acute renal allograft rejection in monkeys who demonstrated clinical and histologic evidence of acute rejection months after initial anti-CD154 administration [140,141]; this would suggest the importance of the CD154:CD40 interaction not only in the prevention of acute allograft rejection, but also in its maintenance.

Interaction of CD154:CD40 induces upregulation of B7 expression on APC membranes [154]. Because of this interaction between the CD28:B7 and CD154:CD40 costimulatory pathways, studies have examined the efficacy of coadministration of CTLA-4-Ig with anti-CD154 mAb. Studies involving the rat pancreatic islet allotransplantation model have suggested that the ability of anti-CD154 mAb to induce long-term graft acceptance is dependent upon the CD154:CD40 interaction with CTLA4:B7. Whereas rats treated prior to transplantation with anti-CD154 mAb combined with donor specific transfusion demonstrate long-term tolerance to islet allografts, B7 blockade by co-administration with CTLA-4-Ig eliminates any development of tolerance [146]. It has therefore been hypothesized that, at least in this model, blockade of the CD154-mediated costimulatory signal is necessary but insufficient without the negative signal mediated by CTLA4:B7 interaction upon the T cell. Interestingly, however, in the mouse model, coadministration of anti-CTLA-4 mAb does not appear to hinder the ability of anti-CD154 mAb to induce the induction of allograft tolerance [147].

The possible interrelationship between the CD28:B7 and CD154:CD40 costimulatory systems is highlighted by observations in the murine cardiac allotransplantation model which demonstrate a potential synergy between CD28:B7 and CD154:CD40 blockade. Mice undergoing blockade of either system alone showed no significant prolongation of allograft survival; however, co-blockade of both produced not only long-term survival, but prevention of coronary arteriosclerotic changes suggestive of chronic allograft rejection [155]. Similarly, treatment of mice undergoing aortic allotransplantation with both CTLA-4-Ig and anti-CD154 mAb demonstrated significantly less post-transplant arteriopathy than did mice receiving either agent alone [156]. In nonhuman primates, however, CTLA-4-Ig does not appear to add any significant prolongation in renal allograft survival to that which is routinely achieved after administration of anti-CD154 mAb alone [140,141].

CD45 blockade

In the murine model, blockade of CD45 has been shown to reproducibly induce allograft tolerance. Thus, perioperatively administered anti-CD45 mAb produced indefinite survival of both pancreatic islet and renal allograft [157,158]. Even when given after the onset of acute rejection in previously untreated mice, anti-CD45 mAb was effective in reversing acute rejection of renal allograft [157]. Furthermore, experience with CD45 blockade provides additional support for the immunoregulatory model of the maintenance of tolerance. Histologic examination of long-surviving pancreatic islet allografts in mice treated with anti-CD45 mAb demonstrates the presence of a marked, prolonged peri-islet inflammatory infiltration which is similar to that observed in non-treated controls. However, unlike control recipients, anti-CD45 mAb-treated allografts did not demonstrate any signs of insulitis or disruption of islet integrity, again suggesting the presence of an immunoregulatory influence of the alloantigen-directed immune response [158]. In addition, spleen cells from anti-CD45 mAb-tolerized mice can adoptively transfer tolerance to naïve recipients [159]. It has also been shown that treatment with anti-CD45 mAb is associated with an increase in intragraft expression of IL-4 and IL-10, suggesting the promotion of immunoregulatory TH2 cells [158].

CD2 blockade

In a similar fashion, costimulatory blockade directed against CD2 has successfully induced tolerance in some small animal models. Anti-CD2 mAb has induced prolonged survival of cardiac and pancreatic islet allografts in mice [160-161]. This survival benefit is prolonged in a synergistic fashion when anti-CD2 treatment is combined with CD28 blockade using CTLA-4-Ig, to a point where reproducible tolerance may be achieved [162]. Tolerance has also been produced in a rat cardiac allotransplantation model [163]. Of note, in the latter study, analysis of mRNA transcripts in the allografts of tolerant rats has shown the specific induction of cytokines compatible with both TH1 and TH2 cell populations. When transferred to nonhuman primate studies, administration of anti-CD2 mAb in baboon cardiac allotransplantation studies confers a significant but only temporary prolongation of allograft survival from 10.6 days in controls to 18.0 days in treated recipients, albeit with significantly less endothelialitis observed in the allografts of treated baboons [164].

A rat anti-CD2 mAb named BTI-322 was synthesized and utilized in small clinical trials in Belgium. In a brief prospective randomized series, 20 patients undergoing cadaveric renal transplantation with a standard immunosuppressive regimen of cyclosporine, azathioprine and predisone were compared to 20 patients receiving the same regimen plus BTI-322 for a ten day course of treatment. Data compiled after nine months exhibited a significant decrease in the number of acute rejection episodes observed (25% in BTI-322-treated subjects vs. 60% in controls) [165]. The same group also administered BTI-322 to patients experiencing either first or refractory acute rejection. They reported clinical "complete responses" in 64% and clinical "partial responses" in 27.3%; histologically, they recorded "complete responses" in 54% and "partial responses" in 36% [166].

LFA-1 blockade

Studies in LFA-1:ICAM blockade have been motivated by the central role these adhesion molecules appear to play in cell:cell interaction. As described earlier, LFA-1:ICAM-1 interactions have been shown to facilitate TCR-mediated T cell activation in vitro and in vivo. However, the role of LFA-1 in providing costimulatory signals to T cells remains controversial. Thus, it is not clear whether LFA-1:ICAM-1 interactions are mediating their effect on T cell activation entirely through adhesion or through a combination of adhesion and costimulation. In vitro studies have shown that although engagement of LFA-1 can provide sufficient costimulatory signals to induce T cell activation and IL-2 gene expression, it cannot protect against anergy induction or provide for T cell survival [167]. This is in contrast to CD28, which has been shown to effectively protect against anergy induction.

In murine heart allotransplantation models, co-administration of anti-LFA-1 and anti-ICAM-1 mAb appears to mediate the induction of tolerance [168,169]. Attempts to reproduce true tolerance with these antibodies in rat cardiac allotransplantation models have been unsuccessful [170]. Some significant but temporary prolongation of cardiac allograft survival has been achieved in rat models with LFA-1 blockade, and this survival time is lengthened when both LFA-1 and ICAM-1 are blocked with mAb [171]. In the mouse model, tolerance could also be induced in some recipients who did not receive LFA-1 and ICAM-1 blockade until post-transplant days four and five [172]. Inspection of gene expression within tolerated cardiac allografts in the murine models has confirmed the selective expression of TH2-type cytokines (IL-4 and IL-10) with concomitant downregulation of TH1-type cytokines (IL-2) [173], an effect not seen in untreated or FK506-treated mice [168]. Furthermore, induction of this experimental tolerance was prevented by administration of exogenous IL-2 [168], which is compatible with the possibility that TH2-mediated immunoregulation is involved in anti-LFA-1 and anti-ICAM-1 mAb-induced tolerance. In a French clinical trial, anti-LFA-1 mAb was compared to rabbit antithymocyte globulin (ATG) among human recipients of primary renal transplantations. Although anti-LFA-1 mAb was better tolerated by patients than was the rabbit ATG, there were no significant clinical advantages to its administration with regard to incidence of acute rejection episodes or frequency of infectious complications [174].

CD44 blockade

Comparatively less work has been directed at the blockade of CD44. It has been shown that CD44-expressing T cells are found in higher concentrations in rejecting small bowel allografts [175]. Similarly, CD44 expression localizes specifically to the portal areas of rejecting rat liver allografts, where lymphocyte infiltration typically tends to concentrate [176]. These data suggest a role of CD44 in the induction or maintenance of allograft rejection. The first experimental evidence confirming this finding has emerged from rat cardiac allotransplantation studies demonstrating that recipients treated with both cyclosporine and soluble hyaluronate (a major binding target which could potentially saturate and block CD44) show both longer graft survival clinically and milder lymphocyte infiltration and architectural changes histologically than recipients treated with cyclosporine alone. The possible role of CD44 in chronic rejection was raised by the observation that the addition of hyaluronate treatment also significantly lessened the extent of graft arteriosclerosis observed in this study [177].

CONCLUSIONS

Recent progress in the field of transplantation immunology has revealed significant insights into the cellular and molecular mechanisms of T cell activation. In particular, the identification of several surface costimulatory molecules critical for TCR function has revolutionized the design of therapeutic regimens to control the natural immune response of the transplant recipient to the allograft. Numerous in vitro and in vivo analyses have demonstrated the potential usefulness of intentionally blocking these necessary costimulatory signals for prolonging allograft survival and, in some cases, for inducing immunologic tolerance. Direct application of these experimental manipulations to the clinical setting is premature in many cases, and will require more comprehensive characterization of the molecular and cellular consequences of costimulatory blockade. However, it is becoming evident that costimulatory blockade may likely be one of the most promising therapeutic avenues toward the successful induction of allograft tolerance.

REFERENCES

1. Berridge MJ. Lymphocyte activation in health and disease. Crit Rev Immunol 1997;17:155-178.
2. Clevers H, Alarcon B, Wileman T, Terhorst C. The T cell receptor/CD3 complex: a dynamic protein ensemble. Annu Rev Immunol 1988;6:629-662.
3. Alberolaila J, Takaki S, Kerner JD, Perlmutter RM. Differential signaling by lymphocyte antigen receptors. Ann Rev Immunol 1997;15:125-154.
4. Qian D, Weiss A. T cell antigen receptor signal transduction. Curr Opin Cell Biol 1997;9:205-212.
5. Cantrell D. T cell antigen receptor signal transduction pathways. Ann Rev Immunol 1996;14:259-274.
6. Irving BA, Chan AC, Weiss A. Functional characterization of a signal transducing motif present in the T cell antigen receptor zeta chain. J Exp Med 1993;177:1093-1103.
7. Su B, Karin M. Mitogen-activated protein kinase cascades and regulation of gene expression. Curr Opin Immunol 1996;8:402-411.
8. Schaeffer HJ, Weber MJ. Mitogen-activated protein kinases: Specific messages from ubiquitous messengers. Mol Cell Biol 1999;19:2435-2444.
9. Klee CB, Ren H, Wang XT. Regulation of the calmodulin-stimulated protein phosphatase, calcineurin. J Biol Chem 1998;273:13367-13370.
10. Crabtree GR. Generic signals and specific outcomes: Signaling through Ca2+, calcineurin, and NF-AT. Cell 1999;96:611-614.
11. Crabtree GR. Contingent genetic regulatory events in T lymphocyte activation. Science 1989;243:355-361.
12. Hanissian SH, Frangakis M, Bland MM, Jawahar S, Chatila TA. Expression of a Ca2+/calmodulin-dependent protein kinase, CaM kinase- Gr, in human T lymphocytes. Regulation of kinase activity by T cell receptor signaling. J Biol Chem 1993;268:20055-20063.
13. Park IK, Soderling TR. Activation of Ca2+/calmodulin-dependent protein kinase (CaM-kinase) IV by CaM-kinase kinase in Jurkat T lymphocytes. J Biol Chem 1995;270:30464-30469.
14. Nghiem P, Ollick T, Gardner P, Schulman H. Interleukin-2 transcriptional block by multifunctional Ca2+/calmodulin kinase. Nature 1994;371:347-350.
15. Sun P, Enslen H, Myung PS, Maurer RA. Differential activation of CREB by Ca2+/calmodulin-dependent protein kinases type II and type IV involves phosphorylation of a site that negatively regulates activity. Genes Dev 1994;8:2527-2539.
16. Sugimoto T, Stewart S, Guan KL. The calcium/calmodulin-dependent protein phosphatase calcineurin is the major Elk-1 phosphatase. J Biol Chem 1997;272:29415-29418.
17. Zwilling S, Dieckmann A, Pfisterer P, Angel P, Wirth T. Inducible expression and phosphorylation of coactivator BOB.1/OBF.1 in T cells. Science 1997;277:221-225.
18. Granelli-Piperno A, Nolan P, Inaba K, Steinman RM. The effect of immunosuppressive agents on the induction of nuclear factors that bind to sites on the interleukin 2 promoter. J Exp Med 1990;172:1869-1872.
19. Zamoyska R. CD4 and CD8: modulators of T-cell receptor recognition of antigen and of immune responses? Curr Opin Immunol 1998;10:82-87.
20. Rudd C, Helms S, Barber EK, Schlossman SF. The CD4/CD8:p56lck complex in T lymphocytes: a potential mechanism to regulate T-cell growth. Biochem Cell Biol 1989;67:581-589.
21. Veillette A, Bookman MA, Horak EM, Bolen JB. The CD4 and CD8 T cell surface antigens are associated with the internal membrane tyrosine-protein kinase

p56lck. Cell 1988;55:301-308.

22. Chan PY, Takei F. Molecular cloning and characterization of a novel murine T cell surface antigen, YE1/48. J Immunol 1989;142:1727-1736.

23. Aruffo A, Seed B. Molecular cloning of a CD28 cDNA by a high-efficiency COS cell expression system. Proc Natl Acad Sci USA 1987;84:8573-8577.

24. Boussiotis VA, Freeman GJ, Gribben JG, Nadler LM. The role of B7-1/B7-2:CD28/CLTA-4 pathways in the prevention of anergy, induction of productive immunity and down-regulation of the immune response. Immunol Rev 1996;153:5-26.

25. Sperling AI, Bluestone JA. The complexities of T-cell co-stimulation: CD28 and beyond. Immunol Rev 1996;153:155-182.

26. Chambers CA, Allison JP. Costimulatory regulation of T cell function. Curr Opin Cell Biol 1999;11:203-210.

27. Green JM, Noel PJ, Sperling AI, et al. Absence of B7-dependent responses in CD28-deficient mice. Immunity 1994;1:501-508.

28. Shahinian A, Pfeffer K, Lee KP, et al. Differential T cell costimulatory requirements in CD28-deficient mice. Science 1993;261:609-612.

29. Linsley PS, Ledbetter JA. The role of the CD28 receptor during T cell responses to antigen. Annu Rev Immunol 1993;11:191-212.

30. June CH, Bluestone JA, Nadler LM, Thompson CB. The B7 and CD28 receptor families. Immunol Today 1994;15:321-331.

31. Bluestone, JA. New perspectives of CD28-B7-mediated T cell costimulation. Immunity 1995;2:555-559.

32. Lenschow DJ, Walunas TL, Bluestone JA. CD28/B7 system of T cell costimulation. Ann Rev Immunol 1996;14:233-258.

33. Yu X, Abe R, Hodes RJ. The role of B7-CD28 co-stimulation in tumor rejection. Int Immunol 1998;10:791-797.

34. Townsend SE, Allison JP. Tumor rejection after direct costimulation of CD8+ T cells by B7-transfected melanoma cells. Science 1993;259:368-370.

35. Melero I, Bach N, Chen L. Costimulation, tolerance and ignorance of cytolytic T lymphocytes in immune responses to tumor antigens. Life Sci 1997;60:2035-2041.

36. Boise LH, Minn AJ, Noel PJ, et al. CD28 costimulation can promote T cell survival by enhancing the expression of Bcl-XL. Immunity 1995;3:87-98.

37. Shi Y, Radvanyi LG, Sharma A, et al. CD28-mediated signaling in vivo prevents activation-induced apoptosis in the thymus and alters peripheral lymphocyte homeostasis. J Immunol 1995;155:1829-1837.

38. Boussiotis VA, Lee BJ, Freeman GJ, Gribben JG, Nadler LM. Induction of T cell clonal anergy results in resistance, whereas CD28-mediated costimulation primes for susceptibility to Fas- and Bax-mediated programmed cell death. J Immunol 1997;159:3156-3167.

39. Lu P, Wang YL, Linsley PS. Regulation of self-tolerance by CD80/CD86 interactions. Curr Opin Immunol 1997;9:858-862.

40. Sayegh MH, Turka LA. T cell costimulatory pathways: promising novel targets for immunosuppression and tolerance induction. J Am Soc Nephrol 1995;6:1143-1150.

41. LaSalle JM, Hafler DA. T cell anergy. FASEB J 1994;8:601-608.

42. Schwartz RH. Models of T cell anergy: is there a common molecular mechanism? J Exp Med 1996;184:1-8.

43. Fields P, Fitch FW, Gajewski TF. Control of T lymphocyte signal transduction through clonal anergy. J Mol Med 1996;74:673-683.

44. Powell JD, Ragheb JA, Kitagawa-Sakakida S, Schwartz RH. Molecular regulation of interleukin-2 expression by CD28 co-stimulation and anergy. Immunol Rev 1998;165:287-300.

45. Waterhouse P, Marengere LE, Mittrucker HW, Mak TW. CTLA-4, a negative regulator of T-lymphocyte activation. Immunol Rev 1996;153:183-207.

46. Saito T. Negative regulation of T cell activation. Curr Opin Immunol 1998;10: 313-321.
47. Oosterwegel MA, Greenwald RJ, Mandelbrot DA, Lorsbach RB, Sharpe AH. CTLA-4 and T cell activation. Curr Opin Immunol 1999;11:294-300.
48. Krummel MF, Allison JP. CTLA-4 engagement inhibits IL-2 accumulation and cell cycle progression upon activation of resting T cells. J Exp Med 1996;183: 2533-2540.
49. Walunas TL, Bakker CY, Bluestone JA. CTLA-4 ligation blocks CD28-dependent T cell activation. J Exp Med 1996;183:2541-2550.
50. Leach DR, Krummel MF, Allison JP. Enhancement of antitumor immunity by CTLA-4 blockade. Science 1996;271:1734-1736.
51. Karandikar NJ, Vanderlugt CL, Walunas TL, Miller SD, Bluestone JA. CTLA-4: a negative regulator of autoimmune disease. J Exp Med 1996;184:783-788.
52. Tivol EA, Boyd SD, McKeon S, et al. CTLA4Ig prevents lymphoproliferation and fatal multiorgan tissue destruction in CTLA-4-deficient mice. J Immunol 1997; 158:5091-5094.
53. Raab M, Cai YC, Bunnell SC, Heyeck SD, Berg LJ, Rudd CE. p56Lck and p59Fyn regulate CD28 binding to phosphatidylinositol 3-kinase, growth factor receptor-bound protein GRB-2, and T cell-specific protein-tyrosine kinase ITK: implications for T-cell costimulation. Proc Natl Acad Sci USA 1995;92:8891-8895.
54. August A, Gibson S, Kawakami Y, Kawakami T, Mills GB, Dupont B. CD28 is associated with and induces the immediate tyrosine phosphorylation and activation of the Tec family kinase ITK/EMT in the human Jurkat leukemic T-cell line. Proc Natl Acad Sci USA 1994;91:9347-9351.
55. Lu Y, Granelli-Piperno A, Bjorndahl JM, Phillips CA, Trevillyan JM. CD28-induced T cell activation. Evidence for a protein-tyrosine kinase signal transduction pathway. J Immunol 1992;149:24-29.
56. Vandenberghe P, Freeman GJ, Nadler LM, et al. Antibody and B7/BB1-mediated ligation of the CD28 receptor induces tyrosine phosphorylation in human T cells. J Exp Med 1992;175:951-960.
57. Hutchcroft JE, Bierer BE. Activation-dependent phosphorylation of the T-lymphocyte surface receptor CD28 and associated proteins. Proc Natl Acad Sci USA 1994;91:3260-3264.
58. Ledbetter JA, Linsley PS. CD28 receptor crosslinking induces tyrosine phosphorylation of PLC gamma 1. Adv Exp Med Biol 1992;323:23-27.
59. Klasen S, Pages F, Peyron JF, Cantrell DA, Olive D. Two distinct regions of the CD28 intracytoplasmic domain are involved in the tyrosine phosphorylation of Vav and GTPase activating protein-associated p62 protein. Int Immunol 1998;10: 481-489.
60. August A, Dupont B. Activation of src family kinase lck following CD28 crosslinking in the Jurkat leukemic cell line. Biochem Biophys Res Commun 1994;199: 1466-1473.
61. Nunes JA, Truneh A, Olive D, Cantrell DA. 1996. Signal transduction by CD28 costimulatory receptor on T cells: B71 and B7-1 regulation of tyrosine kinase adaptor molecules. J Biol Chem 1996;271:1591-1598.
62. Pages F, Ragueneau M, Rottapel R, et al. Binding of phosphatidylinositol-3-OH kinase to CD28 is required for T-cell signalling. Nature 1994;369:327-329.
63. August A, Dupont B. CD28 of T lymphocytes associates with phosphatidylinositol 3-kinase. Int Immunol 1994;6:769-774.
64. Tsuchida M, Manthei ER, Knechtle SJ, Hamawy MM. CD28 ligation induces rapid tyrosine phosphorylation of the linker molecule LAT in the absence of Syk and Zap-70 tyrosine phosphorylation. Eur J Immunol 1999;29:2354-2359.
65. Songyang Z, Shoelson SE, Chaudhuri M, et al. SH2 domains recognize specific phosphopeptide sequences. Cell 1993;72:767-778.

66. Cefai D, Cai YC, Hu H, Rudd C. CD28 co-stimulatory regimes differ in their dependence on phosphatidylinositol 3-kinase: common co-signals induced by CD80 and CD86. Int Immunol 1996;8:1609-1616.

67. Pages F, Ragueneau M, Klasen S, et al. Two distinct intracytoplasmic regions of the T-cell adhesion molecule CD28 participate in phosphatidylinositol 3-kinase association. J Biol Chem 1996;271:9403-9409.

68. Schneider H, Cai YC, Prasad KV, Shoelson SE, Rudd CE. T cell antigen CD28 binds to the GRB-2/SOS complex, regulators of p21ras. Eur J Immunol 1995;25: 1044-1050.

69. Kim HH, Tharayil M, Rudd CE. Growth factor receptor-bound protein 2 SH2/SH3 domain binding to CD28 and its role in co-signaling. J Biol Chem 1998;273: 296-301.

70. Teng JM, King PD, Sadra A, et al. Phosphorylation of each of the distal three tyrosines of the CD28 cytoplasmic tail is required for CD28-induced T cell IL-2 secretion. Tissue Antigens 1996;48:255-264.

71. Truitt KE, Nagel T, Suen LF, Imboden JB. Structural requirements for CD28-mediated costimulation of IL-2 production in Jurkat T cells. J Immunol 1996;156: 4539-4541.

72. Truitt KE, Shi J, Gibson S, Segal LG, Mills GB, Imboden JB. CD28 delivers costimulatory signals independently of its association with phosphatidylinositol 3-kinase. J Immunol 1995;155:4702-4710.

73. Cefai D, Schneider H, Matangkasombut O, Kang H, Brody J, Rudd CE. CD28 receptor endocytosis is targeted by mutations that disrupt phosphatidylinositol 3-kinase binding and costimulation. J Immunol 1998;160:2223-2230.

74. King PD, Sadra A, Teng JM, et al. Analysis of CD28 cytoplasmic tail tyrosine residues as regulators and substrates for the protein tyrosine kinases, EMT and LCK. J Immunol 1997;158:580-590.

75. Gibson S, Truitt K, Lu Y, et al. Efficient CD28 signalling leads to increases in the kinase activities of the TEC family tyrosine kinase EMT/ITK/TSK and the SRC family tyrosine kinase LCK. Biochem J 1998;330:1123-1128.

76. Marengere LE, Okkenhaug K, Clavreul A, et al. The SH3 domain of Itk/Emt binds to proline-rich sequences in the cytoplasmic domain of the T cell costimulatory receptor CD28. J Immunol 1997;159:3220-3229.

77. Okkenhaug K, Rottapel R. Grb2 forms an inducible protein complex with CD28 through a Src homology 3 domain-proline interaction. J Biol Chem 1998;273: 21194-21202.

78. Nunes JA, Collette Y, Truneh A, Olive D, Cantrell DA. The role of p21ras in CD28 signal transduction: triggering of CD28 with antibodies, but not the ligand B7-1, activates p21ras. J Exp Med 1994;180:1067-1076.

79. Kaga S, Ragg S, Rogers KA, Ochi A. Stimulation of CD28 with B7-2 promotes focal adhesion-like contacts where Rho family small G proteins accumulate in T cells. J Immunol 1998;160:24-27.

80. Vojtek AB, Cooper JA. Rho family members: activators of MAP kinase cascades. Cell 1995;82:527-529.

81. Reif K, Cantrell DA.. Networking Rho family GTPases in lymphocytes. Immunity 1998;8:395-401.

82. Su B, Jacinto E, Hibi M, Kallunki T, Karin M, Ben-Neriah Y. JNK is involved in signal integration during costimulation of T lymphocytes. Cell 1994;77:727-736.

83. Nishina H, Bachmann M, Oliveira-dos-Santos AJ, et al. Impaired CD28-mediated interleukin 2 production and proliferation in stress kinase SAPK/ERK1 kinase (SEK1)/mitogen-activated protein kinase kinase 4 (MKK4)-deficient T lymphocytes. J Exp Med 1997;186:941-953.

84. Kaga S, Ragg S, Rogers KA, Ochi A. Activation of p21-CDC42/Rac-activated kinases by CD28 signaling: p21-activated kinase (PAK) and MEK kinase 1

(MEKK1) may mediate the interplay between CD3 and CD28 signals. J Immunol 1998;160:4182-4189.

85. June CH, Ledbetter JA, Gillespie MM, Lindsten T, Thompson CB. T-cell proliferation involving the CD28 pathway is associated with cyclosporine-resistant interleukin 2 gene expression. Mol Cell Biol 1987;7:4472-4481.

86. Bloemena E, Van Oers RH, Weinreich S, et al. The influence of cyclosporin A on the alternative pathways of human T cell activation in vitro. Eur J Immunol 1989;19:943-946.

87. Rafiq K, Kasran A, Peng X, et al. Cyclosporin A increases IFN-gamma production by T cells when co-stimulated through CD28. Eur J Immunol 1998;28:1481-1491.

88. Miyatake S, Nakaseko C, Umemori H, Yamamoto T, Saito T. Src family tyrosine kinases associate with and phosphorylate CTLA-4 (CD152). Biochem Biophys Res Commun 1998;249:444-448.

89. Chuang E, Lee KM, Robbins MD, et al. Regulation of cytotoxic T lymphocyte-associated molecule-4 by Src kinases. J Immunol 1999;162:1270-1277.

90. Chuang E, Alegre ML, Duckett CS, Noel PJ, Vander Heiden M, Thompson CB. Interaction of CTLA-4 with the clathrin-associated protein AP50 results in ligand-independent endocytosis that limits cell surface expression. J Immunol 1997; 159:144-151.

91. Zhang Y, Allison JP. Interaction of CTLA-4 with AP50, a clathrin-coated pit adaptor protein. Proc Natl Acad Sci USA 1997;94:9273-9278.

92. Shiratori T, Miyatake S, Ohno H, et al. Tyrosine phosphorylation controls internalization of CTLA-4 by regulating its interaction with clathrin-associated adaptor complex AP- 2. Immunity 1997;6:583-589.

93. Bradshaw JD, Lu P, Leytze G, et al. Interaction of the cytoplasmic tail of CTLA-4 (CD152) with a clathrin-associated protein is negatively regulated by tyrosine phosphorylation. Biochemistry 1997;36:15975-15982.

94. Lee KM, Chuang E, Griffin M, et al.. Molecular basis of T cell inactivation by CTLA-4. Science 1998;282:2263-2266.

95. Marengere LE, Waterhouse P, Duncan GS, Mittrucker HW, Feng GS, Mak TW. Regulation of T cell receptor signaling by tyrosine phosphatase SYP association with CTLA-4. Science 1996;272:1170-1173.

96. Calvo CR, Amsen D, Kruisbeek AM. Cytotoxic T lymphocyte antigen 4 (CTLA-4) interferes with extracellular signal-regulated kinase (ERK) and Jun NH2-terminal kinase (JNK) activation, but does not affect phosphorylation of T cell receptor zeta and ZAP70. J Exp Med 1997;186:1645-1653.

97. Fraser JH, Rincon M, McCoy KD, Le Gros G. CTLA4 ligation attenuates AP-1, NFAT and NF-kappaB activity in activated T cells. Eur J Immunol 1999;29: 838-844.

98. Olsson C, Riebeck K, Dohlsten M, Michaelsson E. CTLA-4 ligation suppresses CD28-induced NF-kappaB and AP-1 activity in mouse T cell blasts. J Biol Chem 1999;274:14400-14405.

99. Pioli C, Gatta L, Frasca D, Doria G. Cytotoxic T lymphocyte antigen 4 (CTLA-4) inhibits CD28-induced IκBα degradation and RelA activation. Eur J Immunol 1999;29:856-863.

100. Van Gool SW, Vandenberghe P, de Boer M, Ceuppens JL. 1996. CD80, CD86 and CD40 provide accessory signals in a multiple-step T-cell activation model. Immunol Rev 1996;153:47-83.

101. Grewal IS, Flavell RA. The role of CD40 ligand in costimulation and T-cell activation. Immunol Rev 1996;153:85-106.

102. Law CL, Craxton A, Otipoby KL, Sidorenko SP, Klaus SJ, Clark EC. Regulation of signalling through B-lymphocyte antigen receptors by cell- cell interaction molecules. Immunol Rev 1996;153:123-154.

103. Xu J, Foy TM, Laman JD, et al. Mice deficient for the CD40 ligand. Immunity

1994;1:423-431.
104. Aruffo A, Hollenbaugh D, Wu LH, Ochs HD. The molecular basis of X-linked agammaglobulinemia, hyper-IgM syndrome, and severe combined immunodeficiency in humans. Curr Opin Hematol 1994;1:12-18.
105. Schoenberger SP, Toes RM, Vandervoort EH, Offringa R, Melief CM. T-cell help for cytotoxic T lymphocytes is mediated by CD40-CD40L interactions. Nature 1998;393:480-483.
106. van Essen D, Kikutani H, Gray D. CD40 ligand-transduced co-stimulation of T cells in the development of helper function. Nature 1995;378:620-623.
107. Brenner B, Koppenhoefer U, Lepple-Wienhues A, et al. The CD40 ligand directly activates T-lymphocytes via tyrosine phosphorylation dependent PKC activation. Biochem Biophys Res Commun 1997;239:11-17.
108. Koretzky GA. Role of the CD45 tyrosine phosphatase in signal transduction in the immune system. FASEB J 1993;7:420-426.
109. Trowbridge IS, Thomas ML. CD45: an emerging role as a protein tyrosine phosphatase required for lymphocyte activation and development. Annu Rev Immunol 1994;12:85-116.
110. Koretzky GA, Picus J, Thomas ML, Weiss A. Tyrosine phosphatase CD45 is essential for coupling T-cell antigen receptor to the phosphatidyl inositol pathway. Nature 1990;346:66-68.
111. Furukawa T, Itoh M, Krueger NX, Streuli M, Saito H. Specific interaction of the CD45 protein-tyrosine phosphatase with tyrosine-phosphorylated CD3 zeta chain. Proc Natl Acad Sci USA 1994;91:10928-10932.
112. Burns CM, Sakaguchi K, Appella E, Ashwell JD. CD45 regulation of tyrosine phosphorylation and enzyme activity of src family kinases. J Biol Chem 1994; 269:13594-13600.
113. D'Oro U, Ashwell JD. The CD45 tyrosine phosphatase is an inhibitor of Lck activity in thymocytes. J Immunol 1999;162:1879-1883.
114. Pao LI, Bedzyk WD, Persin C, Cambier JC. Molecular targets of CD45 in B cell antigen receptor signal transduction. J Immunol 1997;158:1116-1124.
115. Holter W, Schwarz M, Cerwenka A, Knapp W. The role of CD2 as a regulator of human T-cell cytokine production. Immunol Rev 1996;153:107-122.
116. Davis SJ, van der Merwe PA. The structure and ligand interactions of CD2: implications for T-cell function. Immunol Today 1996;17:177-187.
117. Lin H, Hutchcroft JE, Andoniou CE, Kamoun M, Band H, Bierer BE. Association of p59(fyn) with the T lymphocyte costimulatory receptor CD2. Binding of the Fyn Src homology (SH) 3 domain is regulated by the Fyn SH2 domain. J Biol Chem 1998;273:19914-19921.
118. Bierer BE, Sleckman BP, Ratnofsky SE, Burakoff SJ. The biologic roles of CD2, CD4, and CD8 in T-cell activation. Annu Rev Immunol 1989;7:579-599.
119. Lub M, van Kooyk Y, Figdor CG. Ins and outs of LFA-1. Immunol Today 1995;16: 479-483.
120. Makgoba MW, Sanders ME, Ginther Luce GE, et al. ICAM-1 a ligand for LFA-1-dependent adhesion of B, T and myeloid cells. Nature 1988;331:86-88.
121. Hibbs ML, Xu H, Stacker SA, Springer TA. Regulation of adhesion of ICAM-1 by the cytoplasmic domain of LFA-1 integrin beta subunit. Science 1991;251:1611-1613.
122. Dustin ML, Springer TA. T-cell receptor cross-linking transiently stimulates adhesiveness through LFA-1. Nature 1989;341:619-624.
123. Soede RD, Wijnands YM, Van Kouteren-Cobzaru I, Roos E. ZAP-70 tyrosine kinase is required for LFA-1-dependent T cell migration. J Cell Biol 1998;142: 1371-1379.
124. Tabassam FH, Umehara H, Huang JY, et al. Beta2-integrin, LFA-1, and TCR/CD3 synergistically induce tyrosine phosphorylation of focal adhesion

kinase (pp125(FAK)) in PHA-activated T cells. Cell Immunol 1999;193:179-184.

125. Hynes RO. Integrins: versatility, modulation, and signaling in cell adhesion. Cell 1992;69:11-25.

126. Bachmann MF, McKall-Faienza K, Schmits R, et al. Distinct roles for LFA-1 and CD28 during activation of naive T cells: adhesion versus costimulation. Immunity 1997;7:549-557.

127. Kishimoto H, Cai Z, Brunmark A, Jackson MR, Peterson PA, Sprent J. Differing roles for B7 and intercellular adhesion molecule-1 in negative selection of thymocytes. J Exp Med 1996;184:531-537.

128. Goodison S, Urquidi V, Tarin D. CD44 cell adhesion molecules. J Clin Pathol Mol Pathol 1999;52:189-196.

129. DeGrendele HC, Kosfiszer M, Estess P, Siegelman MH. CD44 activation and associated primary adhesion is inducible via T cell receptor stimulation. J Immunol 1997;159:2549-2553.

130. DeGrendele HC, Estess P, Siegelman MH. Requirement for CD44 in activated T cell extravasation into an inflammatory site. Science 1997;278:672-675.

131. Sayegh MH, Turka LA. The role of T-cell costimulatory activation pathways in transplant rejection. N Engl J Med 1998;338:1813-1821.

132. Motoyama K, Arima T, Lehmann M, Flye MW. Tolerance to heart and kidney grafts induced by nondepleting anti-CD4 monoclonal antibody (RIB 5/2) versus depleting anti-CD4 monoclonal antibody (OX-38) with donor antigen administration. Surgery 1997;122:213-219.

133. Saitovitch D, Bushell A, Mabbs DW, Morris PJ, Wood KJ. Kinetics of induction of transplantation tolerance with a nondepleting anti-CD4 monoclonal antibody and donor-specific transfusion before transplantation. A critical period of time is required for development of immunological unresponsiveness. Transplantation 1996;61:1642-1647.

134. Ito H, Hamano K, Fukumoto T, Wood KJ, Esato K. Bidirectional blockade of CD4 and major histocompatibility complex class II molecules: an effective immunosuppressive treatment in the mouse heart transplantation model. J Heart Lung Transplant 1998;17:460-469.

135. Arima T, Lehmann M, Flye MW. Induction of donor specific transplantation tolerance to cardiac allografts following treatment with nondepleting (RIB 5/2) or depleting (OX-38) anti-CD4 mAb plus intrathymic or intravenous donor alloantigen. Transplantation 1997;63:284-292.

136. Bushell A, Niimi M, Morris PJ, Wood KJ. Evidence for immune regulation in the induction of transplantation tolerance: a conditional but limited role for IL-4. J Immunol 1999;162:1359-1366.

137. Plain KM, Fava L, Spinelli A, et al. Induction of tolerance with nondepleting anti-CD4 monoclonal antibodies is associated with down-regulation of TH2 cytokines. Transplantation 1997;64:1559-1567.

138. Jaques BC, Ahmiedat H, Alastair GJ, et al. Thymus-dependent, anti-CD4-induced tolerance to rat cardiac allografts. Transplantation 1998;66:1291-1299.

139. Orosz CG, Huang EH, Bergese SD, et al. 1997. Prevention of acute murine cardiac allograft rejection: anti-CD4 or anti-vascular cell adhesion molecule one monoclonal antibodies block acute rejection but permit persistent graft-reactive alloimmunity and chronic tissue remodeling. J Heart Lung Transplant 1997;16:889-904.

140. Kirk AD, Harlan DM, Armstrong NN, et al. CTLA4-Ig and anti-CD40 ligand prevent renal allograft rejection in primates. Proc Natl Acad Sci USA 1997;94:8789-8794.

141. Kirk AD, Burkly LC, Batty DS, et al. Treatment with humanized monoclonal antibody against CD154 prevents acute renal allograft rejection in nonhuman primates. Nat Med 1999;5:686-693.

142. Levisetti MG, Padrid PA, Szot GL, et al. Immunosuppressive effects of human CTLA4Ig in a non-human primate model of allogeneic pancreatic islet transplan-

tation. J Immunol 1997;159:5187-5191.

143. Onodera K, Chandraker A, Schaub M, et al. CD28-B7 T cell costimulatory blockade by CTLA4Ig in sensitized rat recipients: induction of transplantation tolerance in association with depressed cell-mediated and humoral immune responses. J Immunol 1997;159:1711-1717.

144. Bolling SF, Lin H, Wei RO, Turka LA. Preventing allograft rejection with CTLA4IG: effect of donor-specific transfusion route or timing. J Heart Lung Transplant 1996;15:928-935.

145. Perez VL, van Parijs L, Biuckians A, Zheng XX, Strom TB, Abbas AK. Induction of peripheral T cell tolerance in vivo requires CTLA-4 engagement. Immunity 1997; 6:411-417.

146. Zheng XX, Markees TG, Hancock WW, et al. CTLA4 signals are required to optimally induce allograft tolerance with combined donor-specific transfusion and anti-CD154 monoclonal antibody treatment. J Immunol 1999;162:4983-4990.

147. Judge TA, Wu Z, Zheng XG, Sharpe AH, Sayegh MH, Turka LA. The role of CD80, CD86, and CTLA4 in alloimmune responses and the induction of long-term allograft survival. J Immunol 1999;162:1947-1951.

148. Dengler TJ, Szabo G, Sido B, et al. Prolonged allograft survival but no tolerance induction by modulating CD28 antibody JJ319 after high-responder rat heart transplantation. Transplantation 1999;67:392-398.

149. Russell ME, Hancock WW, Akalin E, et al. Chronic cardiac rejection in the LEW to F344 rat model. Blockade of CD28-B7 costimulation by CTLA4Ig modulates T cell and macrophage activation and attenuates arteriosclerosis. J Clin Invest 1996;97:833-838.

150. Chandraker A, Azuma H, Nadeau K, et al. Late blockade of T cell costimulation interrupts progression of experimental chronic allograft rejection. J Clin Invest 1998; 101:2309-2318.

151. Larsen CP, Alexander DZ, Hollenbaugh D, et al. CD40-gp39 interactions play a critical role during allograft rejection. Suppression of allograft rejection by blockade of the CD40-gp39 pathway. Transplantation 1996;61:4-9.

152. Parker DC, Greiner DL, Phillips NE, et al. Survival of mouse pancreatic islet allografts in recipients treated with allogeneic small lymphocytes and antibody to CD40 ligand. Proc Natl Acad Sci USA 1995;92:9560-9564.

153. Chang AC, Blum MG, Blair KS, et al. Prolonged anti-CD40 ligand therapy improves primate cardiac allograft survival. Transplant Proc 1999; 31:95

154. Hamawy MM, Knechtle SJ. Strategies for tolerance induction in nonhuman primates. Curr Opin Immunol 1998;10:513-517.

155. Larsen CP, Elwood ET, Alexander DZ, et al. Long-term acceptance of skin and cardiac allografts after blocking CD40 and CD28 pathways. Nature 1996;381: 434-438.

156. Sun H, Subbotin V, Chen C, et al. Prevention of chronic rejection in mouse aortic allografts by combined treatment with CTLA4-Ig and anti-CD40 ligand monoclonal antibody. Transplantation 1997;64:1838-1843.

157. Lazarovits AI, Poppema S, Zhang Z, et al. Prevention and reversal of renal allograft rejection by antibody against CD45RB. Nature 1996;380:717-720.

158. Basadonna GP, Auersvald L, Khuong CO, et al. Antibody-mediated targeting of CD45 isoforms: a novel immunotherapeutic strategy. Proc Natl Acad Sci USA 1998;95:3821-3826.

159. Gao Z, Zhong R, Jiang J, et al. Adoptively transferable tolerance induced by CD45RB monoclonal antibody. J Am Soc Nephrol 1999;10:374-381.

160. Sido B, Dengler TJ, Otto G, Zimmermann R, Muller P, Meuer SC. Differential immunosuppressive activity of monoclonal CD2 antibodies on allograft rejection versus specific antibody production. Eur J Immunol 1998;28:1347-1357.

161. Kapur S, Khanna A, Sharma VK, Li B, Suthanthiran M. CD2 antigen targeting

reduces intragraft expression of mRNA-encoding granzyme B and IL-10 and induces tolerance. Transplantation 1996;62:249-255.

162. Woodward JE, Qin L, Chavin KD, et al. Blockade of multiple costimulatory receptors induces hyporesponsiveness: inhibition of CD2 plus CD28 pathways. Transplantation 1996;62:1011-1018.

163. Krieger NR, Most D, Bromberg JS, et al. Coexistence of Th1- and Th2-type cytokine profiles in anti-CD2 monoclonal antibody-induced tolerance. Transplantation 1996;62:1285-1292.

164. Kaplon RJ, Hochman PS, Michler RE, et al. Short course single agent therapy with an LFA-3-IgG1 fusion protein prolongs primate cardiac allograft survival. Transplantation 1996;61:356-363.

165. Besse T, Malaise J, Mourad M, et al. Prevention of rejection with BTI-322 after renal transplantation (results at 9 months). Transplant Proc 1997;29:2425-2426.

166. Mourad M, Besse T, Malaise J, et al. BTI-322 for acute rejection after renal transplantation. Transplant Proc 1997;29:2353

167. Zuckerman LA, Pullen L, Miller J. Functional consequences of costimulation by ICAM-1 on IL-2 gene expression and T cell activation. J Immunol 1998;160: 3259-3268.

168. Isobe M, Suzuki J, Yamazaki S, et al. Regulation by differential development of Th1 and Th2 cells in peripheral tolerance to cardiac allograft induced by blocking ICAM- 1/LFA-1 adhesion. Circulation 1997;96:2247-2253.

169. Suzuki J, Isobe M, Yamazaki S, Horie S, Okubo Y, Sekiguchi M. Inhibition of accelerated coronary atherosclerosis with short-term blockade of intercellular adhesion molecule-1 and lymphocyte function- associated antigen-1 in a heterotopic murine model of heart transplantation. J Heart Lung Transplant 1997;16: 1141-1148.

170. Brandt M, Steinmann J, Steinhoff G, Haverich A. Treatment with monoclonal antibodies to ICAM-1 and LFA-1 in rat heart allograft rejection. Transpl Int 1997;10: 141-144.

171. Harrison PC, Madwed JB. Anti-LFA-1 alpha reduces the dose of cyclosporin A needed to produce immunosuppression in heterotopic cardiac transplanted rats. J Heart Lung Transplant 1999;18:279-284.

172. Isobe M, Suzuki J, Yamazaki S, Horie S, Okubo Y, Sekiguchi M. Assessment of tolerance induction to cardiac allograft by anti-ICAM-1 and anti-LFA-1 monoclonal antibodies. J Heart Lung Transplant 1997; 16:1149-1156.

173. Xu XY, Honjo K, Devore-Carter D, Bucy RP. Immunosuppression by inhibition of cellular adhesion mediated by leukocyte function-associated antigen-1/ intercellular adhesion molecule- 1 in murine cardiac transplantation. Transplantation 1997;63:876-885.

174. Hourmant M, Bedrossian J, Durand D, et al. A randomized multicenter trial comparing leukocyte function-associated antigen-1 monoclonal antibody with rabbit antithymocyte globulin as induction treatment in first kidney transplantations. Transplantation 1996;62:1565-1570.

175. Uff CR, Reid SD, Wood RF, Pockley AG. CD44 expression in rejecting rat small bowel allografts. Transplantation 1995;60:985-989.

176. Fujisaki S, Miyake H, Amano S, Nakayama H, Oida T, Takizawa H. Expression of CD44 in rat liver allografts during rejection. J Hepatobil Pancreat Surg 1998;5: 196-199.

177. Knoflach A, Magee C, Denton MD, et al. Immunomodulatory functions of hyaluronate in the LEW-to-F344 model of chronic cardiac allograft rejection. Transplantation 1999;67:909-914.

178. Cooperative Clinical Trials in Transplantation Research Group. Murine OKT4A immunosuppression in cadaver renal allograft recipients: a cooperative clinical trial in transplantation pilot study. Transplantation 1997;67:392-398.

7 ORAL TOLERANCE

Howard L. Weiner
Center for Neurologic Diseases
Brigham & Women's Hospital and Harvard University
Boston, Massachusetts, USA

A majority of the contacts with foreign antigenic materials occur at mucosal surfaces, which is larger than the area of the skin. The mucosal surface is constantly and physiologically exposed to a large variety of antigenic materials. Orally administered antigen encounters the gut associated lymphoid tissue (GALT) which has inherent property of not only to protect the host from ingested pathogens but also to prevent the host from reacting to ingested proteins. Thus, orally administered antigens induce systemic hyporesponsiveness to the fed proteins and this phenomenon termed oral tolerance. It was first described in 1911 when Wells fed hen egg proteins to guinea-pigs and found them resistant to anaphylaxis when challenged [1]. In 1946, Chase fed guinea pigs the contact-sensitizing agent dinitrochlorobenzene (DNCB) and observed that animals had decreased skin reactivity to DNCB [2]. It has also been observed in human fed and immunized with KLH [3]. There have been many studies trying to elucidate the mechanisms of oral tolerance [4, 5] and now it is clear that oral tolerance is mediated by T cells through different mechanisms depending on the dose of antigen fed. Low dose antigen favors the induction of regulatory T cells which suppress Th1 cell mediated response and high dose antigen induce T cell clonal anergy or deletion. In recent years, oral tolerance has been used successfully to treat autoimmune diseases in animal models and is now being applied to the treatment of human diseases.

A. W. Thomson (ed.), Therapeutic Immunosuppression, 159–182.
© 2001 *Kluwer Academic Publishers.*

MECHANISM OF ORAL TOLERANCE

Inductive phase

The GALT consists of villi which contain epithelial cells, intraepithelial lymphocytes (IELs), lamina propria lymphocytes (LPLs) and Peyer's patches which are lymphoid nodules interspersed among the villi (Figure 1). Peyer's patches are one of the primary areas in the GALT where specific immune responses are generated. It has been attempted to use the GALT as a vaccination route, but it is difficult due to the systemic hyporesponsiveness that is generated. Although dietary antigens are degraded by the time they reach

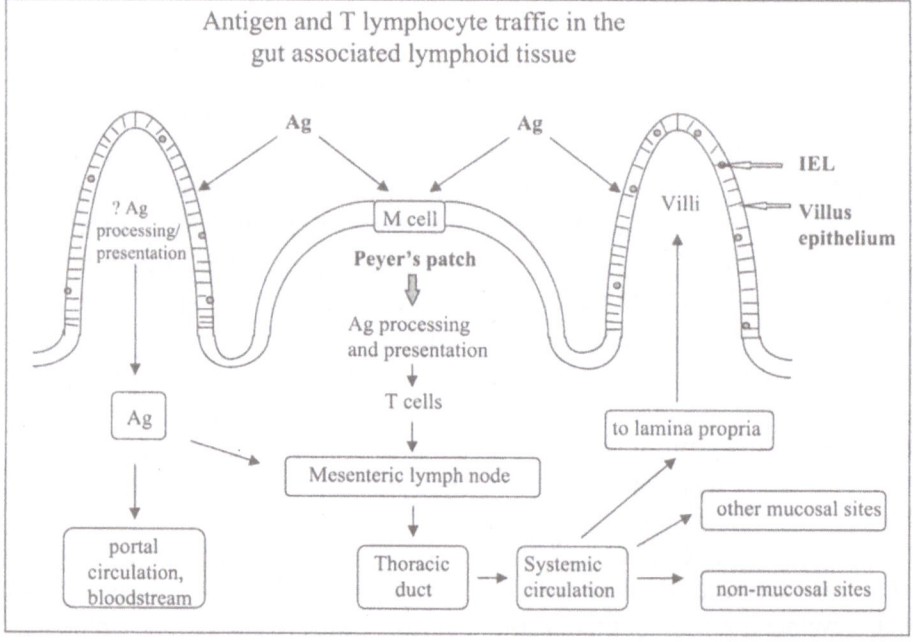

Figure 1
Antigen and T cell traffic in the GALT. Antigen is taken up either via M cells into lymphoid nodules termed Peyer's patches or into the villus epithelium. Particulate antigen is preferentially taken up by M cells and soluble antigen by the villus epithelium. Antigen presentation results in the induction of cells that traffic to the systemic circulation via the mesenteric lymph node and thoracic duct, and then migrate back to the lamina propria and to other mucosal and nonmucosal sites. The villi contain IELs, which are CD8+ T cells unique to the gut. T cells in the lamina propria are in a different state of activation to those in Peyer's patches. Peyer's patches also contain B-cell rich, poorly formed, germinal centers where induction of antibody responses occurs.

the small intestine, studies in humans and rodents have indicated that degradation is partial and that some intact antigen is absorbed into the systemic circulation. [6-8]. High dose oral antigen may result in systemic antigen presentation, which induces hyporesponsiveness either via clonal T cell anergy or clonal deletion.

It is generally believed that in low dose antigen fed animals, oral tolerance is induced in the GALT. Several cells capable of antigen presentation exist in the GALT. These include macrophages, dendritic cells, B cells and epithelial cells. Macrophages-enriched cells obtained from mice fed OVA are able to stimulate antigen-primed lymph node T cells in vitro in an antigen-specific fashion without further exposure to antigen [9]. Dendritic cells have been shown as the major intestinal antigen presenting cells (APC) which can acquire and process orally administered antigen [10]. Epithelial cells may preferentially trigger the activation of CD8+ regulatory T cells. In the rat, these epithelial cell-induced CD8+ T cells are antigen specific [11] whereas in the human they were found to be antigen non-specific [12]. MHC class II positive intestinal epithelial cells from 2, 4-dinitrochlorobenzene (DNCB)-fed mice could induce anergy of DNCB-primed T cells [13]. Lamina propria cells (LPC) also may be involved as antigen presenting cells for oral tolerance. Antigen pulsed splenic APC stimulated Ag specific Th0 cytokine production while PP APC induced a profile consistent with the provision of T cell help for IgA production. Presentation of Ag by LPC stimulated high level of IFN-γ and TGF-β and adoptive transfer of Ag pulsed LPC induced oral tolerance to that Ag in the recipients [14]. However, the type of APC responsible for the effect of LPC was not clear.

T helper cells which are preferentially generated in the GALT are Th2 cells [15, 16]. Th2 cell differentiation depends on the cytokine microenvironment or cytokine milieu the Th precursor cells are exposed to during their activation [17]. If IL-12 is present during activation, Th1 cells are differentiated while IL-4 induce Th2 cell differentiation. Microenvironment of intestinal mucosa may be crucial for the induction of Th2 or Th3 (TGF-β secreting cells). We have shown that dendritic cells, when exposed to IL-10, can drive Th2 cell differentiation of naive OVA TCR CD4+ transgenic T cells [18]. The influence of the cytokine milieu on antigen presentation by DC has also been demonstrated in vivo. Thus, DC exposed to IL-10 in vitro, when injected into the footpad of mice, can prime for Th2 cell type responses [19]. It has also been shown in the human system that PGE-2 treated DC can produce IL-10 and can prime naive human T cells for Th2 cell differentiation [20]. DC from PP preferentially stimulate Th0 clones to produce huge amounts of IL-4 while DC from spleen induce high IFN-γ production [21] [22]. There is also evidence that DC may be involved in oral tolerance induction in that expansion of DC in vivo with Flt3 ligand enhances oral tolerance [23]. It is possible that DC, the most potent APC in activating resting T cells, under the influence of gut cytokine milieu, present antigen for Th2 or Th3 cell differentiation.

APC provide co-stimulatory signals required for the activation of T cells. B7.1 and B7.2 are the most important co-stimulatory molecules. B7.2 has been shown to be critical for Th2 type cell differentiation [24]. To determine the role of co-stimulatory molecules in the induction of oral tolerance, we have tested the effect of anti-B7.1 or anti-B7.2 mAb on the induction of tolerance by both high and low dose antigen feeding [25]. In experimental allergic encephalomyelitis (EAE) model, anti-B7.2 mAb, but not anti-B7.1 mAb inhibited the induction of oral tolerance induced by low dose MBP feeding. We also found that CTLA-4 molecules on the APC appear to be critical for the induction of oral tolerance [26]. CD40-CD40 ligand interactions are also important for high dose oral tolerance [27]. Class II molecules on the APC also appear to be critical for the induction of oral tolerance since oral tolerance can not be induced in class II deficient mice [28].

Recently, it was reported that Cyclooxygenase-2 (Cox-2) dependent arachidonic acid such as PGE2 is produced by lamina propria mononuclear cells and involved in oral tolerance [29]. Although it is antigen non-specific, it is possible that this mechanism, which is not dependent on the cytokines, is important for generating immunoregulatory T cells.

Effector phase

It has become clear that there are two primary effector mechanisms of oral tolerance: the induction of regulatory T cells which mediate active suppression and the induction of clonal anergy or deletion. Depending on the dose of the antigen fed, it is determined which form of peripheral tolerance develops following oral administration of antigen. Low doses of antigen favor the generation of active suppression or regulatory-cell driven tolerance whereas high doses of antigen favor anergy-driven tolerance (Figure 2). However, they are not mutually exclusive and may occur simultaneously and general definitions of "low" and "high" doses need to be established for each antigen.

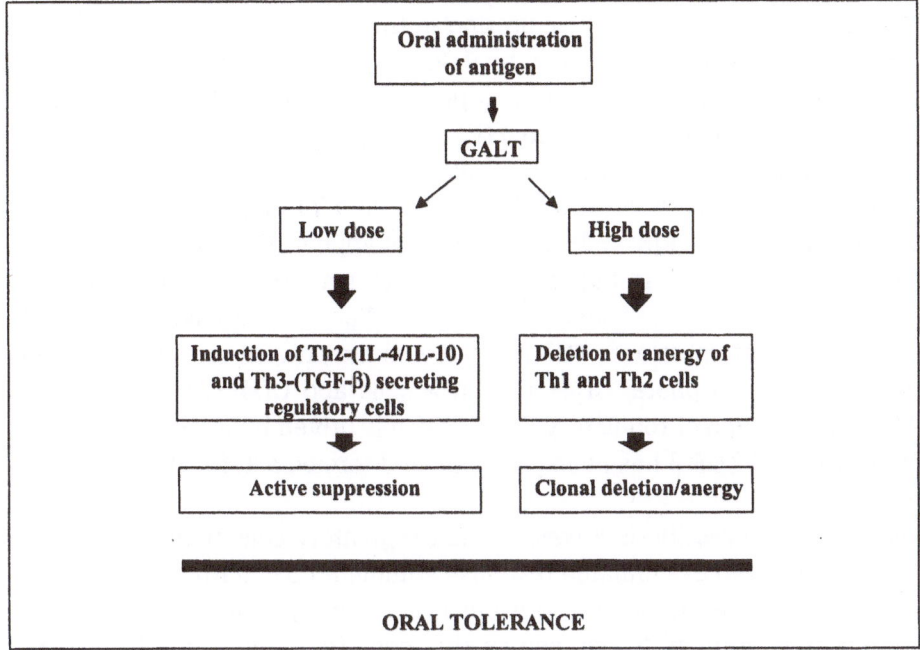

Figure 2
The different mechanisms of oral tolerance are determined by the dose of fed antigen. Abbreviations: GALT, gut-associated lymphoid tissue; IL, interleukin; TGF-ß, transforming growth factor ß; Th, T helper.

1. Active suppression

Many early studies demonstrated that active suppression is an important mechanism for oral tolerance [4]. After feeding antigens, transferable suppression to cell-mediated immune responses was demonstrated using T cells from Peyer's patches, mesenteric lymph node, and spleen as sources of cells for adoptive transfer experiments. Active suppression is believed to be mediated by the induction of regulatory T cells in the GALT such as Peyer's patches [30], which then migrate to the systemic immune system. Several reports indicate that one of the primary mechanisms of active cellular suppression is via the secretion of suppressive cytokines such as TGF-β, IL-4, IL-10 following antigen specific triggering. TGF-β is produced both by CD4+ and CD8+ GALT derived T cells and is an important mediator of the active suppression component of oral tolerance [31, 32]. TGF-β secreting CD4+ cells specific for MBP were cloned from the mesenteric lymph nodes of SJL mice [31]. These clones were found to be structurally identical to Th1- disease-inducing clones with respect to TCR usage, major histocompatibility complex (MHC) restriction and epitope recognition, but suppressed rather than induced disease. TGF-β secreting CD4+ cells were also cloned from

MBP-TCR transgenic mice by culturing in the presence of IL-4 but not IL-2 [33]. These clones did not secrete IL-2, IFN-γ, IL-4 or IL-10. Thus, CD4+ cells that primarily produce TGF-β appear to be a unique T cell subset that includes mucosal helper T cell function and down-regulatory properties for Th1 and other immune cells. These cells have been termed Th3 cells. In contrast to Th1 and Th2 cells, Th3 cells provide help for IgA production and primarily secrete TGF-β [31, 34]. Th3 type cells appear distinct from Th2 cells since CD4+ TGF-β secreting cells that suppress a form of colitis have been generated from IL-4 deficient mice [35]. Studies on rats have also demonstrated an essential role for TGF-β and IL-4 in the prevention of autoimmune thyroiditis by peripheral CD4+ CD45RC- cells and CD4+CD8- thymocytes [36]. Another type of regulatory T cell which is driven by IL-10 and secretes both IL-10 and TGF-β has been proposed and termed a Tr1 cell [37].

Bystander suppression is a concept that regulatory cells induced by a fed antigen can suppress immune response stimulated by an irrelevant antigen as long as the fed antigen is present in anatomic vicinity. It was demonstrated in vitro when it was shown that cells from animals fed MBP suppressed proliferation of an OVA-specific cell line across a transwell, but only when triggered by the fed antigen [38]. The soluble factor shown to be responsible for the suppression was TGF-β. Bystander suppression has since been demonstrated in several autoimmune disease models (Table 1).

Table 1
Models of Autoimmune and Other Diseases that Demonstrate Bystander Suppression

Autoimmune disease	Immunizing antigen	Oral antigen	Target organ
Arthritis	BSA, mycobacteria	Type II collagen	Joint
EAE	PLP	MBP	Brain
EAE	MBP peptide 71–90	MBP peptide 21–40	Brain
EAE	MBP	OVA	Lymph node, DTH response
Diabetes	LCMV	Insulin	Pancreatic islets
IBD	CD4+CD45RBhi T cell transfer	OVA	Intestine
Stroke	None	MBP	Brain

Abbreviation:
BSA, bovine serum albumin; DTH, delayed-type hypersensitivity; EAE, experimental allergic encephalomyelitis; LCMV, lymphocytic choriomeningitis virus; MBP, myelin basic protein; OVA, ovalbumin; PLP, proteolipid. IBD, inflammatory bowel disease.

Bystander suppression solves a major conceptual problem in the design of antigen- or T cell-specific therapy for inflammatory autoimmune diseases such as MS, type 1 diabetes and rheumatoid arthritis (RA), in which the autoantigen is not clear or where there are reactivities to multiple autoantigens in the target tissue. During the course of chronic inflammatory autoimmune processes in animals, there is intra- and inter-antigenic spread of autoreactivity in the target organ [39-43]. Similarly, in human autoimmune diseases, there are reactivities to multiple autoantigens in the target tissue. For example, in MS, there is immune reactivity to at least three myelin antigens: MBP, PLP and myelin oligodendrocyte glycoprotein (MOG) [44, 45]. In type 1 diabetes, there are multiple islet-cell antigens that could be the target of autoreactivity, including glutamic acid decarboxylase (GAD), insulin and heat shock proteins [46]. Because regulatory cells induced by oral antigen secrete antigen-nonspecific cytokines after being triggered by the fed antigen, they suppress inflammation in the microenvironment where the fed antigen is localized. Thus, for a human organ-specific inflammatory disease, it is not necessary to know the specific antigen that is the target of an autoimmune response, but only to administer orally an antigen capable of inducing regulatory cells, which then migrate to the target tissue and suppress inflammation. Bystander suppression has also been shown for IL-10 secreting Tr1 cells in which an OVA-specific Tr1 clone could suppress a murine model of inflammatory bowel disease in vivo when fed [37]. Although bystander suppression was initially described in association with regulatory cells induced by oral antigen, the process could in principal be induced by any immune manipulation that induces Th2-Tr1 or Th-3-type regulatory cells. Bystander suppression mediated by TGF-β secretion has also been reported in a mouse model of transplantation tolerance [47].

2. Anergy and Clonal deletion

Anergy is defined as a state of T lymphocyte unresponsiveness characterized by absence of proliferation, IL-2 production, and diminished expression of IL-2R [48]. Anergy as a mechanism for oral tolerance has been shown indirectly or directly [49, 50]. A single feeding of 20mg OVA induced a state of anergy in OVA specific T cells [51]. T cell clones derived from high dose MBP-fed rats were characterized and following several cell divisions in the presence of IL-2, they undergo a reversal of unresponsiveness [52]. Anergy as a mechanism has also been shown in transfer systems with OVA-TCR transgenic T cells [50]. All above studies associated with anergy as a tolerance-inducing mechanism used relatively high dose antigen. Studies on the cells rendered anergic have raised the possibility that these cells do not function in a totally passive fashion in the tolerance they evoke. Recent reports have suggested that anergic cells can actively suppress T cell responses either through modulation of the T-cell activating capacity of the APC (APC/T cell interaction) [53] or by inhibition of T cells recognizing their ligand in close proximity on the same APC ("linked suppression" through T/T cell interactions) [54]. In these cases described above, the so called anergic cells serve as regulatory cells which mediate tolerance via an active mechanism.

Feeding very high dose antigen induced T cell clonal deletion in the OVA TCR transgenic model [55]. Mowat and co-workers also showed that lymphocytes from these animals die rapidly when cultured *in vitro* in the absence of antigen [56]. Other investigators did not find deletion in wild type mice transferred with T cells from OVA TCR transgenic mice when they fed 25 mg OVA [50]. Oral tolerance to high doses of ovalbumin is reported to be normal in fas-deficient lpr mice [57, 58]. It is also reported that IL-12 is required to prevent an induction of Fas-mediated apoptosis after high dose feeding of OVA to OVA-TCR transgenic mice [59]. Thus, clonal deletion occurs in transgenic mice fed a very high dose of antigen, but its role in high dose tolerance in normal animals is unclear.

MODULATION OF ORAL TOLERANCE

A number of factors have been reported to modulate oral tolerance. As oral tolerance has usually been defined in terms of Th1 responses, anything that suppress Th1 and/or enhances Th2 or Th3 cell development would enhance oral tolerance (Table 2). Th3 cells appear to use IL-4 as one of their growth /differentiation factors [33]. Seder have also found that IL-4 and TGF-β may serve to promote growth of TGF-β secreting cells [60]. Thus, IL-4 administration i.p. enhances low-dose oral tolerance to MBP in the EAE model and is associated with increased fecal IgA anti-MBP antibodies. Oral IL-10 and IL-4 can also enhance oral tolerance when co-administered with antigen [61]. Cytokines have also been administered by the nasal route [62]. Large doses of IFN-γ given intraperitoneally abrogate oral tolerance [63] anti-IL-12 enhances oral tolerance and is associated both with increased TGF-β production and T cell apoptosis [64] and subcutaneous administration of IL-12 reverses mucosal tolerance [65]. In the uveitis model, intraperitoneal IL-2 potentates oral tolerance and is associated with increased production of TGF-β, IL-10 and IL-4 [66]. Oral but not subcutaneous lipopolysaccaride (LPS) enhances oral tolerance to MBP [67] and is associated with increased expression of IL-4 in the brain. Oral IFN-β synergizes with the induction of oral toler-

Table 2
Modulation of Oral Tolerance

Augments	Decreases
IL-2	IFN-γ
IL-4	IL-12
IL-10	CT
Anti-IL-12 Ab	Anti-MCP-1
TGF-β	Anti-γδ Ab
INF-β	GVH
CTB	Anti-B7.2 mAb (low dose tolerance)
Flt-3 ligand	
LPS	
Multiple emulsions	

Abbreviations:
Ab, antibody; CT, cholera toxin; CTB, cholera toxin B subunit; GVH, graft-versus-host; IFN, interferon; IL, interleukin; LPS, lipopolysaccharide; MCP-1, monocyte chemotactic protein 1

ance in SJL/PLJ mice fed low doses of MBP [68]. Cholera toxin (CT) is one of the most potent mucosal adjuvants, and feeding CT abrogates oral tolerance when fed with an unrelated protein antigen [69]. However, when a protein is coupled to recombinant cholera toxin B subunit (CTB) and given orally, there is enhancement of peripheral immune tolerance [70]. Oral administration of corneal epithelial cells coupled to CTB markedly enhanced corneal allograft survival [71]. Antibody to monocyte chemotactic protein 1 (MCP-1) abrogates oral tolerance [72]. Oral antigen delivery using a multiple emulsion system also enhances oral tolerance [73]. γδ T cells may have an important role in oral tolerance induction since it is more difficult to induce oral tolerance in animals depleted of such cells [74, 75] or in delta chain deficient animals [76]. The steroid hormone dehydroepiandrosterone (DHEA) breaks intranasally induced tolerance [77] and diesel exhaust particles block induction of oral tolerance in mice [78]. In the arthritis model, administration of TGF-β or dimaprid (a histamine type 2 receptor agonist) i.p., both of which are believed to promote the development of immunoregulatory cells, enhances the induction of oral tolerance to collagen II even after the onset of arthritis [79].

TREATMENT OF AUTOIMMUNE DISEASES IN ANIMALS

Several studies have demonstrated the effectiveness of orally administered myelin antigens in rat and mouse models of autoimmune disease (Table 3).

EAE

In the Lewis rat, high doses of MBP can suppress EAE via the mechanism of T cell clonal anergy [80], whereas multiple lower doses prevent EAE by transferable active cellular suppression [81]. In the nervous system of low-dose-fed animals, inflammatory cytokines such as TNF-α and IFN-γ are downregulated and TGF-β is upregulated [82]. Oral MBP partially sup-

Table 3
Suppression of autoimmunity by oral tolerance

(a) Animal models

Model	Protein fed
EAE	MBP, PLP, MOG
Arthritis (CIA, AA, AIA)	CII, HSP, gp39
Uveitis	S-Ag, IRBP
Myasthenia gravis	AchR
Diabetes (NOD mouse)	Insulin, GAD
Transplantation	Alloantigen, MHC peptide
Thyroiditis	Thyroglobulin
Colitis	Haptenized colonic proteins

(b) Human disease trials

Disease trial	Protein fed
Multiple sclerosis	Bovine myelin, glatiramer acetate
Rheumatoid arthritis	Chicken and bovine CII
Uveitis	Bovine S-Ag
Type I diabetes	Human insulin
Systemic sclerosis	Type 1 collagen

Abbreviations:
AA, adjuvant arthritis; AIA, antigen-induced arthritis; AchR, acetylcholine receptor; CII, type II collagen; CIA, collagen-induced arthritis; EAE, experimental allergic encephalomyelitis; GAD, glutamic acid decarboxylase; gp39, glycoprotein 39; HSP, heat shock protein; IRBP, interphotoreceptor retinoid-binding protein; MBP, myelin basic protein; MHC, major histocompatibility complex; NOD, non-obese diabetic; PLP, proteolipid protein; S-Ag, S antigen.

presses serum antibody responses, especially at higher doses [83]. Administration of myelin to sensitized animals in the chronic guinea pig model or larger doses of MBP in the murine EAE model is protective and does not exacerbate disease [12, 84] and long term (6 month) administration of myelin in the chronic EAE model was beneficial [85]. EAE can also be suppressed in animals transgenic for an MBP specific TCR following feeding with MBP [86]. Nasally administered MBP peptides have been reported to suppress EAE [87]. The latest approach in animal models has been to utilize glatiramer acetate (Cop-1, Copaxone), a drug approved for therapy of multiple sclerosis, which is given to patients by injection. There are reports that Cop-1 suppresses EAE in both mouse and rat [88, 89] [90] [91].

Arthritis

Oral administration of cartilage antigens such as type II collagen suppress several models of arthritis including collagen- induced arthritis (CIA) [92-94], adjuvant arthritis [95, 96], pristine arthritis [97], and antigen-induced arthritis [98]. One of the first studies to demonstrate that an orally administered autoantigen can suppress an autoimmune disease was the use of oral type II collagen in CIA [99]. Oral type I collagen has also been shown to suppress adjuvant arthritis by bystander suppression [95]. Oral administration of an immunodominant human collagen peptide modulates CIA in mice [100] and type II collagen peptides given nasally also suppresses CIA in mice [101, 102]. Oral mycobacterial 65-kDA heat shock protein has also been shown to suppress adjuvant arthritis or avridine-induced arthritis [96, 103]. One interesting observation in treating arthritis models with collagen is that the suppression was observed at as low doses as 3 and 30 micrograms, suggesting the mechanism involved is the generation of suppressive regulatory T cell rather than clonal anergy.

Diabetes

Oral insulin has been shown to delay and, in some instances, prevent diabetes in the non-obese diabetic (NOD) mouse model. Such suppression is transferable [104], primarily with $CD4^+$ cells [105]. Immunohistochemistry of pancreatic islets of Langerhans isolated from insulin fed animals demonstrates decreased insulitis associated with decreased IFN-γ, as well as increased expression of TNF, IL-4, IL-10, TGF-β and prostaglandin (PGE_2) [106]. Recently, it was also reported that nasal administration of the insulin B chain or GAD and aerosol insulin suppresses diabetes in the NOD mouse

[107-109]. Under special experimental conditions, large doses of OVA given to OVA double transgenic mice resulted in diabetes mediated by OVA specific CTL [110]. These animals expressed OVA on the islets under the rat insulin promoter and were made chimeric to enrich for OVA specific transgenic TCR CTL. Oral insulin suppressed diabetes in a viral induced model of diabetes in which LCMV was expressed under the insulin promoter and animals infected with LCMV to induce diabetes [111]. Protection was associated with protective cytokine shifts (IL-4 / IL-10, TGF-β) in the islets. Oral administration of B-chain of insulin, a 30-amino-acid peptide slowed the development of diabetes and prevented diabetes in some animals [112]. This effect was associated with a decrease IFN-γ and an increase in IL-4, TGF-β and IL-10 expression. Oral administration of recombinant GAD from transgenic plants plant suppresses the development of diabetes in NOD mouse [113] as does oral administration of a plant-based CTB-insulin fusion protein [114].

Uveitis

Oral administration of S antigen (S-Ag), a retinal autoantigen that induces experimental autoimmune uveitis (EAU), or S-Ag peptides prevents or markedly diminishes the clinical appearance of S-Ag-induced disease as measured by ocular inflammation [115-117]. S-Ag-induced EAU can also be suppressed by feeding an HLA peptide [118]. Feeding interphotoreceptor binding protein (IRBP) suppresses IRBP-induced disease and is potentiated by IL-2 [119]. Oral feeding of retinal antigen can not only prevent acute disease but can also effectively suppress second attack in chronic-relapsing EAU, showing that oral tolerance may have practical clinical implications in uveitis, which is predominantly a chronic-relapsing condition in humans [120, 121].

Other models

Although myasthenia gravis is an antibody-mediated disease, oral and nasal administration of the Torpedo acetylcholine receptor (AchR) to Lewis rats prevented or delayed the onset of myasthenia gravis [122-124]. Purified AchR was found more effective than an unpurified mixture [125]. Experimental autoimmune myasthenia gravis (EAMG) can also be suppressed by nasally administered AchR [122, 126], AchR peptides [127], and human AchR fragments [128]. It is recently reported that nasal tolerance for EAMG by AchR is mediated by TGF-β secreting CD4 cells using CD8 knock-out mice [129].

It has been shown that oral feeding of haptenized colonic protein (HCP) effectively prevents 2,4,6-trinitrobenzene sulfonic acid (TNBS) induced granulomatous colitis via the generation of TGF-β secreting T cells [130]. Oral administration of allogeneic cells prevents sensitization by skin grafts and changes accelerated rejection of vascularized cardiac allografts to an acute form typical of unsensitized recipients [131]. Orally administered allopeptide in the Lewis rat reduces DTH responses to the peptide [132]. Oral, but not intravenous, alloantigen was accompanied by elevation of intragraft levels of IL-4 [133]. Oral alloantigen enhanced corneal allograft survival even in pre-immune hosts [71]. Oral thyroglobulin has been shown to suppress autoimmune thyroiditis [134] and feeding peptides of the Der p I allergen suppressed responses to the whole allergen [135]. Experimental granulomatous colitis in mice is abrogated by TGF-β mediated oral tolerance after administration of haptenized colonic proteins [130]. Oral tolerization to adenoviral antigens permitted long-term gene expression using recombinant adenoviral vectors [136].

TREATMENT OF AUTOIMMUNE DISEASES IN HUMANS

Investigators have shown that exposure to a contact-sensitizing agent via the mucosa prior to subsequent skin challenge led to unresponsiveness in a portion of patients studied [137]. KLH administered orally to human subjects has been reported to decrease subsequent cell-mediated immune responses although antibody responses were not affected [3]. Nasal KLH has also been reported to induce tolerance in humans [138].

On the basis of the long history of oral tolerance and the safety of the approach, human trials have been initiated in MS, RA, uveitis and diabetes (Table 3). These initial trials suggest that there has been no systemic toxicity or exacerbation of disease, although reproducible clinical efficacy has yet to be demonstrated. Results in humans however, have paralleled several aspects of what has been observed in animals.

In MS patients, MBP- and PLP- specific TGF-β- secreting Th3- type cells have been observed in the peripheral blood of patients treated with an oral bovine myelin preparation and not in patients who were untreated [139]. There was no increase in MBP- or PLP-specific IFN-γ secreting cells in treated patients. These results demonstrate that it is possible to immunize via the gut for auto-antigen- specific TGF-β-secreting cells in a human autoimmune disease by oral administration of the autoantigen. However, a recently completed 515 patient, placebo-controlled, double-blind Phase III trial of single-dose bovine myelin in relapsing-remitting MS did not show differences between placebo and treated groups in the number of relapses – a large placebo effect was observed (AutoImmune, Inc., Lexington, MA, USA). The dose of myelin was 300mg given in capsule form and contained 8mg MBP and 15 mg PLP. Preliminary analysis of magnetic resonance imaging data showed significant changes favoring oral myelin in certain patient subgroups. A new trial of oral tolerance in MS is being undertaken with glatiramer acetate (Cop-1), an MBP analogue, which is currently given by injection to MS patients but has been shown to be effective orally in animals and to induce regulatory cells that mediate bystander suppression [90, 91].

In RA, a 280 patient double-blind phase II dosing trial of chicken type II collagen in doses ranging from 20 mg to 2500 mg for 6 months demonstrated statistically significant positive effects in the group treated with the lowest dose [140]. Oral administration of larger doses of bovine type II collagen (1-10 mg) did not show a significant difference between tested and placebo groups, although a higher prevalence of responders was reported for the groups treated with type II collagen [141]. These results are consistent with animal studies of orally administered type II collagen in which protection against adjuvant- and antigen-induced arthritis and bystander suppression was observed only at the lower doses [95, 98]. An open-label pilot study of oral collagen in juvenile RA gave positive results with no toxicity [142]. This lack of systemic toxicity is an important feature for the clinical use of oral tolerance, especially in children for whom the long-term effects of immunosuppressive drugs is unknown. Recently completed several Phase II trials of oral collagen, which involved 805 patients treated with CII and 296 treated with placebo, showed that 60µg was the most significant dose compared to other doses [140, 143]. Using linear logistic regression, it was found a statistically significant effect favored patients treated on oral CII versus those on the placebo. However, integrated efficacy analysis of predictors of response including HLACII antibodies, tender and swollen joint count showed no predictors. Based on these data, a phase III trial has been carried out administering 60 µg vs. placebo, however no differences were observed between groups as a 51% response rate occurred in the placebo group.

Choy, et al have recently reported a placebo controlled trial in RA of oral tolerance to bovine type II collagen [144]. They examined the therapeutic effect of bovine CII administered as tablets in a lactose base to RA patients in a double blind randomized controlled trial. Patients who had ACR defined RA for ≥ 2 years and had failed at least one slow acting drug were recruited provided they had active arthritis. Patients were randomly assigned to receive either 0.05 mg, or 0.5 mg, 5 mg daily of CII or placebo for 6 months. All slow acting drugs were stopped at least 4 weeks before starting CII but predniso-lone was permitted if doses were < 10mg/day. Disease activity scores (DAS) were calculated and one way analysis of variance was used to compare dif-ferences between treatment groups. The different groups had similar demo-graphic characteristics. At the end of the study, there were 55 evaluable patients. There was no significant difference between the placebo, 0.05 mg and 5 mg groups. In the 0.5 mg group, however, the DAS improved by approximately 15% from week 8 to 24 which was statistically significant when compared with placebo (*p<0.05). Thus, this study demonstrated a positive effect of oral collagen in RA and a similar dose effect as observed in animals and other previous human trials.

In uveitis, a pilot trial of S-Ag and an S-Ag mixture has been completed at the National Eye Institute (Bethesda, MD, USA) and showed positive trends with oral bovine S-Ag but not the retinal mixture [145]. Feeding of peptide derived from patient's own HLA antigen appeared to have effect on uveitis in that patients could discontinue their steroids because of reduced intraocu-lar inflammation mediated by oral tolerance [121].

Trials have been initiated in new-onset diabetes in which recombinant human insulin is administered orally, and trials are underway in subjects at risk for diabetes as part of the diabetes prevention trial (DPT-1). Preliminary analysis of a randomized double-blind placebo-controlled study of oral insu-lin in newly diagnosed type 1 diabetes demonstrated preserved beta cell function as measured by endogenous C-peptide insulin responses in adult new onset diabetics fed 10mg of recombinant human insulin as compared to those fed placebo [146].

Oral desensitization to nickel-allergy in humans induces a decrease in nickel-specific T cells and affects cutaneous eczema [147]. Positive effects were reported in an open-label pilot study of oral type 1 collagen in patients with systemic sclerosis [148]. A pilot immunological study of oral MHC peptides has been initiated in transplantation patients. Based on results to date in humans, it appears that the clinical application of oral antigen for the treat-ment of human conditions will depend on the specific disease, the nature and dosages of proteins administered and may require the use of synergists or mucosal adjuvants to enhance biologic effects. Also, recombinant human proteins may be more efficacious than animal proteins [149].

FUTURE DIRECTIONS

Although it is clear that oral antigen can suppress autoimmunity and inflammatory diseases in animals, much remains to be learned. Under certain experimental conditions worsening of autoimmune diseases in animals by oral antigen has been reported [110, 150-152]. Cell surface molecules and cytokines associated with inductive events in the gut that generate and modulate oral tolerance are not completely understood. Important areas of investigation include cytokine and chemokine milieu, antigen presentation and co-stimulation requirements, routes of antigen processing, form of the antigen, role of the liver, the effect or oral antigens on antibody and IgE responses and on CTLs, and the role of $\gamma\delta$ T-cells or CD4+CD25+ cells. As the molecular events associated with the generation and modulation of oral tolerance are better understood, the ability to apply mucosal tolerance successfully for the treatment of human autoimmune and other diseases will be further enhanced.

REFERENCES

1. Wells, HG. 1911. Studies on the chemistry of anaphylaxis (III). Experiments with isolated proteins, especially those of the hen's egg. J. Infect. Dis. 8:147.
2. Chase, M. 1946. Inhibition of experimental drug allergy by prior feeding of the sensitizing agent. Proc. Soc. Exp. Biol. Med. 61:257.
3. Husby, S, Mestecky, J, Moldoveanu, Z, Holland, S, and Elson, CO. 1994. Oral tolerance in humans. T-cell but not B cell tolerance after antigen feeding. J. Immunol. 152:4663.
4. Mowat, AM. 1987. The regulation of immune responses to dietary protein antigens. Immunol. Today 8:93.
5. Weiner, HL. 1997. Oral tolerance: immune mechanisms and treatment of autoimmune diseases. Immunol. Today 18:335.
6. Bruce, MG, and Ferguson, A. 1986. The influence of intestinal processing on the immunogenicity and molecular size of absorbed, circulating ovalbumin in mice. Immunology 59:295.
7. Husby, S, Jensenius, JC, and Svehag, S-E. 1986. Passage of undergraded dietary antigen into the blood of healthy adults. Further characterization of the kinetics of uptake and the size distribution of the antigen. Scand. J. Immunol. 24:447.
8. Bruce, MG, and Ferguson, A. 1987. Oral tolerance induced by gut-processed antigen. Adv. Exp. Med. Biol. 216A:721.
9. Richman, LK, Graeff, AS, and Strober, W. 1981. Antigen presentation by macrophage-enriched cells from the mouse Peyer's patch. Cell. Immunol. 62:110.
10. Liu, LM, and MacPherson, GG. 1993. Antigen acquisition by dendritic cells: intestinal dendritic cells acquire antigen administered orally and can prime naive T-cells in vivo. J. Exp. Med. 177:1299.
11. Bland, PW, and Warren, LG. 1986. Antigen presentation by epithelial cells of the rat small intestine. II Selective induction of suppressor T-cells. Immunology 58:9.
12. Mayer, L, and Shlien, R. 1987. Evidence for function of Ia molecules on gut epithe-

lial cells in man. J. Exp. Med. 166:1471.

13. Galliaerde, V, Desvignes, C, Peyron, E, and Kaiserlian, D. 1995. Oral tolerance to haptens: intestinal epithelial cells from 2,4-dinitrochlorobenzene-fed mice inhibit hapten-specific T-cell activation in vitro. Eur. J. Immunol. 25:1385.

14. Harper, HM, Cochrane, L, and Williams, NA. 1996. The role of small intestinal antigen-presenting cells in the induction of T-cell reactivity to soluble protein antigens: association between aberrant presentation in the lamina propria and oral tolerance. Immunology 89:449.

15. Daynes, R, Araneo, B, Dowell, T, Huang, K, and Dudley, D. 1990. Regulation of murine lymphokine production in vivo. III. The lymphoid tissue microenvironment exerts regulatory influences over T helper cell function. J. Exp. Med. 171:979.

16. Xu-Amano, J, Aicher, WK, Taguchi, T, Kiyono, H, and McGhee, JR. 1992. Selective induction of Th_2 cells in murine Peyer's patches by oral immunization. Int. Immunol. 4:433.

17. Abbas, AK, Murphy, KM, and Sher, A. 1996. Functional diversity of helper T lymphocytes. Nature 383:787.

18. Liu, L, Rich, BE, Inobe, J-I, Chen, W, and Weiner, HL. 1998. Induction of T helper 2 cell differentiation in the primary immune response: dendritic cells isolated from adherent cell culture treated with interleukin-10 prime naive CD4+ T-cells to secrete interleukin-4. Int. Immunol. 10:1017.

19. DeSmedt, T, Van Mechelen, M, De Becker, G, et al. 1997. Effect of interleukin-10 on dendritic cell maturation and function. Eur. J. Immunol. 27:1229.

20. Kalinski, P, Hilkens, CM, Snijders, A, Snijdewint, FG, and Kapsenberg, ML. 1997. IL-12 deficient dendritic cells, generated in the presence of prostaglandin E2, promote type 2 cytokine production in maturing human naive T helper cells. J. Immunol. 159:28.

21. Everson, MP, Lemak, DG, McGhee, JR, and Beagley, KW. 1997. FACS-sorted spleen and Peyer's patch dendritic cells induce different responses in Th0 clones. Adv. Exp. Med. Biol. 417:357.

22. Iwasaki, A, and Kelsall, BL. 1999. Freshly isolated Peyer's patch, but not spleen, dendritic cells produce interleukin 10 and induce the differentiation of T helper type 2 cells. J. Exp. Med. 190:229.

23. Viney, JL, Mowat, AM, O'Malley, JM, Williamson, E, and Fanger, NA. 1998. Expanding dendritic cells in vivo enhances the induction of oral tolerance. J. Immunol. 160:5815.

24. Freeman, GJ, Boussiotis, VA, Anumanthan, A, et al. 1995. B7-1 and B7-2 do not deliver identical costimulatory signals, since B7-2 but not B7-1 preferentially costimulates the initial production of IL-4. Immunity 2:523.

25. Liu, L, Kuchroo, VK, and Weiner, HL. 1998. B7.2 but not B7.1 costimulation is required for the induction of low dose oral tolerance. FASEB J. I:A597.

26. Samoilova, EB, Horton, JL, Zhang, H, et al. 1998. CTLA4 is required for the induction of high dose oral tolerance. Int. Immunol. 10:491.

27. Kweon, MN, Fujihashi, K, Wakatsuki, Y, et al. 1999. Mucosally induced systemic T cell unresponsiveness to ovalbumin requires CD40 ligand-CD40 interactions. J. Immunol. 162:1904.

28. Desvignes, C, Bour, H, Nicolas, JF, and Kaiserlian, D. 1996. Lack of oral tolerance but oral priming for contact sensitivity to dinitrofluorobenzene in major histocompatibility complex class II-deficient mice and in CD4+ T-cell-depleted mice. Eur. J. Immunol. 26:1756.

29. Newberry, RD, Stenton, WF, and Lorenz, RG. 1999. Cyclooxygenase-2-dependent arachidonic acid metabolites are essential modulators of the intestinal immune response to dietary antigen. Nature Med. 5:900.

30. Santos, LMB, al-Sabbagh, A, Londono, A, and Weiner, HL. 1994. Oral tolerance

to myelin basic protein induces regulatory TGF-β-secreting T-cells in Peyer's patches of SJL mice. Cell. Immunol. 157:439.

31. Chen, Y, Kuchroo, VK, Inobe, J-I, Hafler, DA, and Weiner, HL. 1994. Regulatory T-cell clones induced by oral tolerance: suppression of autoimmune encephalomyelitis. Science 265:1237.

32. Chen, Y, Inobe, J, and Weiner, HL. 1995. Induction of oral tolerance to myelin basic protein in CD8-depleted mice: both CD4+ and CD8+ cells mediate active suppression. J. Immunol. 155:910.

33. Inobe, J, Slavin, AJ, Komagata, Y, et al. 1998. IL-4 is a differentiation factor for transforming growth factor-beta secreting Th3 cells and oral administration of IL-4 enhances oral tolerance in experimental allergic encephalomyelitis. Eur. J. Immunol. 28:2780.

34. Mosmann, TR, and Sad, S. 1996. The expanding universe of T-cell subsets: Th1, Th2, and more. Immunol. Today 17:138.

35. Powrie, F, Carlino, J, Leach, MW, Mauze, S, and Coffman, RL. 1996. A critical role for transforming growth factor-beta but not interleukin 4 in the suppression of T helper type 1-mediated colitis by CD45RB (low) CD4+ T-cells. J. Exp. Med. 183:2669.

36. Seddon, B, and Mason, D. 1999. Regulatory T cells in the control of autoimmunity: the essential role of transforming growth factor beta and interleukin 4 in the prevention of autoimmune thyroiditis in rats by peripheral CD4(+)CD45RC- cells and CD4(+)CD8(-) thymocytes. J. Exp. Med. 189:279.

37. Groux, H, O'Garra, A, Bigler, M, et al. 1997. A CD4+ T-cell subset inhibits antigen-specific T-cell responses and prevents colitis. Nature 389:737.

38. Miller, A, Lider, O, and Weiner, HL. 1991. Antigen-driven bystander suppression following oral administration of antigens. J. Exp. Med. 174:791.

39. McCarron, R, Fallis, R, and McFarlin, D. 1990. Alterations in T-cell antigen specificity and class II restriction during the course of chronic relapsing experimental allergic encephlomyelitis. J. Neuroimmunol. 29:73.

40. Lehmann, P, Forsthuber, T, Miller, A, and Sercarz, E. 1992. Spreading of T-cell autoimmunity to cryptic determinants of an autoantigen. Nature 358:155.

41. Cross, AH, Tuohy, VK, and Raine, CS. 1993. Development of reactivity to new myelin antigens during chronic relapsing autoimmune demyelination. Cell. Immunol. 146:261.

42. Kaufman, DI, Clare-Salzler, M, Tian, J, et al. 1993. Spontaneous loss of T-cell tolerance to glutamic acid decarboxylase in murine insulin-dependent diabetes. Nature 366:69.

43. Tisch, R, Yang, X-D, Singer, SM, et al. 1993. Immune response to glutamic acid decarboxylase correlates with insulitis in non-obese diabetic mice. Nature 366:72.

44. Kerlero de Rosbo, N, Milo, R, Lees, MB, et al. 1993. Reactivity to myelin antigens in multiple sclerosis: peripheral blood lymphocytes respond predominantly to myelin oligodendrocyte glycoprotein. J. Clin. Invest. 92:2602.

45. Zhang, J, Markovic, S, Raus, J, et al. 1993. Increased frequency of IL-2 responsive T-cells specific for myelin basic protein and proteolipid protein in peripheral blood and cerebrospinal fluid of patients with multiple sclerosis. J. Exp. Med. 179:973.

46. Harrison, LC. 1992. Islet cell antigens in insulin-dependent diabetes: Pandora's box revisited. Immunol. Today 13:348.

47. Teng, Y, Gorczynski, R, and Hozumi, N. 1998. The function of TGF-beta-mediated innocent bystander suppression associated with physiological self-tolerance in vivo. Cell. Immunol. 190:51.

48. Schwartz, RH. 1990. A cell culture model for T lymphocyte clonal anergy. Science 248:1349.

49. Whitacre, CC, Gienapp, IE, Orosz, CG, and Bitar, D. 1991. Oral tolerance in experimental autoimmune encephalomyelitis. III. Evidence for clonal anergy. J. Immunol. 147:2155.

50. Van Houten, N, and Blake, SF. 1996. Direct measurement of anergy of antigen-specific T-cells following oral tolerance induction. J. Immunol. 157:1337.

51. Melamed, D, and Friedman, A. 1993. Direct evidence for anergy in T lymphocytes tolerized by oral administration of ovalbumin. Eur. J. Immunol. 23:935.

52. Jewell, S, Dierksheide, J, Curry, A, Shrestha, A, and Waldman, J. 1998. Suppression of experimental autoimmune encephalomyelitis (EAE) by portal vein (PV) injection of myelin basic protein (MBP). FASEB J. 12:A600.

53. Taams, LS, van Rensen, AJML, Poelen, MCM, et al. 1998. Anergic T-cells actively suppress T-cell responses via the antigen-presenting cell. Eur. J. Immunol. 28:2902.

54. Hoyne, GF, and Lamb, JR. 1997. Regulation of T-cell function in mucosal tolerance. Immunol. Cell Biol. 75:197.

55. Chen, Y, Inobe, J, Marks, R, et al. 1995. Peripheral deletion of antigen-reactive T-cells in oral tolerance. Nature 376:177.

56. Mowat, AM, Steel, M, Worthy, EA, Kewin, PJ, and Garside, P. 1996. Inactivation of Th1 and Th2 cells by feeding ovalbumin. Ann. N. Y. Acad. Sci. 778:122.

57. Miller, ML, Cowdery, JS, Laskin, CA, Curtin, M, Jr., and Steinberg, AD. 1984. Heterogeneity of oral tolerance defects in autoimmune mice. Clin. Immunol. Immunopathol. 31:231.

58. Mowat, A. 1998. Putative role of p55 TNF receptor, but not fas in oral tolerance. FASEB J. 12:A598.

59. Marth, T, Zeitz, M, Ludviksson, BR, Strober, W, and Kelsall, BL. 1999. Extinction of IL-12 signaling promotes Fas-mediated apoptosis of antigen-specific T cells. J. Immunol. 162:7233.

60. Seder, RA, Marth, T, Sieve, MC, et al. 1998. Factors involved in the differentiation of TGF-β-producing cells from naive CD4+ T-cells: IL-4 and IFN-γ have opposing effects, while TGF-β positively regulates its own production. J. Immunol. 160:5719.

61. Slavin, AJ, Maron, R, Garcia, G, Gonnella, P, and Weiner, HL. 1998. Oral administration of IL-4 and IL-10 enhance the induction of low dose oral tolerance. FASEB J. II:A599.

62. Xiao, BG, Bai, XF, Zhang, GX, and Link, H. 1998. Suppression of acute and protracted-relapsing experimental allergic encephalomyelitis by nasal administration of low-dose IL-10 in rats. J. Neuroimmunol. 84:230.

63. Zhang, Z, and Michael, JG. 1990. Orally inducible immune unresponsiveness is abrogated by IFN-γ treatment. J. Immunol. 144:4163.

64. Marth, T, Strober, W, and Kelsall, BL. 1996. High dose oral tolerance in ovalbumin TCR-transgenic mice: Systemic neutralization of IL-12 augments TGF-β secretion and T-cell apoptosis. J. Immunol. 157:2348.

65. Claessen, AM, von Blomberg, BM, De Groot, J, et al. 1996. Reversal of mucosal tolerance by subcutaneous administration of interleukin-12 at the site of attempted sensitization. Immunology 88:363.

66. Rizzo, LV, Miller-Rivero, NE, Chan, C-C, et al. 1994. Interleukin-2 treatment potentiates induction of oral tolerance in a murine model of autoimmunity. J. Clin. Invest. 94:1668.

67. Khoury, SJ, Lider, O, al-Sabbagh, A, and Weiner, HL. 1990. Suppression of experimental autoimmune encephalomyelitis by oral administration of myelin basic protein. III. Synergistic effect of lipopolysaccharide. Cell. Immunol. 131:302.

68. Nelson, PA, Akselband, Y, Dearborn, SM, et al. 1996. Effect of oral beta interferon on subsequent immune responsiveness. Ann. N. Y. Acad. Sci. 778:145.

69. Elson, CO, and Ealding, W. 1984. Cholera toxin feeding did not induce oral tol-

erance in mice and abrogated oral tolerance to an unrelated protein antigen. J. Immunol. 133:2892.

70. Sun, J-B, Holmgren, C, and Czerkinsky, C. 1994. Cholera toxin B subunit: an efficient transmucosal carrier-delivery system for induction of peripheral immunological tolerance. Proc. Natl. Acad. Sci. U. S. A. 91:10795.

71. Ma, D, Mellon, J, and Niederkorn, JY. 1997. Oral administration as a strategy for enhancing corneal allograft survival. Br. J. Ophthalmol. 81:778.

72. Karpus, WJ, Kennedy, KJ, Kunkel, SL, and Lukacs, NW. 1998. Monocyte chemotactic protein 1 regulates oral tolerance induction by inhibition of T helper cell1-related cytokines. J. Exp. Med. 187:733.

73. Elson, CO, Tomasi, M, Dertzbaugh, MT, et al. 1996. Oral antigen delivery by way of a multiple emulsion system enhances oral tolerance. Ann. N. Y. Acad. Sci. 778:156.

74. Mengel, J, Cardillo, F, Aroeira, LS, et al. 1995. Anti-γδ T-cell antibody blocks the induction and maintenance of oral tolerance to ovalbumin in mice. Immunolology Letters 48:97.

75. Ke, Y, Pearce, K, Lake, JP, Ziegler, HK, and Kapp, JA. 1997. Gamma delta T lymphocytes regulate the induction and maintenance of oral tolerance. J. Immunol. 158:3610.

76. Spahn, TW, and Weiner, HL. 1998. γδ T-cells are necessary for low dose but not high dose oral tolerance. FASEB J. I2:A597.

77. Wolvers, DA, Bakker, JM, Bagchus, WM, and Kraal, G. 1998. The steroid hormone dehydroepiandrosterone (DHEA) breaks intranasally induced tolerance, when administered at time of systemic immunization. J. Immunol. 89:19.

78. Yoshino, S, Ohsawa, M, and Sagai, M. 1998. Diesel exhaust particles block induction of oral tolerance in mice. J. Pharmacol. Exp. Ther. 287:679.

79. Thorbecke, GJ, Schwarcz, R, Leu, J, Huang, C, and Simmons, WJ. 1999. Modulation by cytokines of induction of oral tolerance to type II collagen. Arthritis Rheum. 42:110.

80. Javed, NH, Gienapp, IE, Cox, KL, and Whitacre, CC. 1995. Exquisite peptide specificity of oral tolerance in experimental autoimmune encephalomyelitis. J. Immunol. 155:1599.

81. Miller, A, al-Sabbagh, A, Santos, L, Das, MP, and Weiner, HL. 1993. Epitopes of myelin basic protein that trigger TGF-β release following oral tolerization are distinct from encephalitogenic epitopes and mediate epitope driven bystander suppression. J. Immunol. 151:7307.

82. Khoury, SJ, Hancock, WW, and Weiner, HL. 1992. Oral tolerance to myelin basic protein and natural recovery from experimental autoimmune encephalomyelitis as associated with downregulation of inflammatory cytokines and differential upregulation of transforming growth factor β, interleukin 4, and prostaglandin E expression in the brain. J. Exp. Med. 176:1355.

83. Higgins, P, and Weiner, HL. 1988. Suppression of experimental autoimmune encephalomyelitis by oral administration of myelin basic protein and its fragments. J. Immunol. 140:440.

84. Brod, SA, al-Sabbagh, A, Sobel, RA, Hafler, DA, and Weiner, HL. 1991. Suppression of experimental autoimmune encephalomyelitis by oral administration of myelin antigens. IV. Suppression of chronic relapsing disease in the Lewis rat and strain 13 guinea pig. Ann. Neurol. 29:615.

85. al-Sabbagh, AM, Goad, EP, Weiner, HL, and Nelson, PA. 1996. Decreased CNS inflammation and absence of clinical exacerbation of disease after six months oral administration of bovine myelin in diseased SJL/J mice with chronic relapsing experimental autoimmune encephalomyelitis. J. Neurosci. Res. 45:424.

86. al-Sabbagh, AM, Garcia, G, Slavin, AJ, Weiner, HL, and Nelson, PA. 1997. Combination therapy with oral myelin basic protein and oral methotrexate

enhances suppression of experimental autoimmune encephalomyelitis. Neurology 48:A421.

87. Metzler, B, and Wraith, DC. 1993. Inhibition of experimental autoimmune encephalomyelitis by inhalation but not oral administration of the encephalitogenic peptide: influence of MHC binding affinity. Int. Immunol. 5:1159.

88. Maron, R, Slavin, A, and Weiner, HL. 1998. Oral tolerance to glatiramer acetate (Copl, Copaxone) in MBPT cell receptor transgenic mice. J. Neuroimmunol. 90:82.

89. Teitelbaum, D, Arnon, R, and Sela, M. 1998. Immunomodulation of experimental allergic encephalomyelitis by oral administration of copolymer 1 (Copaxone®). J. Neuroimmunol. 90:85.

90. Teitelbaum, D, Arnon, R, and Sela, M. 1999. Immunomodulation of experimental autoimmune encephalomyelitis by oral administration of copolymer 1. Proc. Natl. Acad. Sci. U. S. A. 96:3842.

91. Weiner, HL. 1999. Oral tolerance with Copolymer 1 for the treatment of multiple sclerosis. Proc. Natl. Acad. Sci. U. S. A. 96:3333.

92. Thompson, HSG, and Staines, NA. 1986. Gastric administration of type II collagen delays the onset and severity of collagen-induced arthritis in rats. Clin. Exp. Immunol. 64:581.

93. Thompson, HSG, Harper, N, Bevan, DJ, and Staines, NA. 1993. Suppression of collagen induced arthritis by oral administration of type II collagen: changes in immune and arthritic responses mediated by active peripheral suppression. Autoimmunity 16:189.

94. Nagler-Anderson, C, Bober, LA, Robinson, ME, Siskind, GW, and Thorbeke, FJ. 1986. Suppression of type II collagen-induced arthritis by intragastric administration of soluble type II collagen. Proc. Natl. Acad. Sci. U. S. A. 83:7443.

95. Zhang, JZ, Lee, CSY, Lider, O, and Weiner, HL. 1990. Suppression of adjuvant arthritis in Lewis rats by oral administration of type II collagen. J. Immunol. 145:2489.

96. Haque, MA, Yoshino, S, Inada, S, et al. 1996. Suppression of adjuvant arthritis in rats by induction of oral tolerance to mycobacterial 65-kDa heat shock protein. Eur. J. Immunol. 26:2650.

97. Thompson, SJ, Thompson, HSG, Harper, N, et al. 1993. Prevention of pristane-induced arthritis by the oral administration of type II collagen. Immunology 79:152.

98. Yoshino, S, Quattrocchi, E, and Weiner, HL. 1995. Oral administration of type II collagen suppresses antigen-induced arthritis in Lewis rats. Arthritis Rheum. 38:1092.

99. Thompson, HS, and Staines, NA. 1986. Suppression of collagen-induced arthritis with pregastrically or intravenously administered type II collagen. Agents Actions 19:318.

100. Khare, SD, Krco, CJ, Griffiths, MM, Luthra, HS, and David, CS. 1995. Oral administration of an immunodominant human collagen peptide modulates collagen-induced arthritis. J. Immunol. 155:3653.

101. Staines, NA, Harper, N, Ward, FJ, et al. 1996. Mucosal tolerance and suppression of collagen-induced arthritis (CIA) induced by nasal inhalation of synthetic peptide 184-198 of bovine type II collagen (CII) expressing a dominant T-cell epitope. Clin. Exp. Immunol. 103:368.

102. Myers, LK, Seyer, JM, Stuart, JM, and Kang, AH. 1997. Suppression of murine collagen-induced arthritis by nasal administration of collagen. Immunology 90:161.

103. Prakken, BJ, van der Zee, R, Anderton, SM, et al. 1997. Peptide-induced nasal tolerance for a mycobacterial heat shock protein 60 T-cell epitope in rats suppresses both adjuvant arthritis and nonmicrobially induced experimental arthritis. Proc. Natl. Acad. Sci. U. S. A. 94:3284.

104. Zhang, JZ, Davidson, L, Eisenbarth, G, and Weiner, HL. 1991. Suppression of diabetes in NOD mice by oral administration of porcine insulin. Proc. Natl. Acad. Sci. U. S. A. 88:10252.

105. Bergerot, J, Fabien, N, Maguer, V, and Thivolet, C. 1994. Oral administration of human insulin to NOD mice generates CD4$^+$ T-cells that suppress adoptive transfer of diabetes. J. Autoimmun. 7:655.

106. Hancock, WW, Polanski, M, Zhang, ZJ, Blogg, N, and Weiner, HL. 1995. Suppression of insulitis in NOD mice by oral insulin administration is associated with selective expression of IL-4, IL-10, TGF-β and prostaglandin-E. Am. J. Pathol. 147:1193.

107. Harrison, LC, Dempsey-Collier, M, Kramer, DR, and Takahashi, K. 1996. Aerosol insulin induces regulatory CD8 $\gamma\delta$ T-cells that prevent murine insulin-dependent diabetes. J. Exp. Med. 184:2167.

108. Daniel, D, and Wegmann, DR. 1996. Protection of nonobese diabetic mice from diabetics by intranasal or subcutaneous administration of insulin peptide B-(9-23). Proc. Natl. Acad. Sci. U. S. A. 93:956.

109. Tian, J, Atkinson, MA, Clare-Salzler, M, et al. 1996. Nasal administration of glutamate decarboxylase (GAD65) peptides induces Th2 responses and prevents murine insulin-dependent diabetes. J. Exp. Med. 183:1561.

110. Blanas, E, Carbone, FR, Allison, J, Miller, JFAP, and Heath, WR. 1996. Induction of autoimmune diabetes by oral administration of autoantigen. Science 274:1707.

111. Von Herrath, MG, Dyrberg, T, and Oldstone, MBA. 1996. Oral insulin treatment suppresses virus-induced antigen-specific destruction of beta cells and prevents autoimmune diabetes in transgenic mice. J. Clin. Invest. 98:1324.

112. Polanski, M, Blogg, NS, Zhang, J, and Weiner, HL. 1997. Oral administration of the immunodominant B-chain of insulin suppresses diabetes in NOD mice and is associated with a switch from Th1 to Th2 cytokines. J. Autoimmun. 10:339.

113. Ma, SW, Zhao, DL, Yin, ZQ, et al. 1997. Transgenic plants expressing autoantigens fed to mice to induce oral immune tolerance. Nature Med. 3:793.

114. Arakawa, T, Yu, J, Chong, DK, et al. 1998. A plant-based cholera toxin B subunit-insulin fusion protein protects against the development of autoimmune diabetes. Nat. Biotechnol. 16:934.

115. Nussenblatt, RB, Caspi, RR, Mahdi, R, et al. 1990. Inhibition of S-antigen induced experimental autoimmune uveoretinitis by oral induction of tolerance with S-antigen. J. Immunol. 144:1689.

116. Singh, VK, Kalra, HK, Yamaki, K, and Shinohara, T. 1992. Suppression of experimental autoimmune uveitis in rats by the oral administration of the uveitopathogenic S-antigen fragment and a cross-reactive homologous peptide. Cell. Immunol. 139:81.

117. Vrabec, TR, Gregerson, DS, Dua, HS, and Donoso, LA. 1992. Inhibition of experimental autoimmune uveoretinitis by oral administration of S-antigen and synthetic peptides. Autoimmunity 12:175.

118. Wildner, G, and Thurau, SR. 1994. Cross-reactivity between an HLA-B27-derived peptide and a retinal autoantigen peptide: a clue to major histocompatibility complex association with autoimmune disease. Eur. J. Immunol. 24:2579.

119. Wildner, G, and Thurau, SR. 1995. Orally induced bystander suppression in experimental autoimmune uveoretinitis occurs only in the periphery and not in the eye. Eur. J. Immunol. 25:1292.

120. Thurau, SR, Chan, CC, Nussenblatt, RB, and Caspi, RR. 1997. Oral tolerance in a murine model of relapsing experimental autoimmune uveoretinitis (EAU): induction of protective tolerance in primed animals. Clin. Exp. Immunol. 109:370.

121. Thurau, SR, Diedrichs-Mohring, M, Fricke, H, Arbogast, S, and Wildner, G. 1997. Molecular mimicry as a therapeutic approach for an autoimmune disease: oral treatment of uveitis-patients with an MHC-peptide crossreactive with autoanti-

gen—first results. Immunol. Lett. 57:193.

122. Ma, C-G, Zhang, G-X, Xiao, B-G, et al. 1995. Suppression of experimental auto-immune myasthenia gravis by nasal administration of acetylcholine receptor. J. Neuroimmunol. 58:51.

123. Wang, H-M, and Smith, KA. 1987. The interleukin-2 receptor: functional consequences of its bimolecular structure. J. Exp. Med. 166:1055.

124. Wang, ZY, Qiao, J, and Link, H. 1993. Suppression of experimental autoimmune myasthenia gravis by oral administration of acetylcholine receptor. J. Neuroimmunol. 44:209.

125. Okumura, S, McIntosh, K, and Drachman, DB. 1994. Oral administration of acetylcholine receptor: effects on experimental myasthenia gravis. Ann. Neurol. 36:704.

126. Ma, CG, Zhang, GX, Xiao, BG, and Link, H. 1996. Cellular mRNA expression of interferon-gamma (IFN-γ), IL-4 and transforming growth factor-beta (TGF-β) in rats nasally tolerized against experimental autoimmune myasthenia gravis (EAMG). Clin. Exp. Immunol. 104:509.

127. Karachunski, PI, Ostlie, NS, Okita, DK, and Conti-Fine, BM. 1997. Prevention of experimental myasthenia gravis by nasal administration of synthetic acetylcholine receptor T epitope sequences. J. Clin. Invest. 100:3027.

128. Barchan, D, Souroujon, MC, Im, SH, Antozzi, C, and Fuchs, S. 1999. Antigen-specific modulation of experimental myasthenia gravis: Nasal tolerization with recombinant fragments of the human acetylcholine receptor alpha-subunit. Proc. Natl. Acad. Sci. U. S. A. 96:8086.

129. Shi, FD, Li, HL, Wang, HB, et al. 1999. Mechanisms of nasal tolerance induction in experimental autoimmune myasthenia gravis: Identification of regulatory cells. J. Immunol. 162:5757.

130. Neurath, MF, Fuss, I, Kelsall, BL, et al. 1996. Experimental granulomatous colitis in mice is abrogated by induction of TGF-β-mediated oral tolerance. J. Exp. Med. 183:2605.

131. Sayegh, MH, Zhang, ZJ, Hancock, WW, et al. 1992. Down-regulation of the immune response to histocompatibility antigen and prevention of sensitization by skin allografts by orally administered alloantigen. Transplantation 53:163.

132. Sayegh, MH, Khoury, SJ, Hancock, WH, Weiner, HL, and Carpenter, CB. 1992. Induction of immunity and oral tolerance with polymorphic class II major histocompatability complex allopeptides in the rat. Proc. Natl. Acad. Sci. U. S. A. 89:7762.

133. Hancock, W, Sayegh, M, Kwok, C, Weiner, H, and Carpenter, C. 1993. Oral but not intravenous, alloantigen prevents accelerated allograft rejection by selective intragraft Th2 cell activation. Transplantation 55:1112.

134. Guimaraes, VC, Quintans, J, Fisfalen, M-E, et al. 1995. Suppression of experimental autoimmune thyroiditis by oral administration of thyroglobulin. Endocrinology 136:3353.

135. Hoyne, GF, Callow, MG, Kuo, MC, and Thomas, WR. 1994. Inhibition of T-cell responses by feeding peptides containing major and cryptic epitopes: studies with the Der p I allergen. Immunology 83:190.

136. Ilan, Y, Prakash, R, Davidson, A, et al. 1997. Oral tolerization to adenoviral antigens permits long-term gene expression using recombinant adenoviral vectors. J. Clin. Invest. 99:1098.

137. Lowney, ED. 1968. Immunologic unresponsiveness to a contact sensitizer in man. J. Invest. Dermatol. 51:411.

138. Waldo, FB, Van Den Wall Bake, AWL, Mestecky, J, and Husby, S. 1994. Suppression of the immune response by nasal immunization. Clin. Immunol. Immunopathol. 72:30.

139. Fukaura, H, Kent, SC, Pietrusewicz, MJ, et al. 1996. Induction of circulating

myelin basic protein and proteolipid protein-specific transforming growth factor-beta1-secreting Th3 T-cells by oral administration of myelin in multiple sclerosis patients. J. Clin. Invest. 98:70.

140. Barnett, ML, Kremer, JM, St. Clair, EW, et al. 1998. Treatment of rheumatoid arthritis with oral type II Collagen: results of a multicenter, double-blind, placebo-controlled trial. Arthritis Rheum. 41:290.

141. Sieper, J, Kary, S, Sörensen, H, et al. 1996. Oral type II collagen treatment in early rheumatoid arthritis. Arthritis Rheum. 39:41.

142. Barnett, ML, Combitchi, D, and Trentham, DE. 1996. A pilot trial of oral type II collagen in the treatment of juvenile rheumatoid arthritis. Arthritis Rheum. 39:623.

143. Trentham, D, Dynesius-Trentham, R, Orav, E, et al. 1993. Effects of oral administration of type II collagen on rheumatoid arthritis. Science 261:1727.

144. Choy, EH, Scott, DL, Kingsley, GH, et al. 1999. Control of rheumatoid arthritis (RA) by oral tolerance with bovine type II collagen (CH). Arthritis Rheum. 42.

145. Nussenblatt, RB, Gery, I, Weiner, HL, et al. 1997. Treatment of uveitis by oral administration of retinal antigens: Results of a phase I/II randomized masked trial. Am. J. Ophthalmol. 123:583.

146. Coutant, R, Zeidler, A, Rappaport, R, et al. 1998. Oral insulin therapy in newly-diagnosed immune mediated (type I) diabetes. Preliminary analysis of a randomized double blind placebo controlled study. Diabetes 47 (Suppl 1):A97.

147. Bagot, M, Charue, D, Flechet, ML, et al. 1995. Oral desensitization in nickel allergy induces a decrease in nickel-specific T-cells. Eur. J. Dermatol. 5:614.

148. McKown, KM, Carbone, LD, Bustillo, J, et al. 1997. Open trial of oral type I collagen in patients with systemic sclerosis. Arthritis Rheum. 40:S100.

149. Miller, A, Lider, O, al-Sabbagh, A, and Weiner, H. 1992. Suppression of experimental autoimmune encephalomyelitis by oral administration of myelin basic protein. V. Hierarchy of suppression by myelin basic protein from different species. J. Neuroimmunol. 39:243.

150. Meyer, AL, Benson, JM, Gienapp, IE, Cox, KL, and Whitacre, CC. 1996. Suppression of murine chronic relapsing experimental autoimmune encephalomyelitis by the oral administration of myelin basic protein. J. Immunol. 157:4230.

151. Miller, A, Lider, O, Abramsky, O, and Weiner, HL. 1994. Orally administered myelin basic protein in neonates primes for immune responses and enhances experimental autoimmune encephalomyelitis in adult animals. Eur. J. Immunol. 24:1026.

152. Terato, K, Xiu, JY, Miyahara, H, Cremer, MA, and Griffiths, MM. 1996. Induction by chronic autoimmune arthritis in DBA/1 mice by oral administration of type II collagen and Escherichia coli lipopolysaccharide. Br. J. Rheumatol. 35:828.

HEMATOPOIETIC STEM CELL CHIMERISM AND TOLERANCE INDUCTION

8

Haval Shirwan and Suzanne T. Ildstad
Institute for Cellular Therapeutics
University of Louisville
Louisville, Kentucky, USA

INTRODUCTION

The immune system of mammals evolved to discriminate between self- and nonself-antigens. This assures protection from foreign pathogens without eliciting autoimmunity. The process of self/nonself discrimination is primarily acquired via positive and negative selection of T cells during ontogeny in the thymus. Thymic tolerance to self-antigens, however, is not absolute and several peripheral mechanisms have also evolved to reinforce tolerance to self-antigens and promote immunity to foreign antigens.

The mode of antigen recognition and response by T lymphocytes is critical to the establishment of tolerance to self and to the induction of adaptive immune responses to foreign antigens. T cells recognize antigens as peptides bound to the peptide-binding groove of major histocompatibility complex (MHC) molecules via clonally expressed T-cell antigen receptors (TCRs). This antigen-specific interaction transduces a signal designated as "signal 1". Signal 1 is not sufficient on its own to fully activate the T cell. Additional signals, referred to as costimulatory signals or "signal 2", are also required. Signal 2 is antigen-nonspecific and delivered through receptor/coreceptor interactions between the T cell and an antigen-presenting cell (APC). These two signals play a central role in immune regulation and determine the outcome of an antigenic challenge, which can either lead to a nonproductive response, manifested as tolerance, or a productive response to the antigen. A productive immune response can be either protective if mounted against antigens of the invading pathogen or pathogenic if elicited against self-antigens.

A. W. Thomson (ed.), Therapeutic Immunosuppression, 183–213.

Thymic and peripheral tolerance mechanisms have been the subject of intense studies not only for sheer scientific curiosity but also for potential therapeutic strategies through modulation of the immune response. Most conventional therapeutic approaches use non-specific, general immunosuppressive pharmaceuticals to prevent immune activation. Although several of these approaches have been effective in controlling autoimmunity and graft rejection, their efficacy was short lasting and their chronic use was associated with undesirable side effects in the host. More recent studies, therefore, exploited several aspects of T cell activation for the design of more specific immune modulation to prevent autoimmunity and graft rejection. Although these new approaches hold great promise, their routine use in clinical transplantation remains to be fully accomplished. Hematopoietic stem cell (HSC) transplantation represents an alternative approach for prevention of immune response and induction of antigen-specific tolerance. HSC transplantation targets reeducation of the immune system in the presence of antigens of interest so that it does not respond to these antigens. In this chapter we will first briefly discuss the major mechanisms critical to both immune activation and tolerance to self-antigens to better appreciate the potential of HSC transplantation as a clinical regimen to effectively prevent autoimmunity and graft rejection.

ADAPTIVE IMMUNITY

The survival of vertebrates in an environment with copious pathogenic microorganisms is primarily maintained by two types of immune responses; innate and adaptive. The innate immune system is believed to have evolved first and constitutes the first line of defence against pathogenic microorganisms. It employs relatively simple and evolutionary conserved recognition molecules and modes of recognition for responding to foreign pathogens. Innate immunity is rather prompt and efficient in controlling infection before the more effective and antigen-specific adaptive immune response develops [1]. This simplistic view of innate immunity has recently been called into question and there is accumulating evidence in the literature suggesting that the innate immunity plays a critical role in the regulation of adaptive immunity at the level of second signal and cytokine expression [1,2]. Innate immunity has been the subject of several recent reviews [1] and as such will not be discussed further in this chapter.

The adaptive immune system evolved to cope with rapidly changing pathogenic microorganisms [2]. Unlike innate immunity, the adaptive immune

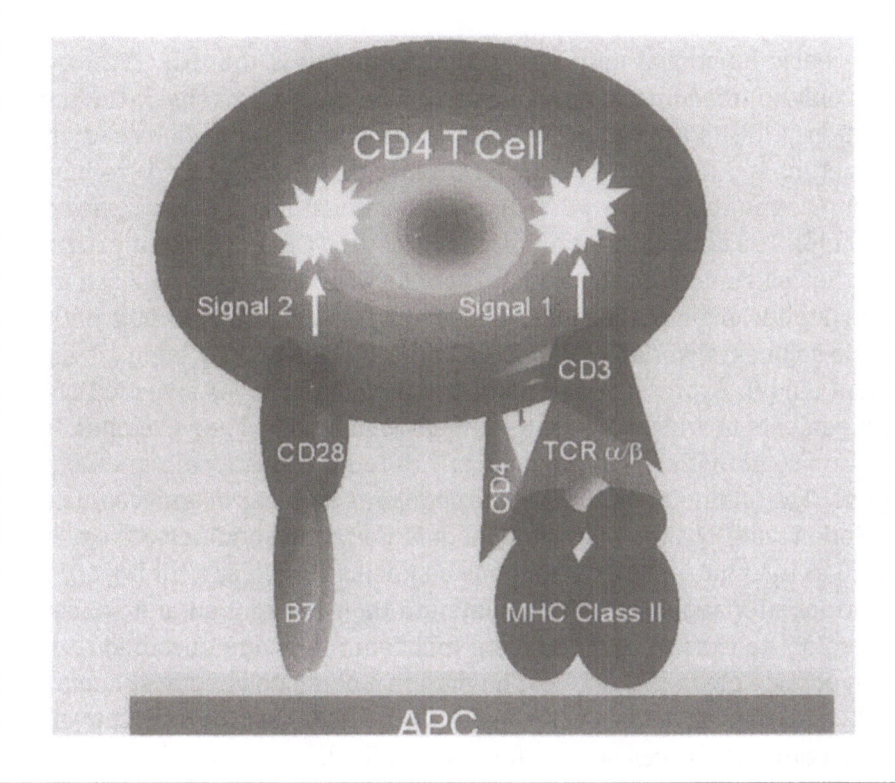

Figure 1
T cell activation. Full activation requires 2 distinct signals; signal 1 is antigen-specific and delivered by the TCR/peptide-MHC interaction whereas signal 2 is antigen-non-specific and delivered by the CD28/B7 interaction.

response employs sophisticated molecules and interactions to discriminate between self- and nonself-antigens. Fundamental to this well-designed and complex reaction, is the mode of antigen recognition and response by T cells. A productive T-cell response requires both the antigen-specific signal 1 and antigen-nonspecific signal 2 (Fig. 1) [3,4]. Transduction of these two signals results in a series of intracellular molecular changes that lead to T-cell activation. Activated T cells in turn synthesize and secret a battery of cytokines that orchestrate effector cells of the immune system for a productive immune response.

Signal 1

The basic functional unit of adaptive immunity is the TCR. TCR evolved not only to transduce signal 1 but also to ensure specificity of the immune response. TCRs are classified into two groups, α/β and γ/δ, based on their structure and function. The α/β TCR plays a key role in adaptive immunity whereas the role of the γ/δ TCR in conventional immune responses is less clear [5]. The antigen recognition chains of the TCR, α/β or γ/δ, are expressed on the cell surface in association with the CD3 complex [5,6]. Each α and β polypeptide chain of the TCR is encoded by several different noncontiguous gene segments; variable (V), diversity (D) (β chain only), joining (J), and constant (C) [7]. Expression of a mature TCR chain involves somatic DNA rearrangements in which a D gene segment joins with a J gene segment which in turn joins with a V gene segment to form a functional variable region gene. The joining of different gene segments involves extensive nucleotide deletion and DNA template independent nucleotide addition (N region addition) at the junctions between gene segments (Vα-Jα and Vβ-Dβ-Jβ). These rearranged V region gene segments are then transcribed and spliced to a C region gene to form a complete functional message encoding a mature polypeptide chain of the TCR. The mature α and β polypeptide chains of the TCR associate with the CD3 complex in the endoplasmic reticulum and are transported to the cell surface for function [5,8].

The hallmark of the vertebrate immune system is its ability to generate a specific immune response to any given antigen. This feature of the immune system is engraved in a vast repertoire of TCRs expressed by T cells. The TCR repertoire of an individual is shaped by: 1) the number of the TCR V, D, and J gene segments; 2) random rearrangement of a given V gene segment to any of D (β-chain) and J gene segments; 3) junctional deletion and addition of nucleotides; and 4) random assortment of α- and β-chain polypeptides. Additional TCR diversity is created by translation of D gene segments in all three reading frames [5,8]. Theoretically, an individual is capable of expressing ~10^{15} different TCRs [5]. The peripheral TCR repertoire, however, is significantly reduced as a result of deletion of T cells expressing self-reactive TCRs in the thymus to maintain tolerance to self-antigens [9-12].

The molecular basis of TCR antigen recognition has recently been elucidated by resolution of several crystal structures for TCR/MHC-peptide complexes [13,14]. Analysis of these structures revealed an Ig-like conformation for the TCR where the CDR1 and CDR2 domains, encoded by V genes, interact primarily with the MHC-encoded determinants. The CDR3 domain encoded by N, D, and J gene segments, on the other hand, dictates interaction with peptide antigen in the peptide-binding groove of the MHC [15-17]. The data from crystal structures is consistent with functional studies demonstrating that the CDR3 domain plays an important role in recognition of peptide antigens [18,19]. Asparagine and aspartic acid residues at defined positions of the CDR3 domain, for example, are important for the recognition of cytochrome c and myelin basic protein by $V\alpha3^+$ and $V\beta8.2^+$ TCRs, respectively [18,19]. Residues 88-103 of cytochrome c serve as an epitope for $V\alpha3/V\beta11^+$ TCRs. Using mice transgenic for the TCR α- or β-chains containing these V molecules, it was possible to demonstrate that immunization with variant cytochrome c peptides results in the selection of TCR containing CDR3 loops with reciprocal charges, thereby providing evidence for a direct physical contact between the TCR and antigen in the peptide-binding groove of the MHC [19].

Although the structural basis of T-cell interaction with peptide antigens is relatively well defined, the molecular nature of the ensuing signals and their mode of transduction are still major unresolved issues. The wealth of information on the TCR structure, antigen recognition, and biochemistry of signal transduction suggests that TCR is a versatile signaling apparatus with an inherent flexibility for antigen recognition that translates into different signaling patterns and functions. As these interactions are further defined, strategies to induce tolerance at the subcellular level may become possible.

Signal 2

Costimulation, or signal 2, is central to the function of adaptive immunity and serves as a link between the adaptive and innate immune systems [2]. Although several molecules such as CD28, CD2, CD154, LFA-1, and HSA have been implicated in the transduction of signal 2, CD28 appears to serve as the primary pathway for costimulation [20]. Engagement of the TCR with its cognate ligand, MHC-peptide complex, and CD28 with B7 molecules on the surface of APCs triggers a series of signaling cascades that act in synergy for full T-cell activation, as manifested by IL-2 synthesis and cell proliferation [21]. Costimulation also prolongs cell survival and sustains cytokine production [20,20-22]. For example, naïve T cells from CD28-deficient mice generate relatively normal responses to antigens with respect to cell proliferation and expression of activation markers, but they cannot sustain the response [23]. Transduction of signal 1 in the absence of costimulation not only results in a failure to induce an immune response but often results in functional inactivation of mature T cells [3]. This feature of adaptive immunity is essential for keeping autoimmune responses in check as well as providing a means for inducing peripheral tolerance to foreign antigens [24].

Costimulation has been exploited as a means of inducing peripheral tolerance in the transplantation setting. Blocking CD28 interaction with B7 molecules using either monoclonal antibody (mAb) or a recombinant fusion protein, CTLA-4Ig, prevents rejection of allogeneic and xenogeneic grafts [25,26]. CTLA-4 is another coreceptor for the B7 molecules and involved in negative regulation of the immune response [27]. Costimulatory blockade has also been effective in preventing graft-versus-host-disease (GVHD) and several autoimmune diseases, including experimental allergic encephalomyelitis, diabetes, and systemic lupus erythematosus [28,29]. Thus, the CD28/B7 pathway can be effectively manipulated for controlling pathologic immune responses, coping with detrimental infections, and inducing transplantation tolerance [30].

IMMUNE TOLERANCE

Tolerance to self-antigens is primarily established in the thymus via clonal deletion of thymocytes that express TCRs with high avidity for self-antigens. Tolerance via clonal deletion alone, however, may generate a significant deficit in the peripheral TCR repertoire that would compromise the response of the host to pathogens. Additional mechanisms, therefore, have evolved to control self-reactive T cells in the periphery. In this section, we will briefly describe major mechanisms that are important for the maintenance of tolerance to self-antigens in order to better understand attempts using HSC transplantation for reeducation of the immune system to prevent graft rejection and induce transplantation tolerance.

Central Tolerance

Tolerance to self-antigens is established in the thymus via positive and negative selection of T cells during ontogeny (Fig. 2). Experimental evidence for these two processes has been provided using congenic or transgenic mice that express both the antigen-specific TCRs and respective antigens. Negative selection of self-reactive T cells in the thymus was first demonstrated in studies investigating the development of T cells reactive to endogenous mouse mammary superantigens in mice. Vβ17⁺ T cells recognize mouse mammary superantigens in the context of class II H-2IE molecule. The cells expressing Vβ17 were shown to be eliminated from both mature thymocytes

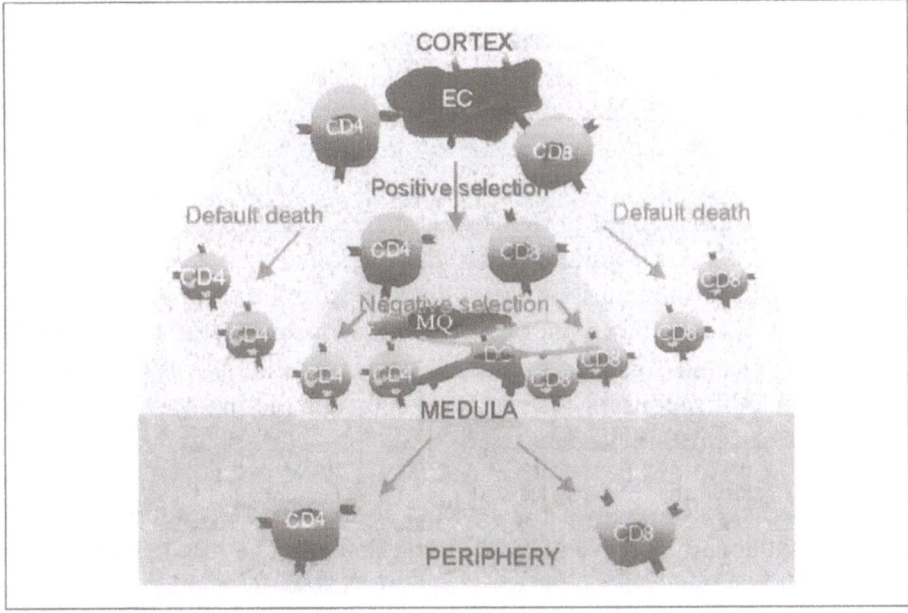

Figure 2
Thymic selection. T cells that react with MHC molecules expressed by epithelial cells in the thymic cortex are rescued by positive selection from the default death pathway. Those expressing receptors with strong avidity for the MHC-peptide complexes presented by bone marrow-derived APCs in the medulla are negatively selected via apoptosis. Cells with low avidity receptors then migrate to the periphery to safeguard the organism against foreign pathogens.

and peripheral T cell populations of mice expressing the IE molecule and the superantigen, providing the first physical evidence for negative selection in the thymus [9]. Positive selection was demonstrated using mice transgenic for a TCR (2C) that has high avidity for the H-2L^d and low avidity for the H-2K^b class I molecules. A large fraction of T cells in the periphery of H-2^b transgenic mice expressed the 2C TCR [31]. In marked contrast, these T cells were deleted in the periphery of transgenic mice expressing H-2L^d at the CD4$^+$CD8$^+$ double positive stage. Most importantly, T cells expressing the 2C TCR were not found in the periphery of mice with a noncrossreactive H-2^s haplotype. Taken together, these data clearly demonstrate that TCR interaction with MHC molecules in the thymus is important for positive selection. This interaction, however, needs to be of low avidity so that T cells can be rescued from negative selection.

Although positive and negative selection in the thymus are well-established phenomena, the nature of cells, molecules, and biochemical events responsible for these selection processes are still the subject of intense debate. It is generally accepted that during ontogeny thymocytes without a productive TCR rearrangement and expression on the cell surface are eliminated via death by neglect. Thymocytes expressing TCR interacting with self-MHC-peptide complexes displayed on cortical thymic epithelial cells are rescued from the default death pathway by positive selection. Positively selected thymocytes then migrate to the thymic medulla where they are subjected to negative selection. Paradoxically, this negative selection also requires interaction with the same self-MHC-peptide complexes [32-34]. Some differences, however, must exist between these two processes that allow the positively selected T cells to escape negative selection in order to form the peripheral TCR repertoire instructed to recognize foreign antigens in the context of self-MHC molecules.

Two hypotheses have been put forward to explain the nature of the processes that govern positive and negative selection. The first hypothesis proposes that positive selection is mediated by TCR/MHC-peptide interactions of lower avidity than those responsible for negative selection or mature T-cell activation [35-37]. This process, therefore, allows survival of T cells whose reactivity with self-MHC-peptide complexes is sufficient enough to drive positive selection without triggering negative selection or activation. In the periphery, these T cells are activated by cross-reaction with MHC-foreign peptide complexes with higher avidity. Ligand density may also play a critical role in the selection process by contributing to overall avidity of TCR for MHC-peptide complexes. Low ligand density may lead to positive selection whereas high ligand density may cause negative selection [36,38]. The alternative hypothesis proposes that positive and negative selections are regulated by kinetics of TCR interaction with the MHC-peptide complex and that the half-life of the TCR/MHC-peptide complex is particularly important [37,39]. Complexes with relatively short half-lives deliver an incomplete signal and trigger positive selection while those with longer half-lives deliver a more complete signal and trigger negative selection.

The nature of APCs and the physiological state of thymocytes and their sensitivity to differential signaling events may also play fundamental roles in the commitment of the cells to positive versus negative selection events. It is generally assumed that cortical epithelial cells expressing self-MHC-peptide complexes mediate positive selection whereas negative selection is mediated in the medulla by endothelial cells and bone marrow-derived APCs [40]. It is presently unknown whether APCs actively participate in the selection processes by transducing differential signals to the interacting thymocytes or if they only serve as cargoes for self-MHC-peptide complexes. An additional factor that may affect positive and negative selection is the developmental stage of thymocytes. It is assumed that early in the development, TCR-mediated signals induce positive selection whereas similar signals lead to negative selection later. This differential effect may be due to the coupling of signaling pathways to different transcriptional and posttranslational events [41,42].

Peripheral Tolerance

Although clonal deletion is the central mechanism responsible for tolerance to self-antigens, it is not sufficient to confer tolerance to all peripheral antigens. First, the thymus is not accessible to all antigens, thus thymocytes are not exposed to all peripheral antigens during ontogeny. Second, clonal deletion of all thymocytes with potential self-reactivity would leave the organism with a restricted TCR repertoire with limited cross-reactivity with foreign antigens. The vertebrate immune system has, therefore, acquired peripheral mechanisms that regulate T-cell responses to self-antigens while assuring immunity to pathogens. Clonal ignorance, anergy, and activation-induced cell death (AICD) are three important peripheral mechanisms that ensure tolerance to self-antigens.

Clonal ignorance

Immunological ignorance is a state of indifference of peripheral T cells to antigens. Numerous studies using transgenic animals that express foreign antigens extrathymically provided basis for our understanding of this form of immunological unresponsiveness [43-45]. Specific expression of the SV40 large T antigen in pancreatic islet beta cells of mice did not result in T-cell activation nor tolerance [43]. T cells in transgenic animals did not respond to the tissue-specific large T antigen in vivo even after priming, but were fully responsive in vitro. This state of immune nonresponsiveness could not be broken by adoptive transfer of antigen-specific immune T cells unless the costimulatory molecule B7-1 was coexpressed in islets. These data provide clear evidence for the role of costimulation in immune ignorance. In a similar study, Ohashi et al. [44] demonstrated that expression of lymphocytic choriomeningitis viral glycoprotein in islets of mice transgenic for virus-specific TCR did not result in immune reactivity or tolerance. Infection of double transgenics with the virus, however, resulted in the destruction of the islets. This type of immune nonresponsiveness is not unique to transgenically expressed antigens and also applies to immune nonresponsiveness to peripheral antigens in adults. For example, transplantation of APC-depleted islet allografts into SCID mice followed by reconstitution of these animals with T-cell-depleted BM cells to reconstitute the peripheral lymphocyte repertoire does not result in rejection nor tolerance to islet allografts [45]. These observations clearly suggest that signal 2 plays a critical role in regulating peripheral immune responses. The nature of APCs and anatomical compartment in which the antigens are expressed may also play a role in immunological ignorance.

Clonal deletion

Deletion of autoreactive mature T cells is another form of peripheral tolerance believed to be mediated by activation-induced cell death (AICD) [46-48]. AICD is induced by repeated stimulation of T cells with antigens in the presence of high levels of IL-2 [46]. IL-2 facilitates AICD by i) upregulating the transcription and surface expression of Fas ligand (FasL) and ii) suppressing the transcription and expression of the Fas-associated death domain-like IL-1β-converting enzyme inhibitory protein, an inhibitor of apoptosis [46]. T cells upregulate both Fas and FasL upon activation. The engagement of Fas with FasL either in an autocrine or paracrine fashion results in apoptosis of the responding T cell [49,50]. The importance of this pathway for the induction of peripheral tolerance to self-antigens is manifested in mice carrying congenital mutation for Fas or FasL or in knockouts for Fas, FasL, or IL-2R [46-48]. All these animals lack AICD and develop severe autoimmune disorders.

It has been known for some time that T cells undergo apoptosis via AICD upon repeated stimulation with specific MHC-peptide complexes [51]. AICD, therefore, plays a critical role in the establishment of immune homeostasis in vivo after any antigenic challenge. For example, systemic infection with lymphocytic choriomeningitis virus was accompanied by cellular expansion of virus-specific CD8+ T cells. The control of viral infection was then followed by a dramatic decrease in the number of virus-specific CD8+ T cells due to apoptosis [52]. In addition, AICD was demonstrated in several transgenic systems expressing TCRs with defined antigenic specificities. Immunization of the transgenics with the cognate antigens led to apoptosis of T cells via AICD [53]. AICD is not only a unique feature of transgenic systems as apoptosis can be induced by selected antigens in normal peripheral T cells. Both CD8+ and CD4+ T cells are susceptible to AICD induced through TCR-mediated recognition of allogeneic class I or class II MHC molecules, respectively [54]. In addition, AICD is triggered in CD4+ T cells by specific antigens, such as tetanus toxoid or myelin basic protein, presented by the appropriate class II molecules [55].

It is believed that peripheral tolerance to self-antigens is induced by chronic stimulation of autoreactive T cells with a large dose of antigens that eventually leads to AICD and the elimination of autoreactive T cells from the system. This contention is consistent with studies demonstrating that the antigen-induced suppression of T cells in vitro required high antigen concentration [56]. These in vitro studies have been corroborated by in vivo studies demonstrating that AICD was preferentially triggered in T cells with high avidity TCR responding to high concentrations of peptide antigens [57]. The development of autoimmunity in animals carrying mutations in molecules involved in apoptosis, taken together with studies demonstrating elimination of antigen-specific T cells by high doses of antigens, provide clear evidence that AICD is a critical component of the mechanisms that establish tolerance to peripheral antigens.

Clonal anergy

Anergy is defined as a state of immune nonresponsiveness to antigen [3]. The anergic state is characterized by T-cell refractoriness to further antigenic stimulation despite normal TCR expression on the cell surface and normal response to exogenous growth factors. A variety of experimental studies indicate that T-cell anergy can develop in response to a heterogeneous set of stimuli under different experimental conditions. Although the molecular mechanisms implicated in this process are not well defined, a series of recent studies using altered peptide ligands showed that anergy develops as a consequence of inadequate stimulation. Anergy can develop either due to inadequate delivery of signal 1 or signal 2 [3]. Occupancy of the TCR by an inappropriate ligand, such as altered peptide ligands that are modified at the TCR contact residues, can lead to inadequate transduction of signal 1 and anergy [58]. These ligands interact with TCR in an unproductive fashion invoking a subset of normal intracellular activation events that lead to anergy, rather than full T-cell activation [59]. Anergy can also develop if both signal 1 and signal 2 are transduced in the absence of IL-2. In variance from deletional tolerance, anergy can be overcome by the provision of cytokines such as IL-2 [60,61].

A large body of data indicates that T-cell anergy is induced in mature T-cell populations when TCR stimulation is not followed by cell proliferation. In this context, clonal anergy develops after an abortive stimulation and therefore may represent a mechanism by which potentially harmful autoreactive T lymphocytes, which have escaped thymic deletion, can be functionally inactivated [62]. Clonal anergy, however, is not restricted to mature peripheral T cells receiving unproductive signals from external stimuli but can also evolve during ontogeny in the thymus. A recent study has demonstrated that the normal thymus produces IL-2R+ CD4+ thymocytes that keep autoreactive T cells in check [63]. These regulatory thymocytes are anergic and can suppress the function of normal T cells. This suppressive effect can be overcome by costimulation with high doses of IL-2 and anti-CD28 antibody. These data, therefore, clearly suggest that anergy, similar to clonal deletion, can develop either centrally via selection of a subset of regulatory T cells in the thymus or peripherally via nonproductive T-cell activation.

Another form of anergy that has recently been described is "activation-induced anergy". This form of anergy has been demonstrated in several experimental systems to develop after full T-cell activation. T-cell response to nominal, viral, or bacterial superantigens in vivo leads to transient T-cell activation ensued by anergy [64-66]. For example, immunization of mice with B7-1-expressing allogeneic tumor cells resulted in activation of CD8+ T cells that was followed by the development of immune nonresponsiveness within 3 or 4 days of initial stimulation [65]. Similarly, administration of mitogenic anti-CD3 antibodies in vivo caused a potent inflammatory response secondary to the secretion of numerous T-cell-derived lymphokines. Following this activation stage, there was a state of T-cell unresponsiveness characterized by defective TCR signaling [67]. This form of anergy may represent a mechanism for down-regulating excessive inflammatory responses that present a potential threat to the integrity of the organism.

In conclusion, mammals evolved several elaborate mechanisms to ensure tolerance to self-antigens and immune reactivity to pathogenic organisms. Positive and negative selection events in the thymus are a critical component of this self-versus-nonself immune regulation. These central thymic events are complemented by several peripheral immunoregulatory mechanisms that further control autoreactive T cells in the periphery without compromising the ability of the host to respond to foreign antigens. Clonal deletion of autoreactive T cells via AICD, clonal ignorance, and clonal anergy are central to these peripheral immunoregulatory mechanisms.

HSC TRANSPLANTATION AND TOLERANCE INDUCTION: MACROCHIMERISM

HSC transplantation has evolved as an effective therapeutic regimen for the treatment of a steadily increasing number of life-threatening hereditary, malignant, hematological, and immunodeficient disorders. Most importantly, it has recently become clear that HSC transplantation leading to macro-chimerism induces immune nonresponsiveness and/or tolerance to foreign cells, tissues, and organ grafts performed within species or interspecies [68]. In addition, the potential use of HSC chimerism to cure autoimmunity has become more obvious in recent years [69]. The efficacy of HSC transplanta-tion as a modality to induce tolerance to self-antigens in case of autoimmu-nity and to foreign antigens in case of foreign grafts stems from its capacity to reeducate the existing peripheral immune system of the host so that it does not respond to selected antigenic stimuli. This approach, therefore, recapitulates in the adult all the central and peripheral immune mechanisms that develop during ontogeny to discriminate between self/nonself antigens. Using HSC transplantation to induce tolerance to foreign transplantation or autoimmune self-antigens obviates the need for chronic use of immuno-suppressive pharmaceuticals that are not only ineffective in preventing the pathogenic conditions, but also have deleterious side effects in the recipi-ent.

HSC transplantation has been effective in inducing tolerance to a series of grafts in several different rodent models [68-73]. Its widespread use in clinics, however, is constrained by four major immunological complications; 1) graft-versus-host disease, 2) failure to engraft because of rejection by the host immune cells, host-versus-graft (HVG), 3) immunoincompetence, and 4) toxicity associated with fully ablative conditioning. Although, sev-eral approaches have been tested in recent years to overcome these com-plications, induction of mixed HSC chimerism in adults is a prerequisite to successful induction of tolerance to donor grafts while preserving the abil-ity of the recipient to respond to unrelated foreign antigens. This approach requires sufficient depletion or inactivation of the host immune system and establishment of conditions that permit donor HSC engraftment. The newly developing lymphocytes in an antigenic milieu consisting of both the donor and recipient histocompatibility antigens are educated to recognize both the host and donor antigens as self while preserving immunocompetence to unrelated foreign antigens. In the following sections, we will discuss the application of mixed chimerism to induction of tolerance to allogeneic and xenogeneic grafts in experimental settings as well as elaborate on the impli-cated mechanisms.

195

HSC chimerism and allotolerance

The notion of using hematopoietic chimerism as a means of inducing tolerance to foreign grafts originated from observations that freemartin cattle
that shared the same placenta exhibited hematopoietic chimerism and
accepted allogeneic skin grafts from their twins [74,75]. Direct experimental
evidence for the role of hematopoietic chimerism in the induction of tolerance to allografts was then provided by Billingham, Brent, and Medawar [76]
who demonstrated that inoculation of homogenized tissues form allogeneic
adult donors into fetal mice led to hematopoietic chimerism and tolerance
to donor organs. Donor BM was then directly used in X-irradiated mice to
induce tolerance to skin allografts [77]. In a series of subsequent studies,
Monaco and coworkers demonstrated that preconditioning of the graft recipients with antilymphocyte serum followed by allogeneic BM infusion led to
tolerance to donor allografts [78]. These initial observations led to a long-
lasting interest and intense studies for application of hematopoietic chimerism to tolerance induction to autoantigens for amelioration of autoimmune
diseases [69] and foreign transplantation antigens for prevention of graft
rejection [68,71,72,79,80].

Tolerance to allografts using HSC chimerism was initially achieved using
fully myeloablative preconditioning regimens followed by reconstitution of
the recipient by transplantation of unmodified donor BM to create a fully
allogeneic chimeric state [81-83]. This fully ablative conditioning was associated with morbidity, mortality, and higher rates of failure in generation of a
chimeric state. It was then established that reconstitution of lethally irradiated mice with a mixture of T-cell-depleted syngeneic and allogeneic bone
marrow cells could facilitate engraftment, generate a durable chimeric state,
and induce tolerance to both donor and recipient antigens [79]. Depletion
of T cells from only syngeneic BM also resulted in durable mixed chimerism
and specific tolerance to donor organs. In marked contrast, removal of T cells
from the allogeneic BM, without manipulation of the host BM, led to engraftment with host-type cells and timely rejection of the allogeneic donor grafts
[80,83].

Reconstitution of a completely myeloablated host with a mixture of T-cell-
depleted host and donor BM cells is effective in producing mixed lymphopoietic chimerism and tolerance to both donor and host antigens. This regimen,
however, is associated with significant morbidity and mortality in the host
that precludes its routine use for tolerance induction in clinics. This limitation led to the development of several nonmyeloablative-conditioning
regimens to achieve durable mixed chimerism. These regimens targeted

the immune system of recipient for downregulation using either nonspecific immunosuppressive regimens or lymphocyte-specific interventions, followed by donor HSC transplantation. Nonspecific lymphoablative regimens included the use of low dose total body and/or thymic irradiation in conjunction with selected immunosuppressive pharmaceuticals. For example, stable mixed allogeneic chimerism and donor-specific transplantation tolerance for skin and heart allografts across multiple histocompatibility barriers was achieved using low dose, total body irradiation (5 Gy) followed by allogeneic BM transplantation and treatment with cyclophosphamide 2 days post BM transplantation [84]. Administration of cyclophosphamide before BM infusion did not facilitate engraftment, suggesting that this drug exerted its effect on newly activated host effector cells. Another nonspecific preconditioning regimen consisted of a single dose of antilymphocyte serum (5 days before transplantation), administration of tacrolimus (days -1 to +10), and a low dose (5 Gy) of total body irradiation (TBI). These conditioned recipients were then given T-cell-depleted donor BM cells that resulted in multilineage hematopoietic chimerism and donor-specific tolerance to cardiac allografts in a rat strain combination disparate for both minor and MHC antigens [85]. Most importantly, long-surviving cardiac allografts showed no evidence of acute or chronic rejection. This regimen also resulted in the induction of tolerance to composite tissue allografts, such as hindlimb, that is even more prone to rejection [86].

T-cell-targeted specific approaches for nonmyeloablative preconditioning regimens include the use of mAbs to selected T-cell markers, such as CD4, CD8, CD3, or TCR, in combination with a low dose of TBI [87-90]. Stable mixed chimerism and donor-specific systemic tolerance could be obtained using a preconditioning regimen consisting of treatment of the host with an anti-TCR α/β mAb and low dose of TBI prior to transfusion with BM cells in a fully disparate mouse strain combination [88]. Similarly, treatment of the host with a single dose of an anti-CD3 mAb and low dose of TBI followed by transfusion with donor BM cells led to high levels of stable mixed chimerism and donor-specific tolerance to skin grafts in a fully disparate mouse model [87]. Pretreatment of the host with a combination of anti-CD4 and anti-CD8 mAbs and low level of TBI (3 Gy) and thymic irradiation (7 Gy) followed by transplantation of unmanipulated fully MHC-disparate BM led to stable mixed chimerism and tolerance to donor and host grafts [90]. The requirement for thymic irradiation could be overcome by further depletion of T cells with two additional doses of anti-CD4 and anti-CD8 mAbs post BM transplantation [89].

Mixed chimerism and tolerance are more readily achieved in semi-allogeneic donor-recipient combinations, suggesting that identity at one MHC haplo-type between the donor and recipient may facilitate the development of mixed chimerism and tolerance. Consistent with this notion is the observation that mixed chimerism and donor-specific transplantation tolerance can be induced in immunologically unmodified rats across a semiallogeneic transplant barrier using vascularized hindlimb bone marrow allografts [91]. The majority of graft recipients remained free of GVHD and developed stable low level mixed T-cell chimerism [91]. This contention is also consistent with observations that BM from transgenic animals expressing one isolated MHC class I molecule is sufficient to induce tolerance to cardiac allografts harboring several different minor and major histocompatibility antigens when used as a treatment regimen [92]. Infusion of 5×10^6 and 5×10^7 BM cells from H-2K^b transgenic CBA into unmanipulated CBA mice on the day of transplantation results in long-term survival of fully allogeneic B10 (H-2^b) cardiac allografts. In contrast, the same doses of fully allogeneic B10 donor BM cells were completely ineffective in prolonging graft survival [92].

The discovery of costimulation for T-cell activation and a better understanding of molecules and interactions involved in transduction of costimulatory signals resulted in the development of milder preconditioning requirements for the establishment of durable mixed HSC chimerism and tolerance. It was initially demonstrated that donor BM cell transplantation accompanied by the treatment of host with the CTLA-4Ig recombinant protein to block costimulation resulted in mixed chimerism and prolonged cardiac and skin allograft survival in a fully allogeneic mouse strain combination [93]. The effect of costimulatory blockade on the establishment of durable mixed allogeneic chimerism and allograft tolerance was much more pronounced when both CD28/B7 and CD40/CD40L pathways were blocked. Preconditioning of mice with a single injection of an anti-CD40L mAb and CTLA-4Ig combined with a low dose (3 Gy) of total body irradiation followed by allogeneic BM transplantation culminated in stable multilineage donor hematopoiesis and donor-specific tolerance to skin grafts in a fully allogeneic murine model [94].

The observations that the presence of allogeneic T cells in donor BM inoculum is critical to engraftment and that purified HSC do not readily engraft in an allogeneic host resulted in the discovery of a unique bone marrow-derived cell type designated as "facilitating cells" (Fig. 3). Cotransplantation of 1,000 allogeneic purified HSC with as few as 30,000 facilitating cells resulted in mixed chimerism and tolerance to several organ allografts in a fully MHC-disparate mouse strain combination [95]. Facilitating cells are phenotypically characterized as CD8$^+$/CD3$^+$/CD45R$^+$/Thy1.2$^+$/TCR$^-$ and are

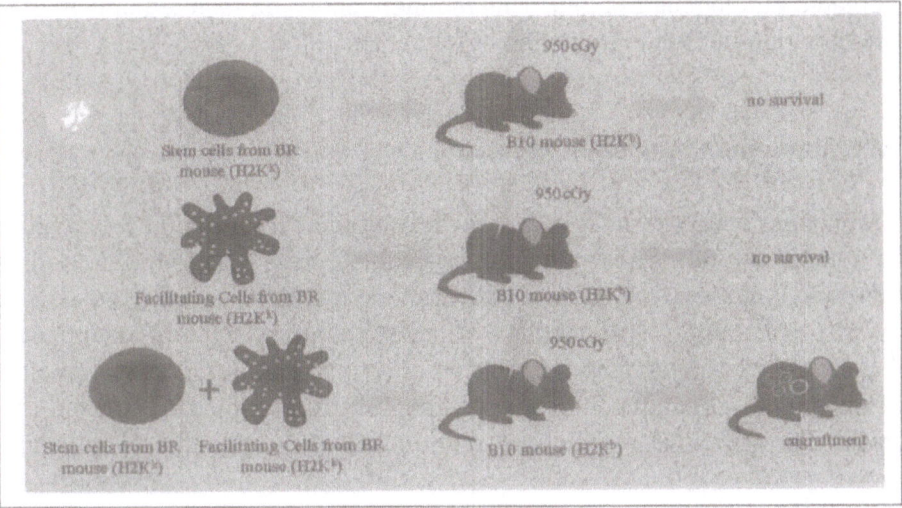

Figure 3
Facilitating cells. Highly purified allogeneic hematopoietic stem cells do not engraft unless cotransplanted with facilitating cells.

distinct from HSCs and other lineages of lymphoid or myeloid origin. Functionally, they enhance HSC engraftment either by protecting the HSC from immune attack or providing them with factors and/or physiological interactions normally found in a syngeneic milieu. A better characterization of this unique cell population and the establishment of in vitro conditions for its expansion are critical to its use for generation of mixed chimerism and tolerance induction in the clinic.

Mixed chimerism has been successfully established in clinical as well as preclinical models. For example, recipients of cadaveric renal allograft treated with antilymphocyte globulin and donor-specific BM transfusion showed augmented, long-lasting donor chimerism and rejection-free graft survival [96]. Similarly, a nonmyeloablative preconditioning regimen that consisted of anti T-cell globulin, TBI (3 Gy) and thymic irradiation (7 Gy) followed by donor BM infusion produced mixed chimerism and tolerance to renal allografts disparate for MHC molecules in nonhuman primates [97]. Stable chimerism and tolerance to kidney allografts, without evidence of GVHD, was also established in chacma baboons using fractionated total lymphoid irradiation and allogeneic BM transfusion [98]. In a similar study using rhesus monkeys, it was shown that donor chimerism induced by allogeneic BM transplantation was critical to the survival of heart allografts in recipients pretreated with myeloablative TBI, followed by constitution with T-cell-depleted autologous BM [99]. This regimen, however, resulted only in graft prolongation but not in induction of tolerance.

HSC chimerism and xenotolerance

HSC chimerism also serves as an effective approach for tolerance induction to xenografts [68]. Unlike allograft rejection that is primarily initiated by adaptive immunity, rejection of xenografts is mediated by adaptive as well as innate immunity that involves xenoantibody-producing T-independent B cells, macrophages, and NK cells as effectors. The fact that tolerance to xenografts can be induced suggests that HSC chimerism is an efficient regimen for downregulating the function of B cells, NK cells, and macrophages [71,100].

Transplantation of lethally irradiated mice with a mixture of rat and mouse BM cells results in mixed xenogeneic chimerism and donor-specific tolerance. Rat T-cell development proceeds as it would for allogeneic T-cell development; including expression of the TCR complex, demonstrable dependence on the thymic environment for development, and normal function in response to T-cell mitogens and transplantation antigens [73]. Rat T cells developing in chimeras display the characteristic phenotypically immature pattern in the thymus (CD4+CD8+TCR+) and mature pattern (CD4+CD8-TCR+ or CD4-CD8+TCR+) in the periphery. Most importantly, xenoantigens in chimeras serve as ligands for the newly developing rat and mouse T cells and as such contribute to the positive and negative selection events in the thymus (Fig. 2) [101]. This was first demonstrated for the mouse mammary tumor virus superantigen system where T cells with selected Vβs are deleted by recognizing superantigens in the context of selected class II molecules [9]. For example, mixed xenogeneic chimeras (mouse + rat → mouse) lacked mouse T cells that express TCRs with Vβs specific for viral superantigens. These T cells are present in unmanipulated mice due to the lack of a permissible class II molecule. This observation suggests that the rat cells contributed to this deletion process by providing the permissible MHC class II molecules for superantigen presentation in chimeras [68].

T cells developing in xenogeneic chimeras (mouse + rat → mouse) recognize antigens presented by mouse, but not rat, APCs. Restriction to the host APCs for antigen recognition results in functional immunocompetence within and across species barriers [102]. Mixed chimeras are tolerant to both the host and donor antigens as they accept cardiac, islet, and skin xenografts from the donor and promptly reject third party either allogeneic or xenogeneic grafts without any sign of GVHD [68,69]. Most importantly, mixed xenogeneic chimerism not only induces tolerance in the T but also in the B cell compartment that curtails xenotransplantation by producing natural preformed antibodies. These antibodies cause hyperacute rejection by interacting with a carbohydrate epitope, $\alpha 1,3$-Gal, expressed by xenoantigens [103]. Transplantation of a mixture of BM from wild type and $\alpha 1,3$-galactosyltransferase knockout mice into knockout mice conditioned with a nonmyeloablative regimen, consisting of depleting mAbs to CD4 and CD8 molecules, 3 Gy TBI and 7 Gy thymic irradiation, led to durable multilineage mixed chimerism associated with a rapid reduction of serum anti-Gal xeno-antibodies [104]. Mixed chimeras were devoid of anti-Gal-producing cells and permanently accepted donor-type heart grafts even after immunization with Gal-bearing xenogeneic cells. More importantly, B cells responsible for the production of natural antibodies for $\alpha 1,3$-Gal were completely absent from the spleens of mixed chimeras, suggesting clonal deletion and/or receptor editing [100].

Humoral tolerance has also been shown in the rat-to-mouse model, which is discordant for BM but concordant for all the other tested tissues and organs. Using either nonmyeloablative or myeloablative preconditioning regimens allo or mixed xenogeneic chimerism are fully induceable. Tolerance induction in F344 rats-to-B10 mice pretreated with an elaborate immunosuppressive regimen consisting of antibodies against CD4, CD8, Thy1, and NK1 markers, a low dose TBI (3 Gy) and a high dose of thymic irradiation (7 Gy) followed by T-cell-depleted BM transplantation resulted in transient mixed chimerism and humoral tolerance as these chimeras did not generate an antibody response upon engraftment with subsequent BM cells or skin grafts [105].

HSC transplantation and mixed xenogeneic chimerism has also been tested for tolerance induction in larger animal models, particularly pig-to-primate, with limited success [106]. Temporary immune nonresponsiveness to pig kidney and heart grafts in baboons has recently been reported using BM transplantation under the cover of a preconditioning regimen that consisted of nonmyeloablative TBI and thymic irradiation, splenectomy, anti-lymphocyte antibody, immunosuppressive pharmaceuticals, and absorption of natural antibodies through the pig liver [107]. Although this rather elaborate regimen prevented hyperacute rejection, all the grafts were rejected in about 15 days. Rejection was accompanied by high titers of natural antibodies against the $\alpha 1,3$-Gal epitope [108]. Suppression of the natural antibody response to xenoantigens in the pig-to-baboon model was reported using a myeloablative regimen accompanied by immunoaffinity depletion of natural antibodies and treatment of autologous BM cells with antibodies to CD2 and CD20 molecules to obtain mixed xenogeneic chimerism [106].

Durable mixed xenogeneic chimerism was accomplished in nonlethally irradiated baboons transplanted with unmodified human BM cells [109]. Intrathymic injection of human CD34+ BM cells into infant baboons resulted in long-term mixed xenogeneic chimerism and specific long-term survival of donor skin graft [110]. In contrast, this regimen was ineffective for mixed xenogeneic chimerism and long-term graft survival in the pig-to-nonhuman primates, suggesting that nonimmunological physiological constrains may also exist for the engraftment of BM across distant species barriers. Consistent with this notion, engraftment of pig BM into nonhuman primates required infusion of pig cytokines [70,111,112]. The data discussed in this section clearly indicate that mixed hematopoietic chimerism can be used as an effective regimen for induction of tolerance in both adaptive as well as innate immunity against xenografts. A better understanding of immunological and nonimmunological factors across distant species, however, will be critical to the application of this regimen to tolerance induction to xenografts in a clinical setting.

HSC chimerism and chronic rejection

Graft loss secondary to chronic rejection remains a major source of morbidity and mortality in solid organ transplantation. Chronic rejection is resistant to most forms of immunosuppressive clinical regimens that effectively control acute rejection [85,113,114]. Mixed hematopoietic chimerism has been successfully used to prevent chronic rejection. For example, mixed chimerism generated by transplantation of T-cell-depleted allogeneic LEW BM into F344 hosts resulted in long-term cardiac allograft survival without sign of graft arteriosclerosis [114]. Similarly, mixed chimerism established in lethally irradiated WF rats reconstituted with a mixture of T-cell depleted syngeneic and allogeneic ACI BM cells resulted in tolerance to cardiac allograft as defined by the lack of chronic rejection [113]. In another detailed study, stable multilineage mixed hematopoietic chimerism was created by a mixture of T-cell-depleted syngeneic and allogeneic BM transplantation into fully myeloablated rat recipients disparate for various combinations of minor and MHC antigens. It was shown that donor chimerism >12% led to true tolerance to skin and cardiac allografts without any sign of chronic rejection and GVHD [115]. Taken together, these experimental data clearly demonstrate that chronic rejection can effectively be treated with mixed hematopoietic chimerism, plausibly inducing true tolerance to donor antigens.

MECHANISMS OF TRANSPLANTATION TOLERANCE INDUCED BY MIXED CHIMERISM

Engraftment of allogeneic or xenogeneic pluripotent HSC in immunomodulated recipients leads to the development of a lymphocyte repertoire in an antigenic milieu consisting of both the host and donor antigens. Lymphocytes developing in such an antigenic environment are tolerant to both the donor and host antigens. Tolerance is thought to be established in the thymus via positive and negative selection processes regulated by both the donor and host hematopoietic cells entering the thymus. Thymic clonal deletion is believed to be the main mechanism that confers tolerance in mixed chimeras. Central deletion per se, however, may not be the sole mechanism of tolerance in mixed chimeras where chimerism is induced using nonmyeloablative regimens as these chimeras have mature T cells in the periphery. Other peripheral mechanisms may, therefore, play a role and these mechanisms may recapitulate the ones that confer self-tolerance in vertebrates. During the past several years significant advances have been made in dissecting the mechanisms responsible for tolerance induced by mixed chimerism. These mechanisms include, but are not limited to, peripheral clonal deletion, clonal anergy, and immunoregulation.

The importance of intrathymic clonal deletion in tolerance induced by mixed hematopoietic chimerism was demonstrated using transgenic recipients expressing a clonotypic TCR specific for a class I, H-2L^d, antigen. 2C TCR transgenic mice (H-2^b), whose transgenic TCR recognizes L^d, were used as recipients of BM cells expressing the L^d molecule after preconditioning with depleting mAbs against CD4 and CD8 molecules combined with whole body (3 Gy) and thymic (7 Gy) irradiation. Intrathymic and peripheral deletion of 2C$^+$/CD8$^+$ T cells was detected in chimeras. Deletion correlated with the presence of donor-type cells in the thymus and tolerance to the donor antigens in vitro and in vivo, as determined by cell-mediated lysis and skin graft acceptance, respectively [116]. Similar thymic and peripheral clonal deletion events have been demonstrated for CD4$^+$ alloreactive T cells. Mixed chimerism established by infusion of class II I-Eα transgenic mice BM cells into C57BL/6 nontransgenics led to clonal deletion of mature, peripheral T cells expressing I-Eα-reactive Vβ11$^+$ TCR and the extent of deletion was proportional to the degree of chimerism [117]. Chimerism >30% resulted in significant deletion of T cells expressing Vβ11 and tolerance to I-E$^+$ skin allografts. In contrast, chimerism <10% was associated with incomplete deletion and prolonged, but not permanent, allograft survival that could also be influenced by the conditioning approach. We have recently shown that partial myeloablation of B10 (H-2^b) mice with 5 Gy TBI followed by BM transplantation from either Balb/c (H-2^d) or B10.BR (H-2^k) and one dose of cyclophos-phamide treatment 2 days after transplantation resulted in mixed allogeneic chimerism and thymic deletion of superantigen-reactive Vβ3$^+$, 5$^+$, and 11$^+$ T cells [118]. These data suggest that the level of BM chimerism is critical to deletion of alloreactive T cells and ensuing transplantation tolerance.

Thymic clonal deletion has also been shown to play a critical role in tolerance induction to xenografts in xenogeneic chimeras. Regardless of the preconditioning regimens used to generate mixed xenogeneic chimeras, chimerism was associated with deletion of xenoreactive T cells and tolerance to donor and recipient antigens as determined by the lack of rejection of donor grafts and GVHD [68]. Engraftment and tolerance are associated with early migration of donor bone marrow-derived cells to the host thymus and positive and negative selection processes, resulting in the deletion of developing thymocytes with reactivity to donor antigens [119]. For example, we demonstrated that mouse and rat T cells developing in mixed chimeras (rat + mouse → lethally irradiated mouse or rat → sublethally irradiated mouse) were tolerant to host and donor antigens and had altered peripheral expression of TCR shaped by positive and negative selection on mouse and rat antigens [101]. Most importantly, rat T cells developing in the mouse were restricted to mouse, but not rat, APCs for class I-restricted responses (Fig. 4) [102]. Stimulation of splenocytes from mixed chimeras with either irradiated mouse or rat splenocytes modified with TNP in vitro resulted in effective TNP response that was restricted to mouse, but not rat, MHC for presentation to both rat and mouse T cells. Host MHC-restricted recognition was confirmed using purified rat or mouse T cells from virally infected chimeras for recognition of virus-infected cells. T cells from chimeras responded only to virus infected fibroblasts in the context of host (mouse) MHC molecules [102].

In addition to central clonal deletion, peripheral clonal anergy has been demonstrated as a mechanism responsible for tolerance to transplantation antigens in mixed chimeras. Mixed chimerism established in B10.A-to-B10 using a nonmyeloablative regimen (consisting treatment of the recipient with anti-CD4 and anti-CD8 mAbs, 7 Gy thymic and 3 Gy whole body irradiation, followed by infusion of the donor BM cells) was associated with central deletion of Vβ11$^+$ T cells that react with superantigens in the context of MHC class II I-E$^+$ of B10.A mice [120]. More importantly, clonal deletion was not complete in these chimeras and mature T cells expressing Vβ11 are detected in the periphery. These T cells, however, were anergic since they did not respond to receptor cross-linking with Vβ11 mAb. The presence of donor class II$^+$ hematopoietic cells in the thymus is shown to be critical to the development of tolerance in chimeras. For example, insufficient depletion of host

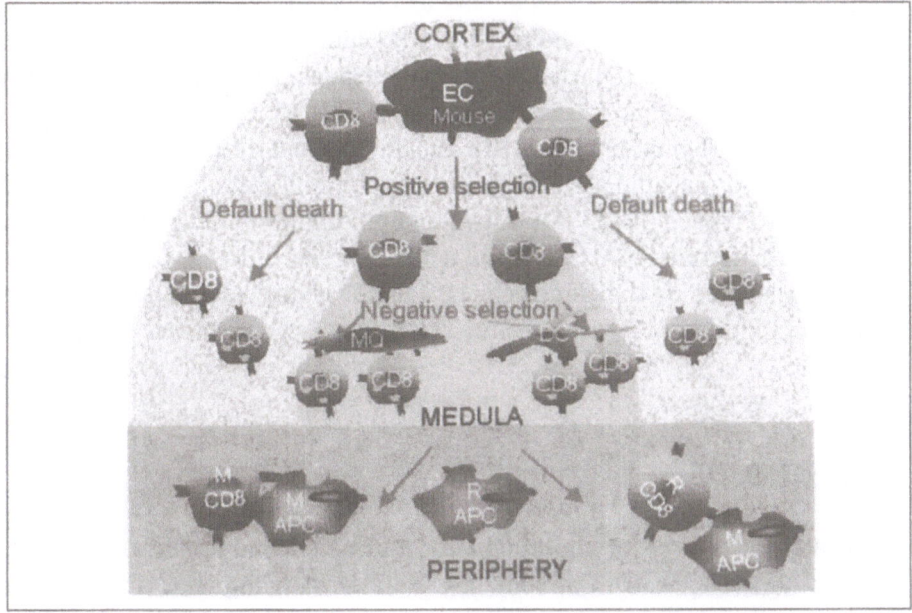

Figure 4
T cell response in xenogeneic chimeras. Both mouse and rat peripheral CD8⁺ T cells developing in chimeras (rat-to-mouse) respond to viral antigens when presented by mouse but not rat APCs.

lymphocytes was associated with the lack of class II⁺ T cells in the thymus and tolerance regardless of the presence of short-lived peripheral chimerism [121]. The presence of class II⁺ cells in the thymus was also required and sufficient for induction of tolerance to heart grafts in mixed xenogeneic chimeras established in the rat-to-mouse model. The analysis of superantigen reactive mouse Vβ5 and Vβ11 TCR in xenogeneic chimeras revealed deletion of T cells expressing these molecules over time. The absence of mature Vβ5⁺ and Vβ11⁺ host T cells in the thymus and periphery was always associated with the presence of rat class II⁺ cells in the thymus, and incomplete deletion of T cells expressing these Vβ families was observed in thymi in which rat class II⁺ cells were not detectable [122].

Peripheral clonal deletion may also play a critical role in tolerance induction in mixed or fully allogeneic chimeras. For example, we have recently demonstrated that reconstitution of adult thymectomized and lethally irradiated B10 mice with T-cell-depleted B10.BR BM cells results in chimerism and tolerance to donor and host antigens [123]. T cells with normal phenotype and function develop in athymic chimeras. These T cells undergo extrathymic positive and negative selection events as indicated by the absence of supe-rantigen-reactive T cells in the periphery of chimeras and restriction to host MHC molecules for recognition of foreign antigens. Although it is presently unknown if extrathymic mechanisms responsible for the development of T cells in these athymic chimeras are similar to those responsible for T-cell ontogeny in normal animals, activation-induced cell death may play a role in peripheral tolerance. AICD is induced by upregulation of Fas and FasL mol-ecules on the surface of T cells upon activation and autocrine interaction of Fas with the FasL on the same cell [124]. AICD is critical to immune homeo-stasis and induction of peripheral tolerance in selected systems [125].

CONCLUSIONS

Regardless of the present limitations of routine clinical application of HSC transplantation for the treatment of a variety of malignant, autoimmune, hereditary disorders, and the induction of tolerance to foreign grafts, there has been overwhelming progress in our understanding of these limitations in recent years. Particularly, the recent advances in our knowledge of adap-tive and innate immune responses, our ability to specifically manipulate these responses under selected conditions combined with the progress in immunobiology of stem cells, provide great promise for the application of HSC chimerism to tolerance induction to allografts as well as xenografts. HSC chimerism also holds great promise for the induction of tolerance to autoimmune antigens. All these will, however, depend upon our comprehen-sive understanding of the host and donor factors that are critical to HSC engraftment and manipulation of the donor and host in selected fashions to facilitate engraftment without significant incidence of morbidity and mortal-ity in the host. If one can reduce the risk:benefit ratio for HSC transplanta-tion, a staggering number of diseases can be potentially treated, including sickle cell disease, thalassemia, a number of autoimmune disease states, and donor-specific tolerance to allografts can be induced. Finally, as is usu-ally the case, HSC chimerism may synergize with genetic modifications of the pig to make xenotransplantation a clinical reality.

REFERENCES

1. Hoffmann JA, Kafatos FC, Janeway CA, Ezekowitz RA. Phylogenetic perspec-tives in innate immunity. Science. 1999; 284:1313-8.
2. Borghans JA, Noest AJ, De Boer RJ. How specific should immunological memory

be? J Immunol. 1999; 163:569-75.

3. Jenkins MK, Schwartz RH. Antigen presentation by chemically modified spleno-cytes induces antigen-specific T cell unresponsiveness in vitro and in vivo. J Exp Med. 1987; 165:302-19.

4. Lafferty KJ, Prowse SJ, Simeonovic CJ. Immunobiology of tissue transplantation: a return to the passenger leukocyte concept. Ann Rev Immunol. 1983; 1:143-73

5. Davis MM, Bjorkman PJ. T cell antigen receptor genes and T cell recognition. Nature. 1988; 334:395-402.

6. Tan L, Turner J, Weiss A. Regions of the T cell receptor alpha and beta chains that are responsible for interaction with CD3. J Exp Med. 1991; 173:1247-56.

7. Kronenberg M, Siu G, Hood LH, Nikblah S. The molecular genetics of the T-cell antigen receptor and T-cell antigen recognition. Ann Rev Immunol. 1986; 4:529-91.

8. Kronenberg M, Goverman J, Haars R, Malissen M, Kraig E, Phillips L, Delovitch T, Suciu-Foca N, Hood L. Rearrangement and transcription of the b-chain genes of the T-cell antigen receptor in different types of murine lymphocytes. Nature. 1985; 313:647-53.

9. Kappler JW, Roehm N, Marrack P. T cell tolerance by clonal elimination in the thymus. Cell. 1987; 49:273-80.

10. Kappler JW, Wade T, White J, Kushir E, Blackman M, Bill J, Roehm N, Marrack P. A T cell receptor V beta segment that imparts reactivity to a class II major histocompatibility complex product. Cell. 1987; 49:273-80.

11. Hugo P, Kappler JW, Godfrey DI, Marrack PC. Thymic epithelial cell lines that mediate positive selection can also induce thymocyte clonal deletion. J Immunol. 1994; 152:1022-31.

12. Surh CD, Sprent J. T-cell apoptosis detected in situ during positive and negative selection in the thymus. Nature. 1994; 372:100-3.

13. Garcia KC, Degano M, Stanfield RL, Brunmark A, Jackson MR, Peterson PA, Teyton L, Wilson IA. An ab T cell receptor structure at 2.5 A° and its orientation in the TCR-MHC complex. Science. 1996; 274:209-19.

14. Ding YH, Baker BM, Garboczi DN, Biddison WE, Wiley DC. Four A6-TCR/peptide/HLA-A2 structures that generate very different T cell signals are nearly identical. Immunity. 1999; 11:45-56.

15. Patten PA, Rock EP, Sonoda T, Fazekas de St.Groth B, Jorgenson JL, Davis MM. Transfer of putative complementarity-determining region loops of T cell receptor V domains confers toxin reactivity but not peptide/MHC specificity. J Immunol. 1993; 150:2281-94.

16. Nalefski EA, Wong JGP, Rao A. Amino acid substitutions in the first complemen-tarity-determining region of a murine T-cell receptor alpha chain affect antigen-major histocompatibility complex recognition. J Immunol. 1990; 265:8842-6.

17. Bentley GA, Boulot G, Karjalainen K, Mariuzza RA. Crystal structure of the b chain of a T cell antigen receptor. Science. 1995; 267:1984-7.

18. Gold DP, Offner H, Sun D, Wiley S, Vandenbark AA, Wilson DB. Analysis of T cell receptor beta chains in Lewis rats with experimental allergic encepha-lomyelitis: conserved complementary determining region 3. J Exp Med. 1991; 174:14677-1476.

19. Jorgensen JL, Esser U, Fazekas de St.Groth B, Reay PA, Davis MM. Mapping T cell receptor-peptide contacts by variant peptide immunization of single-chain transgenics. Nature. 1992; 355:224-30.

20. Schwartz RH. Costimulation of T lymphocytes: the role of CD28, CTLA-4, and B7/BB1 in interleukin-2 production and immunotherapy. Cell. 1992; 71:1065-8.

21. Noel PJ, Boise LH, Green JM, Thompson CB. CD28 costimulation prevents cell death during primary T cell activation. J Immunol. 1996; 157:636-42.

22. Radvanyi LG, Shi YF, Vaziri H, Sharma A, Dhala R, Mills GB, Miller RG. CD28

costimulation inhibits TCR-induced apoptosis during a primary T cell response. J Immunol. 1996; 156:1788-98.

23. Lucas PJ, Negishi I, Nakayama K, Fields LE, Loh DY. Naive CD28-deficient T cells can initiate but not sustain an in vitro antigen-specific immune response. J Immunol. 1995; 154:5757-68.

24. Parijs LV, Ibraghimov A, Abbas AK. The roles of costimulation and Fas in T cell apoptosis and peripheral tolerance. Immunity. 1996; 4:321-6.

25. Lenschow DJ, Zeng Y, Thistlewaite JR, Montag A, Brady W, Gibson MG, Linsley PS, Bluestone JA. Long-term survival of xenogeneic pancreatic islet grafts induced by CTLA4Ig. Science. 1992; 257:789-95.

26. Akalin E, Chandraker A, Russell ME, Turka LA, Hancock WW, Sayegh MH. CD28-B7 T cell costimulatory blockade by CTLA4Ig in the rat renal allograft model: inhibition of cell-mediated and humoral immune responses in vivo. Transplantation. 1996; 62:1942-5.

27. Lenschow DJ, Walunas TL, Bluestone JA. CD28/B7 system of T cell costimulation. Ann Rev Immunol. 1996; 14:233-58.

28. Lenschow DJ, Herold KC, Rhee L, Patel B, Koons A, Qin HY, Fuchs E, Singh B, Thompson CB, Bluestone JA. CD28/B7 Regulation of Th1 and Th2 subsets in the development of autoimmune diabetes. Immunity. 1996; 5:285-93.

29. Judge TA, Wu Z, Zheng XG, Sharpe AH, Sayegh MH, Turka LA. The role of CD80, CD86, and CTLA4 in alloimmune responses and the induction of long-term allograft survival. J Immunol. 1999; 162:1947-51.

30. Denton MD, Magee CC, Sayegh MH. Immunosuppressive strategies in transplantation. Lancet. 1999; 353:1083-91.

31. Sha WC, Nelson CA, Newberry RD, Kranz DM, Russell JH, Loh DY. Positive and negative selection of an antigen receptor on T cells in transgenic mice. Nature. 1988; 336:73-6.

32. Alam SM, Travers PJ, Wung JL, Nasholds W, Redpath S, Jameson SC, Gascoigne NRJ. T-cell-receptor affinity and thymocyte positive selection. Nature. 1996; 381:616-20.

33. Ashton-Rickardt PG, Van Kaer L, Schumacher TNM, Ploegh HL, Tonegawa S. Peptide contributes to the specificity of positive selection of CD8+ T cells in the thymus. Cell. 1993; 73:1041-9.

34. Bill J, Palmer E. Positive selection of CD4+ T cells mediated by MHC class II-bearing stromal cell in the thymic cortex. Nature. 1989; 341:649-54.

35. Baldwin KK, Trenchak BP, Altman JD, Davis MM. Negative selection of T cells occurs throughout thymic development. J Immunol. 1999; 163:689-98.

36. Sebzda E, Wallace VA, Mayer J, Yeung RS, Mak TW, Ohashi PS. Positive and negative thymocyte selection induced by different concentrations of a single peptide. Science. 1994; 263:1615-8.

37. Hogquist KA, Jameson SC, Heath WR, Howard JL, Bevan MJ, Carbone FR. T cell receptor antagonist peptides induce positive selection. Cell. 1994; 76:17-27.

38. Ashton-Rickardt PG, Bandeira A, Delaney JR, Van Kaer L, Pircher HP, Zinkernagel RM, Tonegawa S. Evidence for a differential avidity model of T cell selection in the thymus. Cell. 1994; 76:651-63.

39. Lyons DS, Lieberman SA, Hampl J, Boniface JJ, Chien Y, Berg LJ, Davis MM. A TCR binds to antagonist ligands with lower affinities and faster dissociation rates than to agonists. Immunity. 1996; 5:53-61.

40. Laufer TM, Glimcher LH, Lo D. Using thymus anatomy to dissect T cell repertoire selection. Semin Immunol. 1999; 11:65-70.

41. Finkel TH, Cambier JC, Kubo RT, Born WK, Marrack P, Kappler JW. The thymus has two functionally distinct populations of immature alpha beta + T cells: one population is deleted by ligation of alpha beta TCR. Cell. 1989; 58:1047-54.

42. Guidos CJ, Danska JS, Fathman CG, Weissman IL. T cell receptor-mediated nega-

tive selection of autoreactive T lymphocyte precursors occurs after commitment to the CD4 or CD8 lineages. J Exp Med. 1990; 172:835-45.

43. Soldevila G, Geiger T, Flavell RA. Breaking immunologic ignorance to an antigenic peptide of simian virus 40 large T antigen. J Immunol. 1995; 155:5590-600.

44. Ohashi PS, Oehen S, Buerki K, Pircher H, Ohashi CT, Odermatt B, Malissen B, Zinkernagel RM, Hengartner H. Ablation of "tolerance" and induction of diabetes by virus infection in viral antigen transgenic mice. Cell. 1991; 65:305-17.

45. Coulombe M, Gill RG. T lymphocyte indifference to extrathymic islet allografts. J Immunol. 1996; 156:1998-2003.

46. Refaeli Y, Van Parijs L, London CA, Tschopp J, Abbas AK. Biochemical mechanisms of IL-2-regulated Fas-mediated T cell apoptosis. Immunity. 1998; 8:615-23.

47. Van Parijs L, Biuckians A, Ibragimov A, Alt FW, Willerford DM, Abbas AK. Functional responses and apoptosis of CD25 (IL-2R alpha)-deficient T cells expressing a transgenic antigen receptor. J Immunol. 1997; 158:3738-45.

48. Van Parijs L, Perez VL, Abbas AK. Mechanisms of peripheral T cell tolerance. Novartis Found Symp. 1998; 215:5-14.

49. Suda T, Tanaka M, Miwa K, Nagata S. Apoptosis of mouse naive T cells induced by recombinant soluble Fas ligand and activation-induced resistance to Fas ligand. J Immunol. 1996; 157:3918-24.

50. Suda T, Hashimoto H, Tanaka M, Ochi T, Nagata S. Membrane Fas ligand kills human peripheral blood T lymphocytes, and soluble Fas ligand blocks the killing. J Exp Med. 1997; 186:2045-50.

51. Burrows SR, Silins SL, Moss DJ, Khanna R, Misko IS, Argaet VP. T cell receptor repertoire for a viral epitope in humans is diversified by tolerance to a background major histocompatibility complex antigen. J Exp Med. 1995; 182:1703-15.

52. Christensen JP, Stenvang JP, Marker O, Thomsen AR. Characterization of virus-primed CD8+ T cells with a type 1 cytokine profile. Int Immunol. 1996; 8:1453-61

53. Kyburz D, Aichele P, Speiser DE, Hengartner H, Zinkernagel RM, Pircher H. T cell immunity after a viral infection versus T cell tolerance induced by soluble viral peptides. Eur J Immunol. 1993; 23:1956-62.

54. Kabelitz D, Oberg HH, Pohl T, Pechhold K. Antigen-induced death of mature T lymphocytes: analysis by flow cytometry. Immunol Rev. 1994; 142:157-74.

55. Pelfrey CM, Tranquill LR, Boehme SA, McFarland HF, Lenardo MJ. Two mechanisms of antigen-specific apoptosis of myelin basic protein (MBP)-specific T lymphocytes derived from multiple sclerosis patients and normal individuals. J Immunol. 1995; 154:6191-202.

56. Russell JH, Manning DE, McCulley DE, Meleedy-Rey P. Antigen as a positive and negative regulator of proliferation in cytotoxic lymphocytes. A model for the differential regulation of proliferation and lytic activity. J Immunol. 1988; 140:1796-801.

57. Pearson CI, Gautam AM, Rulifson IC, Liblau RS, McDevitt HO. A small number of residues in the class II molecule I-Au confer the ability to bind the myelin basic protein peptide Ac1-11. Proc Natl Acad Sci U S A. 1999; 96:197-202.

58. Sloan-Lancaster J, Evavold BD, Allen PM. Induction of T-cell anergy by altered T-cell-receptor ligand on live antigen-presenting cells. Nature. 1993; 363:156-9.

59. Sloan-Lancaster J, Shaw AS, Rothbard JB, Allen PM. Partial T cell signaling: altered phospho-zeta and lack of zap70 recruitment in APL-induced T cell anergy. Cell. 1994; 79:913-22.

60. Rocha B, Grandien A, Freitas AA. Anergy and exhaustion are independent mechanisms of peripheral T cell tolerance. J Exp Med. 1995; 181:993-1003.

61. Schwartz RH. A cell culture model for T lymphocyte clonal anergy. Science. 1990; 248:1349-56.

62. Malvey EN, Telander DG, Vanasek TL, Mueller DL. The role of clonal anergy in

the avoidance of autoimmunity: inactivation of autocrine growth without loss of effector function. Immunol Rev. 1998; 165:301-18.

63. Itoh M, Takahashi T, Sakaguchi N, Kuniyasu Y, Shimizu J, Otsuka F, Sakaguchi S. Thymus and autoimmunity: production of CD25+CD4+ naturally anergic and suppressive T cells as a key function of the thymus in maintaining immunologic self-tolerance. J Immunol. 1999; 162:5317-26.

64. Rellahan BL, Jones LA, Kruisbeek AM, Fry AM, Matis LA. In vivo induction of anergy in peripheral V beta 8+ T cells by staphylococcal enterotoxin B. J Exp Med. 1990; 172:1091-100.

65. Deeths MJ, Kedl RM, Mescher MF. CD8+ T cells become nonresponsive (anergic) following activation in the presence of costimulation. J Immunol. 1999; 163:102-10.

66. MacDonald HR, Baschieri S, Lees RK. Clonal expansion precedes anergy and death of V beta 8+ peripheral T cells responding to staphylococcal enterotoxin B in vivo. Eur J Immunol. 1991; 21:1963-6.

67. Smith JA, Tso JY, Clark MR, Cole MS, Bluestone JA. Nonmitogenic anti-CD3 monoclonal antibodies deliver a partial T cell receptor signal and induce clonal anergy. J Exp Med. 1997; 185:1413-22.

68. Ildstad ST, Sachs DH. Reconstitution with syngeneic plus allogeneic or xenogeneic bone marrow leads to specific acceptance of allografts or xenografts. Nature. 1984; 307:168-70.

69. Li H, Kaufman CL, Boggs SS, Johnson PC, Patrene KD, Ildstad ST. Mixed allogeneic chimerism induced by a sublethal approach prevents autoimmune diabetes and reverses insulitis in nonobese diabetic (NOD) mice. J Immunol. 1996; 156:380-8.

70. Sachs DH, Sykes M, Greenstein JL, Cosimi AB. Tolerance and xenograft survival. Nat Med. 1995; 1:969

71. Sharabi Y, Aksentijevich I, Sundt TMI, Sachs DH, Sykes M. Specific tolerance induction across a xenogeneic barrier: production of mixed rat/mouse lymphohematopoietic chimeras using a nonlethal preparative regimen. J Exp Med. 1990; 172:195-202.

72. Zhao Y, Swenson K, Sergio JJ, Arn JS, Sachs DH, Sykes M. Skin graft tolerance across a discordant xenogeneic barrier. Nat Med. 1996; 2:1211-6.

73. Ildstad ST, Wren SM, Boggs SS, Hronakes ML, Vecchini F, Van den Brink MRM. Cross-species bone marrow transplantation: evidence for tolerance induction, stem cell engraftment, and maturation of T lymphocytes in a xenogeneic stromal environment (rat--->mouse). J Exp Med. 1991; 174:467-78.

74. Owen RD. Immunogenic consequences of vascular anastomoses between bovine twins. Science. 1945; 102:400.

75. Billingham RE, Lamphin HG, Medawar PB, Williams HL. Tolerance of homografts, twin diagnosis and the freemartin conditions in cattle. Heredity. 1952; 6:201

76. Billingham RE, Brent L, Medawar PB. Actively acquired tolerance of foreign cells. Nature. 1953; 172:603-6.

77. Main JM, Prehn RT. Fate of skin homografts in x-irradiated mice treated with homologous marrow. J Natl Cancer Inst. 1957; 19:1053.

78. Wood ML, Monaco AP, Gozzo JJ, Liegeois A. Use of homozygous allogeneic bone marrow for induction of tolerance with antilymphocyte serum: dose and timing. Transplant Proc. 1971; 3:676-9.

79. Ildstad ST, Wren SM, Bluestone JA, Barbieri SA, Sachs DH. Characterization of mixed allogeneic chimeras. Immunocompetence, in vitro reactivity, and genetic specificity of tolerance. J Exp Med. 1985; 162:231-44.

80. Ildstad ST, Wren SM, Bluestone JA, Barbieri SA, Stephany D, Sachs DH. Effect of selective T cell depletion of host and/or donor bone marrow on lymphopoietic repopulation, tolerance, and graft-vs-host disease in mixed allogeneic chimeras(

B10 + B10.D2--> B10). J Immunol. 1986; 136:28-33.

81. Markus PM, Selvaggi G, Cai X, Fung JJ, Starzl TE. Induction of donor-specific transplantation tolerance to skin and cardiac allografts using mixed chimerism in (A + B-->A) in rats. Cell Transplant. 1993; 2:345-53.

82. Orloff MS, DeMara EM, Coppage ML, Leong N, Zuo XJ, Prehn J, Jordan SC. Alterations of the interleukin-4 pathway in production of tolerance by mixed hematopoietic chimerism. Surgery. 1995; 118:212-9.

83. Ildstad ST, Wren SM, Oh E, Hronakes ML. Mixed allogeneic reconstitution (A+B-->A) to induce donor-specific transplantation tolerance. Transplantation. 1991; 51:1262-7.

84. Colson YL, Wren SM, Schuchert MJ, Patrene KD, Johnson PC, Boggs SS, Ildstad ST. A nonlethal conditioning approach to achieve durable multilineage mixed chimerism and tolerance across major, minor, and hematopoietic histocompatibility barriers. J Immunol. 1995; 155:4179-88.

85. Gammie JS, Li S, Zeevi A, Demetris AJ, Ildstad ST, Pham SM. Tacrolimus-based partial conditioning produces stable mixed lymphohematopoietic chimerism and tolerance for cardiac allografts. Circulation. 1998; 98:II163-II168

86. Foster RD, Fan L, Niepp M, Kaufman C, McCalmont T, Ascher N, Ildstad S, Anthony JP. Donor-specific tolerance induction in composite tissue allografts. Am J Surg. 1998; 176:418-21.

87. de Vries-van der Zwan A, Besseling AC, van Twuyver E, Boog CJ, de Waal LP. A substantial level of mixed chimerism is required for the induction of permanent transplantation tolerance. Transpl Immunol. 1996; 4:232-40.

88. Nomoto K, Yung-Yun K, Omoto K, Umesue M, Murakami Y, Matsuzaki G. Tolerance induction in a fully allogeneic combination using anti-T cell receptor-alpha beta monoclonal antibody, low dose irradiation, and donor bone marrow transfusion. Transplantation. 1995; 59:395-401.

89. Tomita Y, Sachs DH, Khan A, Sykes M. Additional monoclonal antibody (mAB) injections can replace thymic irradiation to allow induction of mixed chimerism and tolerance in mice receiving bone marrow transplantation after conditioning with anti-T cell mABs and 3-Gy whole body irradiation. Transplantation. 1996; 61:469-77.

90. Sharabi Y, Sachs DH. Mixed chimerism and permanent specific transplantation tolerance induce by a nonlethal preparative regimen. J Exp Med. 1989; 169:493-502.

91. Hewitt CW, Ramsamooj R, Patel MP, Yazdi B, Achauer BM, Black KS. Developement of stable mixed T cell chimerism and transplantation tolerance without immune modulation in recipients of vascularized bone marrow allografts. Transplantation. 1990; 50:766-72.

92. Wong W, Morris PJ, Wood KJ. Syngeneic bone marrow expressing a single donor class I MHC molecule permits acceptance of a fully allogeneic cardiac allograft. Transplantation. 1996; 62:1462-8.

93. Pearson TC, Alexander DZ, Hendrix R, Elwood ET, Linsley PS, Winn KJ, Larsen CP. CTLA4-Ig plus bone marrow induces long-term allograft survival and donor specific unresponsiveness in the murine model. Evidence for hematopoietic chimerism. Transplantation. 1996; 61:997-1004.

94. Wekerle T, Sayegh MH, Hill J, Zhao Y, Chandraker A, Swenson KG, Zhao G, Sykes M. Extrathymic T cell deletion and allogeneic stem cell engraftment induced with costimulatory blockade is followed by central T cell tolerance. J Exp Med. 1998; 187:2037-44.

95. Kaufman CL, Colson YL, Wren SM, Watkins S, Simmons RL, Ildstad S. Phenotypic characterization of a novel bone marrow-derived cell that facilitates engraftment of allogeneic bone marrow stem cells. Blood. 1994; 84:2436-46.

96. McDaniel DO, Naftilan J, Hulvey K, Shaneyfelt S, Lemons JA, Lagoo-Deenadaya-

lan S, Hudson S, Diethelm AG, Barber WH. Peripheral blood chimerism in renal allograft recipients transfused with donor bone marrow. Transplantation. 1994; 57:852-6.

97. Kawai T, Cosimi AB, Colvin RB, Powelson J, Eason J, Kozlowski T, Sykes M, Monroy R, Tanaka M, Sachs DH. Mixed allogeneic chimerism and renal allograft tolerance in cynomolgus monkeys. Transplantation. 1995; 59:256-62.

98. Myburgh JA, Smit JA, Hill RR, Browde S. Transplantation tolerance in primates following total lymphoid irradiation and allogeneic bone marrow injection. II. Renal allografts. Transplantation. 1980; 29:405-8.

99. Moses RD, Orr KS, Bacher JD, Sachs DH, Clark RE, Gress RE. Cardiac allograft survival across major histocompatibility complex barriers in the rhesus monkey following T lymphocyte-depleted autologous marrow transplantation. II. Prolonged allograft survival with extensive marrow T cell depletion. Transplantation. 1989; 47:435-44.

100. Yang YG, deGoma E, Ohdan H, Bracy JL, Xu Y, Iacomini J, Thall AD, Sykes M. Tolerization of anti-Galalpha1-3Gal natural antibody-forming B cells by induction of mixed chimerism. J Exp Med. 1998; 187:1335-42.

101. Huang Y, Ildstad ST, Neipp M, Shirwan H. Mouse xenoantigens contribute to rat T-cell V beta repertoire generation in mixed xenogeneic bone marrow chimeras. Immunology. 2000; 100:317-8.

102. Colson YL, Tripp RA, Doherty PC, Wren SM, Neipp M, Abou EE, Ildstad ST. Antiviral cytotoxic activity across a species barrier in mixed xenogeneic chimeras: functional restriction to host MHC. J Immunol. 1998; 160:3790-6.

103. Platt JL, Vercellotti GM, Dalmasso AP, Matas AJ, Bolman Rm, Najarian jS, Bach FH. Transplantation of discordant xenografts: a review of progress. Immunol Today. 1990; 11:450-7.

104. Ohdan H, Yang YG, Shimizu A, Swenson KG, Sykes M. Mixed chimerism induced without lethal conditioning prevents T cell- and anti-Gal alpha 1,3Gal-mediated graft rejection. J Clin Invest. 1999; 104:281-90.

105. Aksentijevich I, Sachs DH, Sykes M. Humoral tolerance in xenogeneic BMT recipients conditioned by a nonmyeloablative regimen. Transplantation. 1992; 53:1108-14.

106. Kozlowski T, Monroy R, Xu Y, Glaser R, Awwad M, Cooper DK, Sachs DH. Anti-Gal(alpha)1-3Gal antibody response to porcine bone marrow in unmodified baboons and baboons conditioned for tolerance induction. Transplantation. 1998; 66:176-82.

107. Sablinski T, Gianello PR, Bailin M, Bergen KS, Emery DW, Fishman JA, Foley A, Hatch T, Hawley RJ, Kozlowski T, Lorf T, Meehan S, Monroy R, Powelson JA, Colvin RB, Cosimi AB, et al. Pig to monkey bone marrow and kidney xenotransplantation. Surgery. 1997; 121:381-91.

108. Kozlowski T, Shimizu A, Lambrigts D, Yamada K, Fuchimoto Y, Glaser R, Monroy R, Xu Y, Awwad M, Colvin RB, Cosimi AB, Robson SC, Fishman J, Spitzer TR, Cooper DK, Sachs DH. Porcine kidney and heart transplantation in baboons undergoing a tolerance induction regimen and antibody adsorption. Transplantation. 1999; 67:18-30.

109. Fontes P, Rogers J, Rao AS, Trucco M, Zeevi A, Ricordi C, Fung JJ, Starzl TE. Evidence for engraftment of human bone marrow cells in non-lethally irradiated baboons. Transplantation. 1997; 64:1595-8.

110. Allen MD, Weyhrich J, Gaur L, Akimoto H, Hall J, Dalesandro J, Sai S, Thomas R, Nelson KA, Andrews RG. Prolonged allogeneic and xenogeneic microchimerism in unmatched primates without immunosuppression by intrathymic implantation of CD34+ donor marrow cells. Cell Immunol. 1997; 181:127-38.

111. Emery DW, Holley K, Sachs DH. Enhancement of swine progenitor chimerism in mixed swine/human bone marrow cultures with swine cytokines. Exp Hematol.

1999; 27:1330-7.

112. Sablinski T, Emery DW, Monroy R, Hawley RJ, Xu Y, Gianello P, Lorf T, Kozlowski T, Bailin M, Cooper DK, Cosimi AB, Sachs DH. Long-term discordant xenogeneic (porcine-to-primate) bone marrow engraftment in a monkey treated with porcine-specific growth factors. Transplantation. 1999; 67:972-7.

113. Kawaharada N, Shears LL, Li S, Pham SM. Mixed hematopoietic chimerism prevents allograft vasculopathy. J Heart Lung Transplant. 1999; 18:532-41.

114. Orloff MS, DeMara EM, Coppage ML, Leong N, Fallon MA, Sickel J, Zuo XJ, Prehn J, Jordan SC. Prevention of chronic rejection and graft arteriosclerosis by tolerance induction. Transplantation. 1995; 59:282-8.

115. Colson YL, Zadach K, Nalesnik M, Ildstad ST. Mixed allogeneic chimerism in the rat - Donor-specific transplantation tolerance without chronic rejection for primarily vascularized cardiac allografts. Transplantation. 1995; 60:971-80.

116. Manilay JO, Pearson DA, Sergio JJ, Swenson KG, Sykes M. Intrathymic deletion of alloreactive T cells in mixed bone marrow chimeras prepared with a nonmyeloablative conditioning regimen. Transplantation. 1998; 66:96-102.

117. Taniguchi H, Abe M, Shirai T, Fukao K, Nakauchi H. Reconstitution ratio is critical for alloreactive T cell deletion and skin graft survival in mixed bone marrow chimeras. J Immunol. 1995; 155:5631-6.

118. Colson YL, Lange J, Fowler K, Ildstad ST. Mechanism for cotolerance in non-lethally conditioned mixed chimeras: negative selection of the Vβ T-cell receptor repertoire by both host and donor bone marrow-derived cells. Blood. 1996; 88:4601-10.

119. Ildstad ST, Wren SM, Boggs SS, Hronakes ML, Vecchini F, Van den Brink MRM. Cross-species bone marrow transplantation: evidence for tolerance induction, stem cell engraftment, and maturation of T lymphocytes in a xenogeneic stromal environment (rat--->mouse). J Exp Med. 1991; 174:467-78.

120. Tomita Y, Khan A, Sykes M. Role of intrathymic clonal deletion and peripheral anergy in transplantation in mice conditioned with a nonmyeloablative regimen. J Immunol. 1994; 153:1087-98.

121. Tomita Y, Khan A, Sykes M. Mechanism by which additional monoclonal antibody (mAB) injections overcome the requirement for thymic irradiation to achieve mixed chimerism in mice receiving bone marrow transplantation after conditioning with anti-T cell mABs and 3-Gy whole body irradiation. Transplantation. 1996; 61:477-85.

122. Nikolic B, Lei H, Pearson DA, Sergio JJ, Swenson KG, Sykes M. Role of intrathymic rat class II+ cells in maintaining deletional tolerance in xenogeneic rat -->mouse bone marrow chimeras [published erratum appears in Transplantation 1999 Jan 27;67(2):340]. Transplantation. 1998; 65:1216-24.

123. Colson YL, AY AE-E, Gaines BA, Ildstad ST. Positive and negative selection of alpha/beta TCR+ T cells in thymectomized adult radiation bone marrow chimeras. Transplantation. 1999; 68:403-10.

124. Ju S-T, Panka DJ, Cul H, Ettinger R, El-Khatib M, Sherr DH, Stanger BZ, Marshak-Rothstein A. Fas(CD95)/FasL interactions required for programmed cell death after T-cell activation. Nature. 1996; 373:444-8.

125. Kabelitz D, Pohl T, Pechhold K. Activation-induced cell death (apoptosis) of mature peripheral T lymphocytes. Immunol Today. 1993; 14:338-9.

STRATEGIES TO PROMOTE TOLERANCE INDUCTION USING DENDRITIC CELLS

9

Angus W. Thomson and Lina Lu
Department of Surgery,
University of Pittsburgh
Pittsburgh, Pennsylvania, USA

INTRODUCTION

Dendritic cells (DC) are rare but extremely important bone marrow (BM)-derived antigen-presenting cells (APC) that initiate and regulate immune responses [1-4]. Extensive recent investigations [reviewed in refs. 3,4] have improved understanding of DC lineage development, differentiation, activation and function. These studies have revealed that, in addition to the well-recognized immunostimulatory properties of DC that offer potential for therapy of infectious disease and cancer, DC also have potential tolerogenicity [reviewed in refs. 2,5,6]. This capacity of DC is manifested by suppression of T cell responses in experimental models of T cell ontogeny, tumor rejection, autoimmunity, and allograft rejection. Moreover, exposure to a wide variety of agents, e.g. ultraviolet B (UVB) irradiation, IL-10, transforming growth factor β (TGFβ), corticosteroids, prostaglandin E_2 (PGE$_2$), or the chimeric fusion protein cytotoxic T lymphocyte antigen (Ag) 4 immunoglobulin (CTLA4Ig) can confer tolerogenic properties on DC. In addition, genetically-engineered DC expressing immunosuppressive molecules, such as viral (v) IL-10, TGFβ, Fas Ligand (L) (CD95L) or CTLA4Ig may offer potential for the suppression/deletion of auto- or alloAg-specific T cells, with implications for tolerance induction.

The concept of DC tolerogenicity is well-established. A role for DC in the induction of self-tolerance within the thymus was recognized in the mid-late 1980s [7,8]. DC have also been shown to induce peripheral, Ag-specific unresponsiveness in various experimental models. Thus, immature DC that express surface major histocompatibility complex (MHC) class II alloAg

A. W. Thomson (ed.), Therapeutic Immunosuppression, 215–242.
© 2001 *Kluwer Academic Publishers.*

(signal 1) but that lack sufficient surface costimulatory molecules (signal 2), in particular CD40, CD80 (B7-1) and CD86 (B7-2), can induce alloAg-specific anergy *in vitro* [9], and prolong heart [10] or pancreatic islet allograft survival [11] in non-immunosuppressed recipients. The cytokines IL-10 and TGFβ downregulate costimulatory molecule or MHC class II Ag expression on DC. IL-10 suppresses IL-12 production, such that proliferation of CD4$^+$ T helper (Th) cells and the cytotoxic activity of CD8$^+$ T cells induced by these DC is inhibited [12,13]. Moreover, there is evidence that DC derived from either lymphoid [14] or myeloid progenitors, and that express surface Fas L [15] can augment programmed cell death (apoptosis) in activated T cells. One of the challenges of contemporary applied DC biology is to ascertain whether DC can be utilized for the selective prevention/therapy of undesired immune responses, as occur in autoimmune diseases, allograft rejection, and allergic hypersensitivity reactions.

DC AND TOLERANCE INDUCTION

Tolerance is a fundamental property of the immune system and underlies selective unresponsiveness to self-Ags. The induction of permanent, drug-free, Ag-specific immunologic unresponsiveness (tolerance) is the ultimate goal of transplant immunologists/physicians and of those seeking to restore tolerance to autoAgs implicated in the pathogenesis of autoimmune diseases. The principal mechanisms by which tolerance is thought to be induced and maintained are clonal deletion, anergy and suppression by regulatory cells. A major determining factor in these processes is the function of APC that are critical for the initiation of primary immune responses. DC can present Ag in either a tolerogenic or immunogenic fashion [16], depending on the inoculation regimen employed and there is ample evidence, from a variety of studies, that DC may play a key role in determining the balance between tolerance and immunity [17]. Upsetting this balance, as for example, in organ transplantation, by augmenting DC in liver allografts by donor treatment with the hematopoietic growth factor fms-like-tyrosine kinase 3 ligand (Flt3L), can switch tolerance to rejection [18]. Table 1 summarizes observations of the tolerogenic capacity of DC in many diverse experimental systems [7-9, 14,16,19-30]. These findings include reports of roles for DC both in central and peripheral tolerance.

Table 1
Observations of the tolerogenic potential of DC

Dendritic cell type	Tolerogenic effect reported	Reference
Thymic DC	Encephalitogen pulsing and adoptive transfer prevents EAE[1]	Khoury et al, 1995 [19]
	Tolerance acquired to host MHC in chimeric thymi	Jenkinson et al, 1985 [7]
Langerhans cells	Deletion enhances effector phase of CH[2]	Grabbe et al, 1995 [20]
Pancreatic lymph node DC	Transfer reduces incidence of diabetes in NOD[3] mice	Clare-Salzler et al, 1995 [21]
BM-derived DC	Diabetogenic peptide-pulsed/unpulsed DC prevent diabetes in NOD mice	Feili-Hariri et al, 1999 [22]
Splenic DC	IFN-γ stimulated NOD mouse DC exert anti-diabetogenic effects	Shinomiya et al, 1999 [23]
Splenic DC	Reconstitution of DC-depleted thymi restores ability to delete thymocytes in vivo	Matzinger & Guerder, 1989 [8]
	Large numbers of DC reduce local HVG[4] reaction	Knight et al, 1983a [24]
	Large numbers of DC/high antigen load inhibit anti-tumor immunity	Knight et al, 1983a [24]
	CD8[+]/Fas-L[+] DC induce apoptosis in activated T cells	Süss & Shortman, 1996 [14]
	CD8[+] DC downregulate the response of naïve CD8 T cells by limiting their IL-2 production	Kronin et al, 1996 [25]
Costimulator-deficient DC progenitors (BM or blood-derived)	Induction of alloantigen-specific T cell hyporesponsiveness	Lu et al, 1996 [9]; Hayamizu et al, 1998 [26]
CD40-deficient DC (BM-derived)	Induction of alloantigen-specific T cell hyporesponsiveness	Gao et al, 1999 [27]
Renal interstitial DC	Discordant expression of MHC class II and invariant chain may be a regulatory mechanism for peripheral T cell tolerance	Saleem et al, 1997 [28]
Cervical lymph node DC	Adoptive transfer delays the onset of lymphocytic thyroiditis	Delemarre et al, 1995 [29]
Mouse DC	Injection of rat anti-DC mAbs induces rat Ig-specific tolerance	Finkelman et al, 1996 [16]
Mouse DC	Induction of T cell anergy by tumor-associated Ag	Grohmann et al, 1997 [30]

[1]Experimental allergic encephalomyelitis; [2]Contact hypersensitivity; [3]Non-obese diabetic; [4]Host versus graft

Induction of central tolerance by DC

The thymus plays a major role in immune homeostasis by the deletion of self-reactive T cells, thus contributing to the maintenance of self-tolerance. A number of cell types within the thymus, including DC, provide signals responsible for the negative selection of T cells. Matzinger & Guerder [8] outlined the critical role of DC in central tolerance by demonstrating that the tolerogenic properties of the APC-depleted mouse thymus could be restored by reconstitution with purified splenic DC. Intrathymic injection of Mls-incompatible spleen or thymic DC can induce tolerance via clonal anergy [31]. Similar results have been reported in parent → F_1 BM chimeras, and in transgenic mice [32,33]. Strong T cell tolerance in parent → F_1 BM chimeras prepared with supralethal irradiation was evident at the level of mature thymocytes, and presumably occurred in the thymus itself. It was demonstrated that T cell contact with thymic epithelial cells (including DC) induced clonal deletion of most of the host-reactive T cells, but also spared a proportion of low affinity cells. These findings indicate that the role of DC in deletion of autoreactive T cells within the thymus is not dependent upon unique characteristics of thymic DC, but may also be mediated by signaling provided by DC from other tissues.

Since the thymus is the primary site for central tolerance induction, a direct approach to tolerance by clonal deletion is intrathymic Ag injection. Acquired thymic tolerance, induced by intrathymic injection of Ag has been demonstrated in a number of autoimmune diseases [34-37]. Thus, injection of the immunodominant peptide of myelin basic protein (MBP) into the thymus of Lewis rats, protects the animals from experimental allergic encephalomyelitis (EAE) [36]. Thymic DC isolated from these animals can transfer protection to naive recipients, suggesting that DC mediate the effects of acquired thymic tolerance [19]. Moreover, thymic but not splenic DC pulsed ex vivo with the encephalitogenic peptide protect naïve recipients from EAE when injected systemically [19, 38]. Interestingly, animals thymectomized before systemic injection of the ex vivo pulsed APCs were not protected, raising the question of site-specific homing of DC.

The capacity of intrathymic injection of donor spleen cells [39] BM cells, renal glomeruli [40], pancreatic islets [41] or DC [42] to induce tolerance has been reported, indicating that this effect is not restricted to hematopoietic cells. While intrathymic injection has been very effective for tolerance induction in rodents, successful large animal studies have not been reported. In humans, the disadvantages of this approach are that (i), there is no effective method to eliminate mature donor-reactive T cells in large animals, and (ii), the thymus of adult large animals, including humans, is involuted, making it difficult to determine whether it still functions.

Induction of peripheral tolerance by DC, and proposed underlying mechanisms

It is now evident that DC can provide both stimulatory and down-regulatory signals for immune reactions. Recent studies suggest that mouse myeloid DC generated *in vitro* and exhibiting an 'immature' or 'costimulatory molecule-deficient' surface phenotype, or mouse lymphoid (CD8α^+) DC can subvert allogeneic T cell responses. In addition, adoptive transfer of autoAg-pulsed thymic DC [19], or MBP-pulsed splenic DC whose functional expression of costimulatory molecules (CD80 and CD86) has been blocked by CTLA4Ig [38], can inhibit the development of autoimmune disease (EAE). Possible mechanisms involved in DC tolerogenicity are summarized below:

Selective activation of Th2 cell subsets. The mechanism of protection afforded against EAE by Ag-pulsed DC treated with CTLA4Ig is probably a Th2 switch. Immunohistology of the CNS demonstrated almost complete inhibition of Th1 cytokines (IL-2 and IFN-γ), with upregulation of Th2 cytokines (IL-4 and IL-13) [38]. Splenic DC pretreated with TGFβ and encephalitogenic peptide were also tolerogenic (Khoury S. etal; unpublished observations). Thus, non-tolerogenic DC may become tolerogenic by blocking their ability to provide costimulatory signals, or by their modification with suppressive cytokines.

The capacity of diabetogenic, peptide-pulsed or unpulsed BM-derived myeloid DC to prevent the development of type-1 diabetes in non-obese diabetic (NOD) mice has been ascribed to a shift in the balance between regulatory Th2 and effector Th1 cells [22]. Other investigators have observed that Ag-specific suppression of delayed-type hypersensitivity responses can be achieved by i.v. administration of Ag-pulsed Langerhans cells (LC) [43], or splenic DC [44], possibly via a mechanism involving selective activation of Th2-like cells [45].

Induction of regulatory T cells. Pre-diabetic NOD mice can be protected from the development of type-1 diabetes by transfer of DC isolated from pancreatic lymph nodes of diabetic animals [21]. This effect may be mediated by a mechanism involving the enhanced induction of regulatory T cells. Similarly, Delemarre et al [29] have observed that transfer of cervical node DC from autoimmune lymphocytic thyroiditis (LT)-resistant BB/Wor rats to LT-prone BB/Wor recipients delays the onset of LT.

Induction of T cell anergy. Costimulatory signals delivered by APC (e.g. via CD40, CD80, and CD86) have been proposed to regulate the induction of immune responses. Ag-specific tolerance can be achieved when T cell receptor (TCR) triggering (signal 1) occurs without sufficient costimulation (signal 2), a process leading to anergy or apoptosis. Therefore, selective blockade of costimulatory signals is a promising strategy for therapeutic immunosuppression [46, 47]. We and others have demonstrated that DC whose T cell stimulatory function is impaired, either by incomplete maturation, selective blockade of B7 family costimulatory molecules (using CTLA4Ig), the influence of specific cytokines (i.e. IL-10), or UVB irradiation, can either induce Ag-specific hyporesponsiveness or apoptosis *in vitro*, and/or suppress immune reactivity. Table 2 summarizes observations on manipulations that promote DC tolerogenicity [48-55]. Grohmann et al [30] reported that a tumor-associated and self-Ag peptide presented by DC could induce T cell anergy *in vivo*, but that IL-12 could prevent or revert the anergic state.

Intrathymic injection of Ag mediates peripheral tolerance through interaction of thymic DC with activated peripheral T cells that circulate to the thymus. This interaction leads to peripheral T cell anergy [56]. There is also evidence that intrathymic Ag injection leads to apoptosis of T cells, as dem-

Table 2
Manipulations that promote DC tolerogenicity

Dendritic cell type	Tolerogenic effect reported	Reference
CTLA4-Ig-treated splenic DC	Protection from EAE*	Verberg et al, 1996 [48]
IL-10 treated Langerhans cells	Induction of Ag-specific anergy in vitro	Enk et al, 1993 [49]
IL-10 treated splenic DC	Induction of Th2 response in vivo	De Smedt et al, 1997 [50]
Immature DC exposed to IL-10	Induction of alloantigen- or peptide-specific anergy in T cells	Steinbrink et al, 1997 [51]
IL-10 treated DC	Induction of Th2 differentiation	Liu et al, 1998 [52]
DC grown in PGE$_2$	Promotion of Th2 development	Kalinski et al, 1997 [53]
Corticosteroid-induced monocyte-derived DC (DC3)	Promote Th2 responses	De Jong et al, 1999 [54]
Ultraviolet-B irradiated Langerhans cells	Ag-specific unresponsiveness of Th1 cells in vitro	Simon et al, 1991 [55]

* EAE; experimental allergic encephalomyelitis

onstrated in a TCR transgenic mouse system [57].

Induction of activated T cell apoptosis. The expression by DC of molecules associated with the inhibition of T cell growth or the induction of T cell apoptosis (i.e. nitric oxide [NO], or Fas L) may render DC capable of subverting T cell responses. Mouse splenic CD8$^+$ (lymphoid) DC expressing FasL have been reported to induce apoptosis in activated allogeneic CD4$^+$ T cells, resulting in diminished T cell proliferation in mixed leukocyte reactions [MLR] [14]. These DC can also impair IL-2 production by CD8$^+$ T cells [25]. DC exposed to interferon-γ (IFN–γ), bacterial endotoxin (=lipopolysaccharide; LPS), or allogeneic T cells can synthesize NO synthase (NOS). Consequent NO production suppresses allogeneic T cell proliferation in MLR, and also promotes apoptosis, both in the activated T cells and in the DC themselves [58, 59]. Highly-purified myeloid DC grown from mouse BM in GM-CSF + IL-4 have been found to express FasL mRNA by reverse transcriptase polymerase chain reaction (RT-PCR), and to uniformly express surface FasL, by both flow cytometric and immunocytochemical analysis [15]. These cells, but not DC propagated from FasL-deficient (*gld*) mice, induce dose-dependent increases in DNA fragmentation in Fas$^+$ Jurkat T cells. The same DC also induce apoptosis of alloactivated T cells, once the CD28/B7 pathway is blocked by CTLA4Ig [15]. It is tempting to speculate that in organ transplantation, FasL$^+$ donor liver DC trafficking to the host might be responsible for the cytotoxic T cell deletion associated with murine spontaneous liver allograft acceptance and tolerance induction [60]. Apoptosis of immunoreactive host cells is also associated with the marked prolongation of heart allograft survival observed in mice preconditioned with immature donor DC and anti-CD40L mAb [61].

Down regulation of B cell clonal expansion cells by follicular DC. In germinal centers, B lymphocytes are intimately associated with follicular dendritic cells (FDC). It has been hypothesized that FDC are involved in the regulation of B cell growth and differentiation through cell-cell interaction. Highly-enriched preparations of human FDC strongly inhibit mitogen-stimulated B cells, suggesting that FDC may downregulate the clonal expansion of B cells that occurs within lymphoid follicles as part of the normal immune response [62].

Significance of the route of DC administration, cell number and Ag load. Under experimental conditions, DC exhibit a dichotomous potential to regulate immune responsiveness, depending on the source or sub-set of DC, the route of their *in vivo* administration, the number of cells injected, and the amount of Ag presented. Thus, DC loaded with low doses of tumor Ag can enhance tumor rejection in mice, while DC loaded with high doses, or administration of large numbers of tumor Ag- pulsed DC inhibit the anti-tumor effect [24]. BM-derived DC propagated *in vitro* with GM-CSF + IL-4 accelerate donor-specific kidney allograft rejection if delivered i.v., but can prolong graft survival when administrated via the portal vein [63]. Liver-derived immature DC prolong pancreatic islet allograft survival, whereas splenic DC propagated from the same mice, using the same technique, induce rejection of islet allografts in diabetic recipients [11]. There is also considerable evidence that specific components of the local tissue microenvironment, e.g. the anti-inflammatory cytokine TGFβ, may be responsible for imparting tolerogenic activity to DC that migrate from the anterior chamber of the eye to regional lymphoid tissue [64].

Thus, DC are capable of eliciting positive (sensitizing) and negative (tolerizing) responses in the immune system. This reflects the molecular regulation of their immunologic activity, including expression of first and second signals for Th cell activation, stimulatory cytokines (IL-12, IL-6), and death-inducing ligands (reviewed below). The ability to generate immunoregulatory DC in sufficient number has considerable implications for the therapy of cancer, infectious disease, autoimmunity and allograft rejection.

MOLECULAR BASIS OF DC TOLEROGENICITY

The potent capacity of mature DC to activate naïve T cells is related to their high surface expression of MHC class II Ag, and T cell-costimulatory molecules, such as CD40, CD80, and CD86. Deficiency or absence of expression of these molecules reduces the APC function of DC and may render them potentially tolerogenic. DC residing in peripheral tissues (such as epidermal LC of the skin) express relatively low levels of co-stimulatory molecules, and are poor T cell stimulators when freshly isolated [65]. LC precursors in the epidermis function poorly as T cell stimulators [66], and there is even evidence that LC may provide down-regulatory signals during elicitation of cutaneous (contact sensitivity) inflammatory reactions [20]. MHC class II⁻ DC precursors in the airway epithelium of rats [67], freshly-isolated heart or kidney DC [68], and DC progenitors propagated from the mouse liver [69] are also poor allostimulators. It has been suggested that the absence of expression of invariant chain (nonpolymorphic polypeptide associated with MHC class II, and known to play an important role in assembly and peptide loading of class II molecules) by interstitial DC within non-lymphoid tissue [28] may also be a significant factor in the regulation of self-tolerance.

Presentation of Ag to T cells by APC in the absence of co-stimulatory molecules induces T cell anergy [70]. The importance of costimulatory molecule deficiency on DC in peripheral tolerance induction has been emphasized by the fact that CTLA4Ig, a potent blocker of the B7-CD28 pathway, significantly prolongs the survival of experimental organ allografts [71,72]. Studies in our laboratory have demonstrated that myeloid DC propagated from mouse BM or liver in suboptimal concentrations of GM-CSF express only low levels of costimulatory molecules (MHC class II$^+$, CD80^{lo}, CD86$^-$). These cells not only induce alloAg-specific T cell hyporesponsiveness [9], but also extend survival of donor strain cardiac [10] or pancreatic islet allografts [11] when administered systemically one week before transplantation. Likewise, in an autoimmune disease model, MBP-pulsed DC on which the expression of CD80 and CD86 has been blocked by CTLA4Ig protect rats from the induction of EAE [38]. It has also been suggested that rhesus monkey BM-derived DC progenitors (MHC class II$^{-/dim}$) may exert tolerance-promoting activity *in vivo* and *in vitro* [73]. These observations have strengthened the view that immature, costimulatory molecule-deficient DC may play a role in peripheral T cell tolerance induction.

It has been reported that CD8α^+ (lymphoid) DC isolated from mouse spleen express Fas L (CD95L) and are capable of killing activated CD4$^+$ T cells via the Fas/FasL pathway [14]. It has been proposed that Ag presentation by LDC induces deletional tolerance [74]. Expression of the CD8 molecule by these DC [75], was thought initially to enable them to express a 'veto' function [76,77]. However, more recent evidence indicates that CD8 is not important in the "veto" function of murine lymphoid DC [78]. Mouse myeloid DC propagated from BM in GM-CSF + IL-4 (MHC class II^{hi}, CD80^{hi}, CD86^{hi}) also express functional Fas L [15], but induce only low levels of apoptosis in alloactivated T cells. When the B7/CD28 pathway is blocked with CTLA4Ig, however, significant augmentation of T cell apoptosis is detected, indicating that FasL and B7 molecules on DC may play counter-regulatory roles in proliferation and survival of T cells following DC-T cell interaction. Fas/FasL interaction is probably not the only death-inducing pathway that exists in DC-T cell interaction, because a high level of T cell apoptosis can also be induced by DC propagated from the BM of FasL-deficient (*gld*) mice in the presence of CTLA4Ig [15]. Other molecules expressed by DC could contribute to DC-induced apoptosis. Candidate molecular pathways include tumor necrosis factor (TNF)/TNFR, TNFR apoptosis-inducing ligand (TRAIL)/TRAILR, or 4-1BB/4-1BBL [79,80].

Studies of LPS-treated mice have suggested that NO production by presumptive intrathymic DC may be responsible for thymocyte apoptosis, and possibly self-tolerance [81]. These observations are consistent with NO production by a subpopulation of myeloid DC following their exposure to IFN-γ or LPS, or interaction with allogeneic T cells [58,59].

The special properties of DC (expression of MHC and costimulatory/ regulatory molecules, responsiveness to immunosuppressive cytokines, and *in vivo* homing to T-dependent areas of lymphoid tissues to interact with Ag-specific T-cells [82-84]) make manipulation of these cells to maximize their tolerogenic potential an attractive approach to cell-based therapy of immune-mediated disorders (allograft rejection and autoimmune disease). Approaches to the generation of DC with the capacity to inhibit T cell responses will now be discussed.

CULTURE OF "TOLEROGENIC" DC FOR THERAPEUTIC APPLICATION, - THE INFLUENCE OF CYTOKINES, AND OTHER MICROENVIRONMENTAL FACTORS

Only trace numbers of DC can be recovered from normal tissue. The description by Inaba et al [85,86] of a method to propagate DC progenitors from normal mouse BM or blood in response to GM-CSF, has ensured the availability of large numbers of myeloid DC, and opened up possibilities for immunotherapy using DC as vaccines. Numerous groups have subsequently described methods for culture of large numbers of highly stimulatory human, non-human primate, mouse, or rat DC from different tissues using GM-CSF, most often in combination with IL-4. More limited studies have reported the propagation of DC with "tolerogenic" properties.

It is well-recognized that specific cytokines play key roles in the regulation of DC maturation and activation. Thus for example, TNFα enhances the development of mature DC from human progenitors [87,88], whereas IL-1β inhibits the function of LC [89]. Monocytes represent an abundant source of precursors that can polarize towards either DC or macrophages ('dendrophages') depending on the external stimuli. This polarization can be driven *in vitro* by the addition of appropriate cytokines (GM-CSF + IL-4, or macrophage [M]-CSF = colony stimulating factor-1, respectively). Monocyte-derived DC generated in culture with GM-CSF and IL-4 have a very high level of cell surface MHC class II and costimulatory molecules [90].

IL-10 is an excellent example of a cytokine that inhibits DC maturation and function and that confers tolerogenic potential on DC. IL-10 reduces the expression of MHC class II (HLA-DR) or CD86 molecules, but not CD80 or intercellular adhesion molecule-1 (ICAM-1; CD54) on human peripheral blood DC [91], and downregulates both CD80 and CD86 expression on murine LC [92]. It inhibits the upregulation of CD83, CD86 and CD58 on *in vitro* generated human DC [51]. IL-10 also suppresses the production of IL-8 and TNF-α by LPS-activated DC [93]. There is also evidence that IL-10 pretreatment strongly inhibits the DC-induced responses of naive and primed CD4+ T cells in allogeneic MLR and anti-CD3 assays [51]. In addition, IL-10 pretreated immature human DC induce alloAg- or peptide-specific anergy in CD4+ T cells [51]. IL-10 can skew the Th1/Th2 balance to Th2 cells by blocking IL-12 synthesis by DC [93, 94]. It has also been reported that IL-10 accelerates murine LC apoptosis in culture [95]. Interestingly, Kalinski et al have reported that DC grown in the presence of prostaglandin E_2 (PGE_2) are unable to secrete IL-12, and when they present Ag they promote the development of Th2 cells [53].

Several methods for obtaining 'tolerogenic' DC are summarized below. A critical feature of cell propagation for determination of DC function is the removal of contaminating cells, that include granulocytes, macrophages, and B cells. Non-adherent granulocytes can be rinsed away during culture, whereas macrophages remain firmly affixed to the culture plates. Most B cells, which represent a major component of starting BM cell suspensions, can be removed initially by depletion with Ab and complement, or using immunomagnetic beads. Positive selection by cell sorting, or the use of immunomagnetic beads can generally yield DC of very high purity.

Propagation of "tolerogenic"DC

Propagation of "tolerogenic" DC from non-lymphoid tissue (liver). Liver-derived DC progenitors can be propagated in liquid culture in response to GM-CSF [69], using a similar approach to that of Inaba et al [85,86] for the generation of mouse blood or BM-derived DC. The loosely-attached or floating cells with dendritic morphology that can be harvested after 7-10 days of culture are negative for lymphoid lineage markers, positive for the DC markers DEC 205 and CD11c, MHC class II^{lo}, CD86^{lo} and positive for F4/80, and CD32. They are poor allostimulators, elicit low levels of CTL alloresponses *in vitro*, and significantly prolong pancreatic islet allograft survival if given i.v. (2×10^6) 7 days before transplantation in streptozotocin-diabetic mice [11]. Large numbers of DC progenitors can be generated from the livers of mice treated with Flt3L [96].

Table 3
Influence of donor-specific GM-CSF-stimulated immature DC (B7-2⁻) on B10 cardiac allograft survival in C3H mice[a]

Group	Cells injected Day-7	n	Graft survival time (days)	MST
A	None (media control)	8	8(x3), 12, 13(x2), 9, 10	9.5
B	Fresh B10 bone marrow cells (allogeneic)	4	12(x4)	12
Cultured cells				
C	B10 (B7-2⁺) (allogeneic)	17	4 (x5), 5(x3), 7(x2), 8(x2), 9, 10, 14(x2), 15	7[b]
D	B10 (B7-2⁻) (allogeneic)	15	7, 19(x4), 20, 22(x2), 23, 26, 27, 29, 30, 35, 67	22[c,d]
E	C3H (B7-2⁻) (syngeneic)	4	12 (x2), 13 (x2)	12.5
F	BALB/c (B7-2⁻)(third party)	9	7, 12, 16 (x2), 17(x3), 19, 20	16.5

[a]Cells (2×10^6 i.v.) were injected 7 days before heterotopic (B10→C3H) heart transplantation. MST = median survival time. MSTs were compared using the Kruskal-Wallis test. Pairwise comparison was done using the Wilcoxon sum rank test.
[b]$P < 0.01$ compared with groups D and F.
[c]$P < 0.003$ compared with groups C and E.
[d]$P < 0.01$ compared with group F.
For further details, see Fu *et al* [10].

Growth of "tolerogenic" DC from BM using suboptimal concentrations of GM-CSF. GM-CSF is an essential cytokine for the propagation of myeloid DC from proliferating precursors or hematopoietic stem cells. Its effect on DC maturation appears to be dose-related. DC progenitors, deficient in cell surface costimulatory molecules can be grown from the BM of normal or non-obese diabetic (NOD) mice, using an appropriate low concentration of GM-CSF, with removal of contaminating granulocytes by Ab + complement depletion or gradient separation. The cells are characterized as DEC205⁺, MHC class II⁺, CD40^{lo}, CD80^{lo}, CD86$^{-/lo}$, poor stimulators of naive allogenic T cells in MLR, and with a high level of endocytotic activity. These "immature" DC induce alloAg-specific hyporesponsiveness in T cells [9], and prolong heart allograft survival when injected i.v. (2×10^6) 7 days before organ transplantation [10] (Table 3). Treatment of young prediabetic NOD mice with GM-CSF-stimulated, BM-derived 'tolerogenic' DC grown in low concentration GM-CSF, and pulsed with peptides from islet cell Ag, prevents diabetes development [22].

Growth of 'tolerogenic' DC from mouse BM with GM-CSF+TGFβ. TGFβ is a potent immunosuppressive cytokine [97] that affects the proliferation and differentiation of hematopoietic progenitors, including DC. It blocks mouse DC maturation *in vitro* [98,99]. This effect was thought to be mediated via Fc-receptor (CD32) -bearing suppressor cells, presumably macrophages. However, TGFβ1 did not inhibit the production of immature, MHC class II+, CD86- DC, and also did not suppress the differentiation of these cells. Strobl et al [100] found that TGFβ1 promoted GM-CSF, TNF-α and c-kit ligand-induced DC development from CD34+ hematopoietic progenitors in human cord blood. The cord blood-derived DC that developed in the presence of additional TGFβ1 were CD1a+, and did not have strong allo-MLR stimulatory activity. Their surface phenotype and function were similar to those of freshly-isolated epidermal LC (immature DC). We have used TGFβ1 in conjunction with GM-CSF to facilitate the generation of mouse BM-derived DC deficient in costimulatory molecule expression and with tolerogenic potential [99]. Compared with propagation of immature DC in low concentrations of GM-CSF alone, relatively high yields and purity of these cells can be obtained from normal mouse BM using GM-CSF plus TGFβ1. The blocking effect of TGFβ on DC maturation can be reversed, either by adding TNF-α or IL-4, or by removing inhibitory cells (CD32+ adherent cells).

DC propagated in GM-CSF+TGFβ1 and administered i.v. 7 days before organ transplantation can significantly prolong the survival of vascularized heart allografts from the same donor strain [99]. There is also evidence that TGFβ1 impairs the antigen presenting function of human BM-derived APC, including DC [101]. In the context of these and other reports, TGFβ has been implicated strongly as a key microenvironmental factor, acting on APC, in the generation of immune deviation and immunological privilege, such as occurs in the anterior chamber of the eye [64, 102].

THERAPEUTIC APPLICATION OF DC IN EXPERIMENTAL ORGAN TRANSPLANTATION

Using techniques established to propagate DC progenitors from normal mouse liver [69], it was found that DC progenitors of donor origin could be propagated from the BM of mice that spontaneously accepted MHC-mismatched liver allografts [103]. Donor-derived DC could not however, be grown from the BM of mice that acutely rejected heart grafts from the same donor strain [103, 104]. These findings suggested that allogeneic DC might play a role in the induction of allotolerance. Donor-derived DC progenitors can also be propagated from the blood of human liver allograft recipients given adjunctive donor BM in an effort to promote allograft survival [105, 106]. Immunohistochemical studies of Demetris et al [107] suggested that persistence of donor-derived DC in heart allografts might be important in the long-term maintenance of transplantation tolerance, and the prevention of (chronic) allograft rejection.

We have observed that significant prolongation of mouse heart allografts can be achieved by pretreatment of recipients with immature donor-derived DC propagated from mouse BM, using either GM-CSF [10] or GM-CSF + TGFβ1 (TGFβ-DC) [99]. One to eight x 10^6 immature donor (B10; H2^b) DC were injected i.v. into C3H (H2^k) recipients, 7 days before B10 heart transplantation. DC propagated using GM-CSF + IL-4 (mature DC; IL-4-DC) accelerated rejection of subsequent heart grafts from B10 donors. Median graft survival time was strikingly reduced from 10 to 5 days in the IL-4 DC pretreatment group. By contrast, TGFβ-DC (2 x 10^6 i.v., 7 days before organ transplantation) significantly prolonged median heart graft survival time (from 10 to 26 days). This therapeutic effect was correlated with suppression of recipient T cell proliferation in response to alloAg challenge *in vitro*, and with low CTL responses to donor targets cells. If C3H recipients were treated with TGFβ-DC from the BM of either B10 (donor), C3H (recipient) or BALB/c (H2^d; third party), prolongation of graft survival was achieved only using donor strain DC. TGFβ-DC of the B10 strain were unable to prolong BALB/c heart graft (third party) survival. These studies indicated that the effect of the TGFβ-DC was Ag-specific. The inhibition of cardiac allograft rejection by TGFβ-DC was also dependent on the timing of donor DC administration. Two x 10^6 B10 TGFβ-DC were given i.v. once only, on either days -14,-7,-3, or +2 in relation to B10 heart transplantation on day 0. Only administration of the DC on day -7 significantly prolonged subsequent heart graft survival. Furthermore, increases in the number of TGFβ-DC above 2 x 10^6 (to 8 x 10^6) did not significantly affect median graft survival time, indicating the importance of donor-specific Ag, timing, and the amount of Ag delivered by the DC.

THERAPEUTIC APPLICATION OF DC IN EXPERIMENTAL AUTOIMMUNE DISEASE

Evidence that DC can be used or manipulated to exhibit "tolerogenic" effects in autoimmune disease has come predominantly from studies in experimental models of type-1 diabetes or multiple sclerosis. Clare-Salzler etal

[21] showed that pancreatic lymph node DC from diabetic NOD mice could inhibit the development of disease when adoptively transferred to prediabetic NOD recipients. More recently, Feili-Hariri *et al* [22] have reported that BM-derived DC from NOD mice pulsed with pancreatic islet Ag-derived peptides and injected into prediabetic NOD recipients could prevent diabetes development. Moreover, it appeared on the basis of IgG1 Ab responses in the DC-treated mice, that a Th2 response was generated, suggesting that the balance between regulatory Th2 and effector Th1 cells may have been altered. It has also been reported that IFN-γ-stimulated NOD mouse splenic DC exert anti-diabetogenic effects [23]. Adoptive transfer of autoAg (MBP)-pulsed thymic DC or splenic DC (treated with CTLA4Ig) prevents development of EAE in the rat [19,38], also associated with a Th2 switch.

BLOCKADE OF COSTIMULATION POTENTIATES THE THERAPEUTIC EFFECT OF DC

Although costimulatory molecule-deficient DC can prolong allograft survival, most published observations to date indicate that they do not induce permanent allograft acceptance in non-immunosuppressed recipients. Failure of these cells to induce allograft tolerance may be due to the "late" upregulation of costimulatory molecules on the DC following their interaction with host T cells. This hypothesis is supported by the observation that *in vitro* exposure of B10 TGFβ-DC to C3H spleen T cells for 18 hr induces CD40 and B7 molecule expression on the DC [61]. To achieve long-term graft acceptance, it appears important to prevent 'late' upregulation of costimulatory molecules, or to block upregulated costimulatory signal expression with agents such as CTLA4Ig.

The CD40/CD40L (gp 39) pathway has been shown to play an important role in DC activation, and is crucial for the establishment of primary and secondary responses to T-dependent Ags [108,109]. Thus, CD40 engagement upregulates the expression of CD80 and CD86 on DC, providing a link between the CD40/CD40L and CD80:CD86/ CD28:CTLA4 pathways [110, 111]. Ligation of CD40 on DC also induces production/secretion of IL-12, an important Th1 cell activating cytokine. Combination of allogeneic immature DC injection with blockade of the CD40/CD40L pathway using anti-CD40L mAb 7 days before cardiac transplantation results in long-term graft survival, with indefinite (>100 days) graft acceptance in 40% of recipients [99]. A single injection of anti-CD40L mAb alone failed to prolong heart graft survival. This therapeutic effect is not confined to use of DC as the donor cell population. Parker et al [112] have shown in a different model, that anti-CD40L mAb combined with donor small lymphocytes blocks rejection of pancreatic islet allografts. Moreover, Hancock et al [113] found that treatment of recipients with donor spleen cells and anti-CD40L mAb led to indefinite survival of mouse cardiac allografts, although repeated administration of the Ab was required.

The mechanism(s) by which administration of anti-CD40L mAb together with either costimulator-deficient donor DC [99], or resting B cells [114] induces long-term graft survival is not clear. It was noted in the resting B cell studies, that long-term graft survival was associated with striking inhibition of intragraft Th1 cytokine and IL-12 expression, with reciprocal upregulation of Th2 cytokines. Our own studies have shown that the anti-donor CTL activity of freshly-isolated, heart graft-infiltrating cells is dramatically diminished in mice given combined immature DC/anti-CD40L mAb therapy [99]. Generation of anti-donor CTL from recipient spleens is also markedly depressed. More significantly, increased apoptosis of graft-infiltrating cells and spleen cells is associated with comparatively high levels of donor cell microchimerism, found in the combined treatment group, compared with untreated animals, or those given either immature donor DC or mAb treatment alone [61].

In conclusion, the manner in which Ag is presented by DC plays an important role in the regulation of allogeneic DC-T cell interactions *in vivo*. The critical role of CD40 expression on donor DC, and of CD40L in T cell activation, provides a rational basis for blockade of this pathway to augment the tolerogenic potential of donor costimulator-deficient DC in the long-term suppression of organ allograft rejection.

IMMUNOSUPPRESSIVE DRUGS INHIBIT DC MATURATION, AND MAY PROMOTE DC TOLEROGENICITY *IN VIVO*

Evidence has accumulated that immunosuppressive drugs, including costicosteroids, cyclosporine, and deoxyspergualin can inhibit DC maturation, either *in vitro* or *in vivo*. Corticosteroids inhibit the maturation of immature, human monocyte-derived DC, as assessed by lack of expression of CD83, and prevention of loss of Ag-uptake capacity. These corticosteroid-induced DC (termed "tolerogenic DC3") that express low levels of costimulatory molecules, produce reduced levels of IL-12p 70, and induce development of Th2 cells [54]. Studies by Lee etal [115] have shown that cyclosporine also inhibits (murine) DC maturation *in vitro*, and that this effect is associated with inhibition of the nuclear translocation of the gene regulatory protein NFκB, that has been shown to play a significant role in DC maturation. Recent findings by Thomas etal [116] suggest that deoxyspergualin inhibits the maturation of rhesus monkey DC, both *in vitro* and *in vivo*. Thus, administration of deoxyspergualin to anti-CD3 immunotoxin-treated recipients of renal allografts inhibited DC maturation i.e. expression of CD83, CD86 and rel B (an NFκB family member) within lymphoid tissue, in association with the induction of transplant tolerance. Taken together, these findings indicate that a mechanism underlying the immunosuppressive/tolerogenic properties of a diverse group of immunosuppressive drugs may be inhibition of DC cell maturation.

OTHER FORMS OF COMBINATION IMMUNOSUPPRESSIVE THERAPY USING DC

In addition to costimulation blockade or immunosuppressive drugs, other approaches to tolerance induction using donor DC in experimental organ transplantation include their combination with anti-T cell mAbs, or other immunosuppressive agents. Administration of anti-CD4 mAb potentiates the capacity of immature donor DC to prolong heart allograft survival in mice [27], whereas anti-CD4 + anti-CD8 mAb enhances the ability of donor DC to prolong mouse skin graft survival. In the rat, total lymphoid irradiation + anti-thymocyte globulin in combination with immature DC facilitates the long-term acceptance of heart allografts. Strategies using DC to prolong allograft survival are summarized in Table 4 [10,11,26,27,117-121]. These include a recent report of the use of allopeptide-pulsed host DC to induce donor-specific tolerance following their intrathymic injection in ALS-treated, cardiac allografted rats [119].

GENETIC ENGINEERING OF TOLEROGENIC DC

The foregoing information has shown that the antigen-presenting function of DC is impaired and their potential tolerogenicity enhanced, either by their incomplete maturation, the influence of anti-inflammatory cytokines (IL-10, viral IL-10, or TGFβ), blockade of surface costimulatory molecules (CTLA4Ig or anti-CD40L mAb) or immunosuppressive drugs. Since DC maturation is linked to nuclear translocation of NFκB, antagonism of this gene transcrip-

Table 4
Prolongation of allograft survival by DC

Treatment	Graft	Reference(s)
(a) DC alone:		
Costimulator-deficient DC progenitors/immature DC	Cardiac (mouse)	Fu et al, 1996 [10]
	Pancreatic islet (mouse)	Rastellini et al, 1995 [11]
	Cardiac (mouse)	Suri et al, 1998 [117]
CD40-deficient DC	Cardiac (mouse)	Gao et al, 1999 [27]
NFKβ oligodeoxyribo-nucleotide-treated DC	Cardiac (mouse)	Giannoukakis et al, 1999 [118]
Allopeptide-pulsed host DC (intrathymic)	Cardiac (rat)	Garrovillo et al 1999 [119]
(b) DC in combination with:		
Anti-CD40L mAb	Cardiac (mouse)	Lu et al, 1997; 1999 [61,99]
	Skin (mouse)	Markees et al, 1999 [120]
Anti-CD4 mAb	Cardiac (mouse)	Gao et al, 1999 [27]
TLI + ATG	Cardiac (rat)	Hayamizu et al, 1998 [28]
Anti-CD4 + CD8 mAbs	Skin (mouse)	Gozzo et al, 1999 [121]

TLI = total lymphoid irradiation
ATG = anti-lymphocyte globulin

Table 5
Candidate genes as modulators of DC tolerogenicity

Gene	Possible effect
(v) IL-10	Inhibition of expression of CD80, CD86 and MHC II; suppression of IL-12; induction of Th2 response
TGFβ	Inhibition of T cell proliferation
IFN-γdR	Neutralizes IFN-γ
EBI-3	Competitive intracellular binder of IL-12-p35
INOS	Apoptosis-inducing activity for T cells
CTLA4Ig	Blockade of B7 costimulatory signal
CD40Ig	Blockade of CD40-CD40L pathway
Fas Ligand	Apoptosis inducing activity for T cells
TRAIL*	Apoptosis inducing activity for T cells

* TNF receptor apoptosis-inducing ligand

tion regulatory protein by specific antagonist molecules may also enhance DC tolerogenicity. In addition, the expression by DC of key molecules associated with inhibition of T cell growth (NO), or with induction of T cell apoptosis (FasL, or other death-inducing ligands) suggests that transfer of genes encoding one or more of these molecules (summarized in Table 5) either alone or in combination, may render DC tolerogenic in models of transplantation or autoimmune disease.

DC can be genetically modified using retroviral or adenoviral vectors [122,123] or transfected with particulate/plasmid-based vectors that take advantage of the highly phagocytic nature of immature DC/DC progenitors. Thus, Song et al [122], Specht et al [123], and Wan et al [124] have demonstrated that transfer of genes enocoding model Ags renders mouse BM-derived DC capable of inducing protective and/or therapeutic antitumor immunity.

A variety of techniques have been employed to genetically engineer DC to express immunosuppressive molecules including vIL-10 [125,126], TGFβ [127], CTLA4Ig [128,129] and FasL [130-131] (Table 6). DC progenitors from mouse BM transfected with vIL-10-encoding plasmids via gene gun delivery synthesize vIL-10 and exhibit substantially reduced capacity for the induction of allogeneic T cell proliferation (W. Storkus and T. Tueting, personal communication). vIL-10 production by DC is associated with significant reductions in cell surface expression of MHC class II and costimulatory molecules (CD80, CD86). We have also reported [125] that retroviral transduction of mouse BM-derived myeloid DC to produce vIL-10 substantially impairs their allostimulatory activity. Moreover, it renders the DC able to induce alloAg-specific T cell hyporesponsiveness. Production of a "sorting" retroviral vector, encoding both vIL-10 and enhanced green fluorescent protein, permits selection (purification) of positive transfectants (potentially tolerogenic vIL-10-secreting DC) [126].

Adenoviral delivery of CTLA4Ig to myeloid DC results in secretion of the transgene product, blockade of B7 molecule expression, and the capacity of the genetically-modified DC to induce alloAg-specific T cell hyporesponsiveness. These CTLA4Ig-transduced DC traffick *in vivo* to T cell areas of recipient secondary lymphoid tissue, where they survive in enhanced numbers compared with control gene-transduced DC [129]. Interestingly, retrovirally-transduced myeloid DC expressing CTLA4Ig show markedly inhibited ability to prime allogeneic T cells *in vivo*, and skew towards a predominant Th2 cell response (Takayama T. *et al*, submitted for publication). Electroporation of cDNA encoding immunosuppressive molecules into a mouse DC line ren-

Table 6
Genetic manipulation of DC to express immunosuppressive properties

Gene Transferred	Delivery mechanism	Property(ies) observed	Reference
Viral IL-10	Ecotropic retrovirus/ centrifugal trans-duction	Alloantigen-specific T cell hyporesponsiveness	Takayama et al, 1998 [125]
Viral IL-10	Ecotropic retrovirus encoding vIL-10 and EGFP (sorting vector)	Highly-purified (flow-sorted) transfectants exhibit markedly impaired T cell stimulatory activity	Takayama et al, 1999 [126]
TGFβ	Replication-deficient adenovirus	Impaired T cell stimulatory function; enhanced in vivo survival	Lee et al, 1998 [127]
CTLA4Ig	Electroporation (cDNA) of DC line	Prolongation of pancreatic islet allograft survival	O'Rourke et al, 1999 [128]
CTLA4Ig	Replication-deficient adenovirus	Alloantigen-specific hypo-responsiveness; enhanced in vivo survival	Lu et al, 1999 [129]
CTLA4Ig	Ecotropic retrovirus/ centrifugal trans-duction	Alloantigen-specific hypo-responsiveness; inhibition of Th1/augmentation of Th2 cytokine production	Takayama et al, 1999[†]
Fas L (CD95L)	Particle-mediated delivery of cDNA into mature DC line	Antigen-specific immuno-suppression in vivo	Matsue et al, 1999 [130]
Fas L	PBK-CMV phagemid	Alloantigen-specific hypo-responsiveness; prolong-ation of cardiac graft survival	Min et al, 2000 [131]

[*] enhanced green fluorescent protein
[†] submitted for publication

ders the cells capable of prolonging pancreatic islet allograft survival [128]. Particle-mediated delivery of cDNA encoding FasL into a mature murine DC line confers the capacity to induce Ag-specific immunosuppression *in vivo* [130]. In a recent study, Min *et al* [131] have reported that transfer of cDNA encoding human FasL to murine BM-derived DC by lipofection renders the DC capable of inducing apoptosis in Fas[+] target T cells and promoting alloAg-specific hyporesponsiveness *in vivo*. Significantly, repeated i.p. injection of these FasL-transduced DC prolonged vascularized cardiac allograft survival in fully MHC-mismatched recipients. Collectively, these studies indicate the potential of genetically-engineered DC for the regulation of undesired allo- or autoimmune responses.

ACKNOWLEDGMENTS

The authors' work is supported by National Institutes of Health grants DK 49745 and AI 41011, and by grants from the Roche Organ Transplantation Research Foundation, and the Juvenile Diabetes Foundation International. We thank our many colleagues who have made significant contributions to these studies, and Ms. Shelly Lynn Conklin for typing the manuscript.

REFERENCES

1. Steinman, R.M. The dendritic cell system and its role in immunogenicity. Annu Rev Immunol 1991;9:271-296.
2. Banchereau J, Steinman RM. Dendritic cells and the contral of immunity. Nature 1998;392:245-252.
3. Bell D, Young JW, Banchereau J. Dendritic cells. Adv Immunol 1999;72:255-322.
4. Lotze MT, Thomson AW (eds). Dendritic cells. Biology and Clinical Applications. San Diego: Academic Press, 1999:1-733.
5. Steptoe, R.J., Thomson, A.W. Dendritic cells and tolerance induction. Clin Exp Immunol 1996;105:397-402.
6. Thomson AW and Lu L. Dendritic cells as regulators of immune reactivity: implications for transplantation. Transplantation 1999;68:1-8.
7. Jenkinson, E.J., Jhittay, P., Kingston, R., Owen, J.J.T. Studies of the role of the thymic environment in the induction of tolerance to MHC antigens. Transplantation 1985;39:331-333.
8. Matzinger, P., Guerder, S. Does T cell tolerance require a dedicared antigen-presenting cells? Nature 1989;338:74-76.
9. Lu, L., McCaslin, D., Starzl, T.E., Thomson, A.W. Mouse bone marrow-derived dendritic cell progenitors (NLDC145$^+$, MHC class II$^+$, B7-1^{dim}, B7-2-) induce alloantigen- specific hyporesponsiveness in murine T lymphocytes. Transplantation 1995;60:1539-45.
10. Fu, F., Li, Y., Qian, S., Lu, L., Chambers, F., Starzl T.E., Fung, J.J., Thomson, A.W. Costimulatory molecule-deficient dendritic cell progenitors (MHC class II$^+$, B7-1^{dim}, B7-2-) prolong cardiac allograft survival in non-immunosuppressed recipients. Transplantation 1996;62: 659-665.
11. Rastellini, C., Lu, L., Ricordi, C., Starzl, T.E., Rao, A.S., Thomson, A.W. GM-CSF stimulated hepatic dendritic cell progenitors prolong pancreatic islet allograft survival. Transplantation 1995;60:1366-1370.
12. Moore, K.W., O'Garra, A., Malefyt, D.E.W., Vieram P., Mosman, T.R. Interleukin-10. Annu. Rev. Immunol. (1993) 11, 165-190
13. Caux C, Massacrierm B, Dervliet V, Barthelemym C, Liu YJ, Banchereau J. Interleukin-10 inhibits T cell alloreaction induced by human dendritic cells . Int Immunol 1994;6:1177-1185.
14. Süss, G., Shortman, K. A subclass of dendritic cells kills CD4 T cells via Fas/Fas-ligand induced apoptosis. J Exp Med 1996;183:1789-1796.
15. Lu, L., Qian, S., Hershberger, P.A., Rudert, W.A., Li, Y., Chambers, F.G., Lynch, D.H., and Thomson, A.W. Fas ligand (CD95L) and B7 expression on dendritic cells provide counter-regulatory signals for T cell survival and proliferation. J Immunol 1997;158:5676-5684.
16. Finkelman, F.D., Lees, A., Bimbaum, R., Gause, W.C., Morris, S.C. Dendritic cells

can present antigen in vivo in a tolerogenic or immunogenic fashion. J Immunol 1996;157:1406-1414.

17. Thomson, A.W., Lu, L., Steptoe, R.J., Starzl, T.E. Dendritic cells and the balance between transplant tolerance and immunity. In: Banchereau J, Dodet B, Schwartz R, Trannoy E., editors. Immune Tolerance. Elsevier, Paris 1996:173-185.

18. Steptoe, R.J., Fu, F., Li, W., et al. Augmentation of dendritic cells in murine organ donors by treatment with flt-3 ligand alters the balance between transplant tolerance and immunity. J Immunol 1997;159:5483-5491.

19. Khoury, S.J., Gallon, L., Chen, W., Mechanisms of acquired thymic tolerance in experimental autoimmune encephalomyelitis: thymic dendritic-enriched cells induce specific peripheral T cell unresponsiveness in vivo. J Exp Med 1995;182: 357-366.

20. Grabbe, S., Steinbrink, K., Steinert, M., Luger, T.A., Schwarz, T. Removal of the majority of epidermal Langerhans cells by topical or systemic steroid application enhances the effector phase of murine contact hypersensitivity. J Immunol 1995;155:4207-4217.

21. Clare-Salzler, M.J., Brooks, J., Chai, A. K., Anderson, C. Prevention of diabetes in nonobese diabetic mice by dendritic cell transfer. J. Clin. Invest. 1992;90: 741-748

22. Feili-Hariri M, Dong X, Alber SM, Watkins SC, Salter RD, Morel PA. Immunotherapy of NOD mice with bone marrow-derived dendritic cells. Diabetes 1999;48: 2300-2308.

23. Shinomiya M, Fazle Akbar SM, Shinomiya H, Onji M. Transfer of dendritic cells (DC) ex vivo stimulated with interferon-gamma (IFN-γ) down-modulates autoimmune diabetes in non-obese diabetic (NOD) mice. Clin Exp Immunol 1999; 117: 38-43.

24. Knight, S.C., Hunt, R., Dore, C., Medawar, P.B. Influence of dendritic cells on tumor growth. Proc Natl Acad Aci Sci USA 1983;80:6032-6035.

25. Kronin, V., Winkel, K., Suss, G., et al. A subclass of dendritic cells regulates the response of naive CD8 T cells by limiting their IL-2 production. J Immunol 1996; 157:3819-3827.

26. Hayamizu K, Huie P, Sibley RK, Strober S. Monocyte-derived dendritic cell precursors facilitate tolerance to heart allografts after total lymphoid irradiation. Transplantation 1998;66;1285-1291.

27. Gao J-X, Madrenas J, Zeng W et al. CD40-deficient dendritic cells producing interleukin-10, but not interleukin-12, induce T-cell hyporesponsiveness in vitro and prevent acute allograft rejection. Immunology 1999;98:159-170.

28. Saleem, M., Sawyer, G.J., Schofield, R.A., Seymour, N.O., Gustafsson, K., Fabre, J.W. Discordant expression on major histocompatibility complex class II antigen and invariant chain in interstitial dendritic cells. Transplantation 1997;63: 1134-1138.

29. Delemarre, F.G.A., Simons, P.J., Drexhage, H.A. Class II expression and function of dendritic cells from thyroid gland lymph nodes of the BB rat. Thyroid 1995 Suppl. 55, S24

30. Grohmann, U., Bianchi, R., Ayroldi, E., Belladonna, M.L., Surace, D., Fioretti, M.C., Puccetti, P. A tumor-associated and self antigen peptide presented by dendritic cells may induce T cell anergy in vivo, but IL-12 can prevent or revert the anergic state. J Immunol 1997;158:3593-3602.

31. Inaba, M., Inaba, K., Hosono, M., et al. Distinct mechanisms of neonatal tolerance induced by dendritic cells and thymic B cells. J Exp Med 1991;173:549-559.

32. Gao, E.K., Lo, D., Sprent, J. Strong T cell tolerance in parent->F1 bone marrow chimeras prepared with supralethal irradiation. Evidence for clonal deletion and anergy. JExp Med 1990;171:1101-1112.

33. Widera, G., Burkly, L.C., Pinkert, C.A., et al. Transgenic mice selectively lacking

MHC class II (I-E) antigen expression on B cells: an in vivo approach to investigate Ia gene function. Cell 1987;51:175-187.

34. Gerling, I. C., Serreze, D. V., Christianson, S. W., Leiter, E. H. Intrathymic islet cell transplantation reduces β-cell autoimmunity and prevents diabetes in NOD/Lt mice. Diabetes 1992;41:1672-1676.

35. Goss, J. A., Nakafusa, Y., Roland, C. R., Hickey, W. F., Flye, M. W. Immunological tolerance to a defined myelin basic protein antigen administered intrathymically. J. Immunol. 1994;153:3890-3897.

36. Khoury, S. J., Sayegh, M. H., Hancock, W. W., Gallon, L., Carpenter, C. B., Weiner, H. L. Acquired tolerance to experimental autoimmune encephalomyelitis by intrathymic injection of myelin basic protein or its major encephalitogenic peptide. J Exp Med 1993;178:559-566.

37. Koevary, S., Blomberg, M. Prevention of diabetes in BB/Wor rats by intrathymic islet injection. J Clin Invest 1992;89:512-516.

38. Khoury, S. J., Gallon, L., Verburg, R. R., et al. Ex-vivo treatment of antigen presenting cells with CTLA4-Ig and encephalitogenic peptide prevents experimental autoimmune encephalomyelitis in the Lewis rat. J Immunol 1996;157:3700-3705.

39. Ohzato, H., Monaco, A.P. Induction of specific unresponsiveness (tolerance) to skin allografts by intrathymic donor-specific splenocyte injection in antilymphocyte serum-treated mice. Transplantation 1992; 54:1090-1095.

40. Remuzzi, G., Rossini, M., Imberti, O., Perico, N. Kidney graft survival in rats without immunosuppressants after intrathymic glomerular transplantation. Lancet 1991; 337:750-752.

41. Posselt, A.M., Barker, C.F., Tomaszewski, J.E., Markmann, J.F., Choti, M.A., Man, A. Induction of donor-specific unresponsiveness by intrathymic islet transplantation. Science 1990;249:1293-1295.

42. Ridge, J.P., Matzinger, P. Neonatal tolerance revisited: turning on newborn T cells with dendritic cells. Science 1996;271:1723-1726.

43. Morikawa, Y., Furotani, M., Mastsuura, N., Kakudo, K. The role of antigen-presenting cells in the regulation of delayed-type hypersensitivity II. Epidermal Langerhans cells and peritoneal exudate macrophages. Cell Immunol. 1993;152:200-210.

44. Morikawa, Y., Furotani, M., Kuribayashi, K., Marsuura, N., Kakudo, K. The role of antigen-presenting cells in the regulation of delayed-type hypersensitivity. 1. Spleen dendritic cells. Immunology 1992;77:81-87.

45. Morikawa, Y., Tohya, K., Matsuura, N., Kakudo, K. Different migration patterns of antigen-presenting cells correlate with Th1/Th2-type responses in mice. Immunology 1995;85:575-581.

46. Larsen, C.P., Elwood, E.T., Alexander, D.Z., Long-term acceptance of skin and cardiac allografts after blocking CD40 and CD28 pathways. Nature 1996;381:434-438.

47. Kirk, A.D., Harlan, D.M., Armstrong, N.N., et al. CTLA4-Ig and anti-CD40 ligand prevent renal allograft rejection in primates. Proc Natl Acad Sci USA 1997;94:8789-8794.

48. Verberg, R., Chandraker, A., Gallon, L., Hancock, W.W., Sayegh, M.H., Khoury, S.J. Ex-vivo treatment of antigen-presenting cells with CTLA4Ig and peptide prevents EAE in the Lewis rat. J Immunol 1996; 157:3700-3705.

49. Enk, A.H., Angeloni, V.L., Udey, M.C., Katz. S.I. Inhibition of Langerhans cell antigen-presenting function by IL-10. A role for IL-10 in induction of tolerance. J. Immunol. 1993;151:2390-2398.

50. De Smedt T, Van Mechelen M, De Becker G, Urbain J, Leo O, and Moser M. Effect of interleukin-10 on dendritic cell maturation and function. Eur J Immunol 1997;27:1229-1235.

51. Steinbrink, K., Wölfl, M., Jonuleit, H., Knop, J., and Enk, A.H. Induction of toler-

ance by IL-10-treated dendritic cells. J Immunol 1997; 159:4772-4780.

52. Liu L, Rich BE, Inobe J-I, Chen W, Weiner HL. Induction of Th2 cell differentiation in the primary immune response: dendritic cells isolated from adherent cell culture treated with IL-10 prime naïve CD4⁺ T cells to secrete IL-4. Int Immunol 1998;10:1017-1026.

53. Kalinski, P., Hilkens, C. M., Snijders, A., Snijdewint, F. G., Kapsenberg, M. L. IL-12-deficient dendritic cells, generated in the presence of prostaglandin E2, promote type 2 cytokine production in maturing human naive T helper cells. J Immunol 1997;159:28-35.

54. De Jong EC, Vieira L, Kalinski P, Kapsenberg ML. Corticosteroids inhibit the production of inflammatory mediators in immature monocyte-derived DC and induce the development of tolerogenic DC3. J Leukocyte Biol 1999;66:201-204.

55. Simon, J.C., Tigelaar, R.E., Bergstresser, P.R., Edelbaum, D., Cruz, P.D. Ultraviolet B radiation converts Langerhans cells from immunogenic to tolerogenic antigen-presenting cells. Induction of specific clonal anergy in CD4 T helper cells. J. Immunol. 1991;146:485-491.

56. Chen, W., Issazadeh, S., Sayegh, M. H., Khoury, S. J. *In vivo* mechanisms of acquired thymic tolerance. Cell Immunol 1997;179:165-73

57. Chen, W., Sayegh, M. H., Khoury, S. J. Mechanisms of acquired thymic tolerance in vivo: intrathymic injection of antigen induces apoptosis of thymocytes and peripheral T cell anergy. J. Immunol. 1998; 160: 1504-1508.

58. Lu, L., Bonham, C.A., Chambers, F.D., Watkins, S.C., Hoffman, R.A., Simmons, R.L., Thomson, A.W. Induction of nitric oxide synthase in mouse dendritic cells by interferon-γ, endotoxin and interaction with allogeneic T cells: nitric oxide production is associated with dendritic cell apoptosis. J Immunol 1996;157:3577-3585.

59. Bonham CA, Lu L, Li Y, Hoffman RA, Simmons RL, Thomson AW. Nitric oxide production by mouse marrow-derived dendritic cells. Transplantation 1996;62:1709-1714.

60. Qian S, Lu L, Li Y, et al. Apoptosis within spontaneously accepted mouse liver allografts: evidence for deletion of cytotoxic T cells and implications for tolerance induction. J Immunol 1997;158:4654-4661.

61. Lu L, Li W, Zhong C, Qian S, Fung JJ, Thomson AW, and Starzl TE Increased apoptosis of immunoreactive host cells and augmented donor leukocyte chimerism, not sustained inhibition of B7 molecule expression are associated with prolonged cardiac allograft survival in mice preconditioned with immature donor dendritic cells plus anti-CD40L mAb. Transplantation (Rapid Publication) 1999;68:747-757.

62. Freedman, A.S., Munro, J.M., Rhynhart, K., et al. Follicular dendritic cells inhibit human B-lymphocyte proliferation. Blood 1992;80:1284-1288.

63. Gorczynski, R.M., Cohen, Z., Fu, X., Hua, Z., Sun, Y., Chen, Z. Interleukin-13 in combination with anti-interleukin-12, increases graft prolongation after portal venous immunization with cultured allogeneic bone marrow-derived dendritic cells. Transplantation 1996;62:1592-1600.

64. Streilein JW, Wilbanks GA, Cousins SW. Immunoregulatory mechanisms of the eye. J Neuroimmunol 1992;39:185-200.

65. Larsen, C.P., Ritchie, S.C., Hendrix, R., et al. Regulation of immunostimulatory function and costimulatory molecule (B7-1 and B7-2) expression on murine dendritic cells. J Immunol 1994;152:5208-5219.

66. Romani, N., Schuler, G., Frisch, P. Ontogeny of Ia-positive and Thy-1-positive leukocytes of murine epidermis. J Invest Dermatol 1986;86:129-133.

67. Nelson, D.J., Holt, P.G. Defective regional immunity in the respiratory tract of neonates is attributable to hyporesponsiveness of local dendritic cells to activation signals. J Immunol 1995;155:351-357.

68. Austyn JM, Hankins DF, Larsen CP, Morris PJ, Rao AS, Roake JA. Isolation

and characterization of dendritic cells from mouse heart and kidney. J Immunol 1994;52:2401-2410.

69. Lu L, Woo J, Rao AS, et al. Propagation of dendritic cell progenitors from normal mouse liver using granulocyte/macrophage colony-stimulating factor and their maturational development in the presence of type-1 collagen. J Exp Med 1994; 179:1823-1834.

70. Schwartz, R.H. A cell culture model for T lymphocyte clonal anergy. Science 1990; 248:1349-1356.

71. Lin, H., Bolling, S.F., Linsley, P.S., et al. Long term acceptance of major histocompatibility complex mismatched cardiac allografts induced by CTLA4-Ig plus donor-specific transfusion. J Exp Med 1993;178:1801-1806.

72. Sayegh, M.H., Akalin, E., Hancock, W.W., et al. CD28-B7 Blockade after alloantigenic challenge in vivo inhibits Th1 cytokines but spares Th2 J Exp Med 1995; 181:1869-1874.

73. Thomas, J.M., Carver, F.M., Kasten-Jolly, J., et al. Further studies of veto activity in rhesus monkey bone marrow in relation to allograft tolerance and chimerism. Transplantation 1994;57:101-115.

74. Fazekas de St Groth B. The evolution of self tolerance: a new cell arises to meet the channelge of self reactivity. Immunol Today 1998;19:448-454.

75. Vremec, D., Zorbas, M., Scollay, R., et al. The surface phenotype of dendritic cells purified from mouse thymus and spleen: investigation of the CD8 expression by a subpopulation of dendritic cells J Exp Med 1992;176:47-58.

76. Hambor, J.E., Kaplan, D.R., Tykocinskim M.L. CD8 functions as an inhibitory ligand in mediating the immunoregulatory activity of CD8+ cells. J Immunol 1990;145:1644-1652.

77. Sambhara, S.R., Miller, R.G. Programmed cell death of T cells signaled by the T cell receptor and α3 domain of MHC class I. Science 1991;252:1424-1427.

78. Kronin, V., Vremec, D., Winkel, K., et al. Are CD8+ dendritic cells veto cells? The role of CD8 on dendritic cells in the regulation of CD4 and CD8 T cell responses. Int Immunol 1997 In press.

79. Lynch, D.H., Ramsdell, F., and Alderson, M.R. Fas FasL in the homeostatic regulation of immune responses. Immunology Today 1995;16:569-574.

80. Wiley, S.R., Schooley, K., Smolak, P.J., et al. Identification and characterization of a new member of the TNF family that induces apoptosis. Immunity 1995;3: 673-682.

81. Fehsel, K,, Kroncke, K.D., Meyer, K.L., Huber, H., Wahnm V., Kolb-Bachofen, V. Nitric oxide induces apoptosis in mouse thymocytes . J. Immunol. 1995;155: 2858-2865.

82. Austyn JM, Larsen CP. Migration patterns of dendritic leukocytes. Implications for transplantation. Transplantation 1990;49:1-7.

83. Larsen, C.P., Morris, P.J., Austyn, J.M. Migration of dendritic leukocytes from cardiac allografts into host spleens: a novel route for initiation of rejection. J Exp Med 1990;171:307-314.

84. Thomson AW, Lu L, Subbotin VM et al. In vitro propagation and homing of liver-derived dendritic cell progenitors to lymphoid tissues of allogeneic recipients. Transplantation 1995;59:544-551.

85. Inaba, K., Steinman, R.M., Pack, M.W., et al. Identification of proliferating dendritic cell precursors in mouse blood. J. Exp. Med. 1992; 175:1157-1167.

86. Inaba, K., Inaba, M., Romani, N., et al. Generation of large numbers of dendritic cells from mouse bone marrow cultures supplemented with granulocyte/ macrophage colony-stimulating factor. J Exp Med 1992;176: 1693-1702.

87. Caux, C, Dezutter-Dambuyant, C., Schmitt D., Banchereau, J. GM-CSF and TNFα cooperate in the generation of dendritic Laugerhans cells. Nature 1992; 360: 258-26

88. Szabolcs, P., Moore, M.A., Young, J.W. Expansion of immunostimulatory dendritic cells among the myeloid progeny of human CD34$^+$ bone marrow precursors cultured with c-kit ligand, granulocyte-macrophage colony-stimulating factor and TNFα. J Immunol 1995;154:5851-5861.

89. Grabbe, S., Bruvers, S., Granstein, R.D. Interleukin 1β but not transforming growth factor inhibits tumor antigen presentation by epidermal antigen-presenting cells. J Invest Dermatol 1994;102:67-73.

90. Sallusto, F., Cella, M., Danieli, C., Lanzavecchia, A. Dendritic cells use macropinocytosis and the mannose receptor to concentrate macromolecules in the major histocompatibility complex class II compartment: downregulation by cytokines and bacterial products. J Exp Med 1995;182:398-400.

91. Buelens C, Willems E, Delvaux A et al. Interleukin-10 differentially regulates B7-1 (CD80) and B7-2 (CD86) expression on human peripheral blood dendritic cells. Eur. J. Immunol. 1995;25:2668-2672.

92. Kaeamura, T., Furue, M. Comparative analysis of B7-1 and B7-2 expression in Langerhans cells: differential regulation by T helper type 1 and T helper type 2 cytokines. Eur. J. Immunol. 1995;25:1913-1917

93. Buelens C, Verhasselt V, De Groote D, Thielemans K, Goldman M, Willems F. Human dendritic cell responses to lipopolysaccharide and CD40 ligation are differentially regulated by interleukin-10. Eur J Immunol 1997;27:1848-1852.

94. De Smedt T, Van Mechelen M, De Becker G, Urbain J, Leo O, and Moser M. Effect of interleukin-10 on dendritic cell maturation and function. Eur J Immunol 1997; 27:1229-1235.

95. Ludewig, B., Graf, D., Gelderblom, H.R., et al. Spontaneous apoptosis of dendritic cells in efficiently inhibited by TRAP (CD40-ligand) and TNF-α, but strongly enhanced by interleukin-10. Eur J Immunol 1995;25: 1943-1950.

96. Drakes, M.L., Lu, L., Subbotin, V.M., and Thomson, A.W. *In vivo* administration of flt3 ligand markedly stimulates generation of dendritic cell progenitors from mouse liver. J. Immunol. 1997;159:4268-4278.

97. Derynck, R, Choy L. Transforming growth factor-β and its receptors. In Thomson AW, editor. The Cytokine Handbook, Third Edition. Academic Press, San Diego 1998, 593-636.

98. Yasunori, Y., Tsumura, H., Miwa, M., Inaba, K. Contrasting effects of TGFβ1 and TNFα on the development of dendritic cells from progenitors in mouse bone marrow. Stem Cells 1997;15:144-153.

99. Lu, L., Li, W., Fu, F., Chambers, F.G., Qian, S., Fung, J.J., Thomson, A.W. Blockade of the CD40-CD40L pathway potentiates the capacity of donor-derived dendritic cell progenitors to induce long-term cardiac allograft survival. Transplantation. 1997;64:1808-1815.

100. Strobl H, Riedl E, Scheinecker C, et al. TGFβ1 promotes in vitro development of dendritic cells from CD34$^+$ hematopoietic progenitors. J Immunol 1996;157: 1499-1507.

101. Bonham CA, Lu L, Banas AR, Fontes P, Rao AS, Zeevi A, Thomson AW. TGFβ1 impairs the allostimulatory function of GM-CSF stimulated antigen presenting cells propagated from human bone marrow. Transplant Immunol 1996; 4:186-191.

102. Wilbanks, G.A., Streilein, J.W. Fluids from immune privileged sites endow macrophages with the capacity to induce antigen-specific immune deviation via a mechanism involving transforming growth factor-β. Eur J Immunol 1992;22: 1031-1036.

103. Lu, L., Rudert, W.A., Qian, S., et al. Growth of donor-derived dendritic cells from the bone marrow of murine liver allograft recipients in response to granulocyte/ macrophage colony-stimulating factor. J Exp Med 1995;182:379-387.

104. Thomson, A.W., Lu, L., Wan, Y., Qian, S., Larsen, C.P., Starzl, T.E. Identification of

donor-derived dendritic cell progenitors in bone marrow of spontaneously tolerant liver allograft recipients. Transplantation 1995;60:1555-1559.

105. Thomson, A.W., Lu, L., Murase, N., Demetris, A.J., Rao, A.S., Starzl, T.E. Microchimerism, dendritic cell progenitors and transplantation tolerance. Stem Cells 1995;13:622-639.

106. Rugeles, M.T., Aitouche, A., Zeevi, A, et al. Evidence for the presence of multilineage chimerism and progenitors of donor dendritic cells in the peripheral blood of bone marrow-augmented organ transplant recipients. Transplantation 1997;64:735-741.

107. Demetris, A.J., Murase, N., Ye, Q., et al. Analysis of chronic rejection and obliterative arteriopathy. Am. J. Pathol. 1997;150:563-578.

108. Armitage RJ, Fanslow WC, Strockbine L et al. Molecular and biological characterization of murine ligand for CD40. Nature 1992 ;357: 80-82.

109. Yang, Y., Wilson, J.M. CD40 ligand-dependent T cell activation: requirement of B7-CD28 signaling through CD40. Science 1996;273: 1862-1864.

110. Caux, C., Massacrier, C., Vanbervliet, B., et al. Activation of human dendritic cells through CD40 cross-linking. J. Exp. Med. 1994; 180:1263-1272

111. McLellan, A.D., Sorg, R.V., Williams, L.A., Hart, D.N.J. Human dendritic cells activate T lymphocytes via a CD40: CD40 ligand -dependent pathway. Eur J Immunol 1996; 26:1204-1210.

112. Parker, D.C., Greiner, D.L., Phillips, N.E., et al. Survival of mouse pancreatic islet allograft recipients treated with allogeneic small lymphocytes and antibody to CD40 ligand. Proc Natl Acad Sci USA 1995;92:9560-9564.

113. Hancock, W.W., Sayegh, M.H., Zheng, X.G., Peach, R., Linsley, P.S., Turka, L.A. Costimulatory function and expression of CD40 ligand, CD80, and CD86 in vascularized murine cardiac allograft rejection. Proc. Natl. Acad. Sci. USA 1996;93: 139-67.

114. Niimi M, Pearson TC, Larsen CP, et al. The role of the CD40 pathway in alloantigen-induced hyporesponsiveness *in vivo*. J Immunol 1998;161:5331-5337.

115. Lee J-I, Ganster RW, Geller DA, Burckart GJ, Thomson AW, and Lu L. Cyclosporine inhibits the expression of costimulatory molecules on *in vitro* generated dendritic cells: association with reduced nuclear translocation of NF-κB. Transplantation 1999; 68: 1255-1263.

116. Thomas JM, Contreras JL, Jiang XL, et al. Peritransplant tolerance induction in macaques: early events reflecting the unique synergy between immunotoxin and deoxyspergualin. Transplantation 1999;68:1660-1673.

117. Suri RM, Niimi M, Wood KJ, Austyn JM. Immature dendritic cell pretreatment induces cardiac allograft prolongation. J Leukocyte Biol 1998;Suppl.2; 32 Abstract B16.

118. Giannoukakis N, Bonham CA, Qian S, et al. Prolongation of cardial allograft survival using donor dendritic cells treated with NF-κB decoy oligodeoxyribonucleotides. Molecular Therapy 2000; 1: 430-437.

119. Garrovillo M., Ali A, Oluwole SF. Indirect allorecognition in acquired thymic tolerance: induction of donor-specific tolerance to rat cardiac allografts by allopeptide-pulsed host dendritic cells. Transplantation. 1999; 68:1827-1834.

120. Markees TG, Phillips NE, Gordon EJ, et al. Prolonged skin allograft survival in mice treated with Flt3-Ligand-induced dendritic cells and anti-CD154 monoclonal antibody. Transplant Proc 1999;31:884-885.

121. Gozzo J, Masli S, De Fazio S. Extension of graft survival with pulsed administration of donor dendritic cells. Transplant Proc 1999;31:1196.

122. Song, W., Kong, H.-L., Carpenter, H et al. Dendritic cells genetically modified with an adenovirus vector encoding the cDNA for a model antigen induce protective and therapeutic antitumor immunity. J. Exp. Med. 1997;186:1247-1256.

123. Specht, J.M., Wang, G., Do, M.T., et al. Dendritic cells retrovirally transduced

with a model antigen gene are therapeutically effective against established pulmonary metastases. J Exp Med 1997;186:1213-1221.

124. Wan Y, Branson J, Carter R, Graham F, and Gauldie, J. Dendritic cells transduced with an adenoviral vector encoding a model tumor-associated antigen for tumor vaccination. Human Gene Therapy 1997;8:1355-1363.

125. Takayama T, Nishioka Y, Lu L, Lotze MT, Tahara H, and Thomson AW. Retroviral delivery of viral IL-10 into myeloid dendritic cells markedly inhibits their allostimulatory activity and promotes the induction of T cell hyporesponsiveness. Transplantation 1998 (Rapid Publication); 66:1567-1574.

126. Takayama T, Tahara H, and Thomson AW Transduction of dendritic cell progenitors with a retroviral vector encoding viral IL-10 and enhanced green fluorescent protein allows purification of potentially tolerogenic antigen-presenting cells. Transplantation 1999; 68: 1903-1909.

127. Lee W-C, Zhong C, Qian S, Phenotype, function, and *in vivo* migration and survival of allogeneic dendritic cell progenitors genetically engineered to express TGF-β. Transplantation 1998;66:1810-1817.

128. O'Rourke R, Lower J, Kang S-M, et al. A dendritic cell line expressing immunoregulatory molecules as a means to inactivate the alloreactive T cell repertoire. Fifth International Conference on Tolerance Induction. Breckenridge Co, Abstract 1.

129. Lu L, Gambotto A, Lee W-C, et al. Adenoviral delivery of CTLA4Ig into myeloid dendritic cells promotes their *in vitro* tolerogenicity and survival in allogeneic recipients. Gene Therapy 1999;6:554-563.

130. Matsue H, Matsue K, Walters M, Okumura K, Yagita H, Takashima A. Induction of antigen-specific immunosuppression by CD95L cDNA-transfected "killer" dendritic cells. Nature Medicine 1999;5:930-937.

131. Min W-P, Gorczynski R, Huang X-Y, et al. Dendritic cells genetically engineered to express Fas Ligand induce donor-specific hyporesponsiveness and prolong allograft survival. J Immunol 2000;164:161-167.

10 GENE THERAPY FOR AUTOIMMUNE DISEASE AND TRANSPLANTATION

Cristopher H. Evans[1], Angus W. Thomson[2],
Nicholas Giannoukakis[3] and Paul D. Robbins[3]

[1] Center for Molecular Orthopedics
Harvard Medical School
Boston, Massachusetts, USA

[2] Department of Surgery
University of Pittsburgh
Pittsburgh, Pennsylvania, USA

[3] Department of Molecular Genetics and Biochemistry
University of Pittsburgh
Pittsburgh, Pennsylvania, USA

INTRODUCTION

Advances of both a conceptual and technical nature have added inflammatory [1] and degenerative [2] diseases to the list of those conditions potentially treatable by gene therapy. Few diseases of these types are genetic in nature, but gene transfer may nevertheless be of benefit in permitting the controlled expression of therapeutic genes in defined populations of cells. Pre-clinical research into the treatment of such disorders by gene therapy has indeed provided strong evidence that genes may be employed as immunomodulatory agents of potential utility in treating autoimmune conditions such as rheumatoid arthritis and type I diabetes, and for blocking the immune response following transplantation of allogeneic tissues such as islets. The present chapter reviews progress in these areas.

GENE THERAPY

Gene therapy can be most simply defined as the transfer of genes to patients for therapeutic purposes. The genes in question may be wild-type alleles

243

A. W. Thomson (ed.), Therapeutic Immunosuppression, 243–274.
© 2001 Kluwer Academic Publishers.

used to compensate for recessive mutations causing monogenic, Mendelian disorders or, increasingly, genes whose products have therapeutic properties in patients whose diseases have no overriding genetic basis. The latter obtains for the conditions discussed in this review; although there are clearly genetic components to autoimmunity, these are complex, polygenic and confer risk rather than initiating disease progression. In these instances transgenes are used therapeutically to allow the controlled synthesis of immunomodulatory products at strategic locations.

Gene transfer is typically accomplished with the aid of vectors, reviewed in references 3 & 4, which may be viral or non-viral in nature. Several types of viruses have been successfully modified for use as vectors; the salient properties of the most developed of these are summarized in Table 1. Although viral vectors are more efficient for gene transfer than non-viral vectors, they have potential problems with immunogenicity and toxicity. The general strategy for generating replication-defective viral vectors for gene transfer is to remove the genes important for replication from the virus and insert the therapeutic gene or genes. The replication-defective viral vectors are then grown in cell lines where the essential viral proteins, deleted in the vector, are provided.

Retroviral vectors derived from the Moloney murine leukemia virus were the first to be developed, and have been the most widely employed vectors in human clinical trials. Retroviruses are RNA viruses that replicate through a DNA intermediate that integrates into the host cell genome. Largely because of their inability to transduce non-dividing cells, their use has been almost entirely restricted to *ex vivo* protocols where cells are removed from the body, modified extracorporally, and then reimplanted. Such procedures are laborious but, because they do not involve the direct introduction of infectious agents into the body, they bring certain safety advantages. Moreover, because proretroviral genomes are incorporated into the genomic DNA of the host cell, they provide the basis for long term gene expression, should this be required. Novel retroviral vectors derived from lentiviruses insert genes into the host chromosomal DNA without the need for cell division. Such vectors, however, require additional development before human trials can be contemplated.

Adeno-associated virus (AAV) is a parvovirus, a family of single stranded DNA viruses that require a helper virus such as adenovirus or herpes simplex virus for its productive life cycle. Wild-type adeno-associated virus (AAV) also inserts its DNA into the genomic DNA of the host cell in the absence of cell division, but it is unclear whether recombinant AAV does so.

Table 1
Properties of present vectors

Vector	Advantages	Disadvantages
Integrating Viral		
Retrovirus		
• MoMLV-based	Straightforward Production No viral proteins made Extensive use in human trials	Require Target Cell Division Possible Insertional Mutagenesis
• Lentivirus-based	Transduce non-dividing cells	More development required
AAV	Site-specific integration (1) Non-pathogenic Transduce non-dividing cells No viral proteins made	Difficult to produce Small packaging capacity (4kb)
Viral Non-Integrating		
Adenovirus	Straightforward Production High titers Transduce non-dividing cells	Inflammatory Immunogenicity of transduced cells
HSV	Large packaging capacity High titers Transduce non-dividing cells	Difficult to produce Cytotoxic
Non-viral		
naked DNA	Simple Non-immunogenic Inexpensive Safe	Few cells transfect well
Liposomes	As above	Gene expression usually transient and low
Particle bombardment (gene gun)	Used in conjunction with plasmid DNA	Cumbersome; requires specialized equipment
DNA-ligand complexes	May be targetable Receptor-mediated uptake often efficient	Possible antigenicity Low expression

(1) Wild-type AAV integrates in a site-specific fashion. Recombinant virus appears as if it does not. Note that all types of vectors are the subject of considerable research. This table summarizes the present state of development. MoMLV = Moloney Murine Leukemia Virus. AAV = Adeno-Associated Virus. HSV = Herpes Simplex Virus

Nevertheless, there are reports of long term transgene expression following the *in vivo* administration of AAV vectors. There is also literature to suggest that the direct introduction of AAV into the body fails to generate neutralizing antibodies to viral antigens, in which case repeated dosing would be possible. Not all investigators have found this, however, and the issue awaits resolution. The main disadvantages of AAV are its small size and difficult manufacture.

Recombinant adenoviral vectors, in contrast, are straightforward to construct in high titers and show high infectivity towards a wide range of dividing and non-dividing cells. Their main disadvantages are the antigenicity of the viral particles, the synthesis of viral proteins by the cells they transduce and metabolic disturbances in infected cells, including the activation of MAP kinases and NF-kB. Infection with adenoviral vectors *in vivo* is frequently followed by an inflammatory reaction. Removal of increasing amounts of the adenoviral genome has led to newer vectors which do not promote the synthesis of viral proteins in infected cells, but problems of antigenicity and inflammatory responses remain. Because of their ability to infect non-dividing cells, adenoviral vectors are frequently used for *in vivo* gene delivery. This, however, raises safety concerns; indeed, the recent death of a gene therapy patient followed the infusion of recombinant adenoviruses.

Vectors derived from herpes simplex virus (HSV), like adenoviruses, are highly infectious DNA viruses, able to infect both dividing and non-dividing cells, and they can be grown to very high titers. Herpes Simplex Viruses (HSV) are large linear DNA viruses of approximately 150 kilobases that are able to infect cells lytically as well as infect latently certain cell types such as neurons. HSV vectors are able to incorporate exogenous DNA of up to 35 kilobases, allowing for insertion of large fragments of DNA. They have a natural latency in neurons, but tend to be cytotoxic in other types of cells.

Non-viral gene delivery using plasmid DNA, either alone or complexed with carriers such as cationic liposomes, is also possible. In general, viral vectors are more efficient than non-viral systems both in terms of numbers of cells transfected, and the level and duration of transgene expression. Nevertheless, there is evidence that the small amounts of gene transfer and expression obtained with delivery of plasmid DNA is sufficient to effect immune function in rodents with experimental models of lupus, RA and type I diabetes (*vide infra*). Non-viral vectors are usually easier and cheaper to produce than viral vectors, and they are likely to be safer.

GENE THERAPY AND AUTOIMMUNITY

There is clear evidence that immune reactivity can be modulated by gene transfer. Most of the early data came from attempts to develop gene therapies for various cancers. Indeed, the second human gene therapy trial, initiated in 1991, involved the *ex vivo*, retroviral transfer of a tumor necrosis factor (TNF) cDNA to tumor infiltrating lymphocytes. A vast number of experiments have since evaluated the effects of additional genes whose products would be expected to increase the immune response to tumors; examples include interleukins (IL) -2, -4, -10, -12, and -15, granulocyte macrophage colony stimulating factor (GM-CSF), co-stimulatory molecules and MHC molecules [5]. Such genes have been transferred to the tumor cells themselves, to various populations of leukocytes, as well as to cells such as fibroblasts, which are thought to play no role other than to serve as an endogenous source of secreted gene products. Retroviruses, adenoviruses, HSV, liposomes and naked DNA have all been evaluated for these purposes. Numerous clinical trials have developed from such studies and, although cancer has not been cured by these means, good evidence for the immunomodulatory properties of transgenes in humans has been gathered.

A similar logic can be applied to the gene treatment of autoimmunity and treating allograft responses, with the transgenes being immunosuppressive rather than immunostimulatory. Various types of immunosuppressive genes can be envisaged (Table 2). Those whose products interfere with the interactions of co-stimulatory molecules on antigen-presenting cells (APCs) and T-cells, for instance, have the potential to induce anergy and even tolerance. Soluble forms of CTLA-4 are presently of much interest in this regard. Alternative strategies are based upon the use of genes whose products, for example Fas ligand, provoke apoptosis in selected populations of T-cells. The immune system may also be modulated by the transfer of genes whose

Table 2
Candidate Immunomodulatory Genes for Use in Autoimmunity and Allograft Rejection

Gene Product	Comment
Soluble CTLA4, CD 40 etc.	Inhibit co-stimulation of lymphocytes
Fas Ligand, TRAIL, Caspases etc.	Induce apoptosis
Herpes thymidine kinase	Ablative in conjunction with ganciclovir
IL-1Ra, sIL-1R	Antagonize IL-1
sTNFR	Antagonize TNF
IL-4, IL-10, IL-13, vIL-10	Antiinflammatory; Promote Th2 activity
IL-12	Promote Th1 activity (for use in Th1 driven autoimmune diseases)
TGF-β	Immunosuppressive
Transcription factors / signalling molecules	Modulate gene expression
Antibodies	Various uses
Ribozymes, antisense RNA	Regulate gene expression
Oligonucleotides	Decoys

products produce immune deviation. Expression of IL-12, for example, will promote the production of Th-1 cells, of use in Th-2 driven diseases such as lupus, while expression of IL-4 or IL-10 will promote the production of Th-2 cells, of use in Th-1 driven diseases such as rheumatoid arthritis (RA). Cytokines such as IL-10 are of additional interest because they are also anti-inflammatory. Immune deviation may also be accomplished by transfer to CD4+ T-cells of genes encoding transcription factors that promote differentiation along Th-1 or Th-2 lineages; one example is c-maf [6]. Finally, it may be possible to manipulate the activities of cellular components of the immune system by genetic manipulation of key intracellular signalling molecules such as NF-κB; this can be accomplished with decoy oligonucleotides as well as with genes encoding specific inhibitors such as IκB.

Immunomodulatory genes may be targeted to various anatomical sites. In general, it is possible to contemplate the systemic delivery of a gene encoding a secreted immunosuppressive protein, the localized delivery of genes to sites of immune reactivity, such as lymphoid tissues or transplanted organs, and the *ex vivo* return of cells with the ability to home to the desired location. Systemic delivery may be of utility in disseminated diseases, but risks producing generalized immunosuppression. For this reason, local delivery would seem indicated for most purposes. Of particular relevance to the treatment of autoimmunity is the prospect of expressing such products at sites of antigen presentation. The genes in question could be transferred to key cellular components of the immune system, such as antigen presenting cells (APCs) or lymphocytes, or to other cells in the vicinity which would then serve as local sites of transgene production. These principles can be applied

Table 3
Autoimmune Diseases Possibly Treatable by Gene Therapy*
Rheumatoid Arthritis
Systemic Lupus Erythematosis
Sjogren's Syndrome
Multiple Sclerosis
Diabetes
Uveitis
Colitis
Neuritis
Thyroiditis
*Only diseases for which published experimental gene therapy data exist are listed.

to a range of autoimmune disorders (Table 3). Two will be considered here in detail, rheumatoid arthritis and diabetes.

APPLICATION OF GENE THERAPY TO THE TREATMENT OF AUTOIMMUNE DISEASES

Rheumatoid Arthritis

Introduction

RA is a systemic condition whose primary sites of pathology are the joints, particularly knees, wrists, ankles and the small joints of the hands and feet. It affects approximately 1% of the population, and is more common in women than men. RA is considered to be autoimmune in etiology, but the inciting autoantigen has not been identified, although several candidates exist [7].

Rheumatoid joints are characterized by a massive increase in the thickness and cellularity of the synovial lining. The increase in cellularity results from an influx of leukocytes, particularly macrophages and CD4+ T-cells, from the blood stream accompanied by a large expansion of the resident fibroblast population. It is unclear to what degree increased cell division and cell recruitment or decreased cell death account for the accumulation of fibroblasts. The thickened synovium forms a pannus, which grows over and into the adjacent bone and cartilage, as well as intraarticular ligaments, leading to severe erosions, distortion of the joints and loss of function. A variety of cytokines, particularly IL-1 and TNF are thought to orchestrate these pathophysiological changes [8,9,10]. The gene therapy of RA has been the subject of a number of recent reviews [11-13].

Pre-Clinical Findings

Systemic approaches to the genetic treatment of laboratory animals with experimental models of RA have involved the i.v. injection of adenoviral vectors [14-18], the i.m. and s.c. injection of plasmid DNA [19-21], the i.p. injection of AP-1 decoy oligonucleotides [22], and the introduction of genetically modified cells subcutaneously, intraperitoneally, intravenously or within semipermeable chambers [23-27]. In *ex vivo* protocols, both genetically modified fibroblasts and lymphocytes have been evaluated. There is evidence that lymphocytes, unlike fibroblasts, may home to diseased joints thereby increasing their effectiveness while reducing opportunities for side effects. The genes used in various systemic gene therapy strategies include those encoding sTNFR, vIL-10, IL-10, TGF-β, IL-4, IL-13 and galectin. The results have been promising, in that disease activity was suppressed, although some hepatotoxicity has been reported with high doses of adenovirus. In most of these studies, however, gene therapy has been applied prophylactically. In the few instances where therapeutic application has been tested, the results are less impressive.

Greater experimental emphasis has been placed on the local delivery of genes to individual arthritic joints [28]. *Ex vivo* protocols generally employ synovial fibroblasts. Retrovirus, adenovirus, HSV, AAV, liposomes, plasmids and a variety of non-viral formulations have been evaluated as vectors for *in vivo* gene delivery [29-34]. Of these, adenoviruses are the most efficient, and have provided a convenient means to test candidate anti-arthritic genes *in vivo*. Although their inflammatory properties and limitations in the duration of gene expression curtail their human use in protocols other than those involving synovial ablation, they remain experimentally useful. There is presently much interest in the possibility that AAV may permit long term carriage of transferred genes within synovium, with reactivation of gene expression occurring during inflammatory flares [33]. This would be of considerable utility in treating rheumatoid joints, but some investigators have failed to reproduce this phenomenon [34], and the matter awaits clarification.

Because it has not been possible to achieve long-term intraarticular gene expression, there is mounting interest in delivering genes that will ablate the synovium and thereby produce a "genetic synovectomy". Earlier experience with surgical, medical and radiation synovectomy has confirmed the clinical effectiveness of synovectomy which, while not a cure, can improve symptoms for as long as several years. Studies in experimental animals have confirmed that a genetic synovectomy is possible with transfer of the Fas ligand gene [35,36], as well as the herpes thymidine kinase gene used in conjunction with ganciclovir [37,38]. Two human trials based on the latter approach will begin later this year (*vide infra*). A related method includes the use of a gene which promotes the senescence of synovial cells and thus inhibits their ability to proliferate [39]. There is also interest in using genes whose products prevent angiogenesis and thereby interfere with synovial hyperplasia and pannus formation.

Other approaches have involved the delivery to the synovium of a variety of genes, including IL-1Ra, sIL-1R, sTNFR, vIL-10, IL-4, TGF-β, IGF-I, and BMP-2, by *ex vivo* or *in vivo* delivery [17, 29, 41-47]. The latter three growth factors were selected on the basis of their ability to protect and restore articular cartilage. Adenoviral transfer of the TGF-β gene provoked considerable joint pathology, with evidence of cartilage formation within the synovium [Mi et al, unpublished]. IGF-I and BMP-2 genes, however, enhanced matrix synthesis without pathology [46, Mi et al, unpublished). Adenoviral delivery of the IL-4 gene to murine knee joints proved to be inflammatory, but at the same time strikingly protective of bone and cartilage [47]. In contrast, retroviral delivery of IL-4 reduced inflammation, as well as erosion, in rats with adjuvant arthritis [48]. The vIL-10 gene is anti-inflammatory as well as anti-erosive in the knee joints of rabbits with antigen-induced arthritis (a.i.a.), and the paws of mice with collagen-induced arthritis (c.i.a.) [17, 49]. *Ex vivo* delivery of IL-1Ra is also chondroprotective in rabbits with a.i.a., but only partially anti-inflammatory [50]. Adenoviral, *in vivo* delivery of sIL-1R has a stronger anti-inflammatory effect [41], but this may be due to the higher levels of gene expression achieved by this means. Neither the IL-1Ra nor the sIL-1R gene improved the synovitis present in the knee joints of rabbits with a.i.a., but a combination of genes encoding sIL-1R and sTNFR was highly effective in this regard [41].

Makarov and colleagues noted a profound suppression of arthritis in the ankle joints of rats with streptococcal cell wall (scw) arthritis following the intraarticular injection of NF-κB decoy oligonucleotides complex with cationic liposomes [51]. This work has recently been reproduced in rats with c.i.a.[52]. Although the mechanism through which the NF-kB decoy confers a therapeutic effect is not clear, we have shown that administration of NF-kB decoy oligonucleotides to immature dendritic cells in culture blocks their immunostimulatory capacity both in culture and *in vivo*. Thus it is possible that the therapeutic effect observed in the rat models with the NF-kB decoys is due to down modulation of DC function (see below).

The Contralateral Effect

Intraarticular injection of adenovirus carrying the sIL-1R or vIL-10 into one knee joint of a rabbit with bilateral a.i.a.improves the disease in both the injected and uninjected knees [41,49]. This effect has also been seen in scw and adjuvant arthritis in rats following local injection of NF-κB decoys [51] or retrovirus carrying IL-4 [48], and has been reproduced in some studies of mice with c.i.a. [17], but not in others. Evidence from marker gene studies suggests trafficking of transduced cells from joints injected with adenoviral vectors to other joints [41, 49]. Neither the identity of these cells, nor their contribution to the contralateral effect is known. However, after injection of retroviral vectors carrying IL-4 genes in rat joints, elevated IL-4 could be detected in contralteral joints in the absence of the transgene [48]. This could be explained by the generation of Th2 lymphocytes in the injected joint, which then traffick to other joints where they secrete IL-4.

Studies using a delayed-type hypersensitivity (DTH) reaction in mice have shed some light on possible mechanisms for the contralateral effect [53]. Local injection of adenovirus carrying the vIL-10 gene suppresses the DTH reaction and also demonstrates a contralateral effect in this regard. T-lymphocytes recovered from these mice cannot adoptively transfer the DTH reaction, but neither can they suppress the ability of T-lymphocytes from control sensitized animals to do so. Macrophages and dendritic cells recovered from sensitized mice injected locally with adenoviruses carrying the vIL-10 gene inhibit DTH responses following adoptive transfer to sensitized recipients. Finally, dendritic cells grown from bone marrow and transduced with the vIL-10 gene inhibit DTH responses in sensitized, recipient mice. Moreover, dendritic cells transduced with vIL-10 or, especially, IL-4 genes suppress collagen-induced arthritis following injection into recipient mice [our unpublished data]. Thus, it is possible to formulate a working hypothesis that when vectors carrying the appropriate immunomodulatory genes are introduced into an arthritic joint, they transduce APCs, particularly dendritic cells, with the ability to travel to other joints and suppress local disease activity. This hypothesis is testable and, even if incorrect, its experimental examination should provide important new information on the immunopathology of RA.

Clinical Trials

For reasons reviewed elsewhere [54], it was decided to move the intraarticular, retroviral, *ex vivo* delivery of the human IL-1Ra cDNA into a phase I clinical trial. This protocol is described in great detail in reference 55. In 1996 the FDA gave permission for a phase I study in nine post-menopausal women with end-stage RA. The aims of the study were to determine whether the *ex vivo* protocol that had been developed using the knee joints of rabbits could be used safely to deliver the IL-1Ra gene to human, rheumatoid metacarpophalangeal (knuckle) joints with intraarticular expression of the transferred genes. Patients were selected who required surgical management of their condition, including replacement of metacarpophalangeal joints # 2-5 on one hand, and one other joint surgery. The latter provided the opportunity to harvest autologous synovium from which were cultured synovial fibroblasts. The synovial cultures were divided into two, and half were transduced with a retrovirus carrying the IL-1Ra cDNA. After safety testing, in a double blinded fashion two of the four target metacarpophalangeal joints were injected with genetically modified cells and two were injected with naïve cells. One week later, the joints were surgically removed during joint replacement surgery and the retrieved tissues analyzed for evidence of transgene expression. All joints receiving the genetically modified cells expressed transgene mRNA , and most of these also expressed protein. No safety issues arose. The trial thus met its objectives, and a phase II study is being planned. A similar phase I study has started in Germany, with similar preliminary results.

Two additional human trials are about to start in the USA and the Netherlands. Both seek to transfer the herpes thymidine kinase gene to the synovial linings of rheumatoid joints. Upon administration of ganciclovir, cells expressing the transgene should die and cause the death of surrounding cells by the by-stander effect. In this way, a "genetic synovectomy" should be achieved.

Autoimmune diabetes mellitus

IDDM

Autoimmune diabetes mellitus, also called insulin-dependent diabetes mellitus (IDDM), presents a chronic course of immunopathologic development as does rheumatoid arthritis, except that the first clinical signs are seen in early adolescence compared to those of arthritic patients who are first diagnosed at about the fifth decade of life. The immunopathophysiology of IDDM, an autoimmune disorder where the insulin producing β cells of the pancreas are selectively destroyed, is mainly due to the actions of T-lymphocytes [56-58]. Direct cytotoxic effects mediated by CD4+ and CD8+ T-lymphocytes as well as indirect effects via cytokine action on β cells have been demonstrated in a number of studies, in vitro and in vivo [56-58]. Although hyperglycemia can be well controlled by insulin treatment regimens, most patients eventually succumb to complications including nephropathy, neuropathy and heart disease [57,59]. Ideally, the optimal therapeutic option remains the replacement of β cells that secrete insulin in a manner that tightly regulates blood glucose, thereby avoiding the chronic complications. This option, however, has not found common clinical use primarily because of rejection of the cells, which are almost always derived from allogeneic cadaveric donors. Gene therapy offers a tool with which to engineer intact islets of Langerhans, in which the majority of cells are β cells, to resist allorejection. As another approach, once the autoantigens are identified, gene transfer technology can be used to induce tolerance in young individuals deemed to be at high genetic risk thereby obviating transplantation altogether.

IDDM Immunopathophysiology

While there is no doubt that autoreactive T-lymphocytes destroy the β cells, antigen-presenting cells, and macrophages and dendritic cells in particular, are important components of the preinsulitic stage of IDDM, where unknown stimuli result in them acquiring islet antigen and migrating to the peripheral lymphoid organs, most likely the pancreatic lymphoid organs, to engage autoreactive T-lymphocytes. An islet, in which reside roughly 1000 endocrine cells, usually possesses at steady state levels, as many as 15 macrophages. Derived from the monocytic cell lineage, macrophages express class II MHC when activated by cytokines such as tumor necrosis factor alpha (TNF-α). Additionally, macrophages respond to local injury by releasing interleukin-1β (IL-1β) which has been shown to inhibit the release of insulin by β cells in response to glucose [60-63]. The importance of macrophages in IDDM pathogenesis derives from *in vivo* depletion studies in BB rats and CD-1 mice which remained diabetes-free following depletion by silica particle injection [64-65]. Apoptosis of β cells appears to be a very early event in the NOD mouse just prior to the onset of insulitis and IL-1β as well as IL-1α have been shown to sensitize β cells to Fas-triggered apoptosis, both in mouse and human islet culture in vitro [66-67]. The effects of IL-1β on both β cell dysfunction as well as sensitization to Fas-dependent apoptosis appear to be mediated partly by the elaboration of nitric oxide (NO), whose formation from arginine can be inhibited by blocking the inducible nitric oxide synthase (iNOS). In fact, IL-1β activates both iNOS gene expression and enzyme activity [60, 68,69].

T-lymphocytes have long been known to be important effectors of β cell damage and constitute the major cell type of the insulitic infiltrate. T-lymphocytes are detected in the insulitis at disease onset and IDDM was shown to be transferred from a diabetic patient to a non-diabetic recipient by bone marrow transplantation [70-74]. Islet-reactive T-lymphocytes have been detected in newly-diagnosed patients and immunosuppressive therapy has been shown to delay IDDM onset [75 - 77]. Finally, IDDM can be adoptively transferred to normal mice with T-lymphocytes from diabetic donors [78, 79]. The majority of T-lymphocytes at insulitis onset are CD4[+], but progression to destructive insulitis is characterised by an increase in CD8[+] T-cell content [58]. That a variety of autoantigens recognised by autoreactive T-cells in mice and humans have been identified, many of which are not β cell-specific, suggests that a primary lesion results in epitope spreading [80]. In fact, one of the major autoantigens, glutamic acid decarboxylase (GAD) has a six amino acid-long segment that is homologous to a protein of the Coxsackie B virus [81]. This has led to suggestions that GAD may be recognised as a consequence of molecular mimicry following Coxsackie B infection, although other studies have recently challenged this interpretation [80].

Whereas certain studies suggest that either CD4+ or CD8+ T-cells can alone initiate insulitis and IDDM in mice, it appears that both subsets are required [82-86]. Other studies have revealed an imbalance in the CD4+/CD8+ T-cell balance in the peripheral blood of IDDM patients, but the functional significance of this is not clear [87-89]. CD4+ T-cells can be divided into two categories: T_H1 and T_H2, each distinguished by the cytokines they produce upon stimulation. T_H1 cells are mostly associated with cellular immune responses and produce TNFα, interferon γ (IFN γ), and IL-12. T_H2 cells are usually associated with shifting the immune response to a predominantly humoral one that activates B-lymphocytes and antibody production. In response to activation, these cells produce IL-4, IL-10 and transforming growth factor β (TGFβ). In NOD mice, progression to insulitis is associated with increasing IFN γ and monoclonal antibodies against IFNγ have been demonstrated to prevent the autoimmune islet destruction [90, 91]. Immunoregulatory cytokines have profound effects on the outcome of insulitis progression to IDDM in the NOD mouse. Cytokines produced from T_H2 T-cells (IL-4, IL-10 and TGFβ) have been shown to have protective effects [92]. The identification of a suppressor T-cell clone which prevented T-cell-mediated destruction of NOD β cells as well as the destruction of islet transplants in acutely-diabetic syngeneic NOD mice, provided evidence that the suppression was due to TGFβ and IL-10 production by the suppressor cells [92-94]. The importance of IL-10 derives from studies where recombinant IL-10 was shown to delay the incidence and significantly decrease IDDM onset in adult NOD mice [95]. Treatment of young, prediabetic NOD mice with an IL-10-Fc fusion protein resulted in the absence of IDDM even after cessation of treatment [96]. That the expression of TNFα and IFNγ in the islets of these mice was inhibited and that adoptive transfer of diabetogenic splenocytes failed to induce IDDM, suggests the existence of IL-10-modulated suppressor T-cell activity in the host [96]. In another study, daily subcutaneous injection of IL-10 into prediabetic NOD mice was able to delay IDDM onset and incidence. The mechanism by which cytokines derived from T_H2 T-cells affect the onset or the progression of insulitis is not fully defined, however, likely targets include cell survival pathways of both CD4+ and CD8+ autoreactive T-cells, downregulation of class I and II MHC molecules and co-stimulatory, co-activation signals on antigen-presenting cells.

Transplantation of genetically-engineered islets as a therapy for IDDM

Recent advances in methodology of isolation of intact functional human and non-human islets from pancreas has resulted in clinical testing of islet transplantation instead of whole pancreas transplantation. Although there have been some successes with human allografts, where immunosuppressed recipients have remained insulin-independent for a number of years following islet transplantation via the portal vein, most of the patients failed to achieve insulin-independence [97, 98]. Futhermore, immunosuppressive agents in clinical use today, which are used to prevent allograft rejection, especially glucocorticoids, cyclosporin A and FK-506 [97, 98], are toxic and can cause malignancy as well as an induction of diabetes. Autografts have met with better success, but in the majority of cases, the availability of human donors remains an important obstacle [97, 98]. Xenotransplantation is emerging as a potential option and aside from the ethical concerns as well as those for zoonosis, important immunologic hurdles remain to be surmounted [99-101]. Microencapsulated islets in synthetic polymers have been effective in some instances, but their long-term survival has met with obstacles, most likely involving fibrosis of the polymer, islet core damage and death due to ischemic oxygen deprivation and cytokine-induced damage [102-105]. Recent experimental strategies involving the genetic engineering of islets followed by transplantation to allogeneic rodent and non-human primate models have demonstrated that local modulation of the immune response may be sufficient to prevent allograft rejection as well as autoimmunity [106,107].

In order to prevent rejection of the transplanted islets as well as the potential for an autoimmune destruction, a number of approaches delivering immunosuppressive molecules have been tested [106-107] (see Table 4). Adenoviral gene delivery has been the method of choice, primarily because of the ease with which this vector can be grown as well as the simplicity with

Table 4
Gene vectors and genes tested to-date with the aim of facilitating islet allograft survival

Vector	Gene
Adenovirus	IL-4, IL-10, vIL-10, TGFβ, IL-1Ra, CTLA-4Ig, FasL, IL-12(p40), A20, catalase
Herpes Simplex Virus	Bcl-2
Lentivirus	IL-4

which one can introduce transgenes into the adenoviral backbone [108]. More limited use has been made with herpes vectors [109, 110] and much more recently, lentiviruses have demonstrated a certain degree of promise [111-113]. For gene delivery to islets to be successful, the vector of choice should be non-immunogenic, stably-integrating into non-dividing cells and easily grown to high titers. Thus far, lentiviral vectors appear to fulfill all these criteria [114, 115]. Adeno-associated viral vectors also possess non-immunogenic properties and can integrate into the genome under particular conditions, but no report of islet infectivity exists to date.

Immunosuppressive cytokine gene delivery

Islet allograft survival has been achieved in NOD-scid mice transplanted with IL-4-expressing lentiviral vectors, where the recipient mice were subsequently challenged with diabetogenic splenocytes from NOD mice [116]. Moreover, the recipient's endogenous islets were also spared destruction following the adoptive transfer of IDDM by these diabetogenic cells [111]. Other observations, however suggest that IL-4 may not be able to prevent IDDM. Adenoviral gene transfer of IL-4 to islets followed by their transplantation into alloxan-treated syngeneic NOD mice was unable to prevent IDDM onset [116]. It is unclear whether this was due to IL-4, a host response against the adenoviral gene products or to the non-specific effects of alloxan treatment.

IL-10 is another cytokine with immunosuppressive properties, essentially preventing IFNγ production by T_H1-type T-cells, downregulation of class II MHC expression on antigen presenting cells (APC) and the inhibition of IL-12 production by APC. In addition, IL-10 does possess some immunostimulatory capacity on B-lymphocytes, CD8$^+$ T-cells and NK cell activity [62, 63]. In contrast, a homologue of IL-10 isolated from the Epstein-Barr virus, vIL-10, was shown to significantly reduce allogeneic lymphocyte proliferation following infection of human islets *in vitro* using an adenoviral vector [119]. Also, systemic IL-10 production from a DNA plasmid vector was able to prolong the time NOD mice exhibited overt IDDM, following intramuscular injection of the vector [120].

Another cytokine with potent immunosuppressive effects is transforming growth factor β (TGF-β). It inhibits NK cell function, thymocyte proliferation, the induction of T-cell suppressor activity and the inhibition of antibody production [121]. Intramuscular injection of a DNA vector encoding TGFβ1 to NOD mice improved the insulitis grade and decreased IDDM incidence in naturally-occuring diabetes as well as in the cyclophosphamide-accelerated model [122]. More recently, combined transfer of IL-10 and TGFβ by adeno-viral vectors into canine islets, which were subsequently transplanted into xenogeneic rat recipients, led to significant prolongation of graft survival [123].

That IL-1β acts early in the pre-insulitic phase has been demonstrated by a number of studies discussed in an earlier section. Blockade of IL-1β sig-nalling by injection of recombinant interleukin-1 receptor antagonist protein (IL-1Ra) into NOD mice as well as NOD recipients of syngeneic islet trans-plants was shown to protect against autoimmune infiltration, islet destruc-tion and onset of the disease. Other than IL-1Ra, soluble type I receptor exposure to islets proved beneficial in preventing IL-1β-induced, Fas-trig-gered β cell damage [124-126]. IL-1β is at the summit of a pro-inflammatory cascade in response to local perturbations of cell function and survival, espe-cially in response to local viral-mediated trauma. It activates dendritic cells, which then acquire antigen and migrate to the periphery. With this in mind, we have hypothesized that the activation of islet-resident dendritic cells, or antigen-presenting cells of the recipient of islet allografts would be sup-pressed in the absence of IL-1β signalling. As a first approach, we have shown that adenoviral gene transfer of IL-1Ra prevents IL-1β-induced β cell dysfunction, nitric oxide production and sensitisation to Fas-triggered apop-tosis of human islets in culture [127].

Gene transfer to islets to prevent co-stimulatory signals

To become fully activated, a naïve T-cell must, in addition to MHC-peptide :TCR interactions, receive a second signal, usually provided by the CD80 and CD86 co-stimulatory molecules found at the surface of APC, most often den-dritic cells (DC). Blockade of the co-stimulatory signal leads to T-cell anergy or apoptosis [128]. The counter-receptors for CD80 and CD86 are CD28 and CTLA-4. The former is required to promote T-cell activation and prolifera-tion, whereas the latter appears to attenuate or even suppress T-cell activa-tion. Gene transfer of a CTLA-4Ig fusion cDNA to islets has proven effective in achieving significant prolongation of islets in allogeneic recipients [129]. Additionally, prolongation of islet allograft survival was achieved by co-trans-plantation of islets with syngeneic myoblasts expressing CTLA-4Ig [130]. In addition to the co-stimulatory signals, there is also a critical co-activation signal that is required to initiate the activation of T-cells. This interaction occurs between the CD40 molecule at the surface of APC and CD154 on the surface of T-cells. The result of this interaction is the secretion of IL-12 by APC, especially DC. Selective blockade of CD40:CD154 interactions using a humanised antibody against CD154 has proven effective in promoting the survival of islet allografts in non-human primates [131, 132]. That long-term insulin-independence was achieved suggests that blockade of this pathway using soluble CD40-Ig fusion proteins expressed from transplanted islets, may yield the same effect without interfering with the entire immune system of the host, that may have likely happened with the humanised anti-body. IL-12 has also been targeted with encouraging results in NOD mice. IL-12 consists of two subunits: p35 and p40. The active cytokine is a het-erodimer. Adenoviral gene transfer of the p40 subunit to NOD islets followed by transplantation was shown to prolong the time to IDDM onset in synge-neic recipients along with a decrease in IFNγ production and an increase in TGFβ expression at the transplantation site [133]. Additional co-stimulatory signals and counter-receptors that could also serve as targets include the adhesion molecules, like ICAM-1 and ICAM-3. Recombinant soluble ICAM injections into NOD mice were effective in preventing insulitis and IDDM onset [134-136]. Consequently, engineered islets expressing soluble ICAM-1 or ICAM-3 proteins could be spared allograft and perhaps autoimmune rejection.

Anti-apoptotic approaches

Immune rejection of islets is mainly due to apoptotic processes. A variety of interactions between islets and T-cells, NK cells and neutrophils has been shown to culminate in the activation of apoptotic processes within islets. Gene transfer of anti-apoptotic factors could likely contribute in protecting

Table 5
Anti-apoptotic candidate genes to facilitate islet allograft survival

Soluble Fas-Ig
Soluble TRAIL receptors
A20
Dominant-negative FADD/TRADD
Dominant-negative caspases
Bcl-x$_L$
I-FLICE
FLIPs
Heat shock proteins
MnSOD
Cu/ZnSOD
Thioredoxin
IκB

transplanted islets from allo- as well as autoimmune rejection (Table 5). Fas ligand (FasL) is one of the major molecules with which T-cells activate apoptosis of cells. FasL interaction with Fas at the surface of β cells has been shown to result in apoptosis of the β cells [137, 138]. TNFα signalling through the type I TNF receptor also activates an apoptotic cascade within β cells [139]. The intracellular signalling cascades of these two pathways are distinct at the early stages, but converge at common effector pathways, which are attractive candidates with which to interfere as a means of preventing apoptosis of β cells. Signalling through either Fas or the TNF receptor leads to the recruitment of docking proteins to the intracellular domains of the receptors which then, in turn, recruit caspase zymogens activating their catalytic properties and culminating in cell death [140-142]. Fas signalling requires FADD (Fas-associated death domain), a docking protein which then facilitates the interaction of procaspase 9 with the complex. In a similar manner, TRADD (TNF receptor-associated death domain) also interacts with the TNF receptor in recruiting procaspases to the complex. Dominant-negative mutant versions of FADD or TRADD could be useful in perturbing the normal death signals that are transmitted by Fas and the TNFα type I receptor.

Originally identified as an oncogene, Bcl-2 is an anti-apoptotic molecule that can also interfere with Fas-triggered processes [143]. Bcl-2 expression in islets *in vitro*, driven from a herpes vector conferred protection to β cells from apoptosis in the presence of a cytokine cocktail *in vitro*, previously known to induce apoptosis [144]. Moreover, β cell function was not impaired in these cells. Caspase activation is one of the earliest events that follows Fas and TNF signals. One of the earliest caspases, caspase-8 can be inhibited by a naturally-occuring inhibitor called I-FLICE, as well as a group of inhibitory proteins termed FLIPs. Interestingly, one such FLIP is encoded by a herpes virus [144-146]. More recently, an intracellular zinc finger-containing protein, called A20, which is normally expressed in response to pro-inflammatory signals, was shown to inhibit IL-1β-stimulated nitric oxide production and to protect against apoptosis of islets in culture following adenoviral gene transfer [147, 148].

Oxidant stress plays an additional role in priming β cells for apoptotic cell death, and is certainly involved at every stage of islet transplantation, from organ procurement, to mechanical and enzymatic disruption of the pancreas to the time of transplantation. Superoxide and peroxynitrite appear to be key metabolites and their generation could be inhibited by expressing anti-oxidant enzymes within islets to be transplanted. Adenoviral gene transfer of catalase has been shown to reduce the oxidant stress in rodent and human islets in culture [149]. IDDM incidence was significantly reduced in trans-genic NOD mice expressing thioredoxin in β cells [150]. Finally, rodent insu-linoma cells expressing manganese superoxide dismutase (MnSOD) were able to resist the effects of IL-1β *in vitro* [151].

Protection from apoptosis can also be coupled with ways in which islets can be used to deliver death signals to reactive immune cells, as a means of pro-longing islet allograft survival. Upon activation, T-cells are eventually elimi-nated by Fas-mediated apoptosis following the delivery of a FasL signal by other activated T-cells [152-153]. A variety of tissues characterised by their ability to evade immune inflammation and destruction, such as the testis and the cornea of the eye have been shown to eliminate Fas-positive T-cells in a FasL-dependent manner [154]. Transplantation of FasL-express-ing islets would, in principle, protect them from allo- and autoimmune rejec-tion. In fact, early studies were promising, where FasL-expressing myoblasts co-transplanted with allogeneic islets into murine recipients promoted the long-term survival of the islets [155]. Later studies could not confirm the protective role for FasL, as FasL-expressing islet allografts underwent a neutrophil-mediated rejection in murine recipients [156, 157]. More recent data, however, suggest that the form of FasL may be important in confer-ring immune priviledge or in eliciting potent rejection. Soluble FasL expres-sion from allogeneic islets resulted in significant prolongation of allograft survival in rodent recipients [158]. Other potentially important death signals to T-cells could include TRAIL-mediated cell death [159-163], although there is no data yet indicating if TRAIL receptors exist on β cells. On the other hand, TRAIL expression on islets could be effective, in addition to FasL in eliminating autoreactive or alloreactive activated T-cells . Gene transfer of TRAIL to islets could therefore prove helpful.

Tolerance induction: Central and Peripheral

Tolerance can be defined as the permanent acceptance of genetically-mis-matched cell and tissue transplants without the need for any immuno-suppression. In seminal work, long-term prolongation of rat islet allograft survival was achieved following a single injection of anti-lymphocyte serum and inytrathymic injection of donor islets [164]. Additionally, suppression of autoimmunity in spontaneously-diabetic BB rats was also observed using this approach [165]. The interpretation of these observations was that tol-erance occurred consequent to the deletion of islet-reactive thymocytes. In another approach, donor bone-marrow cell injection into the thymus prior to allogeneic islet transplantation in rats resulted in thymic chimerism, donor-specific hyporesponsiveness *in vitro* and long-term islet allograft survival

[166]. Injection of donor class I and II MHC molecules into the thymus as well as putative autoantigens (insulin and GAD) was also able to achieve long-term allograft survival and was effective at preventing IDDM onset in the NOD mouse [168, 169]. Based on these observations, it may be feasible to introduce DNA vectors encoding donor MHC or autoantigens to the thymus as a means of inducing tolerance to allogeneic islet grafts and to prevent autoimmunity in genetically-predisposed individuals.

Antigen presentation is usually carried out by professional APC, such as DC. In the periphery, DC capture antigen, undergo maturation, migrate to the peripheral lymphoid organs and activate naïve T-cells. Full activation of the T-cells requires the DC to provide a co-stimulatory signal through the CD80, CD86:CD28 pathway as well as a co-activation signal via CD40 :CD154 inter-action. DC are the most potent immunostimulatory cells defined to date, but they can also be manipulated to be very powerful tolerogens under defined conditions. These manipulations could be exploited to induce peripheral tolerance to allo and autoantigens in IDDM therapy. DC tolerogenicity has been observed by the suppression of T-cell responses in T-cell ontogeny as well as allo-, tumor and autoimmunity [170]. Exposure of bone-marrow derived DC to UV radiation, IL-10, TGFβ or CTLA-4Ig has been shown to promote tolerogenic characteristics [170, 171]. Adenoviral and retroviral gene delivery of CTLA-4Ig, viral IL-10 or TGFβ to myeloid DC *in vitro* has been shown to elicit alloantigen-specific hyporesponsiveness and enhanced survival in non-immunosuppressed allogeneic hosts [171, 172]. The criterion of tolerogenicity appears to be a low level of co-stimulatory molecule expression at the surface of DC otherwise capable of presenting antigen in both a class I and class II-dependent manner [170]. The injection into allogeneic hosts of DC manipulated in culture to maintain low levels of co-stimulatory molecules has been demonstrated to facilitate long-term survival of allogeneic hearts and islets in mice [170]. Consequently, gene delivery of molecules like CTLA-4Ig or soluble CD40-Ig to DC expressing allo or autoantigens, may promote allograft tolerance. Other attractive co-activation pathways that could be targeted to induce peripheral tolerance could involve OX40, ICAM-1 and ICAM-3 as well as intracellular signalling pathways involved in DC maturation such as NF-κB, STAT5 and STAT6.

Other means to facilitate islet transplantation

Chemokines are a family of soluble immunomodulatory proteins that are involved in the recruitment of different subsets of immune cells to a site of inflammation partly through their promotion of chemotaxis [173-176]. Neutrophils, in particular, appear to be among the primary targets of chemokines [173-177]. Islet-specific T_H1 and T_H2-type T-cells have been shown to produce chemokines where T_H1 T-cells predominantly secrete lymphotactin, monocyte chemoattractant protein (MCP)-1 and macrophage inflammatory protein-1α (MIP-1α) [178]. Additonally, RANTES, MCP-3, IP-10 and MCP-5 production within islets was associated with infiltration of T_H1-type T-cells but not T_H2-type [178]. Transgenic expression of MCP-1 in murine β cells led to the develoment of a chronic monocytic insulitis that was largely devoid of T-cells, although no progression to destructive insulitis or impaired glucose homeostasis was observed in the transgenic mice [179]. It is likely that allogeneic islets could elicit the production of chemokines, either by resident APC or by reactive T-cells. Blockade of chemokine action could be achieved using chemokine antagonist proteins, chemokine binding proteins or soluble chemokine receptors [173, 176, 180, 181].

The understanding of the factors at the feto-placental boundary which prevent the rejection of the fetus are predicted to yield powerful modulators with which an allogeneic immune reaction could be suppressed. Although the absence of HLA antigens on the outermost layer of the placenta spares the organ from T-cell mediated recognition, this stealth mechanism activates NK cells. HLA-G is a non-classical class I MHC molecule that is expressed at the surface of the maternal-fetal interface of the placenta and it has been shown that HLA-G expression is sufficient to protect HLA-deficient cells [182]. Although NK cells are important in rejection of xenogeneic tissues, a role in allogeneic rejection has been demonstrated in autoimmunity of BB rats and allogeneic islet damage *in vitro* [183-187].

Recent data suggest that tryptophan catabolism may play a role in protecting the placenta from T-cell attack [187, 188]. Specifically, fetal rejection is proposed to occur, in part, by the activation of maternal T-cells that are normally suppressed by a tryptophan-depleted environment due to active breakdown of tryptophan by placental cells. Allogeneic concepti were rapidly rejected when pregnant mice were treated with a pharmacologic inhibitor of indoleamine-2,3-dioxygenase (IDO). How tryptophan affects T-cell function remains unclear, but IDO gene transfer to islets may prove beneficial [187, 188].

CONCLUSIONS

It is clear from the information discussed in this chapter that gene therapy has much to offer when seeking to improve the treatment of autoimmune diseases and the success of human allografting. Although these medical conditions differ clinically, their genetic treatments may converge on common approaches, modified only in the technical refinements required by the different circumstances under which they occur. Impressive proof of principle has emerged from studies in experimental animals leading, in the case of RA, to phase I clinical trials. These protocols should serve as a prelude to more ambitious trials leading to the prudent development of new treatments that are safe, effective and affordable.

REFERENCES

1. Evans,C.H. and Robbins, P.D. (eds.) Gene therapy in inflammatory diseases. 272pp. Birkhauser, Basel, 2000.
2. Evans,C.H. and Robbins, P.D. Possible orthopaedic applications of gene therapy. J Bone Jt Surg 77A: 1103-1114, 1995
3. Robbins, PD and Ghivizzani, SC Viral vectors for gene therapy. Pharmacology and Therapeutics 80:35-47, 1997
4. Robbins, PD, Tahara, H, and Ghivizzani, SC Viral vectors for gene therapy. Trends Biotechnology 16:35-40, 1997
5. Tuting T, Storkus WJ and Lotze MT. Gene-based strategies for the immunotherapy of cancer. J Mol Med 75: 478-491, 1997
6. Ho IC, Lo D, and Glimcher LH. c-maf promotes T helper cell type 2 (Th2) and attenuates Th1 differentiation by both interleukin 4-dependent and -independent mechanisms. J Exp Med 188:1859-66, 1998
7. Schumacher HR (ed) Promer on the rheumatic diseases. 10th Edition . 347pp Arthritis Foundation, Atlanta GA, 1993
8. Moreland LW, Heck LW and Koopman WJ. Biological agents for treating rheumatoid arthritis: concepts and progress. Arthrits Rheum 40: 397-409, 1997
9. Feldmann M, Brennan FM, Maini RN. Role of cytokines in rheumatoid arthritis. Ann Rev Immunol.14:397-440, 1996
10. Arend WP, Dayer JM. Cytokines and cytokine inhibitors or antagonists in rheumatoid arthritis Arthritis Rheum 33:305-15,1990
11. Evans CH, Ghivizzani SC, Kang R, Muzzonigro T, Wasko MC, Herndon JH, Robbins PD. Gene therapy for rheumatic diseases. Arthritis Rheum 42: 1-19, 1999
12. Evans, C.H., Rediske, J.J., Abramson, S.B. and Robbins, P.D.: Joint Efforts: Tackling arthritis using gene therapy. Mol Med Today 5:148-151, 1999.
13. Evans, C.H., and Robbins, P.D.: Gene therapy of arthritis. Int Med 38:233-239, 1999
14. Le CH, Nicolson AG, Morales A, Sewell KL. Suppression of collagen-induced arthritis through adenovirus-mediated transfer of a modified tumor necrosis α receptor gene. Arthritis Rheum. 40: 1662-1669, 1997.
15. Ma Y, Thornton S, Duwell LE, Boivin GP, Giannini EH, Leiden M et al. Inhibition of collagen-induced arthritis in mice by viral IL-10 gene transfer. J Immunol 161: 1516-1524, 1998.
16. Apparailly F, Verwaerde C, Jacquet C, Auriault C, Sany J, Jorgensen C. Adenovirus mediated transfer of viral IL-10 gene inhibits murine collagen-induced arthritis. J Immunol 160: 5213-5220, 1998.
17. Whalen JD, Lechman EL, Carlos CA, Weiss K, Glorioso JC, Kovesdi I et al. Adeno-

viral transfer of the viral IL-10 gene periarticularly to mouse paws suppresses development of collagen-induced arthritis in both injected and uninjected paws. J Immunol 162: 3625-3632, 1999.

18. Quattrocchi E, Walmsley M, Browne K, Williams RO, Marinova-Mutafchieva L, Buurman W, Butler DM, Feldmann M. Paradoxical effects of adenovirus-mediated blockade of TNF activity in murine collagen-induced arthritis. J Immunol 163: 1000-1009, 1999.

19. Miyata M, Sato Y, Sato H, Saito A, Irisawa A, Nishimaki T et al. Suppression of murine collagen-induced arthritis by inoculation of plasmid DNA encoding for interleukin 10 (abstract). Arthritis Rheum 40 (suppl 9): S55, 1997.

20. Ragno S, Colston MJ, Lowrie DB, Winrow VR, Blake DR, Tascon R. Protection of rats from adjuvant arthritis by immunization with naked DNA encoding for mycobacterial heat shock protein 65. Arthritis Rheum 40: 277-283, 1997.

21. Song XY, Gu M, Jin WW, Klinman M, Wahl SM. Plasmid DNA encoding transforming growth factor-β uppresses chronic disease in a streptococcal cell wall-induced arthritis model. J Clin Invest 101: 1-7, 1998.

22. Shiozawa S, Shimizu K, Tanaka K, Hino K. Studies on the contribution of c-fos/AP-1 to arthritic joint destruction . J Clin Invest. 99:1210-6, 1997.

23. Chernajovsky Y, Adams G, Podhajcer O, Mueller G, Robbins PD, Feldman M. Inhibition of the transfer of collagen induced arthritis into SCID mice by gene transfer of spleen cells with retrovirus expressing soluble tumor necrosis factor receptor. Gene Ther 2: 731-735, 1995.

24. Chernajovsky Y, Adams G, Triantaphyllopoulos K, Ledda F, Podhajcer OL. Pathogenic lymphoid cells engineered to express TGF-β₁ ameliorate disease in a collagen-induced rarthritis model. Gene Ther 4: 553-559, 1997.

25. Bessis N, Boissier MC, Ferrara P, Blankenstein T, Fradelizi D, Fournier C. Attenuation of collagen-induced arthritis in mice by treatment with vector cells engineered to secrete interleukin-13. Eur J Immunol 26: 2399-2403, 1996.

26. Bessis N, Chiocchia G, Kollias G, Minty A, Fournier C, Fradelizi D, Boissier MC. Modulation of proinflammatory cytokine production in tumor necrosis factor-alpha (TNF-α)-transgenic mice by treatment with cells engineered to secrete IL-4, IL-10 or IL-13. Clin Exp Immunol 111: 391-396, 1998.

27. Triantaphyllopoulos KA, Williams RO, Tailor H, Chernojovsky Y. Amelioration of collagen-induced arthritis and suppression of interferon-gamma, interleukin-12, and tumor necrosis factor alpha production by interferon-beta gene therapy. Arthritis Rheum 42: 90-99, 1999.

28. Bandara G, Robbins PD, Georgescu HI, Mueller GM, Gloriosos JC, Evans CH. Gene transfer to synoviocytes: prospects for gene treatment for arthritis. DNA Cell Biol 11: 227-231, 1992.

29. Bandara G, Mueller GM, Galea-Lauri J, Tindal MH, Georgescu HI, Suchanek MK et al. Intraarticular expression of biologically active interleukin-1 receptor antagonist protein by ex vivo gene transfer. Proc Natl Acad Sci USA 90: 10764-10768, 1993.

30. Roessler BJ, Allen ED, Wilson JM, Hartman JW, Davidson BL. Adenoviral-mediated gene transfer to rabbit synovium in vivo. J Clin Invest 92: 1085-1092, 1993.

31. Nita I, Ghivizzani SC, Galea-Lauri J, Bandara G, Georgescu HI, Robbins PD, Evans CH. Direct gene delivery to synovium: an evaluation of different vectors in vitro and in vivo. Arthritis Rheum 39: 820-828, 1996

32. Yovandich J, O'Malley B, Sikes M, Ledley FD. Gene transfer to synovial cells by intraarticular administration of plasmid DNA. Hum Gene Ther 6: 603-610, 1995.

33. Pan RY, Xiao X, Chen SL, Li J, Lin LC, Wang HJ, Tsao YP. Disease-inducible transgene expression from a recombinant adeno-associated virus vector in a rat arthritis model. J Virol 73: 3410-3417, 1999.

34. Oligino, T.J., Yao, Q., Xiao, X., Glorioso, J.C., Evans, C.H., Robbins, P.D. and

Ghivizzani, S.C.: Intra-articular expression of the IL-1Ra gene following direct delivery with an adeno-associated virus vector. Gene Ther In Press

35. Zhang HG, Yang Y, Horton JL, Samoilva EB, Judge TA, Turka LA et al. Amelioration of collagen-induced arthritis by CD95 (Apo-1/Fas)-ligand gene transfer. J Clin Invest 100: 1951-1957, 1997.

36. Yao,Q., Glorioso,J.C., Evans,C.H., Robbins,P.D., Oligino,T.J. Ghivizzani,S.C: Adenoviral mediated delivery of FAS ligand to rheumatoid synovium results in extensive apoptosis in the synovial lining. Gene Medicine In Press

37. Goossens PH, Schouten GJ, 't Hart BA, Bout A, Brok HP, Kluin PM, Breedveld FC,Valerio D, Huizinga TW. Feasibility of adenovirus-mediated nonsurgical synovectomy in collagen-induced arthritis-affected rhesus monkeys.Hum Gene Ther. 10:1139-49,1999

38. Sant SM, Suarez TM, Moalli MR, Wu BY, Blaivas M, Laing TJ, Roessler BJ. Molecular lysis of synovial lining cells by in vivo herpes simplex virus-thymidine kinase gene transfer. Hum Gene Ther. 9:2735-43, 1997

39. Taniguchi K, Kohsaka H, Inoue N, Terada Y, Ito H, Hirokawa K, Miyasaka N. Induction of the p16INK4a senescence gene as a new therapeutic strategy for the treatment of rheumatoid arthritis. Nat Med 5:760-7, 1999

40. Rabinovich GA, Daly G, Dreja H, Tailor H, Riera CM, Hirabayashi J, Chernojovsy Y. Recombinant galectin-1 and its genetic delivery suppress collagen-induced arthritis via T-cell apoptosis. J Exp Med 190: 385-398, 1999

41. Ghivizzani SC, Lechman ER, Kang R, Tio C, Kolls J, Evans CH, Robbins PD. Direct adenoviral-mediated gene transfer of IL-1 and TNF-a soluble receptors to rabbit knees with experimental arthritis has local and distal anti-arthritic effects. Proc Natl Acad Sci USA 95: 4613-4618, 1998

42. Makarov SS, Olsen JC, Johnston WN, Anderle SK, Brown RR, Baldwin AS et al. Suppression of experimental arthritis by gene transfer of interleukin-1 receptor antagonist cDNA. Proc Natl Acad Sci USA 93: 402-406, 1996

43. Roessler BJ, Hartman JW, Vallance DK, Latta JM, Janich SL, Davidson BL. Inhibition of interleukin-1 induced effects in synoviocytes transduced with the human interleukin-1 receptor antagonist cDNA using an adenoviral vector. Hum Gene Ther 6: 307-316, 1995.

44. Kim,S.H.,Evans,C.H.,Kim,S.,Oligino,T.,Ghivizzani,S.C. and Robbins,P.D.: Gene therapy of established murine collagen-induced arthritis by local and systemic adenoviral mediated delivery of IL-4. Arthritis Res In Press

45. Evans, C.H., Ghivizzani, S.C., Lechman, E., Mi, Z, Jaffurs, D. and Robbins, P.D.: Lessons learned from gene transfer approaches. Arthritis Res http://arthritis research.com/08jul99/ar0101r01

46. Mi, Z, Ghivizzani, SC, Lechman· ER, Jaffurs, D, Glorioso, JC, Evans, CH, and Robbins, PD. Adenoviral mediated gene transfer of IGF-1 stimulates cartilage synthesis in rabbit joints. Submitted.

47. Lubberts E, Joosten LA, van Den Bersselaar L, Helsen MM, Bakker AC, van Meurs JB, Graham FL, Richards CD, van Den Berg WB.Adenoviral vector-mediated overexpression of IL-4 in the knee joint of mice with collagen-induced arthritis prevents cartilage destruction. J Immunol 163:4546-56,1999

48. Boyle DL, Nguyen KH, Zhuang S, Shi Y, McCormack JE, Chada S, Firestein GS.: Intra-articular IL-4 gene therapy in arthritis: anti-inflammatory effect and enhanced T_H2 activity. Gene Ther. 6:1911-8, 1999

49. Lechman, E.R., Jaffurs, D., Ghivizzani, S.C., Gambotto, A., Kovesdi, I., Mi, Z., Evans, C.H. Robbins, P.D.: Direct adenoviral gene transfer of vIL-10 to rabbit knees with experimental arthritis ameliorates disease in both injected and contralateral knees. J Immunol 163: 2202-2208,1999.

50. Otani, K., Nita, I., Macaulay, W., Georgescu, H.I., Robbins, P.D. and Evans, C.H.: Suppression of antigen-induced arthritis by gene therapy. J Immunol

156:3558-3562, 1996.

51. Miagkov AV, Kovalenko DV, Brown CE, Didsbury JR, Cogswell JP, Stimpson SA, Baldwin AS, Makarov SS. NF-kappaB activation provides the potential link between inflammation and hyperplasia in the arthritic joint.Proc Natl Acad Sci U S A. 95:13859-64, 1998

52. Tomita T, Takeuchi E, Tomita N, Morishita R, Kaneko M, Yamamoto K, Nakase T, Seki H, Kato K, Kaneda Y, Ochi T. Suppressed severity of collagen-induced arthritis by in vivo transfection of nuclear factor kappa B decoy oligodeoxynucleotides as a gene therapy. Arthritis Rheum. 42:2532-42, 1999

53. Whalen JD, Thomson AW, Lu L, Robbins PD, Evans CH. Transfer and expression of the viral IL-10 gene in vivo induces a suppressor population of antigen presenting cells which adoptively transfer suppression to soluble antigens. Submitted

54. Evans CH, Ghivizzani SC, Herndon JH, Wasko MC, Reinecke J, Wehling P, Robbins PD. Clinical trials in the gene therapy of arthritis. Clin Orthop Rel Res In Press

55. Evans, C.H., Robbins, P.D., Ghivizzani, S.C., Herndon, J.H., Kang, R., Bahnson, A.B., Barranger, J.A., Elders, E.M., Gay, S., Tomaino, M.M., Wasko, M.C., Watkins, S.C., Whiteside, T.L., Glorioso, J.C., Lotze, M. and Wright, T.M.: Clinical trial to assess the safety, feasibility, and efficacy of transferring a potentially anti-arthritic cytokine gene to human joints with rheumatoid arthritis. Hum Gene Ther 7:1261-1280, 1996.

56. Eisenbarth, G. S. 1993. Molecular aspects of the etiology of type I diabetes mellitus. J Diabetes Complications 7:142.

57. Eisenbarth, G. 1991. Prediction and prevention strategies in type I diabetes. Mt Sinai J Med 58:274.

58. Bach, J. F. 1994. Insulin-dependent diabetes mellitus as an autoimmune disease. Endocr Rev 15:516.

59. Clark, A. P. 1994. Complications and management of diabetes: a review of current research. Crit Care Nurs Clin North Am 6:723.

60. McDaniel, M. L., G. Kwon, J. R. Hill, C. A. Marshall, and J. A. Corbett. 1996. Cytokines and nitric oxide in islet inflammation and diabetes. Proc Soc Exp Biol Med 211:24.

61. Arnush, M., A. L. Scarim, M. R. Heitmeier, C. B. Kelly, and J. A. Corbett. 1998. Potential role of resident islet macrophage activation in the initiation of autoimmune diabetes. J Immunol 160:2684.

62. Arnush, M., M. R. Heitmeier, A. L. Scarim, M. H. Marino, P. T. Manning, and J. A. Corbett. 1998. IL-1 produced and released endogenously within human islets inhibits beta cell function. J Clin Invest 102:516.

63. Corbett, J. A., and M. L. McDaniel. 1995. Intraislet release of interleukin 1 inhibits beta cell function by inducing beta cell expression of inducible nitric oxide synthase. J Exp Med 181:559.

64. Dayer-Metroz, M. D., C. B. Wollheim, P. Seckinger, and J. M. Dayer. 1989. A natural interleukin 1 (IL-1) inhibitor counteracts the inhibitory effect of IL-1 on insulin production in cultured rat pancreatic islets. J Autoimmun 2:163.

65. Hanenberg, H., V. Kolb-Bachofen, G. Kantwerk-Funke, and H. Kolb. 1989. Macrophage infiltration precedes and is a prerequisite for lymphocytic insulitis in pancreatic islets of pre-diabetic BB rats. Diabetologia 32:126.

66. Stassi, G., R. D. Maria, G. Trucco, W. Rudert, R. Testi, A. Galluzzo, C. Giordano, and M. Trucco. 1997. Nitric oxide primes pancreatic beta cells for Fas-mediated destruction in insulin-dependent diabetes mellitus. J Exp Med 186:1193.

67. Yamada, K., N. Takane-Gyotoku, X. Yuan, F. Ichikawa, C. Inada, and K. Nonaka. 1996. Mouse islet cell lysis mediated by interleukin-1-induced Fas. Diabetologia 39:1306.

68. Corbett, J. A., J. L. Wang, T. P. Misko, W. Zhao, W. F. Hickey, and M. L. McDaniel.

1993. Nitric oxide mediates IL-1 beta-induced islet dysfunction and destruction: prevention by dexamethasone. Autoimmunity 15:145.

69. Corbett, J. A., J. L. Wang, M. A. Sweetland, J. R. Lancaster, Jr., and M. L. McDaniel. 1992. Interleukin 1 beta induces the formation of nitric oxide by beta-cells purified from rodent islets of Langerhans. Evidence for the beta-cell as a source and site of action of nitric oxide. J Clin Invest 90:2384.

70. Gepts, W. 1965. Pathologic anatomy of the pancreas in juvenile diabetes mellitus. Diabetes 14:619.

71. Roep, B. O., and R. R. De Vries. 1992. T-lymphocytes and the pathogenesis of type 1 (insulin-dependent) diabetes mellitus. Eur J Clin Invest 22:697.

72. Roep, B. O., A. A. Kallan, and R. R. De Vries. 1992. Beta-cell antigen-specific lysis of macrophages by CD4 T-cell clones from newly diagnosed IDDM patient. A putative mechanism of T-cell- mediated autoimmune islet cell destruction. Diabetes 41:1380.

73. Huang, G. C., J. Tremble, E. Bailyes, S. D. Arden, T. Kaye, A. M. McGregor, and J. P. Banga. 1995. HLA-DR-restricted T cell lines from newly diagnosed type 1 diabetic patients specific for insulinoma and normal islet beta cell proteins: lack of reactivity to glutamic acid decarboxylase. Clin Exp Immunol 102:152.

74. Lampeter, E. F., M. Homberg, K. Quabeck, U. W. Schaefer, P. Wernet, J. Bertrams, H. Grosse-Wilde, F. A. Gries, and H. Kolb. 1993. Transfer of insulin-dependent diabetes between HLA-identical siblings by bone marrow transplantation [see comments]. Lancet 341:1243.

75. Stiller, C. R., J. Dupre, M. Gent, M. R. Jenner, P. A. Keown, A. Laupacis, R. Martell, N. W. Rodger, B. von Graffenried, and B. M. Wolfe. 1984. Effects of cyclosporine immunosuppression in insulin-dependent diabetes mellitus of recent onset. Science 223:1362.

76. Bougneres, P. F., J. C. Carel, L. Castano, C. Boitard, J. P. Gardin, P. Landais, J. Hors, M. J. Mihatsch, M. Paillard, J. L. Chaussain, and et al. 1988. Factors associated with early remission of type I diabetes in children treated with cyclosporine. N Engl J Med 318:663.

77. Sibley, R. K., D. E. Sutherland, F. Goetz, and A. F. Michael. 1985. Recurrent diabetes mellitus in the pancreas iso- and allograft. A light and electron microscopic and immunohistochemical analysis of four cases. Lab Invest 53:132.

78. Wicker, L. S., B. J. Miller, and Y. Mullen. 1986. Transfer of autoimmune diabetes mellitus with splenocytes from nonobese diabetic (NOD) mice. Diabetes 35:855.

79. Bendelac, A., C. Carnaud, C. Boitard, and J. F. Bach. 1987. Syngeneic transfer of autoimmune diabetes from diabetic NOD mice to healthy neonates. Requirement for both L3T4+ and Lyt-2+ T cells. J Exp Med 166:823.

80. Horwitz, M. S., L. M. Bradley, J. Harbertson, T. Krahl, J. Lee, and N. Sarvetnick. 1998. Diabetes induced by Coxsackie virus: initiation by bystander damage and not molecular mimicry [In Process Citation]. Nat Med 4:781.

81. Kaufman, D. L., M. G. Erlander, M. Clare-Salzler, M. A. Atkinson, N. K. Maclaren, and A. J. Tobin. 1992. Autoimmunity to two forms of glutamate decarboxylase in insulin- dependent diabetes mellitus. J Clin Invest 89:283.

82. Santamaria, P., R. E. Nakhleh, D. E. Sutherland, and J. J. Barbosa. 1992. Characterization of T lymphocytes infiltrating human pancreas allograft affected by isletitis and recurrent diabetes. Diabetes 41:53.

83. Santamaria, P., C. Lewis, J. Jessurun, D. E. Sutherland, and J. J. Barbosa. 1994. Skewed T-cell receptor usage and junctional heterogeneity among isletitis alpha beta and gamma delta T-cells in human IDDM [corrected] [published erratum appears in Diabetes 1994 Jul;43(7):954]. Diabetes 43:599.

84. Daniel, D., R. G. Gill, N. Schloot, and D. Wegmann. 1995. Epitope specificity, cytokine production profile and diabetogenic activity of insulin-specific T cell clones isolated from NOD mice. Eur J Immunol 25:1056.

85. Christianson, S. W., L. D. Shultz, and E. H. Leiter. 1993. Adoptive transfer of diabetes into immunodeficient NOD-scid/scid mice. Relative contributions of CD4+ and CD8+ T-cells from diabetic versus prediabetic NOD.NON-Thy-1a donors. Diabetes 42:44.

86. Koike, T., Y. Itoh, T. Ishii, I. Ito, K. Takabayashi, N. Maruyama, H. Tomioka, and S. Yoshida. 1987. Preventive effect of monoclonal anti-L3T4 antibody on development of diabetes in NOD mice. Diabetes 36:539.

87. Buschard, K., C. Ropke, S. Madsbad, J. Mehlsen, T. B. Sorensen, and J. Rygaard. 1983. Alterations of peripheral T-lymphocyte subpopulations in patients with insulin-dependent (type 1) diabetes mellitus. J Clin Lab Immunol 10:127.

88. Buschard, K., C. Ropke, S. Madsbad, J. Mehlsen, and J. Rygaard. 1983. T lymphocyte subsets in patients with newly diagnosed type 1 (insulin- dependent) diabetes: a prospective study. Diabetologia 25:247.

89. Ilonen, J., H. M. Surcel, and M. L. Kaar. 1991. Abnormalities within CD4 and CD8 T lymphocytes subsets in type 1 (insulin-dependent) diabetes. Clin Exp Immunol 85:278.

90. Campbell, I. L., T. W. Kay, L. Oxbrow, and L. C. Harrison. 1991. Essential role for interferon-gamma and interleukin-6 in autoimmune insulin-dependent diabetes in NOD/Wehi mice. J Clin Invest 87:739.

91. Debray-Sachs, M., C. Carnaud, C. Boitard, H. Cohen, I. Gresser, P. Bedossa, and J. F. Bach. 1991. Prevention of diabetes in NOD mice treated with antibody to murine IFN gamma. J Autoimmun 4:237.

92. Han, H. S., H. S. Jun, T. Utsugi, and J. W. Yoon. 1996. A new type of CD4+ suppressor T cell completely prevents spontaneous autoimmune diabetes and recurrent diabetes in syngeneic islet- transplanted NOD mice. J Autoimmun 9:331.

93. Moritani, M., K. Yoshimoto, S. Ii, M. Kondo, H. Iwahana, T. Yamaoka, T. Sano, N. Nakano, H. Kikutani, and M. Itakura. 1996. Prevention of adoptively transferred diabetes in nonobese diabetic mice with IL-10-transduced islet-specific Th1 lymphocytes. A gene therapy model for autoimmune diabetes. J Clin Invest 98:1851.

94. Moritani, M., K. Yoshimoto, S. F. Wong, C. Tanaka, T. Yamaoka, T. Sano, Y. Komagata, J. Miyazaki, H. Kikutani, and M. Itakura. 1998. Abrogation of autoimmune diabetes in nonobese diabetic mice and protection against effector lymphocytes by transgenic paracrine TGF- beta1. J Clin Invest 102:499.

95. Pennline, K. J., E. Roque-Gaffney, and M. Monahan. 1994. Recombinant human IL-10 prevents the onset of diabetes in the nonobese diabetic mouse. Clin Immunol Immunopathol 71:169.

96. Zheng, X. X., A. W. Steele, W. W. Hancock, A. C. Stevens, P. W. Nickerson, P. Roy-Chaudhury, Y. Tian, and T. B. Strom. 1997. A noncytolytic IL-10/Fc fusion protein prevents diabetes, blocks autoimmunity, and promotes suppressor phenomena in NOD mice. J Immunol 158:4507.

97. Weir, G. C., and S. Bonner-Weir. 1997. Scientific and political impediments to successful islet transplantation. Diabetes 46:1247.

98. Ricordi, C. 1996. Human islet cell transplantation: New perspectives for an old challenge. Diabetes Reviews 4:356.

99. Platt, J. L. 1998. New directions for organ transplantation. Nature 392:11.

100. Platt, J. L. 1998. Current status of xenotransplantation: research and technology. Transplant Proc 30:1630.

101. Platt, J. L. 1996. Xenotransplantation: recent progress and current perspectives. Curr Opin Immunol 8:721.

102. Lim, F., and A. M. Sun. 1980. Microencapsulated islets as bioartificial endocrine pancreas. Science 210:908.

103. Sun, A. M., M. F. Goosen, and G. O'Shea. 1987. Microencapsulated cells as hormone delivery systems. Crit Rev Ther Drug Carrier Syst 4:1.

104. Sandler, S., A. Andersson, D. L. Eizirik, C. Hellerstrom, T. Espevik, B. Kulseng, B.

Thu, D. G. Pipeleers, and G. Skjak-Braek. 1997. Assessment of insulin secretion in vitro from microencapsulated fetal porcine islet-like cell clusters and rat, mouse, and human pancreatic islets. Transplantation 63:1712.

105. Sun, Y., X. Ma, D. Zhou, I. Vacek, and A. M. Sun. 1996. Normalization of diabetes in spontaneously diabetic cynomologus monkeys by xenografts of microencapsulated porcine islets without immunosuppression. J Clin Invest 98:1417.

106. Giannoukakis, N., A. Thomson, and P. Robbins. 1999. Gene therapy in transplantation. Gene Ther 6:1499.

107. Giannoukakis, N., W. A. Rudert, P. D. Robbins, and M. Trucco. 1999. Targeting autoimmune diabetes with gene therapy. Diabetes 48:2107.

108. Hardy, S., M. Kitamura, T. Harris-Stansil, Y. Dai, and M. L. Phipps. 1997. Construction of adenovirus vectors through Cre-lox recombination. J Virol 71:1842.

109. Liu, Y., A. Rabinovitch, W. Suarez-Pinzon, B. Muhkerjee, M. Brownlee, D. Edelstein, and H. J. Federoff. 1996. Expression of the bcl-2 gene from a defective HSV-1 amplicon vector protects pancreatic beta-cells from apoptosis. Hum Gene Ther 7:1719.

110. Rabinovitch, A., W. Suarez-Pinzon, K. Strynadka, Q. Ju, D. Edelstein, M. Brownlee, G. S. Korbutt, and R. V. Rajotte. 1999. Transfection of human pancreatic islets with an anti-apoptotic gene (bcl-2) protects beta-cells from cytokine-induced destruction. Diabetes 48:1223.

111. Gallichan, W. S., T. Kafri, T. Krahl, I. M. Verma, and N. Sarvetnick. 1998. Lentivirus-mediated transduction of islet grafts with interleukin 4 results in sustained gene expression and protection from insulitis. Hum Gene Ther 9:2717.

112. Giannoukakis, N., Z. Mi, A. Gambotto, A. Eramo, C. Ricordi, M. Trucco, and P. Robbins. 1999. Infection of intact human islets by a lentiviral vector. Gene Ther 6:1545.

113. Ju, Q., D. Edelstein, M. D. Brendel, D. Brandhorst, H. Brandhorst, R. G. Bretzel, and M. Brownlee. 1998. Transduction of non-dividing adult human pancreatic beta cells by an integrating lentiviral vector. Diabetologia 41:736.

114. Zufferey, R., D. Nagy, R. J. Mandel, L. Naldini, and D. Trono. 1997. Multiply attenuated lentiviral vector achieves efficient gene delivery in vivo. Nat Biotechnol 15:871.

115. Naldini, L., U. Blomer, F. H. Gage, D. Trono, and I. M. Verma. 1996. Efficient transfer, integration, and sustained long-term expression of the transgene in adult rat brains injected with a lentiviral vector. Proc Natl Acad Sci U S A 93:11382.

116. Smith, D. K., G. S. Korbutt, W. L. Suarez-Pinzon, D. Kao, R. V. Rajotte, and J. F. Elliott. 1997. Interleukin-4 or interleukin-10 expressed from adenovirus-transduced syngeneic islet grafts fails to prevent beta cell destruction in diabetic NOD mice. Transplantation 64:1040.

117. MacNeil, I. A., T. Suda, K. W. Moore, T. R. Mosmann, and A. Zlotnik. 1990. IL-10, a novel growth cofactor for mature and immature T cells. J Immunol 145:4167.

118. Chen, W. F., and A. Zlotnik. 1991. IL-10: a novel cytotoxic T cell differentiation factor. J Immunol 147:528.

119. Benhamou, P. Y., Y. Mullen, A. Shaked, D. Bahmiller, and M. E. Csete. 1996. Decreased alloreactivity to human islets secreting recombinant viral interleukin 10. Transplantation 62:1306.

120. Nitta, Y., F. Tashiro, M. Tokui, A. Shimada, I. Takei, K. Tabayashi, and J. Miyazaki. 1998. Systemic delivery of interleukin 10 by intramuscular injection of expression plasmid DNA prevents autoimmune diabetes in nonobese diabetic mice. Hum Gene Ther 9:1701.

121. Gray, J. D., M. Hirokawa, and D. A. Horwitz. 1994. The role of transforming growth factor beta in the generation of suppression: an interaction between CD8+ T and NK cells. J Exp Med 180:1937.

122. Piccirillo, C. A., Y. Chang, and G. J. Prud'homme. 1998. TGF-beta1 somatic gene

therapy prevents autoimmune disease in nonobese diabetic mice. J Immunol 161:3950.

123. Deng, S., R. J. Ketchum, Z. D. Yang, T. Kucher, M. Weber, A. Shaked, A. Naji, and K. L. Brayman. 1997. IL-10 and TGF-beta gene transfer to rodent islets: effect on xenogeneic islet graft survival in naive and B-cell-deficient mice. Transplant Proc 29:2207.

124. Sandberg, J. O., D. L. Eizirik, S. Sandler, D. E. Tracey, and A. Andersson. 1993. Treatment with an interleukin-1 receptor antagonist protein prolongs mouse islet allograft survival. Diabetes 42:1845.

125. Sandberg, J. O., A. Andersson, D. L. Eizirik, and S. Sandler. 1994. Interleukin-1 receptor antagonist prevents low dose streptozotocin induced diabetes in mice. Biochem Biophys Res Commun 202:543.

126. Sandberg, J. O., D. L. Eizirik, and S. Sandler. 1997. IL-1 receptor antagonist inhibits recurrence of disease after syngeneic pancreatic islet transplantation to spontaneously diabetic non-obese diabetic (NOD) mice. Clin Exp Immunol 108:314.

127. Giannoukakis, N., W. A. Rudert, S. C. Ghivizzani, A. Gambotto, C. Ricordi, M. Trucco, and P. D. Robbins. 1999. Adenoviral gene transfer of the interleukin-1 receptor antagonist protein to human islets prevents IL-1beta-induced beta-cell impairment and activation of islet cell apoptosis in vitro. Diabetes 48:1730.

128. Thomson, A. W., L. Lu, N. Murase, A. J. Demetris, A. S. Rao, and T. E. Starzl. 1995. Microchimerism, dendritic cell progenitors and transplantation tolerance. Stem Cells (Dayt) 13:622.

129. Gainer, A. L., G. S. Korbutt, R. V. Rajotte, G. L. Warnock, and J. F. Elliott. 1997. Expression of CTLA4-Ig by biolistically transfected mouse islets promotes islet allograft survival. Transplantation 63:1017.

130. Chahine, A. A., M. Yu, M. M. McKernan, C. Stoeckert, and H. T. Lau. 1995. Immunomodulation of pancreatic islet allografts in mice with CTLA4Ig secreting muscle cells. Transplantation 59:1313.

131. Kenyon, N. S., M. Chatzipetrou, M. Masetti, A. Ranuncoli, M. Oliveira, J. L. Wagner, A. D. Kirk, D. M. Harlan, L. C. Burkly, and C. Ricordi. 1999. Long-term survival and function of intrahepatic islet allografts in rhesus monkeys treated with humanized anti-CD154. Proc Natl Acad Sci U S A 96:8132.

132. Kenyon, N. S., L. A. Fernandez, R. Lehmann, M. Masetti, A. Ranuncoli, M. Chatzipetrou, G. Iaria, D. Han, J. L. Wagner, P. Ruiz, M. Berho, L. Inverardi, R. Alejandro, D. H. Mintz, A. D. Kirk, D. M. Harlan, L. C. Burkly, and C. Ricordi. 1999. Long-term survival and function of intrahepatic islet allografts in baboons treated with humanized anti-CD154. Diabetes 48:1473.

133. Yasuda, H., M. Nagata, K. Arisawa, R. Yoshida, K. Fujihira, N. Okamoto, H. Moriyama, M. Miki, I. Saito, H. Hamada, K. Yokono, and M. Kasuga. 1998. Local expression of immunoregulatory IL-12p40 gene prolonged syngeneic islet graft survival in diabetic NOD mice. J Clin Invest 102:1807.

134. Moriyama, H., K. Yokono, K. Amano, M. Nagata, Y. Hasegawa, N. Okamoto, K. Tsukamoto, M. Miki, R. Yoneda, N. Yagi, Y. Tominaga, H. Kikutani, K. Hioki, K. Okumura, H. Yagita, and M. Kasuga. 1996. Induction of tolerance in murine autoimmune diabetes by transient blockade of leukocyte function-associated antigen-1/intercellular adhesion molecule-1 pathway. J Immunol 157:3737.

135. Martin, S., E. Heidenthal, B. Schulte, H. Rothe, and H. Kolb. 1998. Soluble forms of intercellular adhesion molecule-1 inhibit insulitis and onset of autoimmune diabetes [In Process Citation]. Diabetologia 41:1298.

136. Hasegawa, Y., K. Yokono, T. Taki, K. Amano, Y. Tominaga, R. Yoneda, N. Yagi, S. Maeda, H. Yagita, K. Okumura, and et al. 1994. Prevention of autoimmune insulin-dependent diabetes in non-obese diabetic mice by anti-LFA-1 and anti-ICAM-1 mAb. Int Immunol 6:831.

137. Yamada, K., F. Ichikawa, S. Ishiyama-Shigemoto, X. Yuan, and K. Nonaka. 1999.

Essential role of caspase-3 in apoptosis of mouse beta-cells transfected with human Fas. Diabetes 48:478.

138. Suarez-Pinzon, W., O. Sorensen, R. C. Bleackley, J. F. Elliott, R. V. Rajotte, and A. Rabinovitch. 1999. Beta-cell destruction in NOD mice correlates with Fas (CD95) expression on beta-cells and proinflammatory cytokine expression in islets. Diabetes 48:21.

139. Rabinovitch, A. 1998. An update on cytokines in the pathogenesis of insulin-dependent diabetes mellitus. Diabetes Metab Rev 14:129.

140. Ashkenazi, A., and V. M. Dixit. 1999. Apoptosis control by death and decoy receptors. Curr Opin Cell Biol 11:255.

141. Aravind, L., V. M. Dixit, and E. V. Koonin. 1999. The domains of death: evolution of the apoptosis machinery. Trends Biochem Sci 24:47.

142. Chinnaiyan, A. M., C. G. Tepper, M. F. Seldin, K. O'Rourke, F. C. Kischkel, S. Hellbardt, P. H. Krammer, M. E. Peter, and V. M. Dixit. 1996. FADD/MORT1 is a common mediator of CD95 (Fas/APO-1) and tumor necrosis factor receptor-induced apoptosis. J Biol Chem 271:4961.

143. Kawahara, A., T. Kobayashi, and S. Nagata. 1998. Inhibition of Fas-induced apoptosis by Bcl-2. Oncogene 17:2549.

144. Hu, S., C. Vincenz, J. Ni, R. Gentz, and V. M. Dixit. 1997. I-FLICE, a novel inhibitor of tumor necrosis factor receptor-1- and CD- 95-induced apoptosis. J Biol Chem 272:17255.

145. Thome, M., P. Schneider, K. Hofmann, H. Fickenscher, E. Meinl, F. Neipel, C. Mattmann, K. Burns, J. L. Bodmer, M. Schroter, C. Scaffidi, P. H. Krammer, M. E. Peter, and J. Tschopp. 1997. Viral FLICE-inhibitory proteins (FLIPs) prevent apoptosis induced by death receptors. Nature 386:517.

146. Irmler, M., M. Thome, M. Hahne, P. Schneider, K. Hofmann, V. Steiner, J. L. Bodmer, M. Schroter, K. Burns, C. Mattmann, D. Rimoldi, L. E. French, and J. Tschopp. 1997. Inhibition of death receptor signals by cellular FLIP. Nature 388: 190.

147. Grey, S. T., M. B. Arvelo, W. Hasenkamp, F. H. Bach, and C. Ferran. 1999. A20 inhibits cytokine-induced apoptosis and nuclear factor kappaB- dependent gene activation in islets. J Exp Med 190:1135.

148. Grey, S. T., M. B. Arvelo, W. M. Hasenkamp, F. H. Bach, and C. Ferran. 1999. Adenovirus-mediated gene transfer of the anti-apoptotic protein A20 in rodent islets inhibits IL-1 beta-induced NO release. Transplant Proc 31:789.

149. Benhamou, P. Y., C. Moriscot, M. J. Richard, J. Kerr-Conte, F. Pattou, J. Chroboczek, P. Lemarchand, and S. Halimi. 1998. Adenoviral-mediated catalase gene transfer protects porcine and human islets in vitro against oxidative stress. Transplant Proc 30:459.

150. Hotta, M., F. Tashiro, H. Ikegami, H. Niwa, T. Ogihara, J. Yodoi, and J. Miyazaki. 1998. Pancreatic beta cell-specific expression of thioredoxin, an antioxidative and antiapoptotic protein, prevents autoimmune and streptozotocin-induced diabetes. J Exp Med 188:1445.

151. Hohmeier, H. E., A. Thigpen, V. V. Tran, R. Davis, and C. B. Newgard. 1998. Stable expression of manganese superoxide dismutase (MnSOD) in insulinoma cells prevents IL-1beta- induced cytotoxicity and reduces nitric oxide production. J Clin Invest 101:1811.

152. Nagata, S., and P. Golstein. 1995. The Fas death factor. Science 267:1449.

153. Nagata, S. 1996. Apoptosis mediated by the Fas system. Prog Mol Subcell Biol 16: 87.

154. Stuart, P. M., T. S. Griffith, N. Usui, J. Pepose, X. Yu, and T. A. Ferguson. 1997. CD95 ligand (FasL)-induced apoptosis is necessary for corneal allograft survival. J Clin Invest 99:396.

155. Lau, H. T., M. Yu, A. Fontana, and C. J. Stoeckert, Jr. 1996. Prevention of islet

allograft rejection with engineered myoblasts expressing FasL in mice [see comments]. Science 273:109.

156. Kang, S. M., D. B. Schneider, Z. Lin, D. Hanahan, D. A. Dichek, P. G. Stock, and S. Baekkeskov. 1997. Fas ligand expression in islets of Langerhans does not confer immune privilege and instead targets them for rapid destruction. Nat Med 3: 738.

157. Miwa, K., M. Asano, R. Horai, Y. Iwakura, S. Nagata, and T. Suda. 1998. Caspase 1-independent IL-1beta release and inflammation induced by the apoptosis inducer Fas ligand. Nat Med 4:1287.

158. Suda, T., H. Hashimoto, M. Tanaka, T. Ochi, and S. Nagata. 1997. Membrane Fas ligand kills human peripheral blood T lymphocytes, and soluble Fas ligand blocks the killing. J Exp Med 186:2045.

159. Degli-Esposti, M. 1999. To die or not to die--the quest of the TRAIL receptors. J Leukoc Biol 65:535.

160. Phillips, T. A., J. Ni, G. Pan, S. M. Ruben, Y. F. Wei, J. L. Pace, and J. S. Hunt. 1999. TRAIL (Apo-2L) and TRAIL receptors in human placentas: implications for immune privilege. J Immunol 162:6053.

161. French, L. E., and J. Tschopp. 1999. The TRAIL to selective tumor death. Nat Med 5:146.

162. Mariani, S. M., and P. H. Krammer. 1998. Surface expression of TRAIL/Apo-2 ligand in activated mouse T and B cells. Eur J Immunol 28:1492.

163. Golstein, P. 1997. Cell death: TRAIL and its receptors. Curr Biol 7:R750.

164. Posselt, A. M., C. F. Barker, J. E. Tomaszewski, J. F. Markmann, M. A. Choti, and A. Naji. 1990. Induction of donor-specific unresponsiveness by intrathymic islet transplantation. Science 249:1293.

165. Posselt, A. M., A. Naji, J. H. Roark, J. F. Markmann, and C. F. Barker. 1991. Intrathymic islet transplantation in the spontaneously diabetic BB rat. Ann Surg 214: 363.

166. Posselt, A. M., J. S. Odorico, C. F. Barker, and A. Naji. 1992. Promotion of pancreatic islet allograft survival by intrathymic transplantation of bone marrow. Diabetes 41:771.

167. Singer, S. M., R. Tisch, X. D. Yang, H. K. Sytwu, R. Liblau, and H. O. McDevitt. 1998. Prevention of diabetes in NOD mice by a mutated I-Ab transgene. Diabetes 47:1570.

168. Cetkovic-Cvrlje, M., I. C. Gerling, A. Muir, M. A. Atkinson, J. F. Elliot, and E. H. Leiter. 1997. Retardation or acceleration of diabetes in NOD/Lt mice mediated by intrathymic administration of candidate beta-cell antigens. Diabetes 46:1975.

169. Steptoe, R. J., and A. W. Thomson. 1996. Dendritic cells and tolerance induction. Clin Exp Immunol 105:397.

170. Lu, L., S. Khoury, M. Sayegh, and A. W. Thomson. 1998. Dendritic cell tolerogenicity and prospects for therapy of allograft rejection and autoimmune disease. In Dendritic cells: Biology and Clinical Applications. M. T. Lotze, and A. W. Thomson, eds. Academic Press, San Diego, p. 487-511.

171. Takayama, T., Y. Nishioka, L. Lu, M. T. Lotze, H. Tahara, and A. W. Thomson. 1998. Retroviral delivery of viral interleukin-10 into myeloid dendritic cells markedly inhibits their allostimulatory activity and promotes the induction of T-cell hyporesponsiveness. Transplantation 66:1567.

172. Lu, L., A. Gambotto, W. C. Lee, S. Qian, C.A. Bonham, P.D. Robbins, and A.W. Thomson (1999). Adenoviral delivery of CTLA4-Ig into myeloid dendritic cells promotes their in vitro tolerogenicity and survival in allogeneic recipients. Gene Therapy 6:554.

173. Zlotnik, A., J. Morales, and J. A. Hedrick. 1999. Recent advances in chemokines and chemokine receptors. Crit Rev Immunol 19:1.

174. Mantovani, A. 1999. Chemokines. Introduction and overview. Chem Immunol

72:1.

175. Hedrick, J. A., and A. Zlotnik. 1999. Chemokines and chemokine receptors in T-cell development. Chem Immunol 72:57.

176. Howard, O. M., J. J. Oppenheim, and J. M. Wang. 1999. Chemokines as molecular targets for therapeutic intervention. J Clin Immunol 19:280.

177. Maghazachi, A. A. 1999. Intracellular signalling pathways induced by chemokines in natural killer cells. Cell Signal 11:385.

178. Bradley, L. M., V. C. Asensio, L. K. Schioetz, J. Harbertson, T. Krahl, G. Patstone, N. Woolf, I. L. Campbell, and N. Sarvetnick. 1999. Islet-specific Th1, but not Th2, cells secrete multiple chemokines and promote rapid induction of autoimmune diabetes. J Immunol 162:2511.

179. Grewal, I. S., B. J. Rutledge, J. A. Fiorillo, L. Gu, R. P. Gladue, R. A. Flavell, and B. J. Rollins. 1997. Transgenic monocyte chemoattractant protein-1 (MCP-1) in pancreatic islets produces monocyte-rich insulitis without diabetes: abrogation by a second transgene expressing systemic MCP-1. J Immunol 159:401.

180. Gale, L. M., and S. R. McColl. 1999. Chemokines: extracellular messengers for all occasions? Bioessays 21:17.

181. Dairaghi, D. J., R. A. Fan, B. E. McMaster, M. R. Hanley, and T. J. Schall. 1999. HHV8-encoded vMIP-I selectively engages chemokine receptor CCR8. Agonist and antagonist profiles of viral chemokines. J Biol Chem 274:21569.

182. Pazmany, L., O. Mandelboim, M. Vales-Gomez, D. M. Davis, H. T. Reyburn, and J. L. Strominger. 1996. Protection from natural killer cell-mediated lysis by HLA-G expression on target cells. Science 274:792.

183. Kumagai-Braesch, M., M. Satake, Y. Qian, J. Holgersson, and E. Moller. 1998. Human NK cell and ADCC reactivity against xenogeneic porcine target cells including fetal porcine islet cells. Xenotransplantation 5:132.

184. Karlsson-Parra, A., A. Ridderstad, A. C. Wallgren, E. Moller, H. G. Ljunggren, and O. Korsgren. 1996. Xenograft rejection of porcine islet-like cell clusters in normal and natural killer cell-depleted mice. Transplantation 61:1313.

185. Markmann, J. F., A. M. Posselt, H. Bassiri, K. L. Brayman, M. Woehrle, W. F. Hickey, W. K. Silvers, C. F. Barker, and A. Naji. 1991. Major-histocompatibility-complex restricted and nonrestricted autoimmune effector mechanisms in BB rats. Transplantation 52:662.

186. Nakamura, N., B. A. Woda, A. Tafuri, D. L. Greiner, C. W. Reynolds, J. Ortaldo, W. Chick, E. S. Handler, J. P. Mordes, and A. A. Rossini. 1990. Intrinsic cytotoxicity of natural killer cells to pancreatic islets in vitro. Diabetes 39:836.

187. Munn, D. H., M. Zhou, J. T. Attwood, I. Bondarev, S. J. Conway, B. Marshall, C. Brown, and A. L. Mellor. 1998. Prevention of allogeneic fetal rejection by tryptophan catabolism. Science 281:1191.

188. Munn, D. H., E. Shafizadeh, J. T. Attwood, I. Bondarev, A. Pashine, and A. L. Mellor. 1999. Inhibition of T cell proliferation by macrophage tryptophan catabolism. J Exp Med 189:1363.

11 LOCAL IMMUNOSUPPRESSION: THE EYE

J. Wayne Streilein[1,2] and Andrew W. Taylor[1]

[1] Department of Ophthalmology
[2] Department of Dermatology
The Schepens Eye Research Institute and Harvard Medical School
Boston, Massachusetts, USA

Certain organs and tissues of the body inherently possess the capacity to regulate local immune responses. The term Regional Immunity [1] embraces the concept that each tissue and organ benefits from immune protection, but since immune responses often carry the risk of damaging normal tissues, the type of immune response that is permitted locally is highly regulated. Perhaps the most extreme example of regional immunity is immune privilege. Especially for the eye, immune privilege – as it is studied experimentally – has served to illuminate regulation of immunity within the organ of sight. In many ways this is the most closely studied example of tissue-specific local immunosuppression as a normal physiologic mechanism.

IMMUNE PRIVILEGE IN THE EYE

Definition and Description

During the 1940s, Sir Peter Medawar deduced the principles of transplantation immunology, thereby explaining why grafts of solid tissues from one individual of a species are not accepted by other members, unless donor and recipient are genetically identical [2]. In the course of Medawar's experiments, he placed skin allografts at various body sites, including the eye and the brain. He observed that the rules of transplantation were relaxed, or perhaps even abolished, at these distinctive sites [3]. Whereas skin allografts placed on the body wall were rejected uniformly and acutely, simi-

A. W. Thomson (ed.), Therapeutic Immunosuppression, 275–321.

lar allografts placed in the anterior chamber of the eye (as well as the brain) were often not rejected acutely, and in some instances were accepted indefinitely. Medawar coined the term "immune privilege" to identify this anomalous situation, and he proposed that immune privilege results from a type of immunologic ignorance. He based this proposal on knowledge available at the time, *i.e.* the eye and brain reside behind blood:tissue barriers (at the level of blood vessels), and neither eye nor brain has demonstrable lymphatic drainage pathways to regional lymph nodes. Consequently, Medawar proposed that the immune system remains unaware of the existence of grafts at privileged sites.

Medawar's description of immune privilege preceded his own discovery of immunologic tolerance and antedated the realization that immune responses are susceptible to regulation that can influence both their intensity and character. Fifty years later, we are the beneficiaries of an enormous body of research in immunology, including new information about immune privilege. On the one hand, the early ideas of absent lymphatics and rigid blood:tissue barriers have had to be modified in light of newer information, thereby rendering the immunologic ignorance notion less attractive as a unitary explanation for immune privilege. On the other hand, cells and molecules of the eye have been found to possess remarkable immunomodulatory properties which enable this organ to shape the qualities of systemic immune responses to antigens arising from the eye, and to regulate the expression of immunity directed at antigens within the eye.

Thus, local immunosuppression within the eye has two important dimensions: first, an efferent component in which factors within the eye act to suppress the expression of both innate and adaptive immunity. Second, an afferent component in which the ocular microenvironment shapes the systemic immune response to eye-derived antigens by influencing the functional properties of antigen presenting cells within the eye. Together, local immunosuppression of both the efferent and afferent limbs of the immune reflex arc serves to limit the intraocular expression of immunogenic inflammation. Many believe that the physiologic significance of ocular immune privilege derives from the vulnerability of the visual axis to uncontrolled and intense inflammation. When the eye is inflamed, vision is curtailed, and blindness ensues. Immune privilege acts to prevent that catastrophe.

Immune privilege and the cornea

Allogeneic corneas transplanted orthotopically into normal eyes enjoy considerable immune privilege, *i.e.* in experimental animals a high proportion of these grafts are never rejected despite the absence of immunosuppressive treatment [4-6]; in humans, modest topical immunosuppressive therapy is sufficient to secure the long-term survival of >90% of corneal transplants [7-9]. The cornea itself accounts in part for its success as an allograft. Corneal tissue, especially the stromal cells (fibroblasts) and corneal endothelium (a neuroectodermally-derived epithelium) display reduced MHC class I and no class II expression [10-12]. Corneal tissue is devoid of bone marrow derived cells [13], and lacks both blood vessels and lymphatics. Therefore, as a source of alloantigenic material, and as a target of immune attack, the cornea is deficient, and therefore less susceptible to rejection.

In addition, cells of the cornea, especially the endothelium, secrete immunosuppressive factors, including TGFβ and IL-10, that inhibit activation of T cells, alter antigen presenting cell functions, and suppress macrophage and neutrophil-mediated inflammation [14-17]. Corneal endothelial cells constitutively express three membrane bound inhibitors of complement (CD59, CD46, MCP) [18], as well as apoptosis-promoting CD95 ligand (CD95L)[19]. Formal evidence now implicates the expression of CD95L on corneal endothelium in the privilege that is extended to orthotopic and heterotopic corneal allografts [20-22]. Thus, the cornea is an excellent example of a tissue that possesses inherent immune privilege. Testis, placenta, liver, and certain tumors are additional examples [23]. In all of these instances, immune privileged tissues display attributes that enable them to suppress immunity at the local level.

Immune privilege and the anterior chamber

Another advantage that orthotopic corneal allografts have over other types of solid tissue allografts is that they are placed at the front of the anterior chamber (AC) of the eye. The anterior chamber has long been appreciated to be an immune privileged site [24,25]. Many experiments conducted over the past 25 years have not only re-affirmed the existence of immune privilege in this ocular site, but they have shed light on the responsible cellular and molecular mechanisms [6, 26-29]. Allogeneic tumor cells injected into the anterior chamber have proven to be a particularly convenient and successful approach to studying ocular immune privilege. Using this system, Niederkorn, Streilein and Shadduck [30,31] demonstrated that progressive growth of allogeneic tumor cells injected into the AC of mouse eyes was correlated with a deviant systemic immune response to tumor-derived alloantigens. In this response, delayed hypersensitivity (DH) to tumor alloantigens was impaired systemically, although the sera of mice bearing these tumors contained high levels of alloantigen-specific antibodies. Subsequently, Benson and Niederkorn [32], and Ksander and Streilein [33] demonstrated that the ability of intraocular tumor cells to grow exponentially (eventually killing their hosts) rests with the capacity of the ocular microenvironment to inhibit tumor-specific T cells from acting as effector cells, and from differentiating into immune effector cells *in situ*. More recently, the aqueous humor (AqH) itself has come under scrutiny, and it is now clear that soluble factors within this complex biologic fluid possess immunosuppressive and anti-inflammatory properties to effect local immunosuppression and to promote the induction of systemic deviant immune responses [26]. Thus, there are immune privileged sites (anterior chamber of eye) and immune privileged tissues (cornea) – both of which avoid immune destruction through local immunosuppression.

Local Suppression of adaptive immunity by soluble factors

Effect of aqueous humor on T cell-dependent immunogenic inflammation in vivo

Studies into the ability of the anterior chamber to display local DH reactions [34] have revealed that the ocular microenvironment possesses the inherent capacity to be immunosuppressive. This was demonstrated by Cousins and his colleagues who were unable to elicit DH responses within the AC even when appropriate effector T cells plus antigen and antigen presenting cells (APC) were injected into this ocular compartment. Moreover, DH effector T cells pre-treated with AqH, mixed with antigen and injected into the skin of naïve mice failed to evoke the expected delayed inflammatory response. This result implies that the ocular microenvironment (as represented by AqH) is capable of actively suppressing delayed hypersensitivity and the T cells that mediate it.

It is now known that AqH can affect all stages of DTH induction. The manner by which antigen presenting cells process and present antigen to naïve or previously primed T cells is clearly altered by AqH [35-37]. This effect of AqH on APC function accounts for the ability of the eye to promote systemic immune deviation in response to ocular antigens, a unique response that is discussed in detail below. Since indigenous APC are found between the layers of pigmented and non-pigmented epithelial cells of the ciliary body, as well as adjacent to neurons of the iris and ciliary body [38,39], these cells are in intimate contact with the cellular sources of immunosuppressive factors normally found in AqH. Consequently, ocular APC are always in an environment of immunosuppressive factors. AqH also neutralizes the responses of

Table 1
Ocular factors that regulate adaptive immune response

Adaptive Immune target	Ocular Factors
APC that activate DH T cells	α-MSH
IFN-γ production by T cells	TGF-β2, α-MSH, VIP
IFN-γ-mediated inflammation	α-MSH, CGRP, TGF-β2
T cells that convert to regulators	α-MSH, TGF-β2 Pigment epithelium of iris, ciliary body
C1q binding to IgG, IgM	Low mol.wt. factor of aqueous humor

ocular APC and macrophages to inflammatory mediators. AqH suppresses the ability of macrophages to generate nitric oxide when activated by IFN-γ, a lymphokine produced by DH T cell and NK cells [40]. Therefore, AqH suppresses effector functions of macrophages that might be activated by cytokines produced by adaptive immune cells that enter the eye (see Table 1).

Effects of aqueous humor on T cell activation in vitro

In the presence of AqH *in vivo*-primed T cells that are stimulated with antigen *in vitro* display markedly impaired proliferation [41,42]. However, if the *in vitro* assay is adapted to serum-free culture conditions, to mimic as closely as possible the conditions thought to be present within the normal ocular microenvironment, antigen-stimulated T cell proliferation is not suppressed. However, the consequences of T cell activation in this instance are changed; antigen-stimulated primed T cells exposed to antigen in the presence of AqH secrete reduced amounts of IFN-γ [43]. This result parallels the finding that primed T cells pretreated with AqH can *not* mediate DH in an adoptive transfer into skin [43]. Cultures of T cells and AqH in vitro that are carried out without serum insure that blood-borne proteins (especially proteases) and factors can not interact with and thereby neutralize immunosuppressive factors in AqH [44]. Therefore, the use of serum-free culture conditions allows for examination of the full range of AqH effects on T cells and other inflammatory cells such as macrophages. Identification of immunosuppressive factors in AqH has lead to understanding their role in the mechanisms of AqH suppression of DTH and to their role in ocular immune privilege.

Under serum-free culture conditions, primed T cells stimulated with antigen in the presence of AqH are not only impaired in IFN-γ production - a Th1 cytokine [43], but they are also unable to secrete IL-4 – a Th2 cytokine [45]. More important, when the T cells are harvested from AqH-containing cultures and re-stimulated with antigen *in the absence of AqH* they do not recover either IFN-γ or IL-4 production. Since the cells are capable of re-stimulation under these conditions, there is little to suggest that the reason that T cells fail to secrete IFN-γ and IL-4 in the presence of AqH is that the cells are undergoing apoptosis. Nor do the T cells treated with AqH differentiate into cells with a Th2 phenotype. Instead, the responding T cells in the presence of whole AqH produce TGF-β [45]. Thus, exposure of T cells to a Tcr ligand in the presence of AqH alters the functional program of the cells such that they secrete immunosuppressive cytokines (TGFβ) rather than the expected cytokines – IFN-γ or IL-4.

Aqueous humor promotes development of regulatory T cells

Another important feature of T cells activated in the presence of AqH is that they acquire regulatory properties. That is, if AqH-treated T cells are co-cultured with other T cells being activated via TCR ligation, the latter cells fail to secrete IFN-γ [45]. Much of this suppression is mediated by TGF-β produced by AqH-treated T cells. The induction of regulatory T cells by exposure to AqH indicates that T cells that enter the AC acquires properties that further contribute to the immunosuppressive nature of this ocular microenvironment. Thus, not only is the ocular microenvironment (AqH) directly suppressive to effector T cell activation, but T cells activated in this environment are recruited as regulators that enhance local suppression of immunogenic inflammation.

Local suppression of adaptive immunity by ocular parenchymal cells

AqH is produced by secretory epithelial cells of the ciliary body, and its composition is further influenced by molecules derived from the cornea, iris, lens, and even the vitreous body. Particularly, the epithelial cells of the ocular uveal tract (iris, ciliary body, retinal pigment epithelium and choriocapillaris) are strategically situated to influence adaptive immunity within the eye. Pigment epithelial cells of the iris and retina, and secretory epithelial cells of the iris form a physical barrier (via extensive intercellular tight junctions) through which leukocytes attempting to enter the eye must pass. Experiments initiated more than a decade ago have begun to explain the extent to which these cells, as well as other ocular parenchymal cells (pigment epithelium of ciliary body, corneal endothelium, lens epithelium) contribute to intraocular immunosuppression in addition to providing barrier function.

Suppression of T cell activation in vitro by explants of iris, ciliary body and cornea

Iris and ciliary body (I/CB) tissues and corneas have been removed from normal eyes of mice, rats and humans and cultured as explants [46]. These cultured tissues, or supernatants derived therefrom, have been tested for their capacity to alter lymphocyte activation in vitro. The most common type of experiment has been to conduct mixed lymphocyte reactions (T cells from mouse A stimulated with x-irradiated lymphoid cells from allodisparate mouse B) in cultures containing explanted tissues, or supernatants from I/CB tissues. Whether the explanted tissues or supernatants are of human origin or murine origin, activation of murine alloreactive T cells in these types of cultures is found to be suppressed [47]. Since supernatants proved capable of suppressing mixed lymphocyte reactions, soluble factors must be secreted from cultured explants of I/CB and from explants of cornea. Moreover, the finding that *human* ocular tissue explants, as well as their supernatants, suppress *murine* mixed lymphocyte reactions equally well indicates that no species restriction to the suppression exists. This result implies that soluble factors that are heavily conserved evolutionarily are at work. One such factor has turned out to be transforming growth factor-β[36] However, not all of the immunosuppressive activity observed in these cultures can be ascribed to TGF-β. The identity of other immunosuppressive factors remains to be determined.

Suppression of T cell activation in vitro by cultured pigment epithelial cells.

Yoshida and Streilein have recently cultured pigment epithelial (PE) cells from I/CB (to >95% purity) [48]. When naïve T cells are exposed to these cultured I/CB PE cells in the presence of a ligand for their T cell receptor for antigen, T lymphocyte proliferation was profoundly reduced. Failed proliferation was not the result of programmed cell death among the responding T cells; in fact, stimulation of T cells with anti-CD3 antibodies in the presence of I/CB PE cells actually spared the responder cells from apoptosis. Although supernatants of the cultured I/CB PE cells possessed little inhibitory activity, suppression of T cell activation was intense when contact between T cells and I/CB PE cells was permitted. Thus, I/CB PE cells suppress T cell activation by a mechanism that depends upon direct cell-to-cell contact. Attempts to identify the molecular ligands involved in this contact dependent process have so far been unsuccessful (see Table 1).

Similar studies have been conducted with retinal pigment epithelial (RPE) cells [49-51]. Since RPE cells constitutively express CD95L, the finding that T cell activation was impaired in the presence of RPE cells suggested that interactions between CD95L and CD95 on T cells was involved. In support of this interpretation, T cells activated in the presence of RPE cells are triggered to undergo a high rate of apoptosis. Moreover, this process is dependent upon the integrity of both CD95L and CD95. However, the proximate cause of apoptosis among responding T cells is not CD95 itself, since blocking the CD95 pathway to programmed cell death does not inhibit apoptosis. Instead, interactions between T cells and RPE cells via CD95L cause the latter cells to secrete a soluble molecule (as yet undefined) that is the agent responsible for inducing apoptosis among T cells. Thus, PE cells along the entire uveal tract inhibit T cell activation, a conclusion that suggests that the PE layer of the uvea plays a major role in local immunosuppression.

Induction of regulatory T cells

T cells that encounter PE cells are not merely inhibited from undergoing proliferation. Recent studies have indicated that T cells that are exposed to I/CB PE cells acquire novel regulatory properties, not unlike those displayed by T cells that are treated with AqH (Yoshida and Streilein, Manuscript in preparation). T cells that contact cultured I/CB PE cells display markedly enhanced ability to secrete both latent and active TGFβ. Moreover, their secretion of this immunosuppressive cytokine can have a dramatic influence on bystander T cells in their environment. For example, when T cells exposed to I/CB PE cells are added to cultures containing naïve T cells and anti CD3 antibodies, the latter cells fail to proliferate. Moreover, compared to control T cells, bystander T cells cultured with I/CB PE-exposed T cells secrete reduced amounts of IL-2 and IFN-γ, but enhanced amounts of IL-4 and IL-10. These findings suggest that regulatory T cells generated by exposure to I/CB PE cells bias bystander T cells away from the Th1 phenotype. This suggestion is strengthened by the observations that T cells exposed to I/CB PE cells down-regulate the expression of DH in vivo by adoptively transferred effector T cells. Since delayed hypersensitivity is a prototypic Th1-type response, the evidence points strongly to the conclusion that I/CB PE cells coerce T cells that contact them into regulatory cells, and that these regulatory cells bias bystander T cell responses away from immunogenic inflammation - especially that mediated by Th1 cells.

In summary, the ocular microenvironment, by virtue of soluble factors secreted by, and cell surface molecules expressed on, parenchymal cells alters the circumstances surrounding activation of T cells via the Tcr. Not only are the responding T cells prevented from differentiating into effectors of immunogenic inflammation, but in some instances the responding T cells are converted into regulatory cells that bias bystander T cells toward functional phenotypes more compatible with the maintenance of vision – *i.e.* non inflammatory (see Table 1).

Local suppression of innate immunity by aqueous humor

The classic descriptions of immune privilege paid attention only to those responses generated by adaptive immune T and B lymphocytes. As the study of ocular immune privilege has advanced over the past decade it has become increasingly clear that the phenomenon also modifies the effectors of innate immunity. Perhaps this is not so surprising since, in general, innate immune responses carry a heavy burden of inflammation and tissue injury, and therefore represent significant threats to vision (see Table 2).

Suppression of NK cell activity

Niederkorn and his colleagues have conducted a series of elegant studies to examine the potential influence of the ocular microenvironment on NK cell function [52-53]. They have demonstrated that NK-sensitive tumor cells, that are rejected when injected subcutaneously into immune incompetent (SCID) mice, form progressively growing tumors in the AC of these same mice. This is an example of *innate immune privilege*. As this result predicts, AqH contains factors that inhibit NK cells from lysing susceptible target cells. To date, two factors have been implicated in this inhibition. For quite some time it has been known that NK cell killing can be inhibited by TGFβ, and there is evidence that the TGFβ normally present in AqH prevents NK cell

Table 2
Ocular factors that regulate innate immune response

Innate Immune target	Ocular Factors
Blood-borne molecules and cells	Blood:ocular barriers
NK cell-mediated lysis	TGF-β2, MIF Qa-2 expression
Neutrophil activation/toxicity	TGF-β2, α-MSH
NO production by activated macrophages	CGRP
Alternative complement pathway	Low & high mol.wt. factors Membrane expressed CD55, CD59, CD46

mediated lysis [52]. The lysis that is inhibited by TGFβ is the type detected in vitro in 18-24 hr NK cell lytic assays. However, there is a related NK cell killing mechanism that is maximally effective in 4 hr in vitro assays. This type of killing is impervious to TGFβ, but is inhibited by AqH. Apte and Nie-derkorn [54-56] have discovered that the factor in AqH that is responsible for NK cell killing at the 4 hr time point is macrophage migration inhibitory factor (MIF).

Since AqH contains at least two potent inhibitors of NK mediated lysis, the question arises as to the need for this inhibitory activity. Niederkorn et al have argued that the low expression of MHC class I molecules on ocular cells, especially corneal endothelium, renders these tissues vulnerable to inadvertent NK cell killing [54]. In support of this argument, these workers have demonstrated that transformed cell lines derived from corneal endothe-lium are susceptible to NK cell killing in vitro, and that this susceptibility is abolished in the presence of AqH.

Yet another strategy may exist in the eye to thwart NK cell killing. Nieder-korn and his collaborators have recently reported that ocular parenchymal cells, including corneal endothelium, constitutively express Qa-2, a non-clas-sical class I molecule (58). The possibility exists that Qa-2 expression on class I-deficient corneal endothelium serves as another mechanism to pre-vent NK cells from lysing this critical cell layer. Whether inhibition of NK cell killing by factors in AqH and molecules expressed on ocular cells is an impor-tant mechanism to protect the eye from other aspects of NK cell activity (*e.g.* secretion of IFN-γ) remains to be determined.

Inhibition of neutrophil migration and effector function

The dramatic discovery that CD95L is constitutively expressed on ocular cells [19], especially the corneal endothelium, provoked the interest of immu-nologists in the possibility that CD95L expression, by inducing deletion of CD95+ T cells, might contribute to the success of orthotopic corneal allografts. Similar expression of CD95L on testis allografts was found to promote the acceptance of these grafts beneath the kidney capsule (a conventional, non-immune privileged site) [58]. To the contrary, several laboratories have recently found that cells and tissues transfected with CD95L (in an effort to render them "immune privileged") are swiftly and irrevocably rejected [59,60]. Histology reveals massive accumulation of neutrophils at the site of rejection. Nabel and his colleagues seized on this observation [61]. They transfected tumor cells with CD95L, and then demonstrated that the trans-fected cells were rejected in vivo by a neutrophil-dependent process. More to the point, Nabel et al showed that CD95L-transfected tumor cells were killed by neutrophils in vitro, and that this killing was inhibited by AqH! Their evidence suggests that TGFβ in AqH is responsible for inhibition of neutrophil activation, and therefore for the sparing of tumor cells from lysis. These findings are similar to those reported recently by D'Orazio et al [62].

Very recently, Miyamoto et al [63, and manuscript submitted] have conducted similar experiments using corneal endothelium - which constitutively expresses CD95L. These investigators have shown that murine neutrophils exposed to corneal endothelium are activated via a CD95-dependent mechanism, and that the activated neutrophils release toxic products (nitric oxide, reactive oxygen intermediates) which prove lethal to the endothelium. Similar to the experiments of Nabel et al, AqH prevented neutrophil activation and rendered corneal endothelium less vulnerable to killing. Preliminary evidence suggests that this inhibitory activity within AqH can be ascribed to TGFβ and α-MSH (see Table 2).

Inhibition of complement activation

As early as the 1950s it was observed that AqH appeared to be anti-complementary [64]. Twenty years later, Shimada demonstrated that AqH is profoundly deficient in certain key components of the complement cascade, and that this ocular fluid is strongly inhibitory of complement activation through the classical pathway [65]. More recently, Goslings et al [66] have tried to identify the molecule(s) within AqH that might account for its inhibitory activity. These investigators found that AqH contains at least two types of molecules that inhibit complement. One is a very small molecular weight factor (<1,000 daltons) that is not a peptide and that acts on C1q to inhibit binding to the Fc region of immunoglobulin molecules. There is also evidence that this small molecule inhibits the alternative pathway. In addition, there are one or more large molecules (>30,000 daltons) that inhibit the deposition of C3 on membranes, thereby inhibiting both the alternative and classical pathways.

Ocular parenchymal cells, especially those that surround the AC and the retinal pigment epithelium, express three membrane bound inhibitors of complement activation- CD59, CD46, MCP [18]. To the present there is no compelling experimental evidence to link either the membrane bound or soluble complement inhibitors to a physiologic process in the eye, or to pathologic entities. To this point, Tanaka and Streilein have reported recently that guinea pig corneas grafted orthotopically to eyes of mice do not suffer hyperacute or any other type of antibody-mediated rejection – even though the sera of normal mice contain natural, complement- fixing anti-guinea pig anti-bodies [67]. It is possible that the anti-complement activity of AqH hobbles the deleterious consequences of guinea pig specific antibodies that bind to guinea pig cornea cells in the presence of AqH (see Table 2).

Promotion of systemic immune deviation

The previous section has focused on the ability of the ocular microenvironment to suppress both adaptive and innate immune *effector* responses. As mentioned above, immune privilege also alters the afferent limb of immunity during which antigens are first presented to naïve T and B cells. In general this type of alteration results in a deviant systemic immune response called anterior chamber associated immune deviation (ACAID).

Anterior chamber associated immune deviation

In the mid-1970s Kaplan and Streilein reported that injections of allogeneic lymphoid cells into the AC of rat eyes led to unusual systemic immune responses to alloantigens expressed on the injected cells [27,28]. On the one hand, the recipients developed high titers of allospecific antibodies. But on the other hand, the same recipients accepted orthotopic skin grafts syngeneic with the donor of the injected cells for prolonged (albeit not indefinite) intervals. Similar observations (already discussed above) were made by Niederkorn et al [30] in the early 1980s, using allogeneic tumor cells injected into the AC of mouse eyes. These workers reported that recipients of the tumor cells accepted donor-specific orthotopic skin grafts, and failed to acquire donor-specific DH. At the same time, the recipients developed donor-specific antibodies, and their lymphoid organs contained primed, donor-specific cytotoxic T cells. The term anterior chamber associated immune deviation (ACAID) was applied to this phenomenon [31]. It is worth pointing out that ACAID appears to be regulated in part by a unique set of suppressor T cells that emerge in the spleen [68]. One population of regulatory T cells is CD8+, and inhibits the expression of DH in an antigen specific manner. A second set of regulatory cells is CD4+ and inhibits the induction of immunity among naïve T cells. A third set of T suppressor cells promotes antigen-specific B cell differentiation away from antibodies that fix complement. In the aggregate, these regulatory cells prevent the systemic expression of immunogenic inflammation triggered by delayed hypersensitivity (Th1) cells and complement-fixing antibodies [69].

ACAID has proven to be a universal pattern of immune responses to antigens injected into the AC. Antigens tested to date include minor and major histocompatibility determinants, tumor antigens, viral-encoded antigens, haptens, soluble protein antigens, and certain bacterial antigens. That the eye is central to ACAID induction was revealed by enucleating the eye after injection. Removal of the eye immediately after, or as late as 4 days after injection, curtails the development of ACAID. Considerable effort has been made to understand the cellular and molecular basis for ACAID induction (see below) since the phenomenon has been demonstrated not only in the eyes of rodents and rabbits, but also in primates [70].

Immune deviation from vitreous cavity and subretinal space

The vitreous cavity and the subretinal space resemble the AC in that they lack lymphatic drainage pathways, and are protected from hematogenous cells and molecules by blood:ocular barriers. These intraocular compartments have also proved to be suitable sites for induction of ACAID [71-73]. That is, injection of allogeneic cells (tumor, retinal) into the vitreous cavity or the subretinal space results in acceptance of these grafts, and the emergence of donor-specific immune deviation. Many of the immune features of ACAID are present in animals that receive antigens in the vitreous cavity or the subretinal space, implying that similar mechanisms are involved. There are similarities between AC, vitreous cavity and subretinal space. The vitreous gel is believed to be "immunosuppressive" (similar to AqH), but to date no one has examined the matrix within the subretinal space in this regard.

Immune deviation from brain and other privileged sites

Since the brain is also an immune privileged site, and in certain ways, resembles the eye, it is probably no surprise that antigens injected into the brain also induce systemic immune deviation. Gordon et al [74] injected allogeneic tumor cells into mouse brains and demonstrated a spectrum of immune effectors in the subsequent response that was similar to ACAID. Harling-Berg et al [75] injected myelin basic protein into brains of susceptible rats and found that the rats were protected subsequently from experimental allergic encephalomyelitis, a Th1-type inflammatory disease. Very recently, Wenkel, Streilein and Young (manuscript submitted) have carefully injected soluble antigen (ovalbumin) into the striatum of mouse brains. OVA-specific immune deviation was observed. However, unlike recipients of antigen into the eye, recipients of OVA via the brain developed immune deviation even if their spleen was removed prior to injection. Moreover, unlike the spleens of mice with ACAID, spleens of mice with brain-associated immune deviation (BRAID) contained no regulatory T cells. To the contrary, regulatory cells of this type were found in cervical lymph nodes. These interesting differences between immune deviation of the eye and brain derive in part from differences in the vascular lymphatic drainage pathways available to the two organs. Whereas the AC possesses virtually no lymphatic drainage pathway, the brain enjoys a relatively robust pathway that carries lymph along the olfactory nerves, through the cribriform plate into the submucosa of the nose [76]. As a consequence the cervical lymph nodes represent the secondary lymphoid organs that first receive antigenic signals derived from an injection into the brain. For the AC, antigenic signals can only leave through the trabecular meshwork (the route of resorption of AqH), directly into the venous circulation. As a consequence the spleen serves as the eye's secondary lymphoid organ of choice [77].

Studies to determine whether immune deviation follows introduction of antigenic material into other privileged sites are either rudimentary or non-existent. Shichi et al reported that antigens injected into the testis induced systemic unresponsiveness similar to ACAID [78]. It has been shown by Wilbanks and Streilein that extracellular fluid collections from the eye (AqH), the brain (cerebrospinal fluid) and amniotic cavity (amniotic fluid) contain large amounts of TGFβ and perhaps other similar immunosuppressive factors [35]. Moreover, all three fluids confer ACAID-inducing properties on conventional APCs in vitro (See below).

Local factors that promote immune deviation

The cellular basis for ACAID induction was largely worked out in a series of experiments reported by Wilbanks et al in the early 1990s [36,79,80]. These investigators found that within 24-48 hours of injection of soluble antigen in the AC, a cell-associated signal was found in the blood that induces antigen-specific ACAID when injected intravenously into naïve recipients. The signal proved to be carried by F4/80+ monocytes. Similar F4/80+ cells normally reside (as dendritic cells and macrophages) in the stroma of the I/CB [39], and Wilbanks et al demonstrated that F4/80-bearing cells, harvested within 24 hr from eyes into which antigen had been injected, induced ACAID when injected intravenously into naïve recipients. The implications of these studies are that antigens placed in the AC are captured by resident APC which then migrate across the trabecular meshwork into the blood. Since the spleen is the suspected secondary lymphoid organ of the eye, it is no surprise that cells of this type migrate preferentially to the spleen.

Wilbanks et al materially advanced this line of investigation by demonstrating that conventional APCs (peritoneal exudate cells, peripheral blood monocytes, splenic adherent cells) acquired ACAID-inducing properties if incubated with AqH for 6 or more hours in vitro [36]. When APCs were exposed to AqH and pulsed with an antigen in vitro, they induced immune deviation when injected into naïve recipients. The active factor in AqH appears to be TGF-β2 since identical effects are achieved if this cytokine is substituted for AqH in the in vitro incubation.

Much has been learned recently about the mechanism by which TGF-β2 confers ACAID-inducing properties on APCs [81,82]. First, APCs incubated overnight with TGF-β2 secrete enhanced amounts of active TGF-β. Even though these cells up-regulate B71, B72, ICAM-1 and class II MHC molecules, similar to untreated control APCs, APCs exposed to TGF-β2 secrete significantly less IL-12 and express markedly lower levels of CD40. These co-stimulation deficiencies are relevant because when TGF-β2-treated APCs are pulsed with ovalbumin and used to stimulate OVA-specific Tcr transgenic T cells, the responding cells proliferate, and secrete IL-4, but little or no IFN-γ. Similar deviant T cell responses can be evoked if untreated, OVA-pulsed APCs are used to stimulate OVA-specific T cells in the presence of either anti-IL-12 or anti-CD40 antibodies. Moreover, if IL-12 is added exogenously to cultures containing OVA-pulsed, TGF-β2-treated APCs plus OVA-specific T cells, the latter cells proliferate and differentiate into typical Th1 cells.

The relevance to ACAID of the deviant behavior of T cells stimulated with TGF-β2-treated APCs stems from the functional properties that have been described for the responding T cells. Kezuka and Streilein (manuscript under review) have reported that OVA-specific T cells stimulated in vitro with OVA-pulsed, TGF-β2-treated APCs secrete abundant TGF-β. When these cells are used as regulators in co-cultures containing OVA-pulsed, conventional APCs plus naïve OVA-specific Tcr transgenic T cells or T cells primed to OVA in vivo, the responder T cells fail to proliferate. Moreover, in vitro generated OVA-specific regulator cells inhibit expression of DH in vivo, and they alter the initial activation of Tcr transgenic T cells stimulated with OVA such that the responding T cells secrete Th2, rather than Th1, cytokines. Thus, the T cells activated in vitro by TGF-β2-treated APC acquire functional properties strikingly similar to those displayed by afferent and efferent suppressor T cells found in the spleens of mice with ACAID. While studies of this type remain incomplete, the evidence to date strongly suggests that TGF-β2, a normal constituent of the ocular microenvironment, acts on resident APCs in a manner that forces them to activate T cells in a deviant manner, the result of which is ACAID.

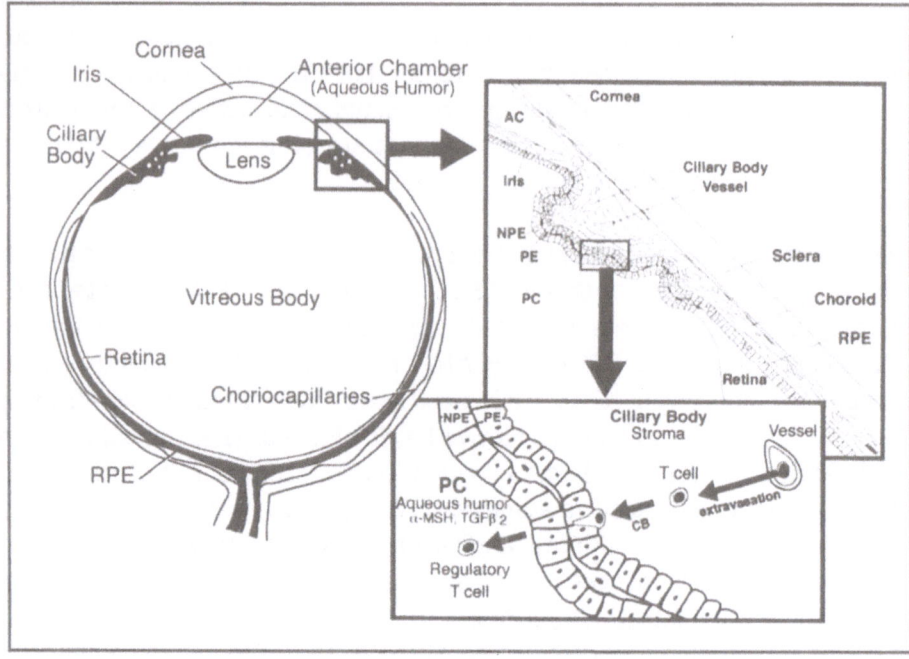

Figure 1
Passive and active mechanisms of ocular immune privilege. AC-anterior chamber,
PE-pigment epithelium, NPE-non-pigmented epithelium, PC - posterior chamber, RPE
- retinal pigment epithelium, CB - ciliary body.

MECHANISMS OF OCULAR IMMUNOSUPPRESSION

The previous section has demonstrated and described the extent to which
the eye, especially the AC, is an immunosuppressive local microenvironment. The creation and maintenance of this site with this functional property is multifactorial in origin. Whereas active mechanisms through secreted
soluble factors and cell surface expressed ligands confer immunosuppression, passive mechanisms which shield the eye from the vicissitudes of the
systemic circulation act to maintain the local state. These forces will be
described separately, but the existence of immune privilege can be neither
created nor maintained by the sole participation of only one, or even merely
a few, factors (see Figure 1).

Passive mechanisms

Anatomical factors that promote local immunosuppression

In the eye, several features of the ocular microanatomy promote the existence of local immunosuppression in a passive manner. First, the ocular compartments (anterior chamber, vitreous cavity, subretinal space) reside behind stringent blood:tissue barriers. The vessels of the iris and of the retina are lined with endothelial cells that maintain extensive tight junctions, similar to microvessels in the brain. In addition, extensive tight junctions connect the epithelial cells lining the posterior surface of the iris, the ciliary body, and the retinal pigment epithelium. Thus, blood-borne cells and molecules gain access into the eye only to the extent that these blood:tissue barriers are permissive. Under normal circumstances the barrier is extremely strict, and so long as it holds, the unique immunosuppressive ocular microenvironment is maintained.

Similar to other tissues, ocular parenchymal cells produce tissue fluids that are turned over each day. The AqH that fills the AC is secreted in large quantities each day and must be resorbed in order to keep the intraocular volume constant. Unlike most other tissues, extracellular fluids of the eye do not normally drain via lymphatics to regional lymph nodes. Instead, ocular fluids collect in the AC and pass through the trabecular meshwork (a baffle of collagen beams covered with neural crest derived epithelium) into the Canal of Schlemm. The Canal is actually a large circumferential vein that drains directly into the veins of the head and neck. Therefore, ocular fluids (and any antigenic material they might contain) are delivered directly into the blood stream. As mentioned previously, this anatomical route proves essential for ocular immune privilege since the eye-derived antigenic signals that induce ACAID pass via the blood directly to the spleen. Thus, immune privilege in the eye depends in part on a unique microanatomic feature which permits ocular fluids to drain into the blood rather than the lymphatics. In fact, if lymphatic drainage from the eye is promoted (as can be accomplished with $PGF_2\alpha$, a prostaglandin that opens the so-called uveoscleral pathway), antigens injected into the AC fail to induce ACAID [70].

Cellular factors that promote local immunosuppression

Immune responses to antigens in peripheral tissues are typically initiated by indigenous antigen presenting cells (typically dendritic cells) that capture and process antigenic material, migrate to parafollicular regions of draining lymph nodes, and up-regulate their co-stimulatory molecules that promote activation of naïve T cells. The eye modifies this paradigm in two distinct ways in order to maintain local immune suppression and privilege. In the first, bone marrow-derived cells (Langerhans cells) are virtually excluded from the cornea [13], and class II-bearing cells are equally rare in the stroma. Thus, in this simple tissue, immunity to cornea-derived antigens is thwarted by the absence of relevant APCs to initiate the afferent limb.

In the second, bone marrow-derived cells are present, but display a deviant functional phenotype. Anatomically, class II+ dendritic cells are deployed in close association with the epithelial layers of the I/CB [39]. Dendritic cells and macrophages are also present in the stromae of the I/CB, the space between the RPE and choriocapillaris, and (as microglia) within the neural retina. When harvested directly from ocular tissues, the class II+ cells of I/CB lack the capacity to activate alloreactive T cells – implying that their constitutive phenotype is deficient in the capacity to activate T cells [46]. Class II+ cells of I/CB can be encouraged to assume potent antigen presenting and co-stimulatory properties if cultured with GM-CSF in vitro for several days, indicating that the cells retain the potential to function as professional APC [83]. Wilbanks et al have demonstrated that bone marrow-derived cells harvested from I/CB of mouse eyes promote ACAID when pulsed with antigen in vitro and injected into naïve mice [80]. Our view is that the capacity of these cells to promote ACAID represents their physiologic phenotype, and that the microenvironment of the eye confers this capacity upon the cells by virtue of its content of immunosuppressive factors. Microglia have also been studied recently, and evidence indicates that although they are able to activate allo-specific T cells in vitro, the responding T cells secrete Th2, rather than Th1, type cytokines [84,85]. It would appear that the eye has developed more than one strategy to direct systemic immune responses to eye-derived antigens, ranging from absence of APCs (cornea), to promotion of ACAID (I/CB) and activation of Th2-type T cells (microglia).

Active Mechanisms

Soluble immunosuppressive factors in aqueous humor

The factors within normal AqH that confer upon this fluid its immunosuppressive properties have been identified (a) by their physical presence in normal AqH, (b) by the similarities of their activities with the *in vitro* immunosuppressive activity of whole AqH, and (c) by the ability of specific antibodies to neutralize the immunosuppressive activity of the factors in AqH. With these approaches, a large number of immunosuppressive have now

Table 3 Immunoregulatory factors in aqueous humor	
transforming growth factor-beta 2	alpha-melanocyte stimulating hormone
vasoactive intestinal peptide	calcitonin gene-related peptide
somatostatin	free cortisol
macrophage migration inhibitory factor	interleukin-1 receptor antagonist
inhibitors of C1q binding to Ig	inhibitors of C3b binding to cell surfaces

been identified. The following discussion will focus on five key factors which we believe to be particularly important in the ability of AqH to suppress T cells, NK cells, and macrophage effector functions: TGF-β2, alpha-melano-cyte stimulating hormone (α-MSH), vasoactive intestinal peptide (VIP), cal-citonin-gene-related peptide (CGRP), and macrophage migration inhibitory factor (MIF) [86-90]. Additional factors with the potential to be immunosup-pressive or immunomodulatory are known to be in the eye, but their precise activities in AqH remain unclear: somatostatin, substance P, and corticoste-roids [91,92]. In addition to these immunosuppressive cytokines, neuropep-tides, and hormones, there is a group of factors that suppress the classical and alternative pathways of complement (see Table 3)

• *Transforming Growth Factor-β2.* The growth factor TGF-β2 was the first immunosuppressive factor identified in normal AqH [87,88,93]. The three mammalian TGF-β isoforms are an evolutionarily conserved family of growth factors with immunoregulatory activity. They exist as a 200 kDa latent com-plex containing the 25 kDa active dimer that is released from its latency-asso-ciated protein by proteolysis [94-97]. Only the freed 25 kDa dimer (active TGF-β) can bind to the three types of TGF-β-receptors. In normal AqH the concentration of TGF-β is between 1-10 ng/ml, and the vast majority (<90%) of the TGF-β is latent [87,88,93]. Although only the TGF-β2 protein has been found in normal AqH, mRNAs for all three TGF-β isoforms are expressed by ocular cells [87,98,99]. The TGF-β2 isoform has also been identified as an important immunosuppressive factor in other immune privileged sites [35], and the same TGF-β2 immunosuppressive activity is observed in all samples of mammalian AqH yet studied (human, bovine, mice, pig, rabbit [87,88,93].

When TGF-β2 in AqH is neutralized with antibodies before adding it to T cell cultures, there is significant recovery (80 - 90%) of antigen-stimulated T cell proliferation [87]. However, as mentioned above, under serum-free *in vitro* conditions AqH does not normally suppress antigen-stimulated T cell prolif-eration. Instead, AqH suppresses IFN-γ production. Neutralization of TGF-β2 under these conditions fails to restore IFN-γ secretion by T cells [43]. This shift in the spectrum of T cell activities suppressed by AqH supports the view that TGF-β2 is normally latent in this fluid, and that when serum proteins are present, the latent molecule is activated by serum proteases. Therefore, in the absence of serum factors the activation rate of TGF-β2 in AqH is very slow and may not mediate any direct suppression of T cell function [100,101]. Recently it has been found that TGF-β2 acts as a cofactor when AqH promotes the generation of regulatory T cells *in vitro* (See below) [102]. It is our view that the most important constitutive function of TGF-β2 in the eye is in the process by which indigenous APCs capture antigen and carry a signal to the spleen that induces ACAID. TGF-β2 influences the ability of APC to activate T cells in vitro, and this influence may take place within the eye as well [36]. TGF-β2-treated APC fail to activate Th1-type T cells, in part because the APC fail to secrete sufficient IL-12 or express enough CD40, and in part because they secrete their own TGFβ. Therefore, APC that establish themselves within the ocular microenvironment come under the influence of TGF-β2 and are unable to promote inflammatory activity among responding T cells.

APC, especially macrophages, can also serve as target cells of factors that mediate inflammation. TGF-β2-treated macrophages are unable to secrete inflammatory cytokines and their bacteriocidal and cytotoxic activities are impaired [103-105]. Therefore, TGF-β2 in the ocular microenvironment probably inhibits macrophages from playing their central role in inflammation. The collective effects of TGF-β2 on APC and T cells indicate that the ocular microenvironment through TGF-β2 can suppress each stage of a T cell mediated inflammatory response. However, TGF-β2 can not be the only immunosuppressive factor in AqH since its neutralization does not permit AqH to allow proliferation of thymocytes exposed to IL-1 [88]. Moreover, under serum-free conditions neutralization of TGF-β2 does not prevent AqH from suppressing IFN-γ production by antigen-stimulated T cells [43].

■ *Alpha-Melanocyte Stimulating Hormone (α-MSH)*. When AqH was fractionated by HPLC in an effort to define different molecular sizes of immunosuppressive factors, one fraction of >3.5 kDa suppressed both antigen-stimulated effector T cell proliferation and IL-1/TNF-induced thymocyte proliferation [87,88,106]. The low molecular size suggested the possibility that neuropeptides might contribute to AqH's immunosuppressive activity, and the first neuropeptide detected in AqH was α-MSH. α-MSH, a protein of thirteen amino acid (1.6 kDa), is encoded within the pro-opiomelanocortin (POMC) gene and is derived from the POMC molecule through two endoproteolytic cleavage steps - one that releases ACTH and a second that releases α-MSH from ACTH [107,108]. α-MSH was originally described for its melanin-inducing activity in amphibians, but it is now appreciated to have a fundamental role in modulating inflammatory responses in mammals [109,110]. Systemic (intravenous) and central (into the brain) injections of α-MSH suppress inflammation and fever induced by endotoxin, IL-1 and TNF [111-113]. α-MSH suppresses macrophage generation of reactive oxygen intermediates, nitric oxide, and inflammatory cytokines induced by LPS and IFN-γ [114-116]. In addition α-MSH enhances its own production and that of its receptor on macrophages, thereby promoting an autocrine suppression of macrophage inflammatory activities. Also, α-MSH suppresses the migration of macrophages and neutrophils [114,117]. Macrophages, keratinocytes, and centrally derived neurons are the typical sources of α-MSH, although other cells that can synthesize POMC and ACTH - such as T cells [116,118,119], may also contribute. Normal mammalian AqH contains on average 20 pM of α-MSH [89].

Primed T cells that are stimulated with antigen in the presence of α-MSH within its ocular concentration range are able to proliferate, but they fail to secrete IFN-γ [89]. Some of the IFN-γ activity released by antigen-stimulated primed T cells can be recovered if α-MSH activity in the low molecular weight fraction of AqH is neutralized [89]. This latter result suggests that other immunosuppressive factors are also present in the low molecular weight fraction. Neutralization of α-MSH in AqH relieves suppression of IFN-γ production by antigen-stimulated primed T cells [43]. Since α-MSH suppresses IFN-γ production by activated T cells while having no affect on proliferation, it appears to alter signaling within the T cell, and beyond the signal arising from the Tcr. T cells activated in the presence of α-MSH produce TGF-β1, but not IFN-γ, IL-4 or IL-10. Such T cells suppress IFN-γ-production by other inflammatory T cells, suggesting that α-MSH is able to confer regulatory properties on T cells activated in its presence [102]. Similarly, AqH confers regulatory properties on T cells, in part by inducing them to produce TGF-β [45,102]. These regulatory T cells suppress bystander T cells through antigen-specific stimulation, but the bystander T cells need not be responding to the same antigen. Only proximity of the regulators to the bystander T cells is required for suppression to take place. TGF-β2 acts as a cofactor in generating regulatory T cells in that it enhances the ability of α-MSH to induce these T cells [102]. These findings suggest that the ocular microenvironment permits the activation of primed T cells – but only those that further contribute to its immunosuppressive features. Intraocular generation of regulatory T cells carries with it the potential for seeding the periphery with regulatory T cells. Thus, it is possible that regulatory T cells that acquire this property within the eye can disseminate systemically and, in so doing, produce peripheral tolerance to the antigen in question. To the present, this is not a possibility that has been subjected to experimental inquiry.

• *Vasoactive Intestinal Peptide (VIP)*. Another immunosuppressive neuropeptide in the eye is VIP [120]. Its immunoreactivity is abundantly present in the nerves of the I/CB [121-127]. Normal rabbit AqH contains approximately 12 nM of immunoreactive VIP [127]. Whole synthetic VIP suppresses IFN-γ production by antigen-stimulated primed T cells [90]; however, unlike whole AqH, VIP at its normal concentration in AqH suppresses (50%) antigen-stimulated primed T cell proliferation [90]. Since it has been suggested that VIP may affect selected populations of T cells [128], AqH may select for activation a T cell sub-population that is nonresponsive to (not inhibitable by) VIP. It has also been reported that VIP regulates T cell expression of adherence molecules such as those needed for migration [128]. It is possible that the anti-proliferative effects observed in vitro with VIP alone may be due to suppression of adherence molecules needed for in vitro activation of inflammatory T cells. One might speculate that the role of VIP in the eye is to prevent not only the activation of inflammatory T cells but their migration through the ocular microenvironment. There is nothing known about the effects of VIP on antigen presentation even though VIP receptors have been found on monocytes [129,130]. It has been demonstrated that VIP suppresses respiratory bursts within inflammatory macrophages [131.132], and, therefore, VIP could suppress activation of inflammatory T cells and the response of macrophages to inflammatory factors in the eye.

• *Calcitonin Gene Related Peptide (CGRP)*. CGRP is present in AqH [133]. Although mature T cells are unresponsive to CGRP [134], this neuropeptide can influence the activity of APC and inflammatory macrophages [135,136]. Constitutive levels of CGRP in normal AqH are in the is 0.5 µM range [86], but in AqH from inflamed eyes, CGRP concentrations are 20-fold greater [137-139]. At its normal constitutive levels, but not at its inflammatory concentrations, CGRP suppresses nitric oxide generation by IFN-γ/LPS-activated macrophages [86]. The ability of normal AqH to suppress nitric oxide production by IFN-γ/LPS-induced macrophages is neutralized by anti-CGRP antibodies [86]. It is also known that CGRP suppresses IFN-γ-induced peroxide generation by macrophages (66). Therefore, under normal conditions in the ocular microenvironment CGRP, along with TGF-β2 and α-MSH, contributes to the suppression of inflammatory macrophages. CGRP also reduces the number of class II MHC-expressing APC, resulting in suppressed antigen presenting abilities of macrophages and dendritic cells [135,136,140,141].

• *Other Neuropeptides*. Two other immunomodulating neuropeptides, somatostatin (SOM), and substance-P (SP), are present in ocular tissue [142-144] and may regulate immune responses within the ocular microenvironment. SOM is considered to be immunosuppressive, while SP is considered to be pro-inflammatory [145]. SOM and mRNA for pro-SOM are found in the iris, ciliary body [144], and in the neural layers of the retina [144]. SOM resembles VIP in suppressing activated T-cell proliferation and IL-2 production [146]. Of the ocular neuropeptides, only SOM has actually been shown to be synthesized in the eye [144]. Preliminary examination of AqH has revealed SOM to be present, although its concentration is some how related to how long the eye is exposed to light. SOM concentration in rabbit AqH that had been kept in subdued light reached a maximal level within fifteen minutes after the donors were exposed to normal light, with SOM concentration falling to nominal levels thereafter (unpublished observations, A.W.Taylor).

In contrast to the other neuropeptides so far discussed, SP is pro-inflammatory. The cornea, I/CB, and the retina are immunoreactive for SP [142.143]. But SP is not found in normal AqH. In dark-adapted mice who are acutely exposed to light, significant amounts of SP appear in AqH [147]. The amount of SP in AqH is inversely proportional to the amount of VIP. When mice are readapted to diurnal light cycles, VIP levels returned to normal and SP concentrations declined. This study demonstrates that the eye selectively regulates the release of neuropeptides, and that changes in ocular neuronal activity could render the eye vulnerable to immunogenic inflammation because of changes in neuropeptide levels in the ocular microenvironment.

In addition to neuropeptides, glucocorticoids [corticosterone (1 - 3 ng/ml), hydrocortisone (10 - 20 ng/ml)] have also been found to be constitutively present in AqH from humans, rats and mice [148]. At these concentrations, corticosterone and hydrocortisone were found to suppress TNF-α induced thymocyte proliferation. Since cortisol binding globulin is absent from AqH, it has been suggested that glucocorticoids are more potent as immunosuppressants than in serum [148].

• *Macrophage Migration Inhibitory Factor (MIF).* Certain ocular cells, especially corneal endothelium, are deficient in expression of MHC class I molecules which, in principle, makes them potential targets of NK cell killing. It has recently been found that AqH suppresses NK cell cytotoxicity through its content of TGF-β2 and the cytokine, macrophage migration inhibitory factor (MIF) [55,57]. MIF is a 12 kDa glycoprotein that was originally described for its capacity to prevent macrophages from migrating away from an inflammatory immune site [149]. MIF mRNA is expressed in various cells within the eye and brain [150]. Neutralization of MIF activity in AqH prevents this fluid from suppressing NK cell killing in 4 hr in vitro assays; by contrast TGF-β2 suppresses NK cell killing that is evident at 18 – 24 hr incubation [55]. The presence of these inhibitors of NK cells in AqH is relevant, on the one hand, because (as mentioned above) corneal endothelium can be lysed by NK cells, and AqH prevents this from occurring. On the other hand, the presence of these inhibitors of NK cell activity makes it possible for NK-sensitive tumor cell lines to grow progressively in eyes of SCID mice, whereas such tumor cells are readily rejected when placed subcutaneously.

- *Interleukin-1 receptor antagonist (IL-1ra).* Corneal cells and RPE cells produce high levels of IL-1 receptor antagonist (IL-1ra), a unique member of the IL-1 gene family [151,152]. IL-1ra competes with IL-1α and β for IL-1 receptors, but unlike the other isoforms, IL-1ra does not induce signal transduction through the IL-1 receptor. IL-1 is central to the pathology of many inflammatory responses, promoting the activation and migration of leukocytes, monocytes, and T cells. IL-1 induces inflammatory cells to produce other pro-inflammatory cytokines, and it induces hepatocytes to produce acute phase reactants. IL-1 promotes expression of adherence molecules and matrix proteins, and it is responsible for the induction of fever. In response to infection, endotoxin, complement activation and clotting, IL-1 is secreted by a variety of cell types: activated lymphocytes, neutrophils and monocytes. IL-1 has been implicated in the pathology of corneal graft rejections, endotoxin-induced uveitis, and inflammation due to surgery. The constitutive production of IL-1ra by ocular cells means that the activity of IL-1α or β released in response to an inflammatory stimulus can be neutralized within the ocular microenvironment. As such, IL-1ra serves to abort the initial phases of inflammation within the eye.

- *Inhibitors of Complement.* Non-immune cell mediated inflammatory responses can be initiated by complement, and its by-products can mediate smooth muscle cell relaxation, chemotaxis and activation of neutrophils. Complement proteins deposited on cell surfaces promote phagocytosis and, if the cascade is allowed to continue to completion, cell lysis. Activation of the complement cascade occurs through binding to immunoglobulins (classical pathway), to permissive cell surfaces (alternative pathway) and to high mannose structures [153]. AqH suppresses activation of the classical pathway through a unique factor (<1.3 kDa) that prevents C1q binding to immunoglobulin, and through the presence of C1 inhibitor [66]. In addition, AqH contains inhibitors that suppress the complement pathway at the C3-applification level, thereby suppressing all three activation pathways. AqH also contains soluble decay accelerating factor (DAF, CD55), factors I and H [154-156]. In addition, membrane-bound complement inhibitors are differentially expressed by ocular parenchymal cells: DAF (CD55), homologous restriction factor (CD59) and membrane cofactor (CD46) [18,157,158]. In aggregate, virtually all facets of complement activation and function are curtailed in the eye.

Surface molecules expressed by ocular parenchymal cells

As described above, ocular parenchymal cells express a variety of surface molecules that influence cells of the lymphoreticular system. Some of these molecules have been identified, such as CD95L and the complement inhibitors. Others, such as the ligands expressed on PE cells of I/CB bind to lymphocyte surface molecules and convert the cells into regulatory cells; but the nature of these ligands is unknown. In general, the net effect of cell surface interactions between T lymphocytes and ocular parenchymal cells is to render the T cells non-inflammatory and suppressive. But this does not appear to be the rule for other types of leukocytes, especially since CD95L on corneal endothelium triggers neutrophil activation and subsequent death of corneal endothelium [62,63]. It is anticipated that this area of research will grow in importance in succeeding years, and that molecules expressed on ocular cells will be appreciated to play a major role in local immunosuppression and privilege.

IMPAIRED LOCAL IMMUNOSUPPRESSION IN THE EYE

The mechanisms of immunosuppression within the eye are very effective and most people will never suffer from ocular inflammation, the clinical term for which is uveitis. Moreover, due to immune privilege, corneal transplants are very successful. However, despite this favorable situation, uveitis does occur and some transplants are rejected. While the causes of uveitis and graft rejection are complex and not completely understood, defining the mechanisms responsible for ocular immunosuppression will lead to the development of therapies to re-impose immunosuppression within uveitic eyes and to prevent corneal graft rejection.

Clinical circumstances where ocular immunosuppression is apparently lost

Uveitis

A brief survey of clinical uveitis helps to place the results of experimental ocular inflammations in perspective. Uveitis is an inflammation of the uveal tract, i.e. the vascular tunic of the eye that contains the arteries, veins and capillaries of the organ [159]. When the uveal tract is inflamed, the disorder may involve the iris, ciliary body, pars plana, and choriocapillaris. When intense, uveitis extends to tissues not directly in contact with the vessels: the endothelial lining of the cornea, the anterior chamber, the lens, the vitreous (intermediate uveitis), the layers of neural retina and the retinal pigment epithelium. Clinicians recognize several forms of uveitis, depending upon which segment of the eye is inflamed. Thus, uveitis may be "anterior", involving the structures in the anterior segment of the eye (cornea, iris, ciliary body, anterior surface of lens), it may be "intermediate", involving the pars plana (posterior extension of the ciliary epithelium just anterior to the oro serrata) and the vitreous body, or it may be "posterior", involving the RPE and choriocapillaris. In some instances the inflammation may spread throughout the eye, yielding a pan-uveitis. Even the vessels of the neural retina may become involved in the inflammatory process. When prolonged and unrelenting, uveitis can lead to extensive ocular injury that is reversible, and associated with reduced vision during the acute phase of the disease. In severe cases, uveitis can lead to permanent loss of vision, through cataract formation, glaucomatous neuropathy, and retinal scars.

Infectious agents induce uveitis due to their ability to damage and infect ocular cells, and in so doing, trigger intraocular inflammation. Many ocular pathogens appear to take advantage of the immune privileged state of the eye [160-162]. The lack (due to local suppression) of immediate innate immune responses allows pathogens to reproduce and establish a foothold in ocular tissues. Moreover, the deficits of delayed hypersensitivity and complement fixing antibodies (immune deviation) that are characteristic of systemic immune responses to pathogens in the eye may rob the eye of critical pathogen-eliminating adaptive immune effector mechanisms.

It has been proposed that certain systemic autoimmune diseases render ocular tissues susceptible to attack by T cells specific for ocular antigens - a proposal that presupposes that affected eyes have lost their normal immunosuppressive microenvironment [163]. Autoimmune uveitis, of which sympathetic ophthalmia is a good example, is characterized by infiltration of lymphocytes into the I/CB and/or into the retina [164]. The sheer mass of this eye-directed immune response results in cellular necrosis, fibrosis, and even blindness. But not all non-infectious intraocular inflammation is thought to be autoimmune. In many instances, no clear etiology has been identified. As an example, Fuchs' heterochromic iridocyclitis is a chronic low-grade inflammation associated with depigmentation of the iris often leading to cataract formation or glaucoma. Regardless of the nature and cause of non-infectious uveitis, the treatment is limited to steroids and non-specific immunosuppressive therapies, which may suppress intraocular inflammation, but the toxicities include glaucoma, cataracts, and further vulnerability of the eye to complicating ocular disease.

Immunosuppressive microenvironment in eyes inflamed with uveitis

Sampling AqH to assess the immunosuppressive properties of the ocular microenvironment has received some experimental attention over the past few years. In general, AqH from human eyes with uveitis contains expected pro-inflammatory cytokines, such as IL-1, TNFα, IL-6, and has been reported to be depleted of transforming growth factor-beta. However, only within the last year has AqH from uveitic eyes been examined for its capacity in vitro to suppress T cell activation. Taylor et al [165] have found that, irrespective of type or cause of uveitis, AqH obtained from uveitic eyes retains its capacity to inhibit T cells stimulated with anti-CD3 antibodies - a finding that is distinctly unexpected. More interestingly, the reasons for T cell inhibition by AqH from uveitic eyes were not the same. In AqH samples with high protein content (indicating sustained breakdown of the blood:ocular barrier), inhibition of T cell activation was due to a high content of PGE_2. Samples in which PGE_2 was neutralized no longer prevented anti-CD3 from inducing T cell proliferation in vitro. In AqH samples with low protein content, the molecular basis of immune suppression is unclear – except that it is does not appear to be due to TGF-β. It is relevant to point out that AqH collected from eyes inflamed secondary to both infectious and presumed non-infections processes displayed similar degrees of inhibitory activity. Although these results must be viewed with caution, since they are preliminary, they suggest that even inflamed eyes act to impose an immunosuppressive microenvironment. Understanding the molecular means by which the eye restores suppression even in the face of inflammation will undoubtedly lead to new therapeutic approaches to intraocular inflammation.

Experimental models where ocular immunosuppression is lost

The ability of the eye to create and maintain local immunosuppression is not absolute. In clinical ophthalmology, numerous infectious, inflammatory and immunopathogenic diseases attack the cornea and the tissues of the intraocular compartments. These disorders represent the failure of the eye to maintain its privileged status. Experimental models have been created to mimic these diseases and, to a certain extent, these models serve to illuminate immunosuppressive mechanisms that maintain immunosuppression, or are generated during ocular inflammation as the eye's putative attempt to restore a non-inflamed condition. Three experimental examples are described as representative.

Experimental Autoimmune Uveitis (EAU)

EAU is induced by immunizing certain genetically susceptible strains of rats and mice with retinal autoantigens: arrestin (retinal S antigen), inter-photoreceptor retinoid binding protein (IRBP), rhodopsin [166,167]. During the course of this disease, the retina becomes infiltrated with immunopatho-genic T cells and inflammatory cells. Not surprisingly, as EAU begins to be expressed in the eye, AqH loses its immunosuppressive properties [168,169]. Loss of activity correlates with local production of large amounts of IL-6 by cells of the I/CB. If IL-6 activity is neutralized in AqH of this type, the fluid still displays profound immunosuppressive properties, and active TGF-β2 is primarily responsible for this inhibitory activity. As the experimental eye disease continues to mount in intensity, AqH re-acquires its immunosuppressive features, in part because IL-6 disappears. Of interest is the observation that high amounts of active TGF-β2 are responsible primarily for the suppression of T cell activation that is observed. Perhaps this helps to explain why these experimentally induced autoimmune diseases are self-limited. Typically, ocular inflammation arises within 2 weeks, then subsides within 4 – 5 weeks after immunization with retinal autoantigens. The important lesson from these studies is that the ocular microenvironment transiently – but only transiently – loses its capacity to suppress immunogenic inflammation in autoimmune eye disease. When immunosuppression is re-exerted by the eye, the molecular basis of suppression is different (active TGF-β2) from the normal ocular microenvironment (α-MSH, VIP, CGRP). Thus, the eye can use more than one molecular strategy to create and maintain local immunosuppression. The details of how these nested layers of immunosuppression are achieved are only now being elucidated.

Endotoxin–induced uveitis (EIU)

Endotoxin, the lipopolysaccharide derived from gram negative bacteria (LPS), is a potent inducer of inflammation in all tissues, including the eye [170]. Direct injection of LPS into the eyes of rodents and rabbits produces intense, destructive intraocular inflammation. In addition, injection of LPS into the footpads of genetically susceptible mice and rats also induces acute inflammation of the anterior uveal tract (iris, ciliary body, anterior chamber), and this inflammation bears certain similarities to acute anterior uveitis in humans. Several laboratories have described the histopathologic and clinical changes evoked in eyes of rodents that received footpad injections of LPS, a disease termed Endotoxin-Induced Uveitis (EIU). Our laboratory and those of Rosenbaum and others have attempted to define the changes in intraocular immunosuppression in this disease. In general, the blood:ocular barrier decompensates within a few hours of LPS injection, leading to leakage of plasma proteins and leukocytes into the eye. AqH removed at this time fails to suppress T cell activation in vitro, a failure that correlates with extremely high levels of IL-6 [169,170]. Comparably high levels of IL-6 mRNA in I/CB tissues from eyes with EIU suggest that IL-6 is being produced intraocularly. Neutralization of IL-6 in EIU AqH restores to the fluid its capacity to suppress T cell activation in vitro. Recent evidence suggests that large amounts of active TGFβ-2 are responsible for the restoration of T cell suppression by anti-IL-6 treated EIU AqH . While normal AqH contains TGFβ-2, virtually all of it is in the latent form; therefore, the normal ability of AqH to suppress T cell activation is due to other factors (α-MSH, VIP). In EIU, the appearance of large amounts of active TGFβ-2 probably reflects conversion of the latent form within the eye by proteases delivered from plasma via the breached blood aqueous barrier, and by proteases expressed on the surfaces of infiltrating leukocytes and perhaps even on ocular parenchymal cells. Even as the inflammation is progressing in EIU, AqH becomes immunosuppressive, largely by the elevated content of active TGFβ-2.

These findings make an important point about the eye and its need to have local immunosuppression. As stated previously, the normal eye creates and maintains an immunosuppressive microenvironment. When the eye is assaulted with an inflammatory insult, eye-derived forces are brought into play that act to restore immunosuppression, even using strategies not present in the normal state. In the case of EIU, the responsibility for suppression in AqH shifts from inhibitory neuropeptides to active TGF-β2. It has been proposed that this shift occurs because IL-6 acts on macrophages present in the inflamed eye, inducing these cells to express cell surface proteases that cleave latent TGF-β2 into its active form. Thus, by rapidly mobilizing IL-6, the eye converts infiltrating inflammatory macrophages into the instruments that restore local immunosuppression, and thereby thwart further inflammation.

Experimental manipulations of ocular tissues

Immune privilege of the cornea and the anterior chamber is abolished if the cornea is manipulated or damaged experimentally [171,172]. Our laboratory has examined two types of manipulation, each of which produces a change in local immunosuppression that is pertinent to this chapter. First, the corneal surface of mouse eyes has been exposed to mild cauterization [173]. Similar maneuvers by Niederkorn and his colleagues include placing small polystyrene beads into the central corneal stroma, or injecting IL-1 directly into the stroma [174,175]. Within a few days of these manipulations, Langerhans cells migrate from the cornea limbus into the corneal epithelium, and macrophages similarly migrate into the corneal stroma. Over the next several weeks these manipulated corneas contain significant numbers of APCs in the epithelium and stroma. Corneas of this type are highly vulnerable to blinding keratitis if the mice are infected with herpes simplex virus on the snout of the same side of the face as the traumatized cornea [176]. This result dramatically demonstrates that the absence of APCs in the normal cornea is important in the tissue's resistance to this type of infectious agent. Moreover, injection of antigen into the anterior chamber of an eye with a cornea containing APCs fails to induce ACAID [173,175]. Thus, the physiologic integrity of the cornea is directly linked not only to its own immune privileged status, but to privilege within the anterior chamber.

A second corneal manipulation that alters local immunosuppression involves severing all afferent nerves to the cornea [174]. Carrying out an orthotopic corneal allograft routinely accomplishes this end. Surprisingly, injection of antigen into the anterior chamber of eyes in which the corneal nerves have been severed circumferentially fails to induce ACAID – until the nerves regenerate (typically within 8 – 12 weeks). Lack of ACAID correlates with the inability of explants of I/CB obtained from eyes with severed corneal nerves to secrete immunosuppressive factors in vitro. Based on these observations, it has been proposed that afferent nerves in the cornea send tonic influences to the brain stem, and that these tonic influences govern the secretion of immunosuppressive factors from I/CB cells. Interruption of this tonic influence leads inevitably to the failure of I/CB cells to secrete the factors that maintain an immunosuppressive intraocular microenvironment. Although the evidence is indirect, it suggests that local immunosuppression in the eye is under neural control – a suggestion already inherent in the presence of immunoinhibitory neuropeptides in normal AqH.

APPROACHES TO RESTORING OCULAR IMMUNOSUPPRESSION

There are both experimental and clinical reasons for trying to restore immunosuppression to the ocular environment once it is lost. Approaches to achieving this end form the closing segment of this chapter. In clinical ophthalmology, the usual treatments for uveitis are steroids and anti-pro-liferative (immunosuppressive) drugs delivered through eye-drops, by sub-conjunctival, intravitreal or intraorbital injections, and, in desperate cases, by systemic administration. If anti-viral and anti-bacterial medications are required, their delivery is determined by the location of the infection in the eye. The cornea can be treated topically with eye-drops, whereas reti-nal infections benefit from injections into the posterior segment (vitreous cavity), or they must be treated systemically. If the blood-ocular barrier is broken these medications may be rendered ineffective because of their sen-sitivity to serum proteases. Their half-life in the eye following intraocular injection may be curtailed if the blood:ocular barrier is breached. These ther-apeutic problems have spawned the development of unique drug delivery systems that can maintain prolonged and effective levels of immunosuppres-sive medications within the eye. As we begin to understand the molecular mechanisms of ocular immunosuppression it may also become possible to re-establish and re-impose immunosuppression by treating uveitic eyes with the immunosuppressive factors that normally regulate immunity and inflam-mation, rather than using steroids and toxic immunosuppressive drugs. In addition, if the eye is predisposed to inflammation by a loss in production of specific ocular immunosuppressive factors, then gene therapy can be imag-ined to re-express these factors within the ocular microenvironment in a pro-longed or permanent manner.

Slow release systems

In order to maintain effective drug concentrations locally, delivery systems have been designed to release drugs in a measured manner within or on the eye [177,178]. The materials used in making newer delivery systems are bioadhesive hydrogel, in-situ gel-forming polymers; colloidal liposome sys-tems, microspheres, cyclodextrins, intra-ocular-lens-bound sustained drug delivery systems, and porous polymer-containing chambers. In each case the drug or therapeutic agent is entrapped in a lattice structure that allows for diffusion of the drug out of the structure at a predictable rate, or that releases the drug as the structure itself dissolves. Some delivery devices are applied to the surface of the cornea, delivering drugs to the ocular surface as if it were continuous eye drops. Colloidal delivery systems can be deliv-ered as eye drops onto the corneal surface. Other devices require surgical insertion into the anterior chamber or vitreous cavity. Therefore, the ideal delivery system would be one that releases the drug at a predictable and sustained rate within the eye, and that does not itself interfere with vision or cause inflammation.

The benefit of drug delivery systems is that the medications are delivered into a limited region, the ocular microenvironment, avoiding the toxicity and side effects that follow systemic administration. Although a number of delivery systems have been shown to be very effective in delivering high concentrations of drugs into the eye, very few of them are commercially available or approved for standard treatment regimes. There is also a limitation as to the types of drugs that can be delivered by these systems. Most systems have used the standard immunosuppressive and anti-proliferative drugs such as prednisolone, pilocarpine, cyclosporine, and the anti-viral acyclovir, but only a few reports use a delivery system for the release of proteins [179]. Although these reports demonstrate an effect caused by the released growth factor protein, they inadvertently demonstrate the limitations in releasing bioactive proteins from these systems. The released bioactive proteins appear to be limited to affecting only the tissues that are in physical contact with the device and have little or no effects on distant tissues within the same microenvironment. This suggests that not enough bioactive protein is released to saturate nearby receptors, and to allow the protein to accumulate within the microenvironment. Progress in this area is rapid, however, so effective new drug delivery systems for uveitis treatments are inevitable.

Gene therapy

Gene therapy has the potential to deliver locally temporary or permanent expression of cytokines and other immunomodulatory molecules within the ocular microenvironment. Cells of the ocular microenvironment appear to be very permissive to transfection, and they usually stably express the transfected gene products [180,181]. In addition, presumably because of the immune privileged nature of the eye, immune responses to antigens expressed by viral vectors has proven not be a major problem [180-182]. Genes have been successfully delivered into the ocular microenvironment through adenoviral and adeno-associated viruses, and through non-viral delivery systems. The goals of recent experiments have been to use gene transfection therapy to deliver genes that encode (a) factors that correct ocular genetic defects or rescue photoreceptor cells threatened by these defects, (b) regulatory proteins that inhibit growth of retinoblastomas, and (c) cytokines that suppress intraocular inflammation [183-186].

Because of the lack of a demonstrable immune response to viral proteins, it has been possible to stably transfect ocular cells using adenoviral delivery systems. Adenoviral delivery of basic fibroblast growth factor (bFGF) into the retina of RCS rats results in photoreceptor rescue by the sustained production of bFGF by RPE cells [183]. RPE cells have also been transfected by adenoviral delivery of glucuronidase to correct for the congenital defect of this enzyme that leads to mucopolysaccharidosis, a disorder associated with photoreceptor cell loss [187]. Injections of adenoviral vectors into the ocular microenvironment of mice have shown that RPE cells, corneal epithelium and endothelial cells, cells of the ciliary body, lens, and iris, and even the cells of the trabecular meshwork cells can stably express the transfected gene [182,188]. In addition, it has been found that adenoviral vectors delivered into the eye remain confined locally, meaning that ocular gene therapy can be treatment-site specific, and pose little threat to systemic spread of the vector [188].

Naked or lipid coated DNA delivery systems have also been successfully used to stably transfect ocular cells [189]. Direct applications of liposomes containing DNA plasmids coding for IL-10 onto HSK-infected corneas suppress the inflammatory response that leads to corneal blindness [185]. This gene transfer treatment has been shown to promote mucosal tolerance due to local expression of IL-10. Lipid transfection delivered by the direct application of the plasmid onto the cornea, usually as drops, effectively transfects cells of the cornea, I/CB. By changing the lipid constitution of DNA plasmid-containing liposomes, it is even possible to transfect retinal cells by corneal application [190]. Because of the fluidity of the lipid structure, it is also possible to include adherence proteins in the liposomes which thereby target the vector to particular ocular cell types. Liposomes assembled with hemagglutinating virus was shown to target trabecular meshwork cells, but not other cell of the ocular microenvironment [191]. Also, naked DNA plasmids coated with fusogenic proteins with binding sites specific to corneal endothelial integrins and to DNA (polylysine regions) target corneal endothelial cells specifically [192]. It is important to acknowledge that the ease of creating and delivering lipid and naked DNA plasmids is mitigated by the fact that lipid/naked DNA delivery places the plasmid episomally. By contrast, with adenoviral transfections, the plasmid is inserted into the cellular genome. Consequently, lipid/naked DNA delivery leads to gene expression that is limited in time and therefore may only be beneficial for diseases where acute treatments are required. One of our interests is to use gene therapy to suppress uveitis by delivering into the ocular microenvironment genes coding for immunosuppressive cytokines and neuropeptides.

Topical applications of natural cytokine regulators

Immune privilege in the cornea and in the anterior chamber is incompatible with the presence of IL-1. Injection of IL-1 into either the cornea or the anterior chamber leads to intense inflammation, and IL-1 plays central roles in the rejection of orthotopic corneal allografts and in neovascularization of the cornea secondary to a variety of traumatic and inflammatory insults. It has recently been demonstrated that topical IL-1 receptor antagonist (applied to the ocular surface) can suppress neovascularization of the cornea in response to sutures placed through its center [193], and can suppress the emigration of Langerhans cells into the corneal epithelium following cautery to the central corneal surface [194]. More impressively, topical IL-1ra therapy has been reported to inhibit the acquisition of donor-specific alloimmunity in recipients of orthotopic corneal allografts [195]. In fact, topical IL-1ra promotes acceptance of orthotopic corneal allografts in normal mouse eyes, as well as in eyes considered to be "high-risk" for acute rejection. Finally, topical IL-1ra has been demonstrated to restore ACAID induction in eyes with neovascularized corneas and in eyes that recently suffered circumferential severance of their corneal nerves [194].

These results indicate that topical application of immunosuppressive agents to the ocular surface can, as expected, directly promote local immunosuppression within the cornea itself. More importantly, these results suggest that topical application of immunosuppressive agents may also promote suppression and privilege within the eye itself (anterior chamber).

Application of ocular immunosuppression to regulate immunity

Since the eye (and other immune privileged sites) has developed elaborate and successful strategies to create and maintain local immunosuppressive and anti-inflammatory microenvironments, one goal of research in this area is to harness ocular mechanisms to re-create and sustain local immunosuppression when it has been lost due to disease or trauma. The following approaches have emerged from relatively new understanding of ocular immune privilege mechanisms, and offer an approach to solving harmful ocular inflammation, as well as potential approaches to solid organ transplantation and cancer (see Table 4)

Ex-vivo generation of ACAID inducing signals

The capacity of the normal eye to promote ACAID when antigens arise or

Table 4
Eye-derived pathways to regulatory lymphocytes

Protocol	Effect
Primed T cells activated by Tcr ligation in presence of AqH, or α-MSH and TGF-β2	Secrete TGF-β Suppress activation of bystander T cells in vitro and EAU in vivo
Naive T cells activated by Tcr ligation in contact with pigment epithelium	Secrete TGF-β, IL-4, IL-10 Suppress activation of bystander T cells in vitro and DH in vivo
OVA-specific Tcr tg T cells activated by OVA-pulsed, TGF-β2-treated APC	Secrete TGF-β, IL-4 Suppress induction and expression of delayed hypersensitivity

are placed intraocularly has led to the speculation that induction of ACAID might be a useful approach to achieving systemic immunologic unresponsiveness. A singular advance in this idea occurred when Wilbanks et al [35] demonstrated that an ACAID-inducing signal could be generated in vitro by incubating conventional APCs in the presence of TGF-β. As mentioned previously, injections of antigen-pulsed, TGF-β-treated APCs intravenously into naïve (or even pre-sensitized) mice induced an antigen-specific suppression of T cells that mediate delayed hypersensitivity. To prove the worthiness of this approach, our laboratory has used in vitro generated ACAID-inducing signals to promote orthotopic corneal allografts survival in mice, and to suppress the induction and expression of experimental autoimmune uveoretinitis [197,198]. Thus, in principle, pre-emptive induction of ACAID to an antigen can suppress or prevent recipients from mounting delayed hypersensitivity to the same antigen. For destructive immunogenic inflammation that results from delayed hypersensitivity, this approach has considerable merit. However, for other forms of inflammation, ACAID may not be appropriate. This has already been demonstrated for other types of solid tissue allografts for which cytotoxic T cells are a threat to acceptance. In the case of skin and heart allografts, induction of ACAID to alloantigens expressed on the graft does not interfere with generation of cytotoxic T cells; thus, pre-emptive ACAID induction to donor alloantigens has no capacity to prevent acute rejection of orthotopic skin or heart allografts. Nonetheless, ex vivo-generation of ACAID-inducing signals may find its way into the therapeutic armamentarium because delayed hypersensitivity remains the immune effector modality most closely associated with destruction of innocent bystander tissues such as that which occurs in autoimmune diseases, and viral diseases with immunopathogenic aspects.

Ex vivo induction of antigen-specific regulatory T cells

The finding that α-MSH and TGF-β2 can convert T cells into regulatory cells that DTH through bystander mechanisms has suggested that if regulatory T cells could be generated against autoantigens they could suppress autoimmunity and possibly re-establish immune-tolerance of the targeted autoantigens. To accomplish this goal, based on animal experiments, a patient's autoreactive-peripheral T cells could be stimulated in vitro with autoantigen-presenting autologous APC in the presence of α-MSH and TGF-β2. After incubation, the T cells can be harvested and returned to the patient's peripheral circulation. The possibility of such procedures working in suppressing autoimmunity is now being tested in the mouse model of experimental autoimmune uveoretinitis. As expected, the procedure yields regulatory T cells that suppress uveitis only if the antigen they were activated against originally is present in the eye. Importantly, it is not necessary for the destructive, autoreactive inflammatory T cells and the protective, regulatory T cells to be specific for the same antigen.

The drawback of this procedure is that in most cases of autoimmune disease the antigen target is unknown. In addition, there may not be enough autoreactive T cells in the periphery. It is relevant that in uveitis and multiple sclerosis, elevated levels of autoreactive T cells have been detected in the blood. Fortunately, since in vitro-generated regulatory T cells suppress inflammation through bystander mechanisms, regulatory T cells could be prepared from T cells specific for antigens included in previous vaccinations. The vaccine antigen could then be purposefully placed within the autoimmune diseased tissue site. There is also the possibility that regulatory T cells of this type may not only suppress expression of immune inflammation, but inhibit the clonal expansion of autoreactive inflammatory T cells. If this is the case, then autoreactive regulatory T cells could be used to re-establish self-tolerance in patients suffering from a specific autoimmune disease by reducing the burden of destructive, autoreactive T cells. In a similar manner, graft rejection could be suppressed by the tolerance induced by alloantigen-reactive regulatory T cells. Together, the ex vivo strategies for creating APCs that promote ACAID to a particular antigen and the ex vivo strategies for generating regulatory T cells make use of recent understanding of the molecular mechanisms of ocular immunosuppression.

Acknowledgments
Some of the experimental work described in this chapter was supported by USPHS grants EY-05678 (JWS), EY-10765 (JWS), EY-09595 (JWS), EY-10752 (AWT).

Dr Streilein is a recipient of a Research to Prevent Blindness Senior Scientific Investigator Award.

REFERENCES

1. Streilein JW Regional Immunology. In: Encyclopedia of human biology. Second Edition, Volume 4. San Diego, Academic Press, 1997, 767-776.
2. Medawar PB. A second study of the behavior and fate of skin homografts in rabbits. J Anat Lond 1945; 79: 157-172.
3. Medawar PB. Immunity to homologous grafted skin. III. The fate of skin homografts transplanted to the brain, to subcutaneous tissue, and to the anterior chamber of the eye. Br J Exp Pathol 1948; 29: 58-69.
4. Sonoda Y, Streilein JW. Orthotopic corneal transplantation in mice. Evidence that the immunogenetic rules of rejection do not apply. Transplantation 1992; 54: 694-703.
5. Joo C-K, Pepose JS, Stuart PM.T cell mediated responses in a murine model of orthotopic corneal transplantation. Invest Ophthalmol Vis Sci 1995; 36: 1530-1540.
6. Niederkorn J Y. Immune privilege and immune regulation in the eye. Adv Immunol 1990; 48: 199-226.
7. Council on Scientific Affairs. Report on the Organ Transplant Panel: Corneal Transplantation. JAMA 1988; 259: 719-722.
8. Wilson SE, Kaufman HE. Graft failure after penetrating keratoplasty. Surv Ophthalmol 1990; 34: 325-356.
9. Stark W, Stulting D, Maguire M, Streilein JW. The Collaborative Corneal Transplantation Studies (CCTS): Effectiveness of histocompatibility matching of donors and recipients in high risk corneal transplantation. Arch Ophthal 1992; 110: 1392-1403.
10. Fujikawa LS, Colvin RB, Bhan AK, FullerTC, Foster CS. Expression of HLA/B/C and DR locus antigens on epithelial, stromal and endothelial cells of the human cornea. Cornea 1982; 1: 213-224.
11. Treseler PA, Foulks GN, Sanfilippo F. The expression of HLA antigens by cells in the human cornea. Am J Ophthlamol 1984; 98: 763-772.
12. Wang H., Kaplan H., Chan C, Johnson M.) The distribution and ontogeny of MHC antigens in murine ocular tissues. Invest Ophthalmol Vis Sci 1987; 28: 1383-1389.
13. Streilein JW, Toews GB, Bergstresser PR. Corneal allografts fail to express Ia antigens. Nature 1979; 282: 325-327.
14. Streilein JW. Immune privilege and the cornea. In: Pleyer U, Hartmann C, Sterry W, editors. Proceedings of Symposium: Bullous Oculo-Muco-Cutaneous Disorders, Buren, The Netherlands, Aeolus Press, 1997, 43-52.
15. Donnelly JJ, Xi MS, Rockey JH. A soluble product of human corneal fibroblasts inhibits lymphocyte activation. Exp Eye Res 1993; 56: 157–165.
16. Kawashima H, Prasad SA, Gregerson DA. Corneal endothelial cells inhibit T cell proliferation by blocking IL-2 production. J Immunol 1994; 153: 1982-1989.
17. Jager MJ, Bradley D, Streilein JW. Immunosuppressive properties of cultured human cornea and ciliary body in normal and pathological conditions. Transplant Immunol 1995; 3: 135–142.
18. Bora NS, Gobleman CL, Atkinson JP, Pepose JS, Kaplan HJ. Differential expression of the complement regulatory proteins in the human eye. Invest Ophthal Vis

Sci 1993;34:3579-3584.

19. Griffith TS, Brunner T, Fletcher SM, Green DR, Ferguson TA. Fas ligand-induced apoptosis as a mechanism of immune privilege. Science 1995; 270: 1189-1192.

20. Stuart PM, Griffith TS, Usui N, Pepose J, Yu X, Ferguson TA. CD95 ligand (FasL)-induced apoptosis is necessary for corneal allograft survival. J Clin Invest 1997; 99: 396-402.

21. Yamagami S, Kawashima H, Tsuru T. Role of Fas-Fas ligand interactions in the immunorejection of allogeneic mouse corneal transplants. Transplantation 1997; 64: 1107-1111.

22. Hori J, Joyce N, Streilein JW. Corneal allografts devoid of epithelium placed beneath the kidney capsule display inherent immune privilege. Invest Ophthalmol Vis Sci 2000; 41: 443-452.

23. Streilein JW. Unraveling immune privilege. Science 1995; 270: 1158-1159.

24. Van Dooremall JC. Die entwicklung der in fremden grund versetzten lebenden gewebe. Albrecht Van Graefes Arch ophthalmol 1873; 19: 358 – 373.

25. Barker CF, Billingham RE. Immunologically privileged sites. Adv Immunol 1977; 25: 1-54.

26. Streilein JW. Immune privilege as the result of local tissue barriers and immunosuppressive microenvironments. Curr Opinion in Immunology 1993; 5: 428 – 432.

27. Kaplan HJ, Streilein JW. Immune response to immunization via the anterior chamber of the eye: I. F_1 lymphocyte-induced immune deviation. J Immunol 1977; 118: 809-814.

28. Kaplan HJ, Streilein JW. Immune response to immunization via the anterior chamber of the eye: II. An analysis of F_1 lymphocyte induced immune deviation. J Immunol 1977; 120: 689-693.

29. Streilein JW. Immune privilege in the eye: a dangerous compromise. FASEB J 1987; 1: 199-208.

30. Niederkorn JY, Streilein JW, Shadduck JA. Deviant immune responses to allogeneic tumors injected intracamerally and subcutaneously in mice. Invest Ophthal Vis Sci 1980; 20: 355-363.

31. Streilein JW, Niederkorn JY, Shadduck JA. Systemic immune unresponsiveness induced in adult mice by anterior chamber presentation of minor histocompatibility antigens. J Exp Med 1980; 152: 1121-1125.

32. Benson J, Niederkorn JY. *In situ* suppression of delayed-type hypersensitivity: another mechanism for sustaining the immune privilege of the anterior chamber. Immunology 1991; 74: 153-159.

33. Ksander BR, Streilein JW. Failure of infiltrating precursor cytotoxic T cells to acquire direct cytotoxic function in immunologically privileged sites. J Immunol 1990; 145: 2057-1063.

34. Cousins SW, Trattler WB, Streilein JW. Immune privilege and suppression of immunogenic inflammation in the anterior chamber of the eye. Curr Eye Res 1991; 10: 287-297.

35. Wilbanks GA, Streilein JW. Fluids from immune privileged sites endow macrophages with the capacity to induce antigen-specific immune deviation via a mechanism involving transforming growth factor-beta. Eur J Immunol 1992;22: 1031-1036.

36. Wilbanks GA, Mammolenti M, Streilein JW. Studies on the induction of anterior chamber-associated immune deviation (ACAID). III. Induction of ACAID depends upon intraocular transforming growth factor-beta. Eur J Immunol 1992;22: 165-173.

37. Taylor AW, Streilein JW, Cousins SW: Alpha-melanocyte-stimulating hormone suppresses antigen-stimulated T cell production of gamma-interferon. Neuroimmunomodulation 1994;1:188-194.

38. Knisely TL, Anderson TM, Sherwood ME, Flotte TJ, Albert DM, Granstein RD. Morphologic and ultrastructural examination of I-A⁺ cells in murine iris. Invest Ophthalmol Vis Sci 1991;32:2423-2531.
39. McMenamin PG, Holthouse I, Holt PG. Class II major histocompatibility complex (Ia) antigen-bearing dendritic cells within the iris and ciliary body of the rat eye: distribution, phenotype, and relation to retinal microglia. Immunology 1992;77: 385-393.
40. Taylor AW, Yee DG, Streilein JW. Suppression of nitric oxide generated by inflammatory macrophages by calcitonin gene-related peptide in aqueous humor. Invest Ophthalmol Vis Sci 1998;39:1372-1378.
41. Kaiser C, Ksander BR, Streilein JW. Inhibition of lymphocyte proliferation by aqueous humor. Regional Immunol 1989;2:42-49.
42. Streilein JW, Cousins SW. Aqueous humor factors and their effects on the immune response in the anterior chamber. Curr Eye Res 1990;9:175-182.
43. Taylor AW. Immunoregulation of the ocular effector responses by soluble factors in aqueous humor. Regional Immunol 1994;6:52-57.
44. Wilson JF, Harry FM: Release, distribution and half-life of α-melanotrophin in the rat. Endocrinology 1980;86:61-67.
45. Taylor AW, Alard P, Yee DG, Streilein JW. Aqueous humor induces transforming growth factor-beta (TGF-beta)-producing regulatory T-cells. Curr Eye Res 1997; 16:900-908.
46. Williamson JSP, Bradley D, Streilein JW. Immunoregulatory properties of bone marrow derived cells in the iris and ciliary body. Immunology 1989; 67: 96-102.
47. Jager MJ, Streilein JW. Regulators of immunological responses in the cornea and anterior chamber of the eye. In: Zierhuit, M., editor. Autoimmunity and the Eye, Amsterdam, The Netherlands, Aeolus Press (IN PRESS).
48. Yoshida M, Takeuchi M, Streilein JW. Participation of pigment epithelium of iris and ciliary body in ocular immune privilege. 1. Inhibition of T cell activation in vitro by direct cell to cell contact. Invest Ophthalmol Vis Sci 2000; 41: 811-821.
49. Liversidge J, McKay D, Mulalen G, Forrester JV. Retinal pigment epithelial cells modulate lymphocyte function at the blood-retina barrier by autocrine PGE₂ and membrane-bound mechanisms. Cell Immunol 1993; 149: 315 – 330.
50. Jorgensen A, Wiencke AK, la Cour M et al. Human retinal pigment epithelial cell-induced apoptosis in activated T cells. Invest Ophthalmol Vis Sci 1998;39: 1590-1599.
51. Farrokh-Siar L, Rezai KA, Semnani RT et al. Human fetal retinal pigment epithelial cells induce apoptosis in the T cell line Jurkat. Invest Ophthalmol Vis Sci 1999; 40: 1503-1511.
52. Ma D, Niederkorn JY. Transforming growth factor-β down-regulates major histocompatibility complex class I antigen expression and increases the susceptibility of uveal melanoma cells to natural killer cell-mediated cytolysis. Immunology 1995; 86: 263 – 269.
53. Ma D, Luyten GP, Luider T M, Niederkorn JY. Relationship between natural killer cell susceptibility and metastasis of human uveal melanoma cells in a murine model. Invest Ophthamol Vis Sci 1995; 36: 435 – 441.
54. Apte RS, Sinha D, Mayhew E, Wistow GL, Niederkorn JY: Role of macrophage migration inhibitory factor in inhibiting NK cell activity. J Immunol. 1998;160:5693-5696
55. Apte RS, Mayhew E, Niederkorn JY. Local inhibition of natural killer cell activity promotes the progressive growth of intraocular tumors. Invest Ophthal Vis Sci 1997; 38: 1277 – 1282, 1997.
56. Apte RS, Niederkorn JY: Isolation and characterization of a unique natural killer cell inhibitory factor present in the anterior chamber of the eye. J Immunol. 1996;156:2667-2673.

57. Li X-Y, Niederkorn JY, Chiang E, Ungchusri T, Stroynowski I. Expression of QA-2 non-classical class I MHC antigen in the mouse eye. Invest Ophthal Vis Sci 1999; 40: S861.
58. Bellgrau D, Gold D, Selawry H, Moore J, Franzusoff A, Duke RC. A role of CD95 ligand in preventing graft rejection. Nature 1995; 377: 630-632.
59. Kang SM et al. Fas ligand expression in islets of Langerhans does not confer immune privilege and instead targets them for rapid destruction. Nature Medicine 1997; 3: 738-743.
60. Allison J, Georgiou HM, Strasser A, Vaux DL. Transgenic expression of CD95 ligand on islet B cells induces a granulocytic infiltration but does not confer immune privilege upon islet allografts. Immunology 1997; 94: 3943-3947.
61. Chen J-J, Sun Y, Nabel GJ. Regulation of the proinflammatory effects of Fas ligand (CD95L). Science 1998; 282: 1714 – 1717.
62. D'Orazio TJ, DeMarco BM, Mayhew ES, Niederkorn JY. Effect of aqueous humor on apoptosis of inflammatory cell types. Invest Ophthal Vis Sci 1999; 40: 1418 – 1426.
63. Miyamoto KI, Taylor AW, Ksander BR. Immune privilege microenvironment modulates proinflammatory function of Fas ligand on the cornea. Invest Ophthal Vis Science 1999; 40: S986.
64. D'Erma F, Lanziera M, Cricchi M, Ovary Z. Research into the complementary and anticomplementary power of aqueous humor and vitreous of guinea pigs. Boll Ocul 1960; 39: 643-549.
65. Shimada K. The complement components and their inhibitors in the intraocular fluids of the guinea pig. Invest. Ophthalmol. 1970;9:304-315.
66. Goslings WRO, Prodeus AP, Streilein JW, Carroll MC, Jager MJ, Taylor AW. A small molecular weight factor in aqueous humor acts on C1q to Prevent antibody-dependent complement activation. Invest Ophthal Vis Sci 1998;39:989-995.
67. Tanaka K, Yamada J, Streilein JW. Xenoreactive CD4+ T cells, but not CD8+ T cells or antibodies, are responsible for acute rejection of orthotopic guinea pig corneas in mice. Invest Ophthal Vis Sci 2000; 41: 1827-1832.
68. Wilbanks GA, Streilein JW. Characterization of suppressor cells in Anterior Chamber-Associated Immune Deviation (ACAID) induced by soluble antigen. Evidence of two functionally and phenotypically distinct T-suppressor cell populations. Immunology 1990; 71: 383 – 389.
69. Wilbanks GA, Streilein JW. Distinctive humoral responses following anterior chamber and intravenous administration of soluble antigen. Evidence for active suppression of IgG2a-secreting B cells. Immunology 1990; 71: 566-572.
70. Eichorn M, Horneber M, Streilein JW, Lutjen-Drecoll E. Anterior chamber associated immune deviation elicited via primate eyes. Invest Ophthal Vis Sci 1993; 34: 2926-2930.
71. Jiang LQ, Streilein JW. Immune privilege extended to allogeneic tumor cells in the vitreous cavity. Invest Ophthal Vis Sci 1991; 32: 224 – 228.
72. Jiang LQ, Jorquera M, Streilein JW. Subretinal space and vitreous cavity as immunologically privileged sites for retinal allografts. Invest. Ophthal Vis Sci 1993; 34: 3347 – 3354.
73. Wenkel H, Chen PW, Ksander BR, Streilein JW. Immune privilege is extended, then withdrawn, from allogeneic tumor cell grafts placed in the subretinal space. Invest Ophthal Vis Sci 1999; 40: 3202-3208.
74. Gordon LB, Nolan SC, Cserr HF, Knopf PM, Harling-Berg CJ. Growth of P511 mastocytoma cells in BALB/c mouse brain elicits CTL response without tumor elimination. J Immunol 1997; 159: 2399 – 2408.
75. Harling-Berg CJ, Knopf PM, Cserr HF. Myelin basic protein infused into cerebrospinal fluid suppresses experimental autoimmune encephalomyelitis. J Neuroimmunol 1991; 35: 45 – 55.

76. Cserr HF, Knopf PM. Cervical lymphatics, the blood-brain barrier and the immunoreactivity of the brain: a new view. Immunology Today 1992; 13: 507 – 511.

77. Kaplan HJ, Streilein JW. Do immunologically privileged sites require a functioning spleen? Nature 1974; 251: 553-554.

78. Yotsukura J, Huang H, Singh AK, Shichi H. Regulatory cells generated by testicular tolerization to retinal S-antigen. Cell Immunol 1997; 182: 89-98.

79. Wilbanks GA, Streilein JW. Studies on the induction of anterior chamber associated immune deviation (ACAID). I. Evidence that an antigen-specific, ACAID-inducing , cell-associated signal exists in the peripheral blood. J Immunol 1991; 146: 2610-2617.

80. Wilbanks GA, Streilein JW. Studies on the induction of anterior chamber associated immune deviation (ACAID). II. Eye-derived cells participating in generating blood borne signals that induce ACAID. J Immunol 1991; 146: 3018-3024.

81. Takeuchi M, Kosiewicz MM, Alard P, Streilein JW. On the mechanisms by which TGF-β2 alters antigen presenting abilities of macrophages on T cell activation. Eur J Immunol 1997; 27: 1648 – 1656.

82. Takeuchi M, Alard P, Streilein JW. TGFβ promotes immune deviation by altering accessory signals of antigen presenting cells. J Immunol 1998; 160: 1589 – 1597.

83. Steptoe R, Holt PG, McMenamin PG. Functional studies of major histocompatibility class II-positive dendritic cells and resident tissue macrophages isolated from the rat iris. Immunology 1995; 85: 630-637.

84. Ma N, Streilein JW. Microglia, as passenger leukocytes, contribute to the fate of intraocular neuronal retinal grafts. Invest Ophthal Vis Sci 1998; 39: 2384 – 2393.

85. Ma N, Streilein JW. T cell immunity induced by allogeneic microglia in relation to neuronal retina transplantation. J Immunol 1999; 162: 4482 – 4489.

86. Taylor AW, Yee DG, Streilein JW. Suppression of nitric oxide generated by inflammatory macrophages by calcitonin gene-related peptide in aqueous humor. Invest Ophthalmol Vis Sci 1998;39:1372-1378.

87. Granstein R, Staszewski R, Knisely TL et al. Aqueous humor contains transforming growth factor-β and a small (<3500 daltons) inhibitor of thymocyte proliferation. J Immunol 1990;144:3021-3026.

88. Cousins SW, McCabe MM, Danielpour D, Streilein JW. Identification of transforming growth factor-beta as an immunosuppressive factor in aqueous humor. Invest Ophthalmol Vis Sci 1991;32:33-43.

89. Taylor AW, Streilein JW, Cousins SW. Identification of alpha-melanocyte stimulating hormone as a potential immunosuppressive factor in aqueous humor. Curr Eye Res 1992;11:1199-1206.

90. Taylor AW, Streilein JW, Cousins SW. Immunoreactive vasoactive intestinal peptide contributes to the immunosuppressive activity of normal aqueous humor. J Immunol 1994;153:1080-1086.

91. Knisely TL, Hosoi J, Nazareno R, Grandstein RD. The presence of biologically significant concentrations of glucocorticoids but little or no cortisol binding globulin with aqueous humor: relevance to immune privilege in the anterior chamber of the eye. Invest Ophthalmol Vis Sci 1994;35:3711-3723.

92. Nicolai J, Larsen B, Bersani M, Olcese J, Holst JJ, Moller M. Somatostatin and prosomatostatin in the retina of the rat: an immunohistochemical, in-situ hybridization, and chromatographic study. Vis Neurosci 1990;5:441-452.

93. Jampel HD, Roche N, Stark WJ, Roberts AB. Transforming growth factor-β in human aqueous humor. Curr Eye Res 1990;9:963-969.

94. Roberts AB, Sporn MB. Transforming growth factor β. Adv Can Res 1988;51: 107-145.

95. Miyazono K, Olofsson A, Colosetti P, Heldin CH. A role of the latent TGF-β1-binding protein in the assembly and secretion of TGF-β1. EMBO J 1991;10: 1091-1101.

96. Flaumenhaft R, Kojima S, Abe M, Rifkin DB. Activation of latent transforming growth factor beta. Adv Pharmacol 1993;24:51-76.
97. Flaumenhaft R, Abe M, Sato Y et al. Role of the latent TGF-β binding protein in the activation of latent TGF-β by co-cultures of endothelial and smooth muscle cells. J Cell Biol 1993;120:995-1002.
98. Pasquale LR, Dorman-Pease ME, Lutty GA, Quigley HA, Jampel HD. Immunolocalization of TGF-β1, TGF-β2, and TGF-β3 in the anterior segment of the human eye. Investi Ophthalmol Vis Sci 1993;34:23-30.
99. Knisely TL, Bleicher PA, Vibbard CA, Granstein RD. Production of latent transforming growth factor-beta and other inhibitory factors by cultured murine iris and ciliary body cells. Curr Eye Res 1991;10:761-771.
100. Nunes I, Shapiro RL, Rifkin DB. Characterization of latent TGF-beta activation by murine peritoneal macrophages. J Immunol 1995;155:1450-1459.
101. Munger JS, Harpel JG, Gleizes PE, Mazzieri R, Nunes I, Rifkin DB. Latent transforming growth factor-beta: structural features and mechanisms of activation. Kidney Int 1997;51:1376-1382.
102. Nishida T, Taylor AW. Specific aqueous humor factors induce activation of regulatory T cells. Invest Ophthalmol Vis Sci 1999; 40:2268-2274.
103. Bogdan C, Paik J, Vodovotz Y, Nathan C. Contrasting mechanisms for suppression of macrophage cytokine release by transforming growth factor-β and interleukin-10. J Biol Chem 1992;267:23301-23308.
104. Chantry D, Turner M, Abney E, Feldmann M. Modulation of cytokine production by transforming growth factor-β. J Immunol 1989;142:
105. Tsunawaki S, Sporn M, Ding A, Nathan C: Deactivation of macrophages by transforming growth factor-β. Nature, 1988;334:260-262.
106. Cannon JG, Tatro JB, Reichlin S, Dinarello CA. α-melanocyte stimulating hormone inhibits immunostimulatory and inflammatory actions of interleukin 1. J Immunol 1986;137:2232-2236.
107. Lee TH, Lerner AB, Buettner-Janusch V. The isolation and structure of α- and β-melanocyte-stimulating hormones from monkey pituitary glands. J Biol Chem 1961;236:1390-1394.
108. Nakanishi S, Inoue A, Kita T et al. Nucleotide sequence of cloned cDNA for bovine corticotropin-b-lipotropin precursor. Nature, 1979;278:423-427.
109. Lipton JM, Catania A. Anti-inflammatory actions of the neuroimmunomodulator α-MSH. Immunol Today 1997;18:140-145.
110. Lipton JM. Modulation of host defense by the neuropeptide α-MSH. Yale J Bio Med 1990;63:173-182.
111. Holdeman M, Khorram O, Samson WK, Lipton JM. Fever-specific changes in central MSH and CRF concentrations. Amer J Pysiol 1985;248:R125-R129.
112. Watanabe T, Hiltz ME, Catania A, Lipton JM. Inhibition of IL-1β-induced peripheral inflammation by peripheral and central administration of analogs of the neuropeptide α-MSH. Brain Res Bull 1993;32:311-314.
113. Martin LW, Catania A, Hiltz ME, Lipton JM. Neuropeptide alpha-MSH antagonizes IL-6- and TNF-induced fever. Peptides 1991;12:297-299.
114. Chiao H, Foster S, Thomas R, Lipton J, Star RA. α-Melanocyte stimulating hormone reduces endotoxin-induced liver inflammation. J Clin Invest 1996;97:2038-2044.
115. Rajora N, Ceriani G, Catania A, Star RA, Murphy MT, Lipton JM. α-MSH production, receptors, and influence on neopterin in a human monocyte/macrophage cell line. J Leukoc Biol 1996;59:248-253.
116. Star RA, Rajora N, Huang J, Chavez R, Catania A, Lipton JM. Evidence of autocrine modulation of macrophage nitric oxide synthase by α-MSH. Proc Natl Acad Sci USA 1995;90:8856-8860.
117. Catania A, Rajora N, Capsoni F, Minonzio F, Star RA, Lipton JM. The neuropeptide α-MSH has specific receptors on neutrophils and reduces chemotaxis in

vitro. Peptides 1996;17:675-679.

118. Chakraborty AK, Funasaka Y, Slominski A et al. Production and release of proopiomelanocortin (POMC) derived peptides by human melanocytes and keratinocytes in culture: regulation by ultraviolet B. Biochim Biophys Acta 1996;1313:130-138.

119. O'Donohue TL, Dorsa DM. The opiomelanotropinergic neuronal and endocrine systems. Peptides 1982;3:353-395.

120. Uddman R, Alumets J, Ehinger B, Håkanson R, Lorén I, Sundler F. Vasoactive intestinal peptide nerves in ocular and orbital structures of the cat. Invest Ophthalmol Vis Sci 1980;19:878-885.

121. Muscettola M, Grasso G. Somatostatin and vasoactive intestinal peptide reduce interferon gamma production by human peripheral blood mononuclear cells. Immunobiology 1990;180:419-430.

122. O'Dorisio MS, Wood CL, O'Dorisio TM. Vasoactive intestinal peptide and neuropeptide modulation of the immune response. J Immunol 1985;135:792-796.

123. Ottaway CA. Vasoactive intestinal peptide as a modulator of lymphocyte and immune function. Ann NY Acad Sci 1988;527:486-500.

124. Stanisz AM, Scicchitano R, Bienenstock J. The role of vasoactive intestinal peptide and other neuropeptides in the regulation of the immune response in vitro and in vivo. Ann NY Acad Sci 1988;527:478-485.

125. Tseng J, O'Dorisio MS. Mechanism of vasoactive intestinal peptide (VIP)-mediated immunoregulation. In: Goetzl EJ, Spector NH, editors. Neuroimmune networks: physiology and diseases. New York, NY, Alan R Liss, Inc, 1989: 105-111.

126. Boudard F, Bastide M. Inhibition of mouse T-cell proliferation by CGRP and VIP: effects of these neuropeptides on IL-2 production and cAMP synthesis. J Neurosci Res 1991;29:29-41.

127. Ganea D, Sun L. Vasoactive intestinal peptide downregulates the expression of IL-2 but not of INF-γ from stimulated murine T lymphocytes. J Neuroimmun 1993;47:147-158.

128. Ottaway CA. Selective effects of vasoactive intestinal peptide on the mitogenic response of murine T cells. Immunology 1987;62:291-297.

129. Segura JJ, Guerrero JM, Goberna R, Calvo JR. Characterization of functional receptors for vasoactive intestinal peptide (VIP) in rat peritoneal macrophages. Regul Pept 1991;33:133-143.

130. Wiik P, Opstad PK, Boyum A. Binding of vasoactive intestinal polypeptide (VIP) by human blood monocytes: demonstration of specific binding sites. Regul Pept 1985;12:145-153.

131. Wiik P, Haugen AH, Lovhaug D, Boyum A, Opstad PK. Effect of VIP on the respiratory burst in human monocytes ex vivo during prolonged strain and energy deficiency. Peptides 1989;10:819-823.

132. Wiik P. VIP inhibition of monocyte respiratory burst ex vivo during prolonged strain and energy deficiency. Int J Neurosci 1990;51:195-196.

133. Terenghi G, Polak JM, Ghatei MA et al. Distribution and origin of calcitonin gene-related peptide (CGRP) immunoreactivity in the sensory innervation of the mammalian eye. J Comp Neurol 1985;233:506-516.

134. Kurz B, VonGaudecker B, Kranz A, Krisch B, Mentlein R. Calcitonin gene-related peptide and its receptor in the thymus. Peptides 1995;16:1497-1503.

135. Asahina A, Moro O, Hosoi J et al. Specific induction of cAMP in Langerhans cells by calcitonin gene-related peptide: relevance to functional effects. Proc Natl Acad Sci USA 1995;92:8323-8327.

136. Asahina A, Hosoi J, Biessert S, Stratigos A, Granstein RD. Inhibition of the induction of delayed-type and contact hypersensitivity by calcitonin gene-related peptide. J Immunol 1995;154:3056-3061.

137. Hanesch U, Pfrommer U, Grubb BD, Schaible HG. Acute and chronic phases of

unilateral inflammation in rat's ankle are associated with an increase in the proportion of calcitonin gene-related peptide-immunoreactive dorsal root ganglion cells. Eur J Neurosci 1993;5:154-161.

138. Unger WG, Terenghi G, Ghatei MA et al. Calcitonin gene-related polypeptide as a mediator of the neurogenic ocular injury response. J Ocul Pharmacol 1985;1: 189-199.

139. Wahlestedt C, Beding B, Ekman R, Oksala O, Stjernschantz J, Håkanson R. Calcitonin gene-related peptide in the eye: release by sensory nerve stimulation and effects associated with neurogenic inflammation. Regul Pept 1986;16:107-115.

140. Nong YH, Titus RG, Ribeiro JMC, Remold HG. Peptides encoded by the calcitonin gene inhibit macrophage function. J Immunol 1989;143:45-49.

141. Niizeki H, Alard P, Streilein JW. Calcitonin gene-related peptide is necessary for ultraviolet B-impaired induction of contact hypersensitivity. J Immunol 1997;159: 5183-5186.

142. Beckers H, Klooster J, Vrensen G, Lamers W. Substance P in the rat cornea and iridial nerves: an ultrastructural immunohistochemical study. Ophthalmic Res 1993;25:192.

143. Unger WG, Butler JM, Cole DF, Bloom SR, McGregor GP:.Substance P, vasoactive intestinal peptide (VIP) and somatostatin levels in ocular tissue of normal and sensorily denervated rabbit eyes. Exp Eye Res 1981;32:797-801.

144. Wahlestedt C, Beding B, Ekman R, Oksala O, Stjernschantz J, Håkanson R. Calcitonin gene-related peptide in the eye: release by sensory nerve stimulation and effects associated with neurogenic inflammation. Regul Pept 1986;16:107-115.

144. Nicolai J, Larsen B, Bersani M, Olcese J, Holst JJ, Moller M. Somatostatin and prosomatostatin in the retina of the rat: an immunohistochemical, in-situ hybridization, and chromatographic study. Vis Neurosci 1990;5:441-452.

145. Goetzl EJ, Adelman DC, Sreedharan SP. Neuroimmunology. Adv Immunol 1990; 48:161-190.

146. Muscettola M, Grasso G. Somatostatin and vasoactive intestinal peptide reduce interferon gamma production by human peripheral blood mononuclear cells. Immunobiology 1990;180:419-430.

147. Ferguson TA, Fletcher S, Herndon J, Griffith TS. Neuropeptides modulate immune deviation induced via the anterior chamber of the eye. J Immunol 1995; 155:1746-1756.

148. Knisely TL, Hosoi J, Nazareno R, Grandstein RD. The presence of biologically significant concentrations of glucocorticoids but little or no cortisol binding globulin with aqueous humor: relevance to immune privilege in the anterior chamber of the eye. Invest Ophthalmol Vis Sci 1994;35:3711-3723.

149. Bloom BR, Bennett B. Mechanisms of a reaction in vitro associated with delayed-type hypersensitivity. Science 1966;153:80-82

150. Wistow GL, Shaughnessy MP, Lee DC, Hodin J, Zelenka PS. A macrophage migration inhibitory factor is expressed in the differentiating cells of the eye lens. Proc Nat Acad Sci 1993;90:1272-1275.

151. Kennedy MC, Rosenbaum JT, Brown J, et al. Novel production of interleukin-1 receptor antagonist peptides in normal human cornea. J Clin Invest 1995;95: 82-88.

152. Holtkamp GM, DeVos AF, Kijlstra A, Peek R. Expression of multiple forms of IL-1 receptor antagonist (IL-1ra) by human retinal pigment epithelial cells: identification of a new IL-1ra exon. Eur J Immunol 1999; 29: 215-224.

153. Janeway CA Jr, Travers P. Immunobiology: The Immune System in Health and Disease, New York, Garland Publishing, 1997.

154. Lass JH, Walter EI, Burris TE, et al. Expression of two molecular forms of the complement decay-accelerating factor in the eye and lacrimal gland. Invest Ophthalmol Vis Sci 1990; 31:1136-1148.

155. Mondino BJ, Sumner H. Compliment inhibitors in normal cornea and aqueous humor. Invest. Ophthalmol. Vis. Sci. 1984; 25:483-486.
156. Liao HR, Minta JO, Basu PK. Anticomplementary activity of cornea, vitreous and chorioretina in rabbits. Can J Ophthalmol 1979; 14:270-273.
157. Lass JH, Walter EI, Burris TE et al. Expression of two molecular forms of the complement decay-accelerating factor in the eye and lacrimal gland. Invest Ophthal Vis Sci 1990; 31:1136-1148.
158. Bora NS, Kabeer NH, Kim MC, Paryjas S, Atkinson JP, Kaplan HJ. Expression of the complement regulatory proteins in the normal and diseased (EAU) rat eye. In: Nussenblatt RB, Whitcup SM, Caspi RR, Gery J., editors. Advances in ocular immunology. Amsterdam:Elsever; 1994:83-86.
159. Rao NA, Forrester DJ: General approach to the uveitis patient. IN Textbook of Ophthalmology, Vol. 2, Eds: Podos SM, Yanoff M. Gower Medical Publishing, NY, NY. 1992; pp 2.1-2.18.
160. Cooper PJ. Guderian RH. Proano R. Taylor DW: Absence of cellular responses to a putative autoantigen in onchocercal chorioretinopathy. Cellular autoimmunity in onchocercal chorioretinopathy Invest Ophthal Vis Sci 1996; 37:405-412.
161. Streilein JW , Dana MR, Ksander BR. Immunity causing blindness: Five different paths to herpes stromal keratitis. Immunology Today 1997, 18: 443-449.
162. Akiba M, Yoshida I, Suzutani T, Ogasawara M, Azuma M. Relationship of the strain and the intraocular amount of herpes simplex virus types 1 and 2 in the induction of anterior-chamber-associated immune deviation. Ophthal. Res. 1996; 28:289-295.
163. Gery I, Streilein JW. Autoimmunity in the eye and its regulation. Curr Opin Immunol. 1994; 6:938-945.
164. Albert DM, Diaz-Rohena R. A historical review of sympathetic ophthalmia and its epidemiology. Surv Ophthalmol 1989; 34:1-14.
165.Taylor AW, Bloch-Michel E, Dana MR, Labetoulle M, Streilein, JW. Human uveitic aqueous humor is still immunosuppressive. Invest Ophthal Vis Sci 1999; 40: S592.
166. McMenamin PG, Broekhuyse RM, Forrester JV. Ultrastructural pathology of experimental autoimmune uveitis: a review. Micron 1993; 24:521-546.
167. Caspi RR, Roberge FG, Chan CC et al. A new model of autoimmune disease: experimental autoimmune uveoretinitis induced in mice with two different retinal antigens. J Immuno. 1988; 140:1490-1495.
168. Ohta K, Wiggert B, Taylor AW, Streilein JW. Effects of experimental ocular inflammation on ocular immune privilege. Invest Ophthal Vis Sci 1999; 46: 2010-2013.
169. Ohta K, Wiggert B, Yamagami S, Taylor AW, Streilein JW. Analysis of immunomodulatory activities of aqueous humor from eyes of mice with experimental autoimmune uveitis. J Immunol 2000; 164: 1185-1192.
170. Rosenbaum JT, McDevitt HO, Guss RB, Egbert PR. Endotoxin-induced uveitis in rats as a model for human disease. Nature 1980; 286:611-613.
171. Sano Y, Ksander BR, Streilein JW. Fate of orthotopic corneal allografts in eyes that cannot support ACAID induction. Invest Ophthal Vis Sci 1995; 36: 2176 – 2185.
172. Streilein JW, Bradley D, Sano Y, Sonoda Y. Immunosuppressive properties of tissues obtained from eyes with experimentally manipulated corneas. Invest Ophthal Vis Sci 1996; 37: 413 - 424.
173. Williamson JSP, DiMarco S, Streilein JW. Immunobiology of Langerhans cells on the ocular surface. I. Langerhans cells within the central cornea interfere with induction of Anterior Chamber Associated Immune Deviation. Invest Ophthal Vis Sci 1987; 28: 1527 – 1532.
174. Niederkorn JY, Peeler JS, Mellon J. Phagocytosis of particulate antigens by corneal epithelial cells stimulates interluekin-1 secretion and migration of Langer-

hans cells into the central cornea. Regional Imm 1989; 2: 83 – 89.

175. Niederkorn JY. Effect of cytokine-induced migration of Langerhans cells on corneal allograft survival. Eye 1995; 9:215-218.

176. McLeish W, Rubsamen P, Atherton SS, Streilein JW. Immunobiology of Langerhans cells on the ocular surface. II. Role of central corneal Langerhans cells in stromal keratitis following experimental HSV-1 infection in mice. Regional Immunol 1989; 2: 236 – 243.

177. Le Bourlais C, Acar A, Zia H, Sado PA, Needham T, Leverge R. Ophthalmic drug delivery systems – recent advances. Prog Retin Eye Res 1998; 17:33-58.

178. Lightman S. New therapeutic options in uveitis. Eye 1997;11:222-226.

179. Grant MB, Mames RN, Fitzgerald C, Ellis EA, Aboufriekha M, Guy J. Insulin-like growth factor I acts as an angiogenic agent in rabbit cornea and retina: comparative studies with basic fibroblast growth factor. Diabetol 1993;36:282-291.

180. Hoffman LM, Maguire AM, Bennett J. Cell-mediated immune response and stability of intraocular transgene expression after adenovirus-mediated delivery. Invest Ophthalmol Vis Sci 1997; 38:2224-2233.

181. Bennett J, Duan D, Engelhardt JF, Maguire AM. Real-time, non-invasive in vivo assessment of adeno-associated virus-mediating retinal transduction. Invest Ophthalmol Vis Sci 1997; 38:2857-2863.

182. Budenz DL, Bennett J, Alonso L, Maguire A. In vivo gene transfer into murine corneal endothelial and trabecular meshwork cells. Invest Ophthalmol Vis Sci 1995; 36:2211-2215.

183. Akimoto M, Miyatake SI, Kogishi JI et al. Adenovirally expressed basic fibroblast growth factor rescues photoreceptor cells in RCS rats. Invest Ophthalmol Vis Sci 1999; 40:273-279.

184. Chau KY, Ono SJ. Gene transfer into retinoblastoma cells. Biotechniques 1999; 26:444-446.

185. Daheshia M, Kuklin N, Kanangat S, Manickan E, Rouse BT. Suppression of ongoing ocular inflammatory disease by topical administration of plasmid DNA encoding IL-10. J Immunol 1997; 159:1945-1952.

186. Murata T, Kimura H, Sakamoto T, Osusky R, Spee C, Stout TJ, Hinton DR, Ryan SJ. Ocular gene therapy: experimental studies and clinical possibilities. Ophthalmic Res 1997; 29:242-251.

187. Li T, Davidson BL. Phenotype correction in retinal pigment epithelium in murine mucopolysaccharidosis VII by adenovirus-mediated gene transfer. Proc Natl Acad Sci 1995; 92:7700-7704.

188. Abraham NG, DaSilva JL, Lavrovsky Y et al. Invest Ophthalmol Vis Sci 1995; 36: 2202-2210.

189. Masuda I, Matsuo T, Yasuda T, Matsuo M. Gene transfer with liposomes to the intraocular tissues by different routes of administration. Invest Ophthalmol Vis Sci 1996; 37:1914-1920.

190. Matsuo T, Masuda I, Yasuda T, Matsuo N. Gene transfer to the retina of rat by liposome eye drops. Biochem Biophys Res Com 1996; 219:947-950.

191. Hangai M, Tanihara H, Honda Y, Kaneda Y. Introduction of DNA into the rat and primate trabecular meshwork by fusogenic liposomes. Invest Ophthalmol Vis Sci 1998; 39:509-516.

192. Shewring L, Collins L, Lightman SL, Hart S, Gustafsson K, Fabre JW. A non-viral vector system for efficient gene transfer to corneal endothelial cells via membrane integrins. Transplantation 1997; 64:763-769.

193. Dana MR, Yamada J, Streilein JW. Topical IL-1 receptor antagonist promotes corneal transplant survival. Transplantation 1997; 63: 1501-1507.

194. Yamada J, Dana MR, Zhu S-N, Alard P, Streilein JW. Interleukin-1 receptor antagonist suppresses allosensitization in corneal transplantation. Arch Ophthal 1998; 116: 1351 – 1357.

195. Dana MR, Dai R, Yamada J, Streilein JW. Interleukin-1 receptor antagonist suppresses Langerhans cell activity and promotes immune privilege. Invest Ophthal Vis Sci 1998; 39: 70 – 77.
196. Sano Y, Okamoto S, Streilein JW. Induction of donor-specific ACAID can prolong orthotopic corneal allograft survival in "high-risk" eyes. Curr Eye Res 1997; 16: 1171 – 1174.
197. Streilein JW. ACAID: A treatment option for the immunological ocular disorders. In: Ohno S, Oaki K, Usui M, Uchio E, editors. Uveitis Today, Proceedings of the Fourth International Symposium on Uveitis, Amsterdam, The Netherlands, 1998, 297 – 302.

12

TOPICAL SKIN IMMUNE SYSTEM RESPONSE MODIFIERS

Jan D. Bos
Department of Dermatology
Academic Medical Center
University of Amsterdam
Amsterdam, The Netherlands

INTRODUCTION

In dermatological diseases, both systemic and topical therapeutic options are available. The choice between them depends on a variety of factors, of which severity and spread of disease are among the obvious. Topical therapy is restrained by the physical and chemical properties of skin. Immunomodulation is possible but can only be understood with some knowledge of the skin immune system (SIS) [1]. Thus, an introduction to the physicochemical characteristics of skin and the essentials of the SIS is needed here first.

PHYSICOCHEMICAL CHARACTERISTICS OF SKIN

The skin is continuously exposed to the external world. During evolution, it has evolved into an organ which is difficult to penetrate from outside. The human integument is composed of three layers, from outside inwards: epidermis, dermis and subcutis. The epidermis is a regenerating tissue primarily consisting of keratinocytes, but melanocytes, Langerhans cells, Merkel cells, and some T lymphocytes are also present in normal human epidermis. Keratinocytes divide in the basal and suprabasal layers of epidermis, then migrate outwards, differentiate and undergo natural cell death, ending their cell cycle as corneocytes. These corneocytes do not contain a nucleus and are mainly composed of lipids and keratin-type proteins.

The physicochemical skin barrier is mainly formed by this corneal layer, a

A. W. Thomson (ed.), Therapeutic Immunosuppression, 323–332.
© 2001 *Kluwer Academic Publishers.*

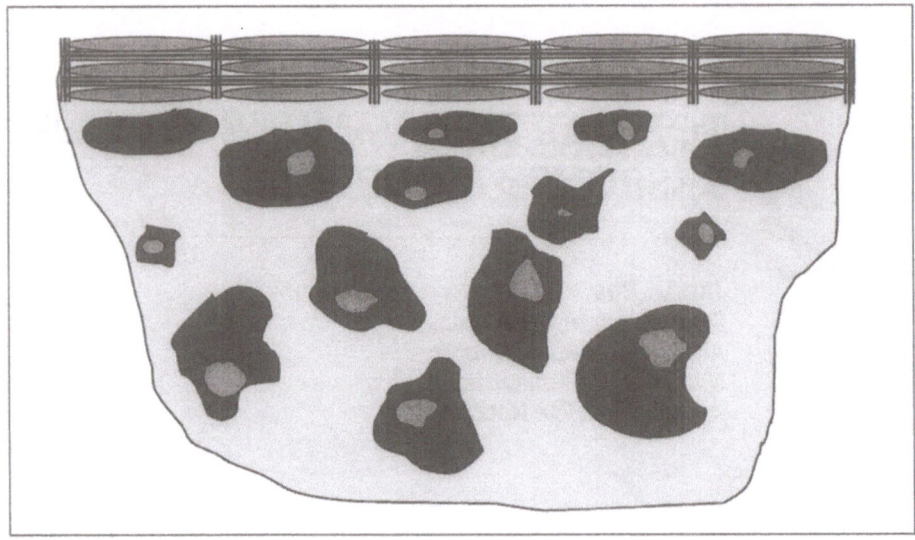

Figure 1
The epidermis when analyzed at the electron microscopic level shows that it is externally characterized by the presence of flattened anuclear keratinocytes (corneocytes), intertwined with a bilaminar lipid membrane.

complex structure consisting of these transformed keratinocytes intertwined with a bilaminar lipid layer (Figure 1). Its physical characteristics provide a primary protecting function which on first contact prevents penetration of substances varying from small water molecules to microbial agents. It also reflects light and part of ultraviolet irradiation.

However, there are a number of compounds that can reach the living tissues of the integument and such a phenomenon is used when topical drugs are developed for their subsequent use in dermatological disease. Since many of the known skin diseases are inflammatory, the most important topical drugs used in dermatology are the broad acting anti-inflammatory corticosteroids. In view of their side effects which vary from induction of irreversible skin atrophy to the facilitation of infections, there is an obvious need for more specific immunomodulating compounds.

It must be emphasized that the human skin has a particular threshold for the inroad of chemical compounds. The main barrier is formed by the corneal layer which allows penetration of only small molecules. Thus, biological response modifiers such as interferons, interleukins, and other cytokines or glycoprotein-type cytokine antagonists are not of interest for subsequent development in topical therapy. The exceptions are diseases in which the corneal layer is absent, such as in wounds. Platelet derived growth factor (PDGF) is indeed of use for enhancing wound healing in certain types of leg ulcers.

We have proposed the *"500 dalton rule for the penetration of drugs and chemical compounds"*, reflecting the relative impermeability of the human skin for molecules larger then 500 dalton [2]. An exception can be made for mucosal surfaces such as in the mouth and genitalia, where larger molecules can penetrate due to the absence of the corneal layer. Another exception seems to exist in patients with atopic dermatitis, whose eczema responds to drugs with a molecular weight of approximately 800 dalton, where other skin diseases cannot be managed with such compounds (*vide infra*).

THE SKIN IMMUNE SYSTEM (SIS)

Many dermatological diseases are related to interferences in the normal function of the skin immune system (SIS). The most widely known model is that of allergic contact dermatitis, which is a form of T-cell mediated delayed hypersensitivity. Normal persons do not react to hapten type chemical compounds, such as nickel salts, fragrances and preservatives that they are normally exposed to. Some individuals do get sensitized and upon repeated skin contact they develop a dermatitis or eczema. Since this is not what fits with normality, it might be studied as an imbalance of SIS. Many other diseases including psoriasis, atopic dermatitis and lichen ruber planus are thought to be dysregulations of SIS, often with a general background of abnormal reactivity.

The term SIS was coined to outline the complexity of cellular and humoral immune response-related elements that are normally present in human skin. In Table 1, they are summarized. The complexity of SIS also makes it possible to pharmacologically attack dysregulations, i.e. skin diseases, from various perspectives. Antihistamines block the histamine receptors on a variety of cells, but may be seen as drugs primarily directed at the mast cells, which produce histamine as well as a wide variety of other mediators after different types of stimulation. Cyclosporine is assumed to be primarily effective because it inhibits further activation of T cells, which play a central role in a number of common skin diseases. Knowledge of SIS is thus essential for the development of new therapeutical concepts in dermatology, including the development of topical compounds.

Table 1
Cellular and humoral constituents of the skin immune system.

cellular constituents	humoral constituents
keratinocytes	antimicrobial peptides, defensins
dendritic antigen presenting cells	complement and complement regulatory proteins
monocytes / macrophages	immunoglobulins
granulocytes	cytokines, neuropeptides
mast cells	fibrinolysins
lymphatic / vascular endothelial cells	eicosanoids and prostaglandins
T lymphocytes	free radicals

(adopted from [1])

CLASSICAL TOPICAL AGENTS IN DERMATOTHERAPY

Topical tar preparations have been in use for over 100 years. They are mentioned here because they are effective in a variety of dermatological diseases which all are thought to be immune-mediated. Although cosmetically unpleasant, they are still used because of their relative safety, although in Great Britain, there is serious concern about their possible carcinogenicity. In psoriasis, tar extracts are often used in combination with ultraviolet irradiation. In atopic dermatitis, especially in infants, they are sometimes preferred over corticosteroids or also used in alternate combination. As with most of the older drugs, controlled trials are sparse and the mode of action of tar preparations is not precisely known. Attempts have been made to identify the active ingredient in tar preparations, which contain over 800 different chemical structures.

Cignolin (anthralin) is an extract of a South American tree and has been in use for the topical therapy of psoriasis since the end of the 19th century. It is not effective in other skin diseases. It is toxic but may act by decreasing the expression of adhesion molecules, thereby inhibiting ongoing cell-to-cell contacts, including those necessary for promoting the ongoing immune activity thought to be central in psoriasis pathogenesis.

PHOTOTHERAPY USING VARIOUS FORMS OF ULTRAVIOLET IRRADIATION

Studying the effects of ultraviolet irradiation (UV) on the immune function of skin is known as photoimmunology. It has grown into a complex field in which a number of different modes of actions are studied separately. Ultraviolet irradiation is widely used in the therapy of a number of inflammatory diseases including psoriasis, atopic dermatitis and lichen planus. Biological activity increases with shortening wavelengths, while penetration into skin increases with wavelength. Thus, short wave UV types such as UVB have strong actions but tend to go no deeper than the superficial part of the papillary layer of the dermis. Long wave UV (UVA) is less effective from a biological point of view, but goes deeper. UVA is often used in combination with psoralens, a treatment modality known as PUVA photochemotherapy.

Central in the mode of action of UV is that it induces dimers in DNA, leading to loss of cell function and cell death. Keratinocytes are relatively resistant to such exposure, but T cells are very sensitive. Thus, one of the mode of actions of UV in T-cell mediated dermatoses is that the acting T cells are simply wiped out of the process.

Other effects of UV include photo-isomerization of *trans-* to *cis*-urocanic acid, where increased formation of cis-urocanic acid is known to be associated with immunosuppression, especially in models of delayed hypersensitivity. Furthermore, UV leads to free radical formation in the skin. Subsequently, there is damage to lipids and proteins, which may ad up to the cellular damage following DNA dimer formation.

Extracorporal photopheresis has been developed for the treatment of cutaneous T cell lymphoma (mycosis fungoides). Peripheral blood white cells are collected from patients that have ingested psoralens, and the white cells are irradiated extracorporally with UVA. Subsequently, the cells are reinfused into the patient. The mode of action of this complicated and expensive therapy is unknown. Its efficacy in certain stages of mycosis fungoides is established. It is also used in other diseases such as psoriasis and atopic dermatitis, in some centers, but controlled studies are lacking.

For psoriasis, it has been found that 311 nm is the most desirable part of UVB, and special units have been devised to conform to this. Wavelengths under 311 nm lead increasingly to erythema and sunburn, so that this modality is of great use in the phototherapy of psoriasis patients. In fact, it is replacing broad band UVB (280 - 320) as well as PUVA. In atopic dermatitis, longwave UVA (UVA1: 340 - 400) has recently become available. It has a promising future due to proven effectivity in atopic dermatitis and in morphea, a localized variant of scleroderma. It is a pity that equipment for small range UVB (311 nm) and long wave UVA1 is not generally available in dermatological centers around the world.

CORTICOSTEROIDS

Corticosteroids form the cornerstone of dermatological topical therapy. They are available in many chemical variants. In general, they are divided in 4 groups according to their potency. Topically applied corticosteroids generally have a molecular weight around 450 dalton, and thus are easily absorbed into the corneal layer. From there, they are gradually dispersed into the epidermal and superficial dermal layers. The reservoir function of the corneal layer makes it possible to only apply the corticosteroid once daily. There will be at least 24 hours of continuous influx of steroids from the corneal layer into the deeper parts of the skin.

Corticosteroids bind to cytosolic receptors, as a consequence of which gene promotor NF-κB molecules in the nucleus become diminished in availability. Thus, gene transcription of a large variety of genes is decreased, silencing out cellular activity of all cells of SIS as well as other cellular components of skin. The wide variety of dermatological indications for topical corticosteroid therapy might thus be explained by this broad mode of action. Those cellular components that are hyperactive in a given skin disease are silenced out and activity of the disease process is halted. In inflammatory and immune-mediated skin diseases, it is the keratinocytes, T cells and monocytes that are thought to be the principal targets of corticosteroid therapy.

NON-STEROIDAL ANTI-INFLAMMATORY DRUGS

The NSAIDs have been developed for rheumatic diseases, and at least two have been available as topical agents. Bufexamac is one example, and it has been used in atopic dermatitis. However, controlled studies are sparse and their efficacy is questioned. Other agents that interfere with leukotriene metabolism have been a target of studies for a long time, but until today, there is no such leukotriene inhibitor available for topical therapy in dermatology.

CYCLOSPORINE

The introduction of cyclosporine (CsA) in dermatological therapy has changed the therapeutical protocols in a number of common skin diseases such as psoriasis and atopic dermatitis.

Both CsA, as well as the cyclic macrolactams tacrolimus and ascomycins described below, are inflammatory cytokine inhibitors that inhibit the activation and proliferation of T-cells by interfering, at an early stage in the cell cycle, with the calcium-dependent transduction pathways which lead to gene expression. The cyclic immunosuppressants (Figure 2), as they are also called, become biologically active when they form a complex with their respective cytosolic immunophyllin, enzymes with peptidyl-prolyl cis-trans isomerase activity. The activated immunophyllin-cyclic immunosuppressant complex subsequently binds to calcineurin, a calcium- and calmodulin-dependent protein phosphatase. Calcineurin is required for the calcium-dependent signal transduction pathway which conveys the crucial information, necessary for the initiation of interleukin-2 (IL-2) synthesis, from the cell membrane into the nucleus [3]. Suppression of the phosphatase activity of calcineurin by the immunophyllin-cyclic immunosuppressant complex results in the inhibition of the T-cell specific transcription factor (NF-AT) which regulates IL-2 transcription [4], and so T-cell production is blocked.

CsA is given orally in doses between 3 and 5 mg/kg/day. It is remarkably effective but its side effect profile prevents it from being used commonly. Nephrotoxicity, hypertension and facilitation of the development of (skin) malignancies are of major concern. For severe cases of atopic dermatitis

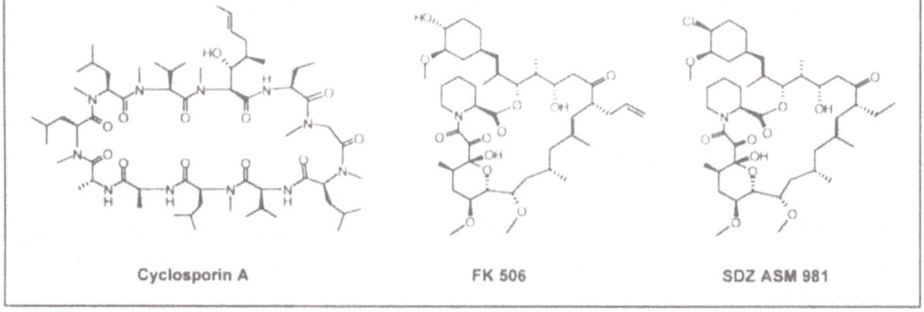

Cyclosporin A   FK 506   SDZ ASM 981

Figure 2
Molecular formulas of cyclosporine A, tacrolimus (FK506), and ascomycin (SDZ ASM 981).

and psoriasis, but also of pyoderma gangrenosum, lichen ruber planus and Behçet disease, systemic application of CsA is however a true advance in dermatotherapy.

The impressive efficacy of CsA has prompted studies into its possible use as a topical agent in dermatological indications. However, in accordance with our 500 dalton rule, topical CsA is not effective in atopic dermatitis, allergic contact dermatitis [5], and only in psoriasis when injected intralesionally [6]. The obvious reason for this lack of efficacy of topical CsA is its relatively large molecular weight, which is 1202 dalton. Topical CsA has been found to be effective in oral and genital diseases, where there is no corneal layer, and larger molecules can penetrate. Controlled studies have been published of topical CsA efficacy in oral lichen planus [7], but have not been easy to confirm [8]. Finally, topical CsA has been observed to have a potential advantage in the treatment of CsA-responsive ulcerating diseases, where there is no epidermis, such as pyoderma gangrenosum [9].

MACROLACTAMS

Tacrolimus (FK506) and ascomycin (SDZ ASM 981) are compounds with a molecular weight of 822 and 811 dalton respectively. As such, they are somewhat large to allow percutaneous absorption (500 dalton rule). Both compounds have a mode of action comparable to that of CsA as described above. The primary target of CsA, tacrolimus and ascomycin thus is the T lymphocyte. A major advantage of the possible use of tacrolimus and ascomycin over corticosteroids, which they are intended to (partially) replace, is that they do not induce skin atrophy [10]. The broad action of corticosteroids as described above also leads to unwanted effects, such as the decrease in collagen synthesis by dermal fibroblasts, ultimately leading to irreversible skin atrophy.

Tacrolimus was originally developed for transplantation medicine. It is now in use as an oral and intravenous agent for prevention of allograft rejection, especially of liver and kidney transplants [11]. It was also found to be very effective orally when given to patients with moderate to severe plaque type psoriasis [12-14]. As with CsA, investigations into the possibility of topical therapy of dermatological T-cell mediated diseases started. It was observed that especially (if not only) atopic dermatitis was responsive to the topical application of tacrolimus [15-18], but it was not effective topically in psoriasis [19]. Tacrolimus is now under development and registration as a topical agent for the use in infant and adult atopic dermatitis.

A similar compound, ascomycin SDZ ASM 981, is one of a series of ascomycins under development for use in man [20] . As a topical agent, it is under development and registration as a topical agent for the treatment of infant and adult atopic dermatitis. The first publication of the efficacy of ascomycin in adults with atopic dermatitis, using a double blind left to right in-patient comparison of active compound versus vehiculum showed an immediate effect on symptom scores including pruritus [21]. This was also observed in tacrolimus studies, and it is essential that pruritus is immediately relieved, because that is the only way to patient compliance and thus to efficacy. Other ascomycins are under study, while oral application is also under investigation. Until now, it has only been found to be useful in atopic dermatitis. It has been observed that ascomycin works topically in psoriasis, but only when used under occlusion, which is impractical [22].

It seems that atopic dermatitis patients have a distinct corneal layer with functional capacities different from those in normal controls or in patients with other skin diseases such as psoriasis.

Acknowledgements. *R. Rodenburg and A. Sibbes are gratefully acknowledged for preparing the Figures.*

REFERENCES

1. Bos JD (Ed.) Skin Immune System (SIS): Cutaneous Immunology and Clinical Immunodermatology. 2nd rev ed. Boca Raton: CRC Press, 1997.
2. Bos JD, Meinardi MMHM. The 500 Dalton rule for the cutaneous penetration of chemical compounds and drugs. Exp Dermatol 2000;9:224-8.
3. Bierer BE, Mattila PS, Standaert RF, Herzenberg LA, Burakoff SJ, Crabtree G, and Schreiber SL. Two distinct signal transmission pathways in T lymphocytes are inhibited by complexes formed between an immunophilin and either FK506 or rapamycin. Proc Natl Acad Sci USA 1990;87:9231-9235.
4. Shaw J-P, Utz PJ, Durand DB, Toole JJ, Emmel EA, Crabtree GR. Identification of a putative regulator of early T-cell activation genes. Science 1988;241:202-205.
5. De Rie MA, Meinardi MMHM, Bos JD. Lack of efficacy of topical cyclosporin A in atopic dermatitis and allergic contact dermatitis. Acta Derm Venereol (Stockh) 1991;71:452-4.
6. Powles AV, Baker BS, McFadden J, Rutman AJ, Griffiths CEM, Fry L. Intralesional injection of cyclosporin in psoriasis. Lancet 1988;351:537.
7. Eisen D, Ellis CN, Duell EA, et al. Effect of topical cyclosporin rinse on oral lichen planus. N Engl J Med 1990;328:290-4.
8. Levell NJ, MacLeod RI, Marks JM. Lack of effect of cyclosporin mouthwash in oral lichen planus. Lancet 1991;337:797-80.

9. Schuppe HC, Homey B, Assmannn T, Martens R, Ruzicka T. Topical tacrolimus for pyoderma gangrenosum. Lancet 1998;351:832.
10. Reitamo S, Rissanen J, Remitz A, Granlund H, Erkko P, Elg P, Autio P, Lauerma AI. Tacrolimus ointment does not affect collagen synthesis: results of a single-center randomized trial. J Invest Dermatol 1998;111:396-398.
11. European FK506 Multicentre Liver Study Group. Randomised trial comparing tacrolimus (FK506) and cyclosporin in prevention of liver allograft rejection. Lancet 1994;344:423-428.
12. Jegasothy BV, Ackerman CD, Todo S, Fung JJ, Abu-Elmagd K, Starzl TE. Tacrolimus (FK 506) - A new therapeutic agent for severe recalcitrant psoriasis. Arch Dermatol 1992;128:781-785.
13. European FK506 Multicentre Psoriasis Study Group. Systemic tacrolimus (FK 506) is effective for the treatment of psoriasis in a double-blind, placebo-controlled study. Arch Dermatol 1996;132 419-423.
14. Bos JD. Tacrolimus (FK506) in the treatment of psoriasis. In: Roenigk HH Jr, Maibach HI, editors. Psoriasis. New York: Marcel Dekker 1998; 743-737.
15. Aoyama H, Tabata N, Tanaka M, Uesugi Y, Tagami H. Successful treatment of resistant facial lesions of atopic dermatitis with 0.1% FK506 ointment. Brit J Dermatol 1995;133:492-500.
16. Ruzicka Th, Bieber Th, Schöpf E et al. A short-term trial of tacrolimus ointment for atopic dermatitis. N Engl J Med 1997;337:816-821.
17. Alaiti S, Kang S, Fiedler VC et al. Tacrolimus (FK506) ointment for atopic dermatitis: A Phase I study in adults and children. J Am Acad Dermatol 1998;38:69-76.
18. Boguniewicz M, Fiedler VC, Raimer S, Lawrence ID, Leung DYM, Hanifin JM. A Randomized, vehicle-controlled trial of tacrolimus ointment for treatment of atopic dermatitis in children. J Allergy Clin Immun 1998; 103:637-644.
19. Zonneveld IM, Rubins A, Jablonska S, Dobozy A, Ruzicka T, Kind P, Dubertret L, Bos JD. Topical tacrolimus is not effective in chronic plaque psoriasis. Arch Dermatol 1998;134:1101-1102.
20. Mollison KW, Fey TA, Gauvin DM et al. Discovery of ascomycin analogs with potent topical but weak systemic activity for treatment of inflammatory skin diseases. Curr Pharm Des 1998;4:367-379.
21. Van Leent EJM, Gräber M, Thurston M, Wagenaar A, Spuls PhI, Bos JD. Effectiveness of the ascomycin macrolactam SDZ ASM 981 in the topical treatment of atopic dermatitis. Arch Dermatol 1998;134:805-809.
22. Mrowietz U, Graeber M, Bräutigam M, Thurston M, Wagenaar A, Weidinger G, Christophers E. The novel ascomycin derivate SDZ ASM 981 is effective for psoriasis when used topically under occlusion. Brit J Dermatol 1998;139:992-996.

13

LOCAL IMMUNOSUPPRESSION: THE LUNG

Aldo T. Iacono[1], Gilbert J. Burckart[2], Adriana Zeevi[3], Erdogan Kunter[1] and Bartley P. Griffith[4]

[1] Department of Medicine
[2] Department of Pharmacy and Therapeutics
[3] Department of Pathology
[4] Department of Surgery
University of Pittsburgh
Pittsburgh, Pennsylvania, USA

INTRODUCTION

Lung transplantation represents an unusual situation in solid organ transplantation in that the graft is accessible to the external environment. In this situation aerosolized pharmacologic agents have direct access to the donor graft, and the technology for delivering medication by the inhalational route is well developed for other pulmonary disorders. In 1988, a team of investigators at the University of Pittsburgh made the decision to pursue aerosolized immunosuppression for lung transplant recipients based upon the belief that other limited models of localized immunosuppression have been successful, and the current pharmacologic regimen was not adequate for managing lung transplant rejection.

The driving force for pursuing new approaches to immunosuppression in lung transplantation was the incidence of chronic rejection in the recipients. Chronic rejection most frequently manifests histologically as obliterative bronchiolitis, a progressive inflammatory process leading to scarring and occlusion of small airways [1,2]. Early in the disease no demonstrable change in pulmonary function may be observed, but the usual course of chronic rejection is progressive deterioration with worsening pulmonary function and increasing symptoms of dyspnea and fatigue [3-5]. Obliterative bronchiolitis is traditionally treated with short term enhancement of immune suppression consisting of pulse corticosteroids and antilymphocyte

333

A. W. Thomson (ed.), Therapeutic Immunosuppression, 333–356.
© 2001 *Kluwer Academic Publishers.*

globulin, after which maintenance immune suppression is increased to tolerance [6-8]. These treatments are associated with significant morbidity and mortality as 49% of the 65 patients in our center with this diagnosis have experienced serious infectious complications following antithymocyte globulin for recurrent graft rejection, with three deaths as a result of their infections. In over 30% of lung transplant patients treated for obliterative bronchiolitis, persistent histological evidence of scarring of small airways and progressive loss of lung function is observed [3, 6-9]. These patients have a dismal prognosis with a life expectancy of less than two years.

Hepatic and renal toxicity often limit the dosing of cyclosporine (CsA, Neoral, Novartis, East Hanover, NJ) in patients with graft rejection [10]. If CsA could be delivered directly into the transplanted lung by aerosol inhalation, higher concentrations of CsA in the graft may be achieved which could result in improvement of rejection with acceptable systemic toxicity. The concept of using CsA as an aerosol was originally proposed by Dr. Rene Duquesnoy, but the task of turning this concept into a clinical reality was larger than anyone in the investigative team imagined at the time.

The clinical use of CsA as an immunosuppressive aerosol in lung transplantation was encouraged by a diverse group of studies that had been conducted by other investigators previously. A sponge matrix allograft model first demonstrated the local development of cells within the graft that are responsive against the donor [11]. Local radiation therapy had been used in canine renal and heterotopic heart allografts with some success [12,13]. Human kidney allografts also have been reported to benefit from local radiation therapy [14]. Regional delivery of steroids by intra-arterial infusion results in downregulation of class II MHC antigen and IL-2 receptors [15] and prolongation of heterotopic cardiac allografts in rats [16]. Intra-arterial CsA has prolonged rat heterotopic heart allograft survival beyond that observed with a similar intravenous or oral CsA dose [17], and demonstrated that the highest CsA tissue concentration in recipient tissue was achieved in the lungs. Therefore, the stage was set for the development of a therapeutic regimen that could directly deliver CsA to the transplanted lung or lungs in our patient population.

ANIMAL STUDIES

Our initial studies with aerosolized CsA were conducted in dogs. Our first attempts to deliver aerosolized CsA were in normal anesthetized and intubated dogs [18]. The CsA was dissolved in ethanol since this appeared to be the only reasonable vehicle for administration to animals or human subjects that could solubilize CsA to the extent necessary. This initial protocol involved dissolving 200 mg of CsA powder in 5 mL of 95% USP ethanol and nebulizing the solubilized drug via a small particle aerosol generator (SPAG-2, ICN Pharmaceuticals, Cosa Mesa, CA). Nebulization was complicated by the precipitation of CsA within the nebulization chamber as the ethanol was volatilized off, which clogged the SPAG-2 generator. Future protocols with ethanol used 100% absolute ethanol in an attempt to overcome this problem.

Five dogs received the 200 mg nebulized CsA daily for eight (8) doses via endotracheal tube, and blood and tissue concentrations were measured. Sufficient tissue was available to distinguish proximal airway, distal airway and lung parenchymal concentrations of CsA. Trough blood levels before the final nebulized dose of CsA were less than 50 ng/mL in all cases while lung parenchymal levels were greater than 700 ng/gm. Whole blood CsA levels did increase following the dose of CsA, and peaked at 100-250 ng/mL 60 minutes following the dose. The CsA concentrations observed in proximal and distal airway (up to 25,000 ng/gm) were 10 to 100 times the concentrations observed in kidney and heart tissue. The aerosolized administration of CsA did not appear to cause any damage as measured by blood gases in the animals or by histologic examination. Therefore, we concluded that while the daily intubation of the dogs was labor-intensive and time-consuming, the model of canine aerosolized CsA delivery was adequate for an initial trial in canine lung transplantation.

The study of aerosolized CsA in canine lung transplantation that followed was reported by Drs. Robert Dowling, Marco Zenati et al in 1990 [19]. The model was a canine single lung transplant model, and 200 mg CsA was aerosolized daily for eight doses to eight animals as in the previous study in non-transplanted animals. Six animals were transplanted but received no immunosuppressive therapy as the control group. Table 1 lists the grade of rejection measured on open lung biopsy on postoperative day #7 in the control and CsA-treated groups.

Over 75% of the trough blood samples obtained in the CsA-aerosol treatment group had whole blood HPLC concentrations less than 100 ng/mL. The average blood concentrations at 20 and 60 minutes after the CsA dose rose to 165 and 185 ng/mL respectively. Mean trough and 60 minutes post aerosol lung parenchymal levels were 2424 and 25,550 ng/gm respectively, but considerable variation existed between animals. Grade 0 histologic rejection

Table 1
Grade of rejection in the CsA-aerosol treated and control groups following canine single lung transplantation.

Histologic Grade of Rejection	Control Group (n=6)	ScA Aerosol Group (n=7)
0	0	1
1+	0	1
2+	0	3
3+	0	2
4+	6	0

was observed in the animals with the highest measured concentrations of CsA in lung tissue. This initial lung transplant study demonstrated that aerosolized CsA was effective in suppressing the rejection process even when very low concentrations of drug could be measured in blood.

The evolution of this therapy required that a greater number of animals be studied to both investigate the toxicologic properties of aerosolized CsA and to further validate its therapeutic effect. The procedures used in the initial dog studies were too difficult to carry out in large numbers of animals. Therefore the next studies were performed using rats and a rat model of lung transplantation.

The rat studies were conducted with the collaboration of Drs. Michelle Schaper and Andrew Duncan using the Pitt generator for the production of the CsA aerosol. The first study in non-transplanted rats involved administering 50 mg/m^3 aerosolized CsA to 15 Lewis rats for 45 minutes [5]. Five rats were sacrificed at 90 minutes, five were sacrificed at 6 hours, and the remaining five rats were sacrificed at 24 hours. Table 2 presents the tissue and blood concentrations observed in these animals. This initial study provided the basis for dosage adjustment in a 30 day toxicology trial and in a rat lung transplant trial that followed.

The toxicology study was conducted in 10 non-transplanted Lewis rats who were exposed to 50 mg/m^3 CsA aerosol for 90 minutes per day [5]. Five animals were exposed for 15 days and sacrificed, and five animals were exposed for 30 consecutive days. Histopathological and microbiologic examination of the lungs, kidneys, livers and hearts of the ten exposed rats revealed no lesions or infections. All whole blood CsA concentrations by HPLC were less than 50 ng/mL in all animals.

Table 2
Tissue and blood CsA levels after a single exposure to aerosolized CsA in rats.

	90 min post (n=5)	6 h post (n=5)	24 h post (n=5)
Lung	7102 ± 756	1670 ± 285	208 ± 35
Liver	1045 ± 68	1668 ± 368	ND
Kidney	639 ± 56	647 ± 71	ND
Heart	248 ± 23	88 ± 11	ND
Blood	93 ± 22.5	71 ± 13	ND

Concentrations by HPLC expressed as ng/mL in whole blood and ng/gm in tissues (mean ± SD)
ND = not detectable (< 50 ng/gm or mL)
Reprinted with permission from [5].

Table 3
Rejection grade and incidence of pneumonia in a rat lung transplant model treated with aerosolized or intramuscular CsA.

	CsA Dose/Route	Mean Rejection Grade	Pneumonia
Group 1	None	4	--
Group 2	25 mg/kg IM x 1	2.2	3/10
Group 3	25 mg/kg IM x 4	1.8	5/10
Group 4	3.6 mg/kg aerosol x 7	1.2	0/6

The rat lung transplant experiment compared a control untreated group to rats given a 25 mg/kg dose of intramuscular CsA and to an aerosolized CsA group [5]. The intramuscular group either received a single injection or received a daily injection for the first four postoperative days. The aerosolized CsA dose was increased from the toxicologic studies to 180 mg/m³ for three hours daily for seven doses. Microbiologic and histologic studies were performed in all groups, and the results of all groups on postoperative day #6 are presented in Table 3.

A question that remained in the previous rat study was whether there was a definite dose-response relationship with aerosolized CsA. This question was addressed in an extension of the previous rat study, where low, intermediate and high dose aerosolized CsA dose groups were added [20]. As can be seen in Table 4, a clear relationship was apparent between the dose of the aerosolized CsA administered to the transplanted rat, the concentrations of CsA that were achieved in blood and lung tissue, and the histologic grade

Table 4
Doses of aerosolized CsA in a rat left lung transplant model in relation to blood/tissue concentrations and grade of histologic rejection.

CsA Aerosol (mg/kg/day)	CsA blood (ng/mL)	CsA lung (ng/gm)		Grade of Rejection
		Left	Right	
0.98	198	1580	2853	3.25
1.94	390	3423	5253	2.3
3.6	1057	7838	10,516	1.3

of rejection after seven days of aerosolized CsA therapy. This observation may be critically important as we attempt to develop dosing regimens in patients with differing needs for immunosuppressive therapy.

A concurrent avenue of investigation with the rat studies was to attempt a different method of administration of the CsA aerosol to dogs. More sophisticated studies of the administration of aerosolized CsA in beagle dogs were conducted in collaboration with Drs. Bruce Muggenberg and Mark Hoover of the Lovelace Inhalation Toxicology Research Institute [21]. These studies included the use of radiolabeling the CsA aerosol by adding ^{99m}Tc as a sulfur colloid to the CsA, and making an assessment of whole body and lung deposition using a gamma camera. The Lovelace nebulizer was used to administer the aerosol via an oral mouthpiece to the dogs, and demonstrated that while 20 to 78% of the aerosolized dose was deposited in the body of the dog, only 5 to 24% was deposited in the lungs. Therefore significant amounts of the CsA given by this method were deposited in the mouth and swallowed or were cleared from large airways by mucociliary action and swallowed. Bronchoalveolar lavage (BAL) was performed 24 hours after the aerosol dose and identified only one biochemical abnormality; lactate dehydrogenase was increased in the BAL fluid after CsA aerosol as compared to the BAL fluid of animals given CsA by other routes of administration.

The most recent study was conducted in a rat ACI to Lewis single lung transplant model. The animals were treated posttransplant with either no therapy, aerosolized CsA in doses of 1 to 3 mg/kg/day, or intramuscular CsA in doses of 2, 5, 10 and 15 mg/kg/day [22]. Lung tissue concentrations were measured after drug administration and lung histopathology was examined at postoperative day 6. Aerosolized CsA was able to control the rejection (grade 1 rejection) at 3 mg/kg/day, and only the highest systemic dose of CsA (15 mg/kg/day) was able to achieve the same biopsy results. Aerosolized

CsA was able to accomplish this immunosuppression at much lower blood concentrations than with an equally effective systemic dose (725 ng/ml for the aerosol, 3306 ng/ml for the intramuscular drug). The expression of mRNA for IL-6, IL-10 and IFN-γ was substantially more suppressed with the highest systemic dosage of CsA than with the aerosolized CsA, but the long term implications of intense cytokine suppression is unclear in relation to the development of chronic rejection. These studies demonstrated that suppression of the immune response to the graft can be achieved with low doses of aerosolized CsA, resulting in a lower systemic exposure which could translate into reduced systemic toxicity.

HUMAN STUDIES

Aerosolized cyclosporine in ethanol

Prior to the first human experiments, cyclosporine aerosols were tested *in vitro* and an aerosol of cyclosporine in ethanol and propylene glycol was produced which was shown to be optimal for pulmonary deposition (mass median aerodynamic diameter 1.2 mm). The addition of a radiolabel (technetium bound to human serum albumin, ^{99m}Tc-HSA) enabled calculation of the dose of cyclosporine deposited in the allograft as summarized below [23].

Prelude to Clinical Studies

In previous Phase I and Phase II clinical trials performed at the University of Pittsburgh and by our collaborators at SUNY-Stony Brook, aerosolized cyclosporine in ethanol was effectively delivered to the lungs of patients with end stage obliterative bronchiolitis. The determinants of the factors that affected the dose deposited in the lung allograft were analyzed [24].

In this study, we have shown that total lung deposition of the inhaled cyclosporine particles is heterogeneous in individual recipients, being dependent on local anatomical (single versus double lung) and physiological factors (presence of obstructive airways disease and obliterative bronchiolitis). Thus, the initial nebulizer charge (milligrams of cyclosporine) does not correlate with deposition (milligrams of cyclosporine) within the transplanted lung. In fact, we found that both disease in the native lung (in single lung transplants) and the extent of rejection in the allograft affected the regional distribution of the deposited aerosolized cyclosporine.

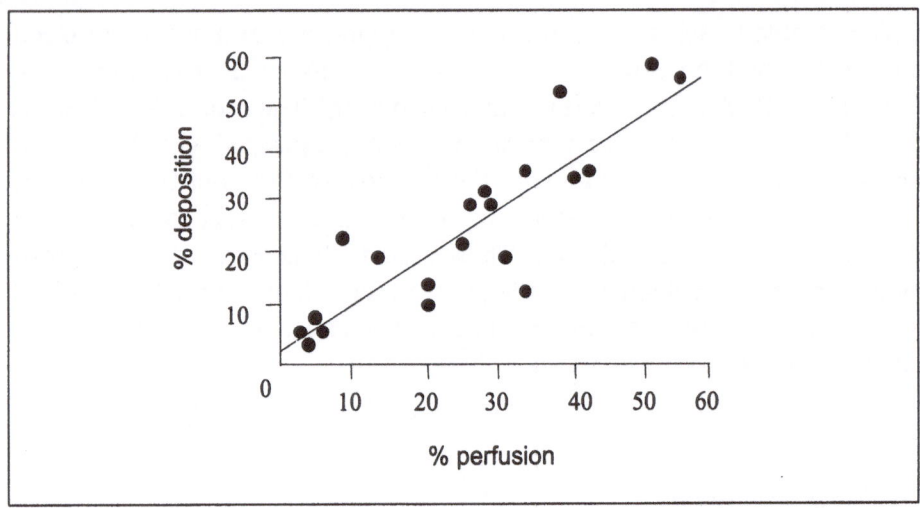

Figure 1
Distribution of deposited aerosolized cyclosporine determined by gamma camera in pulmonary allografts of patients with severe obliterative bronchiolitis.
Reprinted by permission from [24]. *There is a close correlation between deposited drug and preserved lung as indexed by regional perfusion (r=0.891, p<0.0001).

As shown in Figure 1, severe pulmonary disease (as evidenced by diminished parenchymal perfusion) resulted in reduced deposition of aerosolized cyclosporine [24]. These data suggest that patients with advanced lung ejection do not demonstrate predictable patterns of inhaled drug deposition. This is in contrast to some other groups of patients. For example, most patients with AIDS inhaling radiolabeled pentamidine will have peripheral, uniform deposition. Patients with severe COPD inhaling radioaerosols will consistently deposit the aerosol in their central airways. The reason for the lack of predictability of deposition in the allograft probably relates to the asymmetric nature of the disease processes between allograft and native lung in single lung transplants and in non-uniform disease due to obliterative bronchiolitis in double lung patients. These observations suggest that direct measurement of regional deposition will be essential in initial studies of efficacy. These difficulties do not preclude aerosolized cyclosporine therapy, since increasing the quantity of inhaled cyclosporine can subsequently increase the regional dose.

Aerosolized cyclosporine in propylene glycol

In parallel to the deposition study (which was a nested study in a Phase 1 clinical trial), we assessed histologic and functional changes in these

Table 5
Histology Prior to and Within 86 Days of Aerosol cyclosporine and
Radiolabeled Cyclosporine Deposition Measurements[a]

Patient #	Histology[b]		Radiolabeled cyclosporine deposition (mg)	
	Pre (Grade)	Rx Cs (Grade/Day)	Right lung	Left lung
#1	Active OB (C1a) Mild AR (A2a)	Inactive OB (C1b/43) No AR (43)	25.4 (allograft)	9.5 (allograft)
#2	Active OB (C1a)	Mild AR (A2a/21)	15.8 (native)	6.9 (allograft)
#3	Active OB (C1a) Mild AR (A2c)	Minimal AR (A1c/14)[†]	12.3 (native)	20.5 (allograft)
#4	Active OB (C1a)	No OB (86) Moderate AR (A3a/86)	11.0 (allograft)	9.4 (allograft)
#5	Active OB (C1a) Moderate AR (A3a,c)	No OB (14) Minimal AR (A1b/14)	N/A	N/A
#6	Active OB (C1a) Moderate AR (A3)	Inactive OB (C1b/47) Minimal AR (A1b/47)	N/A	N/A
#7	Active OB (C1a)	Active OB (C1a[c]/24)	N/A	N/A
#8	Active OB (C1a)	Lymphocytic bronchitis (B1/65)	N/A	N/A
#9	Active OB (C1a)	Inactive OB (C1b/26)	N/A	N/A

[a] Definition of abbreviations Pre = histology before Aerosol cyclosporine, Rx Cs = Histology during Aerosol cyclosporine treatment.
[b] Chronic rejection (C); 1 = total, a = active, b = inactive; OB = obliterative bronchiolitis. Acute rejection (AR); A1 = minimal, A2 = mild, A3 = moderate, a = with small airways, b = without small airways, c = large airways. [†] = no small airways to assess OB.
[c] The degree of active airway inflammation during Aerosol cyclosporine is diminished when compared to the pre - therapy biopsy. NA = not available.
Reprinted with permission from [25].

patients with obliterative bronchiolitis [25]. Aerosolized cyclosporine was given as rescue in 9 lung transplant recipients with unremitting chronic graft rejection with histologically documented active obliterative bronchiolitis and severe, progressively worsening obstructive airways disease. Improvement in histologic inflammation associated with active obliterative bronchiolitis was seen in 7 patients during aerosolized cyclosporine (see Table 5).

Bronchoalveolar lavage (BAL) and peripheral blood (PBL) cells were analyzed for the presence of mRNA using ^{32}P-labeled primers of cytokines IL-2, IL-6, IL-10 and IFN-γ using reverse transcriptase – polymerase chain reaction (RT-PCR). IL-2 and IL-10 in BAL and PBL was not informative. Upregulation of IL-2 mRNA was seen in a few samples only after antigen stimulation while IL-10 was present in all BAL samples tested during rejection and quiescence.

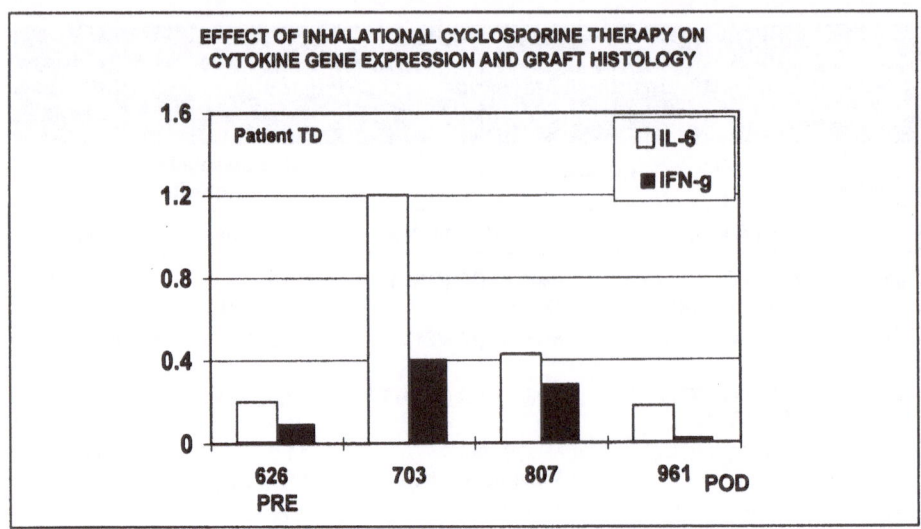

Figure 2
Cytokine gene expression before and after the administration of aerosolized cyclosporine in a lung transplant patient.

Changes in histology correlated with IL-6 and IFN-γ mRNA expression. As seen in Figure 2, the patient's IL-6 and IFN-γ in RNA expressed as a ratio to β-actin diminished following ACsA treatment 6 and 4 fold respectively. Overall in the 9 patients tested post-treatment IL-6 and IFN-γ mRNA expression were significantly ($p < 0.005$) lower, ranging from 2 to 150 and 8-90 fold lower respectively [26].

Lung function was analyzed in the 7 histologic responders and 9 control patients with similar rejection patterns with histologic bronchiolitis obliterans and the individual slopes of the FVC and FEV$_1$ were compared. By regression analysis, both FVC and FEV$_1$ declined significantly in the pre-treatment period in the aerosolized cyclosporine and control group ($p = 0.03$) and the rate of decline in these groups were comparable. In contrast, during aerosolized cyclosporine or a comparable period in controls, the slopes of the FVC and FEV$_1$ continued to decline in the control group ($p = 0.004$) whereas in patients who received aerosolized cyclosporine there was stabilization of pulmonary function ($p = 0.300$).

Changes in Histology In All Those Patients That Received Aerosolized Cyclosporine For Refractory Histologic Bronchiolitis Obliterans

Of 20 patients that had transbronchial biopsy immediately prior to and fol-

Table 6
Changes In Histology In All Patients With Histologic Bronchiolitis Obliterans Treated With Aerosol cyclosporine.

Patient #	Histology Pre-Aerosol cyclosporine	Histology Post Aerosol cyclosporine	Days of Initial TB Bx
1	A_3C_{1a}	$A_{1\ no\ ob}$	25
2	A_2	A_1	93
3	C_{1a}	$A_{3\ no\ ob}$	146
4	A_1	A_1	78
5	A_2C_{1a}	C_{1a}	24
6	A_3C_{1a}	CMV	28
7	A_3C_{1a}	A_3C_{1a}	31
8	A_3	A_3C_{1a}	15
9	A_2	A_2	57
10	A_2	A_2C_{1a}	53
11	C_{1a}	C_{1a}	32
12	B_1	Neg	49
13	C_{1a}	C_{1b}	38
14	C_{1a}	A_1B_1	88
15	C_{1a}	B_1	63
16	C_{1b}	C_{1a}	278
17	C_{1a}	C_{1a}	83
18	B_1	B_1B_2	54
19	C_{1a}	C_{1b}	49
20	C_{1a}	C_{1a}	62

Definition of abbreviations: Histology Pre Aerosol cyclosporine = Histology immediately prior to aerosolized cyclosporine administration; Histology Post Aerosol cyclosporine = Histology immediately after initiation of aerosolized cyclosporine administration; Day of Initial TBBx = Day first transbronchial biopsy performed after initiation of aerosolized cyclosporine, A_0 = No acute rejection; A_1 = Minimal acute rejection; A_2 = Mild acute rejection; A_3 = Moderate acute rejection A_4 = Severe acute rejection; Neg. = no histologic abnormalities; Possible Ar = Possible acute rejection; CMV = Cytomegalovirus pneumonia; DAD = Diffuse alveolar damage; NA = Not available; B1 = lymphocytic bronchitis; B2 = lymphocytic bronchiolitis; C_{1a} = active obliterative bronchiolitis; C_{1b} = inactive obliterative bronchiolitis; no ob = no obliterative bronchiolitis.

lowing aerosolized cyclosporine administration, 10/20 patients whose biopsy results failed to improve by conventional immunosuppression demonstrated a reduction of the mononuclear cell inflammatory infiltrate associated with bronchiolitis obliterans soon after initiation of aerosolized cyclosporine (see Table 6).

These data indicate that aerosolized cyclosporine reverses histologic abnormalities associated with bronchiolitis obliterans which, prior to use of this drug, was refractory to conventional forms of immunosuppression including tacrolimus, anti-lymphocyte globulin and pulsed corticosteroids (methylprednisolone 1gm I.V. for 3 consecutive days, Atgam 15mg/kg I.V. for 15 days).

Protocol # 002: Refractory Acute Rejection

As of February 2, 1998, 59 patients received aerosolized cyclosporine because of acute rejection that failed to respond to conventional immunosuppressive treatments. Most patients failed to improve clinically and by biopsy after having their rejection treated by multiple cycles of corticosteroids and anti-lymphocyte globulin. The average number of rejection events prior to initiation of aerosolized cyclosporine was 4.7±2.7 per patient during 462 days.

Reversal of Refractory Acute Rejection Based On First Biopsy Taken Following Rescue With Aerosolized Cyclosporine

A total of 38/59 (64%) of patients had a reduction in their histologic grade of acute rejection by initial transbronchial lung biopsy usually performed within 30-60 days after initiation of aerosolized cyclosporine. Moreover, 9 of the 59 patients that did not decrease their rejection grade initially, did so by the second biopsy accounting for an 80% early response rate following initiation of aerosol cyclosporine (see Table 7).

Reduction in Histologic and Clinical Acute Rejection Events Occurs During Aerosolized Cyclosporine

Transbronchial lung biopsy is performed at three-month intervals or more frequently should patients receiving aerosolized cyclosporine develop symptoms or signs of rejection prior to this designated interval. On average, the duration between biopsies was 54.3 days prior to initiation of aerosolized cyclosporine versus 74.7 days during aerosol cyclosporine. The total number of rejection events diagnosed histologically decreased by 46% following initiation of cyclosporine aerosol (mean 4.6 number of rejection events/patient/462 days versus 2.5 events/patient/627 days.) The average duration of follow-up after initiation of aerosolized cyclosporine was greater during aerosol cyclosporine maintenance compared to the interval that patients received conventional immunosuppression exclusively (mean 627 days/patient after initiation of treatment versus 462 days prior to aerosol cyclosporine).

Table 7
Histology of Pulmonary Allograft Rejection Immediately Prior to and Following Initiation of Aerosolized Cyclosporine In Patients with Acute Refractory Rejection

Patient #	Histology Pre ACA	Histology Post Aerosol cyclosporine	Days of Initial TB Bx
1	A_2	A_0B_1	29
2	A_3	Neg	32
3	A_3	CMV	26
4	A_2	A_1; B_1	39
5	A_2C_{1a}	(no small airways)	70
6	A_2	Neg.	45
7	A_2	B_1	21
8	A_3	A_1	26
9	A_2	A_2	18
10	A_2	Neg	78
11	A_3	A_3	44
12	A_3	A_3	9
13	A_2	A_3;C_{1a}	63
14	A_3	A_0B_1	38
15	A_3	A_3	42
16	A_2	A_1	57
17	A1 Previous bx A_2	A_1	63
18	A_3C_{1a}	A_2	69
19	A_3	A_3	49
20	A_3	A_2	42
21	A_4	N/A	22
22	A_3	A_1	21
23	A_3C_{1a}	A_4C_{1a}	47
24	A_3;C_{1a}	B_1	657
25	A_2	A_3	56
26	A_3;C_{1a}	A_3C_{1a}	15
27	A_3	A_1	34
28	A_2	A_3	49
29	A_4	A_1	54
30	A_1; C_{1a}	A_1	46
31	A_2	B_1	17
32	A_3	A_1	48
33	A_3	Neg	13
34	A_3	$A_2 C_{1a}$	22
35	B_2	A_1	72

(continued on next page)

Patient #	Histology Pre ACA	Histology Post Aerosol cyclosporine	Days of Initial TB Bx
36	A_2; C_1a	A_3; C_1a	62
37	A_2	A_1	41
38	A_2	B_1	55
39	A_3	A_1	29
40	A_1 (prev. C_{1b})	A_3 ;C_1a	619
41	A_2	A_2	57
42	A_3	A_2 ;C_1a	87
43	A_3	A_3	11
44	Pneum. (BOS)	A_1	52
45	A_2	$C_{1a}A_1$	70
46	A_2	A_0B_1	40
47	DAD	A_4	26
48	A_2C_{1a}	A_1	56
49	A_2	Neg	63
50	A_3	Neg	55
51	A_3C_{1a}	A_1C_{1a}	37
52	A_4	Neg	27
53	A_4	Neg	47
54	A_1 (previous A_3)	A_1	44
55	A_2	CMV	44
56	A_4	A_3	17
57	A_1 (previous A_3)	CMV	45
58	A_3	A_2	19
59	A_3	A_1	22

Definition of abbreviations: Histology Pre Aerosol cyclosporine = Histology immediately prior to aerosolized cyclosporine administration; Histology Post Aerosol cyclosporine = Histology immediately after initiation of aerosolized cyclosporine administration; Day After Initial TBBx = Day first transbronchial biopsy performed after initiation of aerosolized cyclosporine, A_0= No acute rejection; A_1 =Minimal acute rejection; A_2 = Mild acute rejection; A_3 = Moderate acute rejection A_4 = Severe acute rejection; Neg. = no histologic abnormalities; Possible Ar = Possible acute rejection; CMV = Cytomegalovirus pneumonia; DAD = Diffuse alveolar damage; NA = Not available; B1 = lymphocytic bronchitis; B2 = lymphocytic bronchiolitis; C_{1a} = active obliterative bronchiolitis; C_{1b} = inactive obliterative bronchiolitis; no ob = no obliterative bronchiolitis

These data indicate that aerosol cyclosporine reverses rejection which was previously refractory to all forms of conventional immunotherapy and that the rate of histologic acute rejection is substantially reduced when aerosolized cyclosporine is added to the conventional oral immunosuppressive drug regimen.

Table 8
Incidence of Acute and Chronic Rejection Before and During Aerosol cyclosporine[a]

	Number Bx Pre	Number ACR Pre	Number CR Pre	Days Pre	Number Bx Post	Number ACR Post	Number CR Post	Days Post	FUD	% Change ACR Pre vs Post
Mean	8.5	4.6	0.5	462	7	2.5	0.7	523	627	-46%
Median	8	4	0	327	7	2	0	477	554	-50%
S.D.	5.3	2.5	1.1	455	4.2	3	1.7	439	438	
	54.3 days/biopsy									74.7 days/biopsy

[a]Definition of abbreviations: Number Bx Pre., Number of biopsies performed prior to initiation of aerosolized cyclosporine; Number ACR Pre, Number of biopsies showing acute rejection of grade ≥ 2 prior to initiation of aerosol cyclosporine; Number CR Pre, Number of biopsies showing chronic rejection prior to initiation of aerosol cyclosporine; Days Pre, Average number of days after transplantation prior to initiation of aerosolized cyclosporine; Number Bx Post, Number of biopsies performed after initiation of aerosolized cyclosporine; Number ACR Post, Number of biopsies showing acute rejection of grade ≥ 2 after initiation of aerosol cyclosporine; Number CR Post, Number of biopsies showing chronic rejection after initiation of aerosolized cyclosporine; Days Post, Average number of days of therapy on maintenance aerosolized cyclosporine; FUD, total duration of follow up after initiation of aerosol cyclosporine; % Change ACR Pre versus Post, change in rate of acute rejection prior to and after initiation of Aerosol cyclosporine.

Table 8 summarizes the incidence of histologic rejection events and treatments administered with pulsed corticosteroids and anti-lymphocyte globulin before and during, administration of cyclosporine aerosol.

BAL IL-6 and IFN-γ cytokine mRNA expression in 17 recipients with refractory acute cellular rejection was analyzed before and after approximately 180 days of ACsA treatment. With the exception of two histologic nonresponders in each group a decline in cytokine expression was associated with improved lung histology (see Figure 3).

The expression of IL-6 and IFN-γ mRNA in recipients with refractory acute rejection was significantly greater than that in a group of patients with reversible rejection [26]. Although after 50 days of treatment there was a marked reduction in mRNA expression for both IL-6 and IFN-γ in BAL cells it did not reach the baseline level of control patients without rejection. Based on our findings, at least 180 days exposure to ACsA was necessary to achieve stable lung function [27].

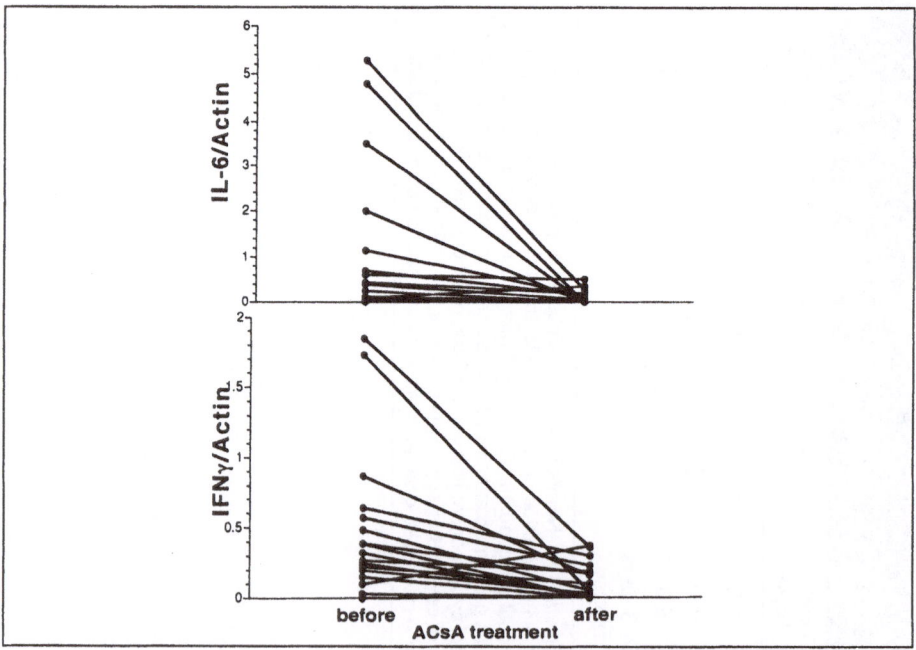

Figure 3
Effect of ACsA on IFN-γ and IL-6 mRNA expression from BAL cells. The cytokine to actin ratio for each recipient is represented before treatment and after approximately 180 days of ACsA. Of 17 recipients, 15 demonstrated a decline in IL-6 and IFN-γ cytokine mRNA expression.

Table 9
Reduction of immunosuppressive therapy for rejection after the initiation of aerosolized cyclosporine

	Number Corticosteroids Pre (Cycles)	Number Corticosteroids Post (Cycles)	% Change	Number ATG/ALG Pre (Cycles)	Number ATG/ALG Post (Cycles)	% Change
Mean	3.7	1.4	-62%	0.7	0.3	-57%
Median	3.0	1.0	-67%	1.0	0.0	-100%
S.D.	2.1	1.4		0.7	0.5	

* 462 days pre versus 627 post

[a]*Definition of abbreviations:* Number Corticosteroids Pre, number of cycles of corticosteroids required to treat rejection prior to aerosol cyclosporine (Solumedrol one gram I.V. x three days or prednisone taper 100→10mg over 10 days); Number Corticosteroids Post, number of cycles of corticosteroids required to treat rejection after initiation of Aerosol cyclosporine; % Change, percent change in steroid cycles before and after initiation aerosolized cyclosporine; Number ATG/ALG Pre, number cycles anti lymphocyte globulin required to treat rejection prior to initiation of Aerosol cyclosporine (OKT3, 5mg I.V. for 5 days, ATGAM (15 mg/kg for 10 days); Number ATG/ALG Post, number cycles anti lymphocyte globulin required to treat rejection after initiation of aerosol cyclosporine (OKT3, 5mg I.V. for 5 days, ATGAM (15 mg/kg for 10 days); % Changes, percent change in cycles anti-lymphocyte globulin before and after initiation of aerosolized cyclosporine

The average number of cycles of augmented immunosuppression (pulsed corticosteroids and anti-lymphocyte globulin) required to control rejection decreases significantly following initiation of aerosolized cyclosporine (See Table 9).

Maintenance therapy with aerosol cyclosporine when added to the maintenance immunosuppressive oral drug regimen substantially reduces systemic immunosuppression requirements and provides superior protection against rejection recurrence. Oral and intravenous immunosuppression, in general, are toxic as they characteristically profoundly depress the hosts' immune response predisposing to opportunistic infection. In addition, they are expensive therapies (in particular OKT3 and ATGAM) and generally require an extended hospital admission and frequent laboratory testing to monitor toxicity (anaphylaxis, serum sickness, fever, leukopenia, nephritis, renal insufficiency, headache, myalgia). Atgam costs about $30,000 per cycle in addition to hospital fees for 10 days. In addition, this treatment is toxic and based on our experience at the University of Pittsburgh, approximately 40% of patients develop serious opportunistic infections after receiving this treatment. The cost of diagnosing and treating each rejection event at our institution is approximately $15,000 since the rejection rate was reduced by 46% during aerosol cyclosporine, we estimate that $30,000 per patient was saved during a 627 day follow-up interval.

Improvement in Survival in Patients Treated with Aerosolized Cyclosporine for Acute Refractory Rejection

Patients treated for acute refractory rejection that failed to improve clinically and histologically with aerosol cyclosporine demonstrated improved survival as compared to historical controls with refractory rejection treated solely by conventional immunosuppression. Figure 4 depicts survival analyzed by the method of Kaplan and Meyer after lung transplantation in 42

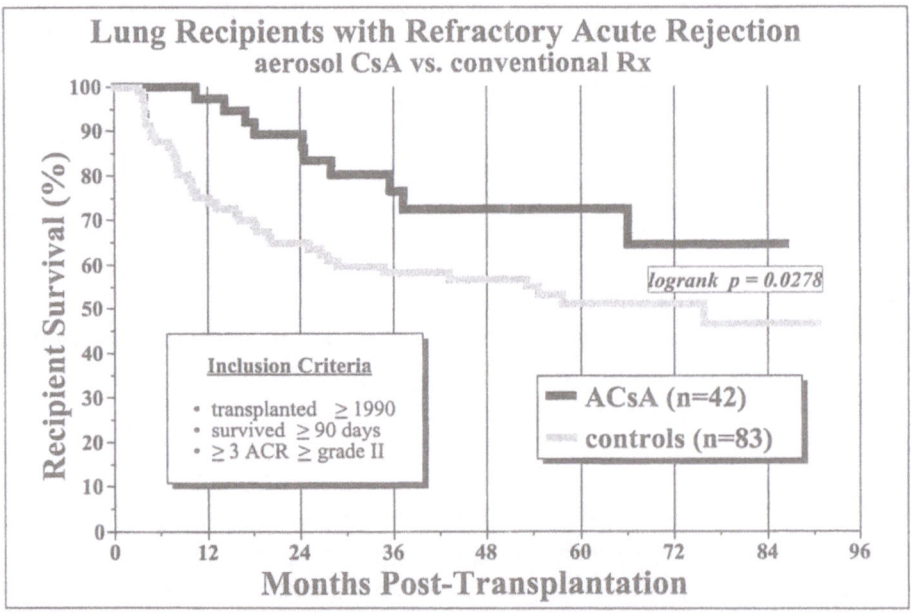

Figure 4
Survival in all patients treated with aerosol cyclosporine with at least 3 histologic rejection events (≥ grade 2) in 1 year after transplantation and matched controls transplanted from 1990 to present with ≥ at least 3 histologic rejection events (≥ grade 2) within 1 year after transplantation that received conventional immunosuppression exclusively.
Abbreviations: ACsA, patients that received aerosolized cyclosporine; controls, patients treated with conventional systemic immunosuppression; Inclusion Criteria All patients that underwent lung transplantation at the University of Pittsburgh from 1990 to present, and survived all at least 90 days and experienced 3 or more histologically documented rejection events of grade 2 or greater within 365 days of transplantation.

patients with persistent acute rejection, defined as 3 histologically distinct documented acute rejection events within 365 days after transplantation that received aerosol cyclosporine and 83 controls that received conventional immunosuppression only but did not receive aerosol cyclosporine because the drug was not available or they refused experimental therapy. All subjects that received aerosol cyclosporine and control patients had greater than or equal to 3 biopsy proven acute rejection events (grade II) within 365 days of lung transplantation (51% of subjects received aerosolized cyclosporine prior to day 365). Patients that underwent single, bilateral and heart-lung transplantation at the University of Pittsburgh since 1990 that met entry criteria based on documented histological rejection events were used as controls in this analysis. Cumulative probabilities of survival in treated versus control patients were computed by the method of Kaplan and Meier and comparison statistics were calculated using the logrank statistic (p=0.027) (see Figure 4).

Protocol # 003: Prevention of Acute Rejection

The following is a brief description of data related to early administration of aerosolized cyclosporine after lung transplantation. We have analyzed the rate of histological acute rejection for pilot patients that received aerosol cyclosporine early after lung transplantation (average day 10) compared to controls that received conventional oral therapy.

The rate of acute rejection early after lung transplantation in treatment versus placebo group is the primary endpoint for the forthcoming prospective randomized placebo controlled study. Bioavailability of aerosolized cyclosporine was measured by monoclonal antibody assay following inhalation of a 300 mg dose. The patient demographics appear in Table 10. A total of three patients underwent double lung transplantation; one underwent heart-lung transplantation, nine, right or left single lung transplantation.

In these 13 patients, administration of aerosolized cyclosporine occurred on average ten days following transplantation. Twelve of the thirteen patients received tacrolimus based immunosuppression. The immunosuppressive drug regimen consisted of tacrolimus (0.3 mg/kg/day), or cyclosporine (2.5–5.0 mg/kg/day), azathioprine (1-2 mg/kg/day), and prednisone (0.3 mg/kg/day). All patients tolerated the aerosolized cyclosporine therapy. The dose was 300 mg for ten consecutive days followed by 300 mg three days per week on Mondays, Wednesdays, and Fridays. The average duration of follow-up was 245 days. Rejection was monitored by serial transbronchial lung biopsies performed at 2-3 month intervals in all 13 patients. Rejection was

Table 10

	Sex	Diagnosis	Age	Tx type	Rec. CMV	Donor CMV	D/C Ims	Init. Day of Aerosol cyclosporine	Days of f/u
1	M	re-transplant/OB	50	DL	positive	negative	CsA	31	422
2	F	CF	23	DL	positive	negative	FK	11	200
3	F	alpha 1 antitrypsin re-transplant	48	LSL	positive	negative	FK	8	294
4	M	emphysema	66	LSL	negative	positive	FK	4	181
5	F	re-transplant/OB	43	RSL	positive	negative	FK	6	358
6	M	emphysema	67	RSL	negative	positive	FK	4	245
7	F	emphysema	58	LSL	positive	positive	FK	9	240
8	M	emphysema	57	LSL	positive	negative	FK	7	249
9	M	emphysema	66	LSL	negative	positive	FK	3	210
10	M	pulmonary htn	37	H-lung	positive	positive	FK	9	265
11	M	IPF	48	LSL	negative	positive	FK	11	199
12	M	emphysema/ re-transplant	57	LSL	positive	positive	FK	18	71
13	M	alpha 1 antitrypsin	44	DL	positive	negative	FK	16	310

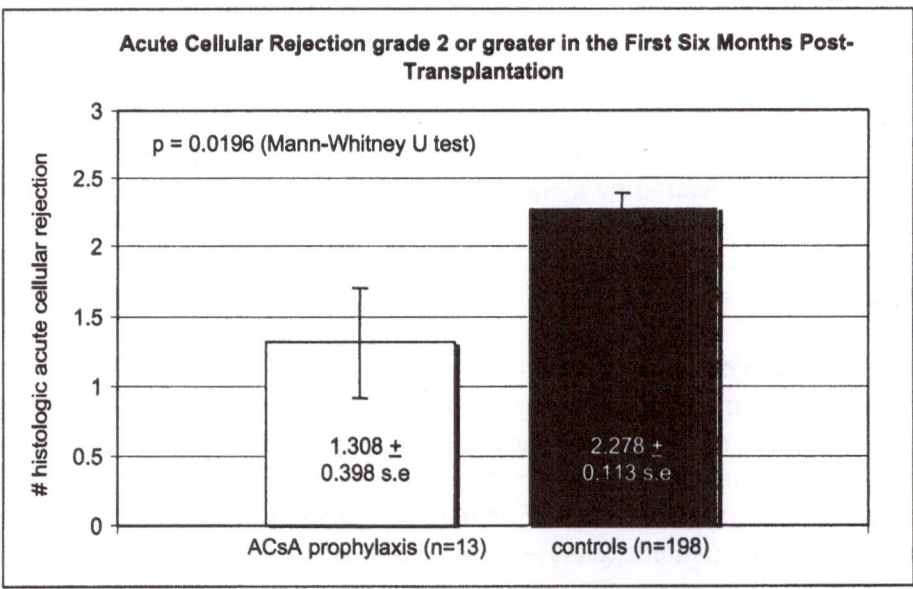

Figure 5
A comparison of the grade of acute histologic rejection during the first six months post transplantation in the aerosol cyclosporine prophylaxis patients versus the control patients.

considered significant if histology showed greater than or equal to grade II acute cellular rejection or active bronchiolitis obliterans. The rate of rejection in the 13 treated subjects was compared to a group of controls consisting of all patients transplanted at University of Pittsburgh between 1990 and 1994 at six months after lung transplantation. The rate of significant acute cellular rejection ($\geq$ Grade II) was decreased in subjects versus controls that received standard triple drug immunosuppression (See Figure 5, 2.278 episodes/rejection/patient±0.113 versus 1.308±0.398, p value=0.0196 Mann-Whitney U test).

None of the subjects developed bronchiolitis obliterans to date. Two of the treatment patients died. Both patients died from cytomegalovirus infection and multi-organ system failure [28].

PHARMACOKINETIC STUDIES

The initial pharmacokinetic studies were difficult to interpret since the patients were receiving CsA orally as their primary immunosuppressant, but

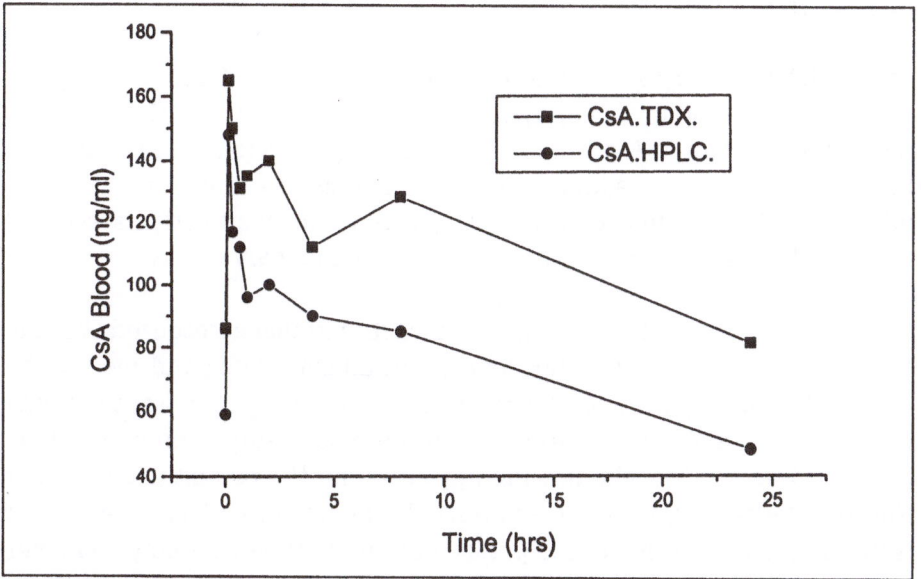

Figure 6
CsA blood concentrations in a lung transplant patient after receiving a 200 mg aerosolized CsA dose. Blood concentrations were measured by high pressure liquid chromatography (HPLC) and by a nonspecific immunoassay (TDX, Abbott Laboratories).

this situation was remedied by using tacrolimus as the primary agent. The trough blood concentrations of CsA did not change significantly in patients receiving oral CsA therapy, but acute changes in concentration following inhalation are more easily recognized in subjects on oral tacrolimus therapy. A rapid increase in CsA blood concentration is observed immediately after the inhalation of the CsA dosage, and then a prolonged return to the pre-inhalation concentration is apparent (see Figure 6). This pattern of change in blood concentration indicates that a small portion of the drug is immediately solubilized in lung and, with its lipid solubility characteristics, readily passes into the blood stream. The remaining portion of the deposited drug may be present in an insoluble form which is slowly absorbed over time, producing a slow decline in blood concentrations. Although intravenous CsA studies were not performed in these patients, the decline in blood CsA concentrations over time is slower than the normal decline in transplant patients observed after an intravenous dose of CsA. In one patient in whom we have sufficient information to calculate drug deposition from both the ^{99m}Tc and from the pharmacokinetic study, both measurements predicted a 20 mg deposition in the patient.

SUMMARY

The modulation of cytokines within the lungs is of value for lung transplant rejection and for other pathophysiologic processes such as asthma. Investigational work with CsA given orally has already been found to be effective both animal models of asthma and in limited clinical trials. The ability to administer CsA by inhalation will benefit lung transplant patients, but will also benefit other patients with inflammatory pulmonary disease.

Our animal and human studies have demonstrated that aerosolized CsA can modify the course of acute rejection in an animal model and modify the course of refractory acute and chronic rejection in lung transplant patients. Considerable refinement in our techniques are necessary to properly adjust patient doses and to make this therapy easier for the patient to administer. Newer anti-cytokine agents may be more amenable to inhalational administration due to their increased potency or due to their solubility characteristics in the propellants used in metered dose inhalers. Animal work with agents such as tacrolimus has demonstrated that this approach is possible [29]. Local immunosuppression in pulmonary transplant patients is a very realistic goal, and the aforementioned studies with aerosolized CsA have taken a major step toward achieving that goal.

REFERENCES

1. Griffith BP, Paradis IL, Zeevi A, et al. Immunologically mediated disease of the airways after lung transplantation. Ann Surg 1988; 208:371.
2. Yousem SA, Berry GJ, Brunt EM, et al. A working formulation for the standardization of nomenclature in the diagnosis of heart and lung rejection: Lung rejection study group. J Heart Lung Transplant 1990; 9:593.
3. Paradis I, Yousem S, Griffith BP. Airway obstruction and bronchiolitis obliterans after lung transplantation. Clin Chest Med 1993; 14:751.
4. Cooper JD, Billingham M, Egan T, et al. C, Yousem S. A working formulation for nomenclature and for clinical staging of chronic dysfunction in lung allografts. J Heart Lung Transplant 1993; 12:713.
5. Zenati M, Duncan AJ, Burckart GJ, et al. Immunosuppression with aerosolized cyclosporin for prevention of lung rejection in a rat model. Eur J Cardiothorac Surg 1991; 5:266.
6. Trulock EP. Management of lung transplant rejection. Chest 1993; 103:1566.
7. Bando K, Paradis IL, Konishi H, et al. Obliterative bronchiolitis after lung and heart-lung transplantation: an analysis of risk factors and management. J Thoracic Cardiovas Surg 1995;110:4-13.
8. Glanville GR, Baldwin JC, Burke CM, Theodure J, Robin E. Obliterative bronchiolitis after heart-lung transplantation: apparent arrest by augmented immunosuppression. Ann Int Med 1987; 107:300.
9. Theodure J, Starnes VA, Lewiston NJ. Obliterative bronchiolitis. Clin Chest Med 1990; 11:309.
10. Kahan BD. Cyclosporine. N Engl J Med 1989; 321:1725.
11. Ascher NL, Chen S, Hofman RA, Simmons RL. Maturation of cytotoxic T-cells within sponge matrix allograft. J Immunol 1983; 131.
12. Wolf JS, McGavic JD, Hume DM. Inhibition of the effector mechanism of transplant immunity by local graft irradiation. Surg Gynecol Obstet 1969; 128:584
13. Gergely NF, Coles JC. Prolongation of heterotopic cardiac allografts in dogs by topical irradiation. Transplantation 1970; 9:193.
14. Fidler JP, Alexander JW, Smith EJ, Miller HC, Muthiah V. Radiation reversal of acute rejection in patients with life threatening infection. Arch Surg 1973; 107:256.
15. Ruers TJM, Buurman WA, van der Linden CJ, Kootstra G. Local inhibition of major histocompatibility complex class II induction within the graft: an effective way to induce immunosuppression. Transplant Proc 1987; 19:246.
16. Ruers T, Daemen M, Thijssen H, van der Linden C, Buurman W. Sensitivity of graft rejection in rats to local immunosuppressive therapy. Transplantation 1988; 46:820.
17. Stepkowski SM, Goto S, Ito T. et al. Prolongation of heterotopic heart allograft survival by local delivery of continuous low-dose cyclosporine therapy. Transplantation 1989; 47:17.
18. Burckart GJ, Dowling R, Zenati M, Yousem SA, Venkataramanan R, Griffith BP. Cyclosporine administration by aerosol. J Clin Pharmacol 1989; 29:832-62.
19. Dowling RD, Zenati M, Burckart GJ, Yousem SA, Schaper M, Hardesty RL, Griffith BP: Aerosolized cyclosporine as single agent immunotherapy in canine lung allografts. Surgery 1990; 108:198-205.
20. Keenan RJ, Duncan AJ, Yousem SA, Zenati M, Schaper M, Dowling RD, Alarie Y, Burckart GJ, Griffith BP: Improved immunosuppression with aerosolized cyclosporine in experimental pulmonary transplantation. Transplantation 1992; 53:20-5.
21. Muggenburg BA, Hoover MD, Griffith BP, Haley PJ, Snipes MB, Wolff RK, Yeh HC, Burckart GJ, Mauderly JL: Administration of cyclosporine by aerosol: A feasibility

study in beagle dogs. J Aerosol Med 1990; 3:1-13.

22. Mitruka SN, Pham SM, Zeevi A, Li S, Cai J, Burckart GJ, Yousem SA, Keenan RJ, Griffith BP. Aerosol cyclosporine prevents acute allograft rejection in experimental lung transplantation. Journal of Thoracic and Cardiovascular Surgery 1998; 115: 28-37.

23. O'Riordan TG, Duncan SR, Burckart GJ, Griffith BP, Smaldone GC: Production of an aerosol of cyclosporine as a prelude to clinical studies. J Aerosol Med 1992; 5: 171-177.

24. O'Riordan TG, Iacono A, Keenan RJ, Duncan SR, Burckart GJ, Griffith BP, Smaldone GC. Delivery and distribution of aerosolized cyclosporine in lung allograft recipients. Am J Resp Crit Care Med 1995; 151:516-21.

25. Iacono A, Keenan RJ, Duncan SR, Smaldone GC, Dauber JH, Paradis IL, Ohori NP, Grgurich WF, Burckart GJ, Zeevi A, Delgado E, O'Riordan TG, Zendarsky MM, Yousem SA, Griffith BP: Aerosolized cyclosporine in lung recipients with refractory chronic rejection. Am J Resp Crit Care Med 1996; 153: 1451-1455.

26. Iacono A, Dauber J, Keenan R, Spichty K, Cai J, Grgurich W, Burckart G, Smaldone G, Pham S, Ohori NP, Yousem S, Griffith B, Zeevi A. Interleukin-6 and interferon-γ gene expression in lung transplant recipients with refractory acute cellular rejection: implications for monitoring and inhibition by treatment with aerosolized cyclosporine. Transplantation 1997; 64:263-269.

27. Dhanjal U, Dauber J, Grgurich W, Raghu S, Keenan R, McCurry K, Griffith B, Smaldone G, Burckart G, Iacono A. Use of aerosol cyclosporine for refractory rejection in lung transplant patients. Am J Respir Crit Care Med 1999; 159:A279.

28. Iacono et.al. Aerosolized Cyclosporine Given as Prophylaxis for Acute Rejection After Lung Transplantation: Safety and Peripheral Lung Deposition Following Early Administration. Am. J. of Resp. and Crit. Care Med., 157:3; 328.

29. Akutsu I, Fukuda T, Majima K, Makino S. Inhibitory effect of inhaled FK-506 on increased bronchial responsiveness and eosinophil infiltration in the airway mucosa. Arerugi 1992; 41: 543-547.

14
THERAPY OF AUTOIMMUNE CONNECTIVE TISSUE DISEASES

Timothy M. Wright and Dana P. Ascherman
Department of Medicine
University of Pittsburgh
Pittsburgh, Pennsylvania, USA

INTRODUCTION

The autoimmune diseases can be divided into two basic categories: *organ specific* and *systemic*. Organ specific autoimmune disease can affect virtually any tissue of the body and is associated most often with evidence of both T and B cell autoimmune responses directed against the cells of the affected organ. Examples of organ specific autoimmune disease include multiple sclerosis, Type I diabetes mellitus, Grave's disease, autoimmune hemolytic anemia, and myasthenia gravis, which affect the central nervous system, pancreatic β-cells, thyroid gland, erythrocytes, and cholinergic neuromuscular junctions, respectively. The systemic autoimmune diseases, also referred to as connective tissue diseases (CTD), comprise a group of illnesses in which multiple organ system damage is a common characteristic. These diseases are also related in that they can share autoantibody specificities and have overlap in organ system involvement as well as in clinical features. The CTD group includes systemic lupus erythematosus (SLE), rheumatoid arthritis (RA), systemic sclerosis (SSc), idiopathic inflammatory myopathies (polymyositis and dermatomyositis), and systemic vasculitides (e.g. Wegener's granulomatosus and polyarteritis nodosa).

The therapy of autoimmune diseases is currently a field in rapid evolution, and specific approaches to therapy differ significantly according to the disease type and severity. However, general strategies apply to all autoimmune diseases, whether organ specific or systemic, and these will be reviewed in this chapter. The focus of this chapter is on the management of CTD; however, recent advances in the treatment of organ specific autoimmune

A. W. Thomson (ed.), Therapeutic Immunosuppression, 357–384.

diseases or animal models of autoimmune diseases that have the potential for broad applicability are included. As shown in Table 1, therapy for auto-immune diseases ranges from very non-specific, "global" immunosuppression to highly targeted immunotherapy. For severe CTD in which there is an extensive expansion of autoreactive T and B cells, an aggressive non-specific approach (e.g. immunoablation and stem cell transplantation, which is currently experimental) may be necessary to induce remission. In such patients, targeted immunotherapy (e.g. toleragens or vaccines) may be helpful in preventing disease recurrence. Although the general trend in research for the treatment of autoimmune diseases is to develop highly targeted immunotherapies, this goal is currently hampered by an incomplete understanding of basic disease mechanisms and a paucity of detailed information regarding autoantigen epitopes and autoreactive T and B cell repertoires. Thus, there continues to be considerable effort in advancing less specific immunotherapies in the hope of increasing efficacy and reducing side effects.

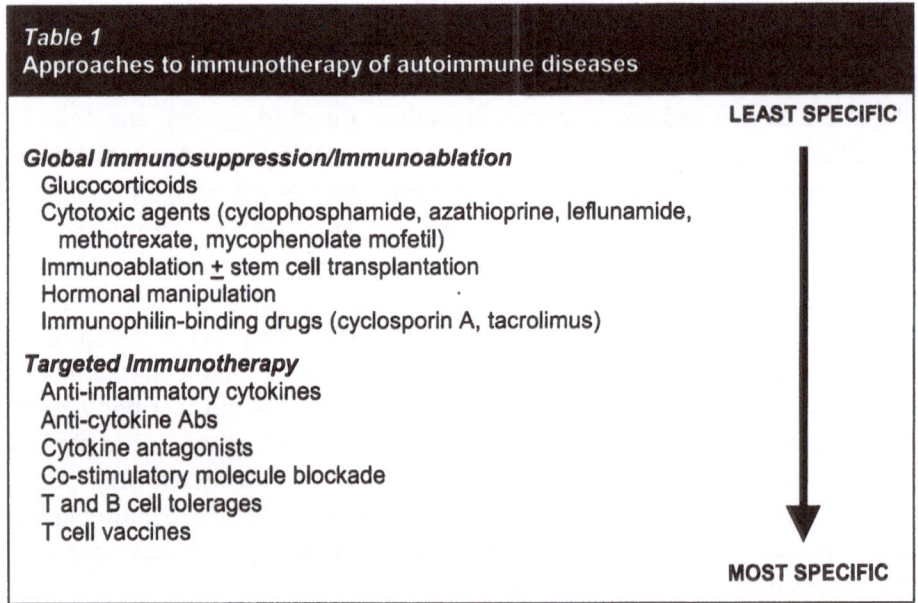

Table 1
Approaches to immunotherapy of autoimmune diseases

LEAST SPECIFIC

Global Immunosuppression/Immunoablation
  Glucocorticoids
  Cytotoxic agents (cyclophosphamide, azathioprine, leflunamide,
    methotrexate, mycophenolate mofetil)
  Immunoablation ± stem cell transplantation
  Hormonal manipulation
  Immunophilin-binding drugs (cyclosporin A, tacrolimus)

Targeted Immunotherapy
  Anti-inflammatory cytokines
  Anti-cytokine Abs
  Cytokine antagonists
  Co-stimulatory molecule blockade
  T and B cell tolerages
  T cell vaccines

MOST SPECIFIC

GLOBAL IMMUNOSUPPRESSION/IMMUNOABLATION

Non-specific immunotherapy

The majority of currently available treatments for autoimmune diseases are relatively non-specific with regard to their mode of immunosuppression. Included in this group of medications are: glucocorticoids, cytotoxic agents, and immunophilin-binding drugs. The choice of drug(s), dosing regimens, and toxicities for this group of medications are beyond the scope of this chapter and have been recently reviewed [1,2].

Glucocorticoids – In general, for the vast majority of CTD manifestations, glucocorticoids are used acutely to control inflammation and chronically to induce immunosuppression. The anti-inflammatory and immune effects of glucorticoids are mediated through inhibition of arachidonate release and metabolism, decreased cytokine gene expression (IL-1, IL-2, IL-6, IL-8, IFN-γ, TNF-α), and suppression of inflammatory cytokine signalling through NF-κB [3,4]. Although they are often highly effective, glucocorticoids can cause significant side effects including hyperglycemia, hypertension, osteoporosis, avascular necrosis (AVN) of bone, cataract formation, obesity, accelerated atherosclerosis, and susceptibility to opportunistic infections [3,5]. In most cases these side effects are dependent on the dose and duration of therapy; therefore, an effort is made to taper the dosage to the lowest effective level, to use alternate day regimens if possible (which are less toxic), and to reduce the dosage by the concurrent use of other immunosuppressive ("steroid-sparing") agents.

Cytotoxic immunosuppressants – Cytotoxic drugs, which include DNA alkylating agents and metabolic inhibitors, are commonly used as steroid sparing agents in the management of CTD. In certain potentially life-threatening or organ-threatening illnesses (e.g. SLE with diffuse proliferative glomeronephritis, polyarteritis nodosa, Wegener's granulomatosus, rheumatoid vasculitis), cyclophosphamide in combination with glucocorticoids is the common approach to therapy [1,2]. Cyclophosphamide is a potent toxin for dividing cells including those of hematopoietic origin, explaining its effects on T cell proliferation and autoantibody production. Unfortunately, cyclophosphamide is non-selective in its toxicity for dividing cells, and its potential for adverse effects is significant. These include hemorrhagic cystitis, leukopenia, mucositis, alopecia, sterility, infections, and malignancy (bladder and leukemias) [2,3]. Another DNA-modifying cytotoxic drug, azathioprine, is metabolized to its active metabolite, 6-mercaptopurine, in the liver. The purine analog

6-mercaptopurine is incorporated into DNA during replication and repair. Its cellular effects are similar to cyclophosphamide, although it is a less potent immunosuppressant and side effects are primarily bone marrow suppression, elevated liver enzymes, and increased risk of lymphoproliferative disorders [2].

Another related group of cytotoxic immunosuppressants is comprised of three inhibitors of nucleotide metabolism: methotrexate, leflunamide, and mycophenolate mofetil. Methotrexate is a folic acid antagonist that inhibits the enzyme dihydrofolate reductase, which is essential for purine and thymidine synthesis [3]. Leflunomide, approved for the treatment of RA in 1998, inhibits de novo pyrimidine synthesis by blocking dihydroorotate dehydrogenase activity [6]. Mycophenolate mofetil is metabolized in the liver to its active form, mycophenolic acid, an inhibitor of inosine monophosphate dehydrogenase. Mycophenolic acid blocks the de novo synthesis pathway of purine synthesis, which is critical for lymphocyte proliferation [7]. All three nucleotide synthesis inhibitors have relatively favorable side effect profiles, with gastrointestinal side effects, leukopenia, thrombocytopenia, and hepatic enzyme elevations being the most frequently observed.

Azathioprine and the nucleotide metabolism inhibitors leflunamide and methotrexate are most often used in the chronic management of moderately active CTD, such as RA, inflammatory myopathies, and non-renal manifestations of SLE. These immunosuppressant drugs are members of a group of medications used to treat erosive RA, referred to collectively as "Disease Modifying Anti-Rheumatic Drugs" or DMARDs [8]. The DMARDs are so named because of their ability to alter disease progression and to retard joint destruction. In multiple longitudinal studies investigating the use of various DMARDs in RA, drug cessation occurred frequently due to inefficacy or serious and/or intolerable side effects. Only methotrexate was found to have reasonable long term efficacy and tolerability in managing RA [8-11], and, therefore, it is regarded as the "gold standard" for monotherapy.

Mycophenolate mofetil, approved for use in the solid organ transplant setting, has also been shown to be effective in patients with pemphigus vulgaris (a potentially life-threatening autoimmune blistering skin disease) refractory to conventional management with glucocorticoids and azathioprine [12]. In the (NZBxW)F1 mouse model of SLE, mycophenolate mofetil significantly delayed the onset of proteinuria, reduced anti-dsDNA antibody levels by 50%, and prolonged survival (from 9 to 13 months compared to control) [13]. Similar results were obtained in the treatment of MRL lpr/lpr mice with mycophenolate mofetil [14]. There has been only limited experience using mycophenolate mofetil in human SLE, but the results thus far are promising [15,16].

Immunoablation and stem cell transplantation – Relatively low (15 to 25%) concordance rates for CTD in monozygotic twins suggests that genetic susceptibility plays only a limited role in the development of disease and that environmental factors and/or stochastic events (e.g. T cell receptor rearrangement) are critical for disease initiation and expression [17-19]. Immunoablation using high dose cytotoxic therapy with or without autologous stem cell rescue for the treatment of patients with CTD, therefore, is based on the premise that intensive immunosuppression will give rise to a reconstituted immune system that will develop new (self-tolerant) T and B cell repertoires. A growing number of case reports and small case series indicate the potential for success in inducing remission of autoimmune disease using immunoablative therapy with [20-25] or without [26,27] autologous stem cell transplantation. Large multicenter trials are ongoing to further investigate the efficacy and toxicity of this aggressive but potentially curative approach to therapy for autoimmune disease.

Hormonal manipulation

Many autoimmune diseases manifest a striking female preponderance. This gender predilection undoubtedly reflects differences in the hormonal milieu, as the skewed disease distribution has not been linked specifically to sex chromosomes. Previous work in humans and autoimmune-prone strains of mice has focused on hormone-related differences in lymphocyte subset distribution, immunoglobulin production, and cytokine profiles. For example, estrogen inhibits suppressor T cell function, leading to an increased CD4/CD8 ratio and enhancing polyclonal B cell activation (particularly CD5+ B cells known to produce "natural" autoantibodies) [28-30]. Despite this extensive body of descriptive work, however, relatively little information has emerged regarding immunoregulatory mechanisms of estrogen-mediated effects in autoimmune diseases. Whether such effects are directly related to immunopathogenesis or merely permissive for disease expression, hormonal manipulation presents a feasible method of autoimmune disease modification.

Selective estrogen receptor modulators (SERMs) – The SERMs represent a class of agents possessing both agonist and antagonist properties, depending on the tissue and estrogen receptor subtype. Perhaps the best known SERM is tamoxifen, a partial agonist used primarily in the treatment of breast cancer. When administered in the 16/6 dsDNA idiotype model of murine lupus, tamoxifen lessens the degree of leukopenia, thrombocytopenia, and proteinuria with a clearcut dose response [31]. These clinical benefits extend to pre-existing disease as well [31], providing the rationale for use in humans with established SLE. To elucidate tamoxifen's mechanism of action, investigators have compared the effect of tamoxifen to that of anti-E2 antibody in a SLE-prone strain of BALB/c mice. Not only does tamoxifen bias the IgG isotype toward IgG2a with potential implications for complement fixation, but this treatment also shifts the cytokine profile from IL-1, IL-10, and TNF-α to IL-2, IL-4, and IFN-γ [32]. Moreover, because tamoxifen and anti-estrogen treatment yield similar clinical benefit, these investigators conclude that tamoxifen must function as an estrogen antagonist [32]. Applying these results to human SLE is not yet possible given the paucity of published trials involving tamoxifen treatment of human SLE. Although a pilot study in 10 patients with SLE demonstrated no clinical benefit from tamoxifen treatment, the trial suffered from limited enrollment in a population with stable baseline disease [33]. Given the safety profile of this drug as well as the convincing preclinical data, future large scale trials in more active disease are warranted.

Dehydroepiandrosterone (DHEA) – Based on a large body of work in murine models of lupus showing the dichotomous impact of estrogens and androgens on disease course, investigators have analyzed the effect of DHEA, a weak androgen. In NZB/W mice, DHEA treatment does result in clinical improvement of spontaneous, lupus-like disease [34]. Combined with human studies showing DHEA-induced alterations in circulating sex hormone levels [35], the NZB/W response to DHEA has prompted trials of this agent in humans with SLE. The results have been somewhat equivocal, however, with marginal clinical benefit and side effects that include acne, hirsutism, and menstrual irregularity [36].

Bromocriptine – Previous work has revealed that elevated prolactin levels in lupus-prone NZB/W mice as well as some human SLE patients correlate with disease activity [35,37,38]. Prolactin affects the production of other sex hormones (including estrogen) and influences both humoral and cell-mediated immune functions through binding of prolactin receptors on circulating lymphocytes [39]. Although these data suggest a possible role for prolactin blockade, a randomized, placebo-controlled trial with bromocriptine (dopamine receptor agonist that downregulates pituitary release of prolactin) has shown only limited reduction of disease activity/flare rate without a concomitant decrease in prednisone requirement [40]. The future role of this drug is therefore uncertain.

Immunophilin-binding drugs

Cyclosporin and tacrolimus (FK 506) block T cell activation and cytokine (e.g. IL-2) production by inhibiting the calcineurin-dependent pathway of transcription activation. These compounds derived from fungi bind to intracellular proteins referred to as immunophilins which form complexes that block the calcium-calmodulin-dependent phosphatase, calcineurin, and prevent it from acting on substrates including the transcription factor NFAT [41]. Both drugs have similar toxicity profiles which include the common side effects of tremor, hypertension, and nephropathy [42]. Cyclosporin and tacrolimus have been highly effective in treating animal models of autoimmune disease [43-47]. Their use in treating human CTD has been limited (presumably due to the potential for serious side effects) to the treatment of refractory disease, in particular RA, SLE, polymyositis and uveitis [48-53].

TARGETED IMMUNOTHERAPY

Cytokines

Functioning as biochemical messengers between different components of the immune system, cytokines play a key role in both physiologic and pathologic processes. Several paradigms have emerged that categorize these cytokines on the basis of function. While cytokines can be generaly divided into "pro-inflammatory" and "anti-inflammatory" mediators, many cytokines also can be classified according to the T cell subset capable of producing them, i.e. TH1 versus TH2. The TH1 cytokines include IFN-γ, IL-2, and Lymphotoxin, all of which play a key role in cell-mediated immune functions such as delayed T cell hypersensitivity (DTH), tumor surveillance, and defense against pathogens that include mycobacteria, viruses, and certain parasites [54]. As a group, these cytokines have been implicated in organ specific autoimmune diseases as well as acute GVHD [54-56]. In contrast, TH2 cytokines play a greater role in humoral immunity, chronic GVHD, and CTD such as SLE. The TH2 cytokines include IL-4, IL-5, IL-6, IL-10, and IL-13 [54-56]. Other distinguishing features of TH2 cytokines include downregulation of macrophage function as well as increased production of IgE and non-complement binding IgG subtypes [56]. Although this classification scheme is somewhat artificial and oversimplified, separating various autoimmune diseases on the basis of TH1 or TH2 predominance has generated the important therapeutic concept of "immune deviation" – diversion of a pathologic immune process through the conversion of TH phenotypes [55,56].

Anti-inflammatory cytokines

IL-10 – A basic concept in cytokine modulation is inhibition of pro-inflammatory cytokines or supplementation of anti-inflammatory cytokines. Of the TH2 or anti-inflammatory cytokines, IL-10 has been the most widely studied in pre-clinical and clinical trials. Synthesized primarily by monocytes, IL-10 downregulates several aspects of the immune response including the expression of MHC Class II molecules, co-stimulatory molecules (B7-1 and B7-2), adhesion proteins (ICAM-1), pro-inflammatory cytokines (IL-1, IL-2, IL-6, IL-8, IL-12, GM-CSF, and TNF-α), and various inflammatory mediators of tissue destruction (NO, free radicals, prostaglandins, and metalloproteases) [57,58]. IL-10 exerts these functions both directly and indirectly through upregulation of molecules including IL-1 receptor antagonist (IL-1ra) and soluble TNF-α receptor (sTNFR) [58]. Ultimately, the net effect is downregulation of macrophages, neutrophils, and CD4+ T cells, decreased antigen presentation, augmented CD8+ T cell cytolytic activity, and enhanced proliferation/differentiation of B cells [57,58].

Coupled with this *in vitro* data, several animal models of autoimmunity suggest that IL-10 may provide beneficial effects in TH1-mediated diseases. For example, not only does IL-10 prevent disease in experimental allergic encephalomyelitis (EAE) and collagen-induced arthritis (CIA) [58-61], but this cytokine also ameliorates existing disease in CIA [60,62]. These models have provided the basis for human trials in diseases such as multiple sclerosis, RA, psoriasis, and Crohn's disease. Although preliminary, phase I clinical trials with rhIL-10 have demonstrated a "trend toward efficacy" in both RA and inflammatory bowel disease [59,63,64].

IL-4 – Like IL-10, IL-4 is an important member of the TH2 family of anti-inflammatory cytokines. Because IL-4 antagonizes the effects of IL-12, a macrophage-derived cytokine promoting TH1 development, IL-4 represents an important regulator of the TH1/TH2 balance [65]. Additional regulatory effects vary depending on tissue type, but include decreased production of pro-inflammatory cytokines, increased expression of IL-1ra, and modulation of cell adhesion molecules (decreased ELAM-1 and ICAM-1 versus increased VCAM-1) [59,66]. *In vitro* application of IL-4 to cultured synoviocytes therefore decreases inflammatory cytokine production and inhibits IL-1-induced proliferation [66]. These *in vitro* effects have translated into therapeutic benefit in several animal models of TH1-mediated autoimmunity, including collagen-induced arthritis (CIA) and streptococcal cell wall-induced arthritis [66,67]. Of note, available evidence suggests that IL-4 synergizes with IL-10 to limit mononuclear cell infiltration of synovial tissue and prevent cartilage degradation [64,68]. Future applications in human autoimmune disease may therefore hinge on similar combinatorial strategies.

IFN-β – Among those cytokines not classified within the TH1/TH2 paradigm, IFN-β has shown great therapeutic promise as an anti-inflammatory cytokine in multiple sclerosis. Large phase III, placebo-controlled trials involving IFN-β administration to MS patients have demonstrated a decrease in disease progression and flare rate, as well as diminished gadolinium-enhancing white matter lesions on MRI [69,70]. Based on *in vitro* and *in vivo* observations, a number of potential mechanisms have emerged that could explain IFN-β's therapeutic effect. While antagonism of IFN-γ leads to impaired antigen presentation, inhibitory effects and decreased expression of IL-2R effectively limit T cell proliferation [71]. IFN-β may also bias the TH balance away from TH1 through enhanced production and secretion of the TH2 cytokine IL-10 [71,72]. Finally, both *in vitro* experiments and *in vivo* data from Lewis rats with EAE have shown IFN-β-induced downregulation of critical adhesion molecules such as ICAM-1 and monocyte VLA-4 that clearly play a role in the pathogenesis of MS by controlling cellular trafficking within the CNS [71].

TGF-β – Produced by multiple cell types including platelets, monocytes/macrophages, lymphocytes, and synovial fibroblasts, TGF-β is a potent inhibitory cytokine responsible for regulating several facets of the immune response [59,66]. Many of these effects that limit both cell-mediated and humoral immunity stem from antagonism of the pro-inflammatory cytokines TNF-α and IL-1 [66]. For example, TGF-β not only decreases expression of Type I and II IL-1 receptors, but this cytokine also upregulates IL-1ra [73,74]. Applied in the animal model experimental allergic encephalomyelitis (EAE), TGF-β delays disease development and decreases the rate of recurrence in established disease [75]. In CIA, on the other hand, TGF-β does not prevent disease but does result in decreased antibody production and altered histopathology with decreased lining membrane hyperplasia and limited mononuclear cell infiltration [75].

Cytokine antagonists

As pro-inflammatory molecules contributing to different stages of autoimmune disease, cytokines such as TNF-α, IL-1, IL-6, and IL-12 represent potential therapeutic targets. In turn, because cytokine function depends on the complex integration of production, secretion, receptor binding, and subsequent intracellular signalling, numerous strategies for interrupting this process have emerged. Examples include monoclonal antibodies directed against cytokines and their receptors, soluble receptors, receptor antagonists, agents designed to disrupt cytokine-mediated signals and blockade of cytokine regulated transcription factors such as NF-κB [66]. While the number of therapeutic strategies available to disrupt a particular cytokine pathway appears promising, the redundancy of pro-inflammatory cytokine function implies that combined approaches targeting multiple cytokines will be required for effective cytokine modulation of autoimmune diseases.

sTNF-R, anti-TNF antibody – Among the proinflammatory cytokines, TNF-α is often referred to as a "primary" cytokine since its action is coupled to the expression of numerous other inflammatory mediators and adhesion molecules including IL-1, IL-6, GM-CSF, chemokines (IL-8, MIP-1α, RANTES, and MCP-1) prostaglandins, nitric oxide, ICAM-1, VCAM-1, and E-selectin [76]. The initial descriptions of TNF-α were based on its cytotoxic affects on certain tumors and its function as a mediator of cachexia ("cachectin") due to inhibition of adipocyte lipoprotein lipase [77,78]. TNF-α is now recognized to play major roles in the chronic inflammation of RA and inflammatory bowel disease (e.g. Crohn's disease) and the acute systemic response to bacterial sepsis [76,79]. TNF-α exerts its effects through interactions with high affinity receptors, p55 TNF-R (CD120a, type I receptor) and p75 TNF-R (CD120b, type II receptor), present on a wide variety of cell types [76].

Because of its position upstream in the cascade of important inflammatory molecules, TNF-α was a logical target for the development of neutralizing therapy. Early animal studies demonstrated the effectiveness of administering anti-TNF therapy in murine models of erosive arthritis [80-82]. Two pharmacologic approaches to neutralize the deleterious effects of TNF-α in humans have led to the development of a soluble TNF-α receptor and the generation of a chimeric anti-TNF-α antibody. Taking advantage of the high affinity of TNF-α for its receptors, a soluble recombinant fusion protein was generated containing the Fc portion of human IgG and the extracellular portion of the human p75 TNF-R (etanercept/Enbrel). The resulting soluble receptor molecule is bivalent (due to its antibody-like structure) which contributes to increased avidity for TNF-α and a longer biologic half-life [83]. The second approach to neutralizing TNF-α for human administration was the generation of a chimeric anti-TNF-α antibody containing constant regions from a human IgG1 molecule and variable regions from a mouse monoclonal anti-TNF-α antibody (infliximab/Remicade) [76].

Clinical trials of both etanercept and infliximab have demonstrated significant improvement of clinical signs, symptoms, and functional status in patients with RA [76,83]. Both agents are FDA approved for use in RA patients who have failed conventional DMARD therapy. Clinical efficacy of these agents appears to be comparable to MTX, the current standard for monotherapy of RA. In addition, patients who respond to MTX may gain added benefit from combined treatment with etanercept [84,85]. Repeated administration of infliximab has been associated with the development of antibodies against the chimeric Ig molecule which can result in hypersensitivity reactions. This was shown to be inhibited by concomitant immunosuppression with low dose methotrexate, which is currently included in the regimen for treating refractory RA [86]. Studies to determine the long term effect of anti-TNF therapy in RA are in progress. Also in the trial stage are additional humanized anti-TNF-α antibodies which should reduce or potentially eliminate the problem of hypersensitivity due to anti-chimeric antibody [76].

IL-1ra, sIL-1R – IL-1 is a critical pro-inflammatory cytokine with pleiotropic functions ranging from T cell activation to macrophage-mediated proteoglycan degradation [87,88]. At the cellular level, these processes reflect upregulation of vascular and cellular adhesion molecules, enhanced expression of IL-2 and IL-2R, downregulation of the TH2 cytokines IL-4 and IL-10, increased synovial production of prostaglandins such as PGE_2, and activation of degradative enzymes including collagenase and stromelysin [66,88]. To counteract these inflammatory and potentially destructive cascades, monocytes/macrophages produce natural antagonists that include IL-1 receptor antagonist (IL-1ra), soluble IL-1 receptors (sIL-1R), and type II membrane bound IL-1R that serves as a non-signalling decoy receptor [57,66]. In cell culture, treatment with IL-1ra decreases synoviocyte-derived collagenase, as well as chondrocyte and synoviocyte production of prostaglandins [89]. Further supporting the therapeutic potential of IL-1ra, transplantion of fibroblasts/synoviocytes transfected with the IL-1ra gene has ameliorated antigen-induced arthritis in several animal models and set the stage for targeted gene therapy of human RA [90,91]. Other therapeutic trials in human RA have focused on the systemic delivery of exogenous IL-1ra; in a 24 week, placebo-controlled trial involving 472 patients, the highest dosing group sustained a statistically significant response in 6 clinical parameters, decreased ESR, and improved Larsen score (measure of radiographic progression) [92]. Corresponding to this clinical effect, histologic analysis on a limited number of biopsy specimens demonstrated a reduction in sublining macrophages, T cell infiltration, and adhesion molecule expression [92]. In contrast, a smaller randomized, placebo-controlled trial involving sIL-1R type I failed to show any dramatic clinical benefit, possibly because type I IL-1R binds IL-1ra as well as IL-1 [93]. Because type II IL-1R preferentially binds IL-1 rather than IL-1ra, the use of sIL-1R type II may represent a more feasible therapeutic strategy in future trials [93].

Anti-IL-6 antibody – Induced by IL-1 and TNF-α, IL-6 plays an integral role in the acute phase response as well as B cell growth/differentiation and T cell activation [35,94]. Not surprisingly, levels of circulating IL-6 correlate closely with erythrocyte sedimentation rate (ESR) and C-reactive protein (CRP) in autoimmune diseases such as RA [94]. Targeting this cytokine with monoclonal antibodies over 10 days in a small open label pilot study resulted in some clinical improvement sustained up to 6 months [95]. Coupled with clinical improvements of CIA in monkeys treated with anti-IL-6R antibodies [96], this result has provided the rationale for larger, controlled trials of anti-IL-6 monoclonal antibody in humans with RA.

Anti-IL-12 antibody – Through stimulation of IFN-γ and counter-regulation of IL-4, IL-12 functions as a key regulator of the TH1/TH2 balance. However, IL-12 not only promotes T cell production of pro-inflammatory, TH1 cytokines, but it also enhances the cytotoxicity of NK cells [65]. A number of factors contribute to IL-12 production by monocytes, including the integration of multiple co-stimulatory signals derived from TNF-α/TNFR, GM-CSF/GM-CSFR, CD58/CD2, CD40/CD40L, and CD28/B7 interactions [65]. In contrast, IL-4, IL-10, and TGF-β synergize to limit the positive feedback loop between IL-12 and IFN-γ [65]. Illustrating the fundamental role of IL-12 in maintaining this delicate balance, a number of TH1-mediated autoimmune diseases fail to develop in IL-12-deficient mice [65,97]. Furthermore, anti-IL-12 monoclonal antibody treatment effectively blocks the development of EAE, CIA, and IBD (inflammatory bowel disease) in different animal models [98-101]. Other novel strategies potentially applicable to human autoimmune diseases include treatment with inhibitors of the transcription factor STAT4 (unique to IL-12 signalling) as well as the administration of receptor-binding, functionally inactive IL-12 p40 *homodimers* (IL-12 normally consists of 35 and 40 kDa *heterodimers*) [65].

ACCESSORY MOLECULES

Co-stimulatory molecules

Over the last decade, the concept of antigen-driven immunity has evolved from the relatively simplistic "tri-molecular complex" consisting of the T cell receptor and MHC-bound peptide to encompass the critical role of costimulatory pathways. In parallel, the so-called "2 signal" hypothesis has emerged as a fundamental tenet of immunology. Products of both TCR- and co-stimulatory receptor/ligand-mediated pathways, these two signals are required for augmented expression of IL-2 and generation of a productive immune response [102,103]. While TCR recognition of antigen (signal 1) in the absence of co-stimulation (signal 2) fails to upregulate IL-2 and leads to anergy (cellular unresponsiveness), co-stimulatory signals alone simply do not generate antigen-specific immunity [102]. Therefore, disrupting these co-stimulatory pathways represents an effective approach for limiting deleterious immune responses, particularly because many of the ligands involved in co-stimulation are specifically upregulated in *activated* immune cells.

B7/CD28, B7/CTLA-4 – Of the co-stimulatory pathways, the interaction between B7 expressed on antigen presenting cells (APCs) and CD28 present on T cells is most directly responsible for generating the 2nd signal needed for augmented IL-2 production [103]. As an immune response develops, however, T cells upregulate expression of CTLA-4, a molecule that competitively binds CD28 to generate negative signals and dampen T cell responses. From this paradigm, investigators have developed two basic strategies to block the B7/CD28 pathway: anti-B7 antibodies and CTLA-4:Ig. In the NZB/NZW model of lupus nephritis, for example, combined treatment with antibodies directed against both B7.1 and B7.2 blocked autoantibody formation and nephritis [104]. Similarly, administration of CTLA-4:Ig to NZB/W mice prevented the development of nephritis [105]. Moreover, CTLA-4:Ig effectively treated established nephritis, a key factor suggesting therapeutic potential in human autoimmune diseases that cannot be predicted prior to disease onset [105]. Validating this concept, a 26 week open label, dose escalation CTLA-4:Ig protocol in patients with psoriasis demonstrated clinically significant benefit most pronounced in patients receiving the highest dosing regimens [106]. Several histologic and immunologic parameters correlated with this clinical effect, including reduced dermal CD3+ (T) cell infiltration, diminished expression of integrins, and decreased epidermal hyperplasia/proliferation [106]. Based on these promising results, additional trials in RA and SLE are currently underway.

CD40/CD40L – Complementing the B7/CD28 co-stimulatory pathway, the binding of CD40L (CD154) with its counterreceptor CD40 plays an important role in the interaction of T cells with monocytes, B cells, and other nonhematopoetic cells such as vascular endothelium [107,108]. In turn, these interactions facilitate immunologic processes ranging from antigen presentation to antibody isotype switching and the development of memory B cells [107,108]. Deficiency of CD40L results in the hyper IgM syndrome characterized by defects in both cellular and humoral immunity [109]. Given the central role played by this molecule that is preferentially expressed by *activated* T cells, investigators have employed monoclonal antibodies directed against CD40L in numerous animal models of autoimmunity. Examples include GVHD, CIA, EAE, diabetes mellitus (DM), and lupus nephritis [110-116]. Not only has anti-CD40L antibody treatment effectively prevented these examples of humoral and cell-mediated diseases, but such therapy has also shown benefit in delaying progression of established disease in certain models such as SNF1 lupus nephritis [117]. These preclinical studies have therefore provided the foundation for human clinical trials in idiopathic thrombocytopenic purpura, SLE, and renal transplantation.

OX40-R/OX40L – Although less well studied, the OX40-R/OX40L co-stimulatory pathway represents an additional target for disruption of autoimmune processes. Because the expression of OX-40R and OX-40L are limited to activated T and B cells [118], respectively, targeting these molecules circumvents the generalized immunosuppression of currently available "disease-modifying" chemotherapeutic agents. When applied in the SJL murine model of EAE, OX-40R:Ig lessens the severity of disease and hastens recovery, though relapses do occur [118]. In vitro transfection experiments comparing the relative co-stimulatory effects of OX-40L and B7.1 demonstrate that OX-40R/OX-40L is operative in memory rather than naive T cells and therefore suggest that OX-40R:Ig selectively targets APCs interacting with previously primed T cells [118]. Overall, beyond serving as a target for immunotherapy, OX-40R defines a limited subset of activated T cells in inflammatory lesions that may ultimately permit characterization of antigen-specific T cell receptors in diseases with unknown autoantigens (such as RA) [118,119].

Adhesion molecules

Analogous to co-stimulatory receptor/ligand interactions, adhesion molecules facilitate communication between different cells of the immune system and promote cellular activation. Because adhesion molecules also mediate interaction between cells and vascular endothelium, they play a critical role in processes such as lymphocyte homing and peripheral migration of leukocytes to inflammatory sites [120]. Family members include selectins (E-selectin, P-selectin), immunoglobulin family proteins (intracellular adhesion molecule [ICAM-1], vascular cell adhesion molecule [VCAM-1]), and integrins (leukocyte function-associated antigen 1 [LFA-1], very late antigen 4 [VLA-4]). Together, these molecules comprise a highly complex and precisely regulated system governed by inflammatory cytokines such as TNF-α and IL-1 [121]. Disruption of these pathways is therefore possible at multiple levels ranging from TNF-α inhibition to monoclonal antibodies against adhesion molecules themselves.

ICAM-1/LFA-1 – A number of preclinical and human studies have focused on ICAM-1 (CD54) and LFA-1 (CD11a), molecules expressed on leukocytes as well as vascular endothelium (in the case of ICAM-1) [120,121]. For example, in a murine model of GVHD and autoimmune glomerulonephritis, combined antibody treatment directed against ICAM-1 and LFA-1 decreased albuminuria and enhanced survival, though effects on autoantibodies were less definitive [122]. Histologic analysis revealed diminished CD11+ leukocyte infiltration of glomeruli and reduced deposition of C3 within capillary walls [122]. Additional trials in antigen-induced arthritis and EAE set the stage for preliminary open label trials in both RA and multiple sclerosis. Although a phase I study of anti-CD11/18 in multiple sclerosis was too small to permit conclusions regarding efficacy [123], two separate open label trials in early as well as refractory RA showed clinical benefit [124,125]. Unfortunately, the murine monoclonal antibodies used in these patients with RA evoked anti-murine antibodies that limited responses upon re-treatment, suggesting that future trials will require chimeric or humanized monoclonal antibodies [126].

VCAM-1/VLA-4 – Regulating the interaction between mononuclear leukocytes and activated endothelium, VCAM-1 and VLA-4 also play a critical role in leukocyte transmigration and subsequent development of inflammatory lesions [120,121]. IL-1 and TNF-α enhance expression of VCAM-1 through induction/activation of NF-κB, while IL-4 and IL-13 specifically upregulate this adhesion protein in a NF-κB-independent fashion [121]. Most importantly, because VLA-4 is not expressed on neutrophils, targeting the VCAM-1/VLA-4 interaction results in more selective immunosuppression than anti-ICAM-1/LFA-1 strategies [120,121]. Numerous animal models employing either anti-VLA-4 antibodies or a soluble VCAM-1:Ig fusion protein have demonstrated therapeutic efficacy in preventing/limiting diseases ranging from allograft rejection to autoimmune diabetes and EAE [127-129]. In a model of viral-induced EAE, for example, anti-VLA-4 antibodies proved more effective than anti-Mac-1 or anti-ICAM-1 antibodies in decreasing the severity of CNS lesions and ameliorating clinical deficits [130]. Moreover, anti-VLA-4 treatment downregulated expression of both VCAM-1 and ICAM-1, suggesting that clinical benefit may result from decreased priming of CNS vascular endothelium by activated T cells. Despite the weight of evidence favoring anti-VLA-4 treatment in preclinical studies, trials in human autoimmune disease are currently lacking.

Cell surface molecules

CD4 – Given the dominant role of cell-mediated immunity in most autoimmune diseases, numerous strategies have evolved to target T cells through cell surface markers such as CD4. This immunoglobulin-like molecule acts as a co-receptor for the peptide-MHC complex, stabilizing the T cell/APC interaction and generating intracellular signals through activation of p56lck kinase and consequent phosphorylation of ZAP-70 kinase associated with the TCR/CD3 complex [131]. Therefore, antibody targeting of CD4 may exert biologic effects through negative signalling and tolerance induction/immune deviation rather than simple blockade of T cells. Although initial trials with depleting anti-CD4 antibodies resulted in potentially unacceptable immunosuppression and were only marginally effective in RA, these studies demonstrated that clinical benefit correlated more with synovial fluid T cell depletion than peripheral lymphopenia [132,133]. Subsequent open label trials with various non-depleting anti-CD4 monoclonal antibodies demonstrated promising results in RA [134,135]; however, larger placebo-controlled trials have yielded conflicting results [136,137]. Among those patients who did respond to a humanized anti-CD4 monoclonal antibody (4162W94), decreased expression of adhesion molecules as well as diminished synovial fluid IL-6 and TNF-α levels occurred [138]. Coupled with additional studies showing reduced TH1 cytokine production following CD4 monoclonal antibody treatment, this data supports the possibility of treatment-induced immune deviation [139].

CD5, CD7 – Additional molecules targeted in T cell-depleting strategies include CD5 and CD7. Unfortunately, neither approach has proved successful in RA patients. While an open label trial of anti-CD5 monoclonal antibody appeared promising, a follow-up placebo controlled trial provided no evidence of therapeutic response, possibly because of insufficient dosing [140]. Treatment with anti-CD7 antibodies did cause peripheral T cell depletion; however, no significant clinical benefit emerged, and subsequent studies revealed the predominance of CD7- T cells within the synovial joints of RA patients [141-143]. Overall, the general approach of T cell depletion has been disappointing in RA and may reflect the enhanced susceptibility of naive peripheral T cells relative to activated synovial T cells [144].

Toleragens and vaccines

T cell tolerance – Perhaps the most sought after, yet controversial, approach to treatment of systemic autoimmune diseases involves the induction of antigen-specific tolerance through the administration of exogenous antigen. Based on a number of animal models, two primary concepts have emerged regarding potential mechanisms of tolerance induction: clonal deletion/ anergy and immune deviation [145]. While tolerance stemming from clonal deletion/anergy is non-transferrable, immune deviation hinges on the production of regulatory cytokines such as TGF-β by antigen-specific T cells that can actively transfer tolerance and dampen surrounding inflammation mediated by T cells with different antigen specificities [145-148]. The latter concept of bystander suppression is particularly intriguing, as this mechanism could permit tissue-targeted treatment of autoimmune diseases with unknown inciting antigens.

In animal models, factors determining the outcome of tolerance induction include the dose and form of antigen, route of administration, and stage of development [145,147,148,149]. For example, feeding low doses of soluble antigen typically generates regulatory, TGF-β-secreting T cells, while high doses of the same antigen favor clonal deletion/anergy [145]. Peptide modification experiments have demonstrated the exquisite sequence specificity of this process, as well as the importance of MHC and TCR contact points in determining tolerance versus immunogenicity [147,150]. In turn, these experiments have fostered the concept of using altered peptide ligands (APLs) that bind the TCR with reduced affinity and thereby induce anergy or divert the immune response toward a TH2 phenotype [147,149]. Proof of principle has been established in different models of EAE in which systemically-administered APLs either prevent or treat established disease [150-152]. Overall, despite the volume of literature showing efficacy of systemic and oral tolerance induction in animals, a number of key questions remain that pertain to use of these approaches in humans - namely, the nature of the APC involved in oral tolerance, the role of γ/δ T cells, the effect of adjuvant co-administration, the effectiveness and safety of peptides compared to intact antigen, and the relative efficacy of systemic versus mucosal administration [145,146,148,149].

Because of these uncertainties as well as the inherent differences between animal models and human disease, devising clinical trials has been problematic. Nevertheless, a pilot experiment involving oral administration of KLH to human volunteers showed a reduction in delayed T cell hypersensitivity to KLH and established the feasibility of antigen-specific tolerance in humans

[153]. Similarly, small phase I/II trials of oral tolerance demonstrated modest clinical benefit in RA (chicken collagen), uveitis (retinal S antigen), and MS (bovine myelin) [154-156]. A subsequent phase III, placebo-controlled trial involving different doses of type II collagen in RA patients supported these results, showing statistically significant benefit in the lowest dose group (20 micrograms daily) [157]. While a large scale trial in MS showed no overall benefit in patients consuming bovine myelin, a subset of patients did experience clinical and radiographic improvement. Furthermore, T cells derived from other myelin-fed patients secreted increased amounts of TGF-β [145,158]. Whether these strategies would be more successful with different dosing regimens or timing relative to disease onset remains unclear, but a large scale diabetes prevention trial (DPT-1) comparing oral insulin to placebo in high risk patients should clarify many of the issues surrounding oral tolerance and prevention of autoimmune disease.

T cell vaccines – In the past several years there have been major advances in the identification and characterization of autoantigen-specific T cells in animal models of autoimmunity and in humans with autoimmune diseases. This work has led to the development of a novel therapeutic approach for autoimmune disease based on vaccines (either irradiated autoimmune T cell clones or TCR peptides) designed to generate a specific regulatory immune response to eliminate or anergize these autoreactive T cells [159,160]. The field of T cell vaccination has advanced the farthest with respect to the therapy of MS, a T cell-mediated autoimmune disease characterized by an autoreactive T cell response directed toward nervous system proteins. Both in animal work and more recently human studies, it has been found that the T cell response to myelin basic protein is oligoclonal, with one or a few dominant T cell clones in a given individual [161-163]. Vaccination with these T cell clones is capable of preventing the autoimmune disease (EAE) in mice and ameliorating the disease (MS) in humans. T cell vaccination was shown to induce sustained remission (> 2y) of disease activity in 6 of 9 MS patients in a pilot study. In these studies the beneficial effect was associated with elimination of the pathogenic clones [163]. In turn, the elimination of the vaccinating clones was associated with the development of regulatory T cells including CD8+ cytotoxic T lymphocytes (CTL) and growth inhibitory CD4+ T cells. TCR peptides corresponding to the autoreactive T cell clones also were successful as vaccines to eliminate disease-causing T cell clones [164].

B cell tolerance – For unclear reasons, TH2 responses characterized by pathogenic autoantibodies may be less amenable to immunomodulation mediated by systemic or mucosal antigen administration [145,148]. To achieve B cell tolerance in disorders such as anti-phospholipid antibody syndrome and SLE, investigators have therefore devised toleragens consisting of peptides or oligonucleotides conjugated to an organic "platform." These hybrid molecules prevent antigen processing and T cell help after binding B cell receptors, thereby inducing a state of B cell anergy. Murine models of anti-phospholipid antibody syndrome and SLE have demonstrated the efficacy of B cell tolerance, with reduced titers of anti-β2-glycoprotein I and dsDNA titers, respectively [165,166]. Unfortunately, this preclinical data has not translated into success with human disease, as a phase II/III trial examining the dsDNA toleragen LJP 394 in SLE failed to show clinical benefit and was prematurely terminated [35]. Because this abbreviated trial focused on "time to renal flare" in a cohort of patients with fairly stable disease, however, future trials with different outcome variables will be critical for assessing the viability of B cell tolerance.

SUMMARY

The therapy of autoimmune CTD is rapidly advancing due to (1) new cytotoxic drugs with improved safety profiles, (2) novel *biologic* agents which target specific immune cells, cytokines, and cell-cell interactions, and (3) innovative approaches directed at specific tolerance induction.

Current management of CTD is based on balancing the required level of immunosuppression, which is determined largely by disease severity and organ system involvement, with drug toxicity. For severe CTD in which there is an extensive expansion of autoreactive T and B cells, an aggressive non-specific approach such as immunoablation and stem cell transplantation (currently experimental) may be necessary to induce remission. In such patients, targeted immunotherapy (e.g. toleragens or vaccines) may be helpful in preventing disease recurrence.

REFERENCES

1. Langford CA, Klippel JH, Balow JE, James SP, Sneller MC. Use of Cytotoxic Agents and Cyclosporine in the Treatment of Autoimmune Disease: Part I Rheumatologic and Renal Diseases. Ann Int Med 1998; 128:1021-1028.
2. Langford CA, Klippel JH, Balow JE, James SP, Sneller MC. Use of Cytotoxic Agents and Cyclosporine in the Treatment of Autoimmune Disease: Part 2: Inflammatory Bowel Disease, Systemic Vasculitis, and Therapeutic Toxicity. Ann Int Med 1998; 129:49-58.
3. Ballow M, Nelson R. Immunopharmacology: Immunomodulation and Immuno-

therapy. JAMA 1997; 278:2008-2017.

4. Angeli A, Masera RG, Sartori ML, Fortunati N, Racca S., Dovio A, Staurenghi A, Frairia R. Modulation by Cytokines of Glucocorticoid Action. Ann N Y Acad Sci 1999; 210-220.

5. Morand EF. Corticosteroids in the treatment of rheumatologic diseases. Curr Opin Rheum 1998; 10:179-183.

6. Fox RI, Herrmann ML, Frangou CG, Wahl GM, Morris RE, Strand V, Kirschbaum BJ. Mechansim of action for leflunomide in rheumatoid arthritis 1999; Clin Immunol 93:198-208.

7. Sievers TM, Rossi SJ, Ghobrial RM, Arriola E, Nishimura P, Kwano M, Holt CD. Mycophenolate mofetil. Pharmacotherapy 1997;17:1178-1197.

8. Li E, Brooks P, Conaghan PG. Disease-modifying antirheumatic drugs. Curr Opin Rheum.1998; 10:159-168.

9. Wolfe F, Hawley DJ, Cathey MA: Termination of slow-acting antirheumatic therapy in rheumatoid arthritis: a 14 year prospective evaluation of 1017 consecutive starts. J Rheumatol 1990; 17: 994-1002

10. Felson DT, Anderson JJ, Meenan RF: Use of short-term efficacy/toxicity tradeoffs to select second-line drugs in rheumatoid arthritis: A meta-analysis of published clinical trials. Arthritis Rheum 1992; 35: 1117-1125

11. Fries JF, Williams CA, Ramey D, Bloch DA: The relative toxicity of disease-modifying antirheumatic drugs. Arthritis Rheum 1993; 36: 297-306

12. Enk AH, Knop J. Mycophenolate is effective in the treatment of pemphigus vulgaris. Arch Derm 1999; 135: 54-56.

13. Corna D, Morigi M, Facchinetti D, Bertani T, Zoja C, Remuzzi G. Mycophenolate mofetil limits renal damage and prolongs life in murine lupus autoimmune disease. Kidney Int 1997; 51:1583-1589.

14. Jonsson CA, Svensson L, Carlsten H. Beneficial effect of the inosine monophosphate dehydrogenase inhibitor mycophenolate mofetil on survival and severity of glomerulonephritis in systemic lupus erythematosus (SLE)-prone MRLlpr/lpr mice. Clin Exp Immunol 1999;116:534-541.

15. Glicklich D, Acharya A. Mycophenolate mofetil therapy for lupus nephritis refractory to intravenous cyclophosphamide. Am J Kid Dis 1998; 32:318-322.

16. Gaubitz M, Schorat A, Schotte H, Kern P, Domschke W. Mycophenolate mofetil for the treatment of systemic lupus erythematosus: an open pilot trial. Lupus 1999; 8:731-736.

17. Jarvinen P, Aho K. Twin studies in rheumatic diseases. Sem Arth Rheum. 1994; 24:19-28.

18. Silman AJ, MacGregor A, Thomson W, et al. Twin concordance rates for rheumatoid arthritis: results of a nationwide study. Br J Rheum 1993; 32: 903-907.

19. Grennan DM, Parfitt A, Manolios N, Huang Q, Hyland V, Dunckley H, Doran T. Gatenby P, Badcock C. Family and twin studies in systemic lupus erythematosus. Dis Markers. 1997;13:93-98.

20. Marmont AM, van Lint MT, Gualandi F, Bacigalupo A. Autologous marrow stem cell transplantation for severe systemic lupus erythematosus of long duration. Lupus. 1997; 6:545-548.

21. Burt RK, Georganas C, Schroeder J, et al. Autologous hematopoietic stem cell transplantation in refractory rheumatoid arthritis. Arth Rheum. 1999; 42: 2281-2285.

22. Burt RK, Traynor AE, Pope R, et al. Treatment of autoimmune disease by intense immunosuppressive conditioning and autologous hematopoietic stem cell transplantation. Blood. 1998; 92:3505-3514.

23. Traynor A, Burt RK. Haematopoietic stem cell transplantation for active systemic lupus erythematosus. Rheumatology. 1999; 38:767-772.

24. Fouillard L, Gorin NC, Laporte JP, Leon A, Brantus JF, Miossec P. Control of

severe systemic lupus erythematosus after high-dose immunusuppressive therapy and transplantation of CD34+ purified autologous stem cells from peripheral blood. Lupus. 1999; 8:320-323.

25. Wulffraat N, van Royen A, Bierings M, Vossen J, Kuis W. Autologous haemopoietic stem-cell transplantation in four patients with refractory juvenile chronic arthritis Lancet. 1999; 353:550-553.

26. Brodsky RA, Petri M, Smith BD, et al. Immunoablative high-dose cyclophosphamide without stem-cell rescue for refractory, severe autoimmune disease. Ann Int Med 1998;129:1031-1035.

27. Nousari HC, Brodsky RA, Jones RJ, Grever MR, Anhalt GJ. Immunoablative high-dose cyclophosphamide without stem cell rescue in paraneoplastic pemphigus. J Am Acad Derm. 1999; 40:750-754.

28. Paavonen T. Hormonal regulation of immune responses. Ann Med 1994; 26: 255-258.

29. Olsen NJ, Kovacs WJ. Gonadal steroids and immunity. Endocrine Rev 1996; 17: 369-384.

30. Cutolo M, Sulli A, Seriolo B, Accardo S, Masi AT. Estrogens, immune response and autoimmunity. Clin Exp Immunol 1995; 13:217-226.

31. Sthoeger ZM, Bentwich Z, Zinger H, Mozes E. The beneficial effect of the estrogen antagonist Tamoxifen, on experimental systemic lupus erythematosus. J Rheumatol 1994; 21:2231-2238.

32. Dayan M, Zinger H, Kalush F, Mor G, Amir-Zaltzman Y, Kohen F. The beneficial effects of treatment with tamoxifen and anti-oestradiol antibody on experimental systemic lupus erythematosus are associated with cytokine modulations. Immunology 1997; 90:101-108.

33. Sturgess AD, Evans DT, Mackay IR, Riglar A. Effects of the oestrogen antagonist tamoxifen on disease indices in systemic lupus erythematosus. J Clin Lab Immunol 1984; 12:11-14.

34. Kanai Y, Takeda O, Miura K, Kurosawa Y. Novel autoimmune phenomena induced by a recombinant nucleobindin that has a long leucine zipper structure. Arthritis Rheum 1992; 35:S207.

35. Strand V. Biologic agents and innovative interventional approaches in the management of systemi lupus erythematosus. Curr Opin Rheumatol 1999; 11: 330-340.

36. Petri M, Lahita R, McGuire J, et al. Results of the GL701 (DHEA) multicenter steroid-sparing SLE study. Arthritis Rheum 1997; 40:S326

37. McMurray RW. Prolactin and systemic lupus erythematosus. Ann Med Interne 1996; 147:253-258.

38. Elbourne KB, Keisler D, McMurray RW. Differential effects of estrogen and prolactin on autoimmune disease in the NZB/NZW F1 mouse model of systemic lupus erythematosus. Lupus 1998; 7: 420-427.

39. Reber PM. Prolactin and immunomodulation. Amer J Med 1993; 95:637-644.

40. Alvarez-Nemegyei J, Cobarrubias-Cobos A, Escalante-Triay F, Sosa-Munoz J, Miranda JM, Jara LJ. Bromocriptine in systemic lupus erythematosus: a double-blind, randomized, placebo-controlled study. Lupus 1998; 7:414-419.

41. Halloran, PF. Molecular mechanisms of new immunosuppressants. Clin Transplant 1996; 10:118-123.

42. Henry M L. Cyclosporine and tacrolimus (FK506): A comparison of efficacy and safety profiles. Clin Transplant 1999; 13:209-220.

43. Blank M. Ben-Bassat M. Shoenfeld Y. The effect of cyclosporin A on early and late stages of experimental lupus. Arthritis Rheum 35:1350-5, 1992;

44. Entani C, Izumino K, Iida H, Fujita M, Asaka M, Takata M, Sasayama S. Effect of a novel immunosuppressant, FK506, on spontaneous lupus nephritis in MRL/MpJ-lpr/lpr mice. Nephron. 1993; 64:471-475.

45. Woo J, Wright TM, Lemster B, Borochovitz D, Nalesnik MA, Thomson AW. Combined effects of FK506 (tacrolimus) and cyclophosphamide on atypical B220+ T cells, cytokine gene expression and disease activity in MRL/MpJ-lpr/lpr mice. Clin Exp Immunol. 1995; 100:118-125.

46. Furukawa F, Imamura S, Takigawa M. FK506: therapeutic effects on lupus dermatoses in autoimmune-prone MRL/Mp-lpr/lpr mice. Arch Derm Res. 1995; 287:558-563.

47. Burkhardt H, Kalden JR. Xenobiotic immunosuppressive agents: therapeutic effects in animal models of autoimmune diseases. Rheum Int. 1997; 17:85-90.

48. Sullu Y, Oge I, Erkan D, Ariturk N, Mohajeri F. Cyclosporin-A therapy in severe uveitis of Behcet's disease. Acta Ophth Scand 1998; 76:96-99.

49. Cush JJ, Tugwell P, Weinblatt M, Yocum D. US consensus guidelines for the use of cyclosporin A in rheumatoid arthritis. J Rheum.1999; 26:1176-1186.

50. Lightman S. New therapeutic options in uveitis. Eye. 1997; 11:222-226.

51. Duddridge M, Powell RJ. Treatment of severe and difficult cases of systemic lupus erythematosus with tacrolimus. A report of three cases. Ann Rheum Dis 1997; 56:690-692.

52. Gremillion RB, Posever JO, Manek N, West JP, van Volen-Hoven RF. Tacrolimus (FK506) in the treatment of severe, refractory rheumatoid arthritis J Rheum. 1999; 26:2332-2336.

53. Oddis CV, Sciurba FC, Elmagd KA, Starzl TE. Tacrolimus in refractory polymyositis with interstitial lung disease. Lancet. 1999; 353:1762-1763.

54. Mosmann TR, Sad S. The expanding universe of T-cell subsets: Th1, Th2 and more. Immunology Today 1996;17:138-146.

55. Wallis WJ, Furst DE, Strand V, Keystone E. Biologic agents and immunotherapy in rheumatoid arthritis. Progress and perspective. Rheum Dis Clin N Amer 1998; 24:537-565.

56. Röcken M, Shevach EM. Immune deviation - the third dimension of nondeletional T-cell tolerance. Immunol Rev 1996;149: 175-194.

57. Jorgensen C, Apparailly F, Sany J. Immunological evaluation of cytokine and anti-cytokine immunotherapy in vivo: what have we learnt? Ann Rheum Dis 1999; 58:136-141.

58. Keystone E, Wherry J, Grint P. IL-10 as a therapeutic strategy in the treatment of rheumatoid arthritis. Rheum Dis Clin N Amer 1998; 24:629-639.

59. Brennan FM, Feldman M. Cytokines in autoimmunity. Curr Opin Immunol 1996; 8:872-877.

60. Persson S, Mikulowska A, Narula S, O'Garra A, Holmdahl R. Interleukin-10 suppresses the development of collagen type II-induced arthritis and ameliorates sustained arthritis in rats. Scand J Immunol 1996; 44:607-614.

61. Crisi GM, Santamgrogio L, Hochwald GM, et al. Staphylococcal enterotoxin B and tumor-necrosis factor-alpha-induced relapses of experimental allergic encephalomyelitis: protection by transforming growth factor-beta and interleukin-10. Euro J Immunol 1995; 25:3035-3040.

62. Walmsley M, Katsikis PD, Abney E, et al. Interleukin-10 inhibition of the progression of established collagen-induced arthritis. Arthritis Rheum 1996; 39:495-503.

63. Heresbach D, Semana G, Gosselin M, Bretagne MG. An immunomodulation strategy targeted towards immunocompetent cells or cytokines in inflammatory bowel diseases. Europ Cytokine Network 1999;10: 7-15.

64. Jorgensen C, Apparailly F, Couret I, Canovas F, Jacquet C, Sany J. Interleukin-4 and interleukin-10 are chondroprotective and decrease mononuclear cell recruitment in human rheumatoid synovium in vivo. Immunology 1998; 93:518-523.

65. Caspi RR. IL-12 in autoimmunity. Clin Immunol Immunopathol 1998; 88:4-13.

66. Weckmann AL, Alcocer-Varela J. Cytokine inhibitors in autoimmune disease. Semin Arthritis Rheum 1996; 26:539-557.

67. Allen JB, Wong HL, Costa GL, Bienkowski MJ, Wahl SM. Suppression of mono-cyte function and differential regulation of IL-1 and IL-1ra by IL-4 contribute to resolution of experimental arthritis. J Immunol 1993; 151:4344-4351.

68. Joosten LAB, Lubberts E, Durez P, et al. Role of interleukin-4 and interleukin-10 in murine collagen-induced arthritis: protective effect of interleukin-4 and inter-leukin-10 treatment on cartilage destruction. Arthritis Rheum 1997; 40: 249-260.

69. Li DKB, Paty DW, The UBC MS/MRI Analysis Research Group, The PRISMS Study Group. Magnetic resonance imaging results of the PRISMS Trial: A randomized, double-blind, placebo-controlled study of interferon-[beta]1a in relapsing-remit-ting multiple sclerosis. Ann Neurol 1999; 46:197-206.

70. Anonymous. Randomised double-blind placebo-controlled study of interferon beta-1a in relapsing/remitting multiple sclerosis. Lancet 1998; 352:1498-1504.

71. Ruuls SR, Sedgwick JD. Cytokine-directed therapies in multiple sclerosis and experimental autoimmune encephalomyelitis. Immunol Cell Biol 1998; 76:65-73.

72. Rep MHG, Schrijver HM, van Lopik T, et al. Interferon (IFN)-β treatment enhances CD95 and interleukin 10 expression but reduces interferon-γ producing T cells in MS patients. J Neuroimmunol 1999; 96:92-100.

73. Turner M, Chantry D, Katsikis P, Berger A, Brennan FM, Feldmann M. Induction of the interleukin 1 receptor antagonist protein by transforming growth factor-beta. Euro J Immunol 1991; 21:1635-1639.

74. Dubois CM, Ruscetti FW, Palaszynski EW, Falk LA, Oppenheim JJ, Keller JR. Transforming growth factor beta is a potent inhibitor of interleukin 1 (IL-1) recep-tor expression: proposed mechanism of inhibition of IL-1 action. J Exp Med 1990; 172:737-744.

75. Kuruvilla AP, Shah R, Hochwald GM, Liggitt HD, Palladino MA, Thorbecke GJ. Protective effect of transforming growth factor beta-1 on experimental autoim-mune diseases in mice. Proc Natl Acad Sci (USA) 1991; 88:18-21.

76. Kavanaugh AF. Anti-tumor necrosis factor-a monoclonal antibody therapy for rheumatoid arthritis. Rheum Dis Clin North Am 1998; 24:593-614.

77. Carswell EA, Old LJ, Kassel RL, Green S, Fiore N, Williamson B. An endotoxin-induced serum factor that causes necrosis of tumors. Proc Natl Acad Sci (USA) 1975; 72:3666-3670.

78. Beutler B, Mahoney J, Le Trang N, Pekala P, Cerami A. Purification of cachectin, a lipoprotein lipase-suppressing hormone secreted by endotoxin-induced RAW 264.7 cells. J Exp Med 1985; 161:984-995.

79 Kollias G, Douni E, Kassiotis G, Kontoyiannis D. On the role of tumor necrosis factor and receptors in models of multiorgan failure, rheumatoid arthritis, multi-ple sclerosis and inflammatory bowel disease. Immunol Rev. 1999; 169:175-194.

80 Piguet PF, Grau GE, Vesin C, Loetscher H, Gentz R, Lesslauer W. Evolution of collagen arthritis in mice is arrested by treatment with anti-tumour necrosis factor (TNF) antibody or a recombinant soluble TNF receptor. Immunology.1992; 77:510-514.

81 Williams RO, Feldmann M, Maini RN. Anti-tumor necrosis factor ameliorates joint disease in murine collagen-induced arthritis. Proc Natl Acad Sci (USA). 1992; 89: 9784-9788.

82 Joosten LA. Helsen MM. van de Loo FA. van den Berg WB. Anticytokine treat-ment of established type II collagen-induced arthritis in DBA/1 mice. Arthritis Rheum. 1996; 39:797-809.

83. Moreland LW. Soluble tumor necrosis factor receptor (p75) fusion protein (ENBREL) as a therapy for rheumatoid arthritis. Rheum Dis Clin North Am 1998; 24:579-591.

84 Moreland LW, Baumgartner SW, Schiff MH, et al: Treatment of rheumatoid arthri-tis with a recombinant human tumor necrosis factor receptor (p75)-Fc fusion pro-tein. New Engl J Med 1997; 337: 141-147.

85 Weinblatt ME, Kremer JM, Bankhurst AD, Bulpitt KJ, Fleischmann RM, Fox RI, Jackson CGT, Lang M, Burge DJ: A trial of etanercept, a recombinant tumor necrosis factor receptor:Fc protein, in patients with rheumatoid arthritis receiving methotrexate. New Engl J Med 1999; 340: 253-259.

86. Maini RN, Breedveld FC, Kalden JR, et al. Therapeutic eff icacy of multiple intravenous infusions of anti-tumor necrosis factor alpha monoclonal antibody combined with low-dose weekly methotrexate in rheumatoid arthritis. Arthritis Rheum 1998; 41:1552-1563.

87 van der Meer JW, Vogels MT, Netea MG, Kullberg BJ. Proinflammatory cytokines and treatment of disease. Ann N Y Acad Sci. 1998; 856:243-251.

88. Warren JS. Cytokines in autoimmune disease. Clin Lab Med 1997; 17:547-557.

89. Arend WP, Welgus HG, Thompson RC, Eisenberg SP. Biological properties of recombinant human monocyte-derived interleukin 1 receptor antagnoist. J Clin Invest 1990; 85:1694-1697.

90. Otani K, Nita I, Macaulay W, Gerogescu HI, Robbins PD, Evans CH. Suppression of antigen-induced arthritis in rabbits by ex vivo gene therapy. J Immunol 1996; 156:3558-3562.

91. Makarov SS, Olsen JC, Johnston WN, et al. Suppression of experimental arthritis by gene transfer of interleukin 1 receptor antagonist cDNA. Proc Nat'l Acad Sci USA 1996; 93:402-406.

92. Bresnihan B, Alvaro-Gracia JM, Cobby M, et al. Treatment of rheumatoid arthritis with recombinant human interleukin-1 receptor antagonist. Arthritis Rheum. 1998; 41:2196-204.

93. Drevlow BE, Lovis R, Haag MA, et al. Recombinant human interleukin-1 receptor type I in the treatment of patients with active rheumatoid arthritis. Arthritis Rheum 1996; 39:257-265.

94. Cohick CB, Furst DE, Quagliata S, Corcoran KA, Steere KJ, Yager JG, Lindsley HB. Analysis of elevated serum interleukin-6 levels in rheumatoid arthritis: correlation with erythrocyte sedimentation rate or C-reactive protein. J Lab Clin Med. 1994; 123:721-7.

95 Wendling D, Racadot E, Wijdenes J. Treatment of severe rheumatoid arthritis by anti-interleukin 6 monoclonal antibody. Journal of Rheumatology. 1993; 20: 259-262.

96. Mihara M, Kotoh M, Oda, et al. Anti-Il-6 receptor antibody suppresses the onset of collagen arthritis in monkeys. Arthritis Rheum 1997;40: S133.

97. McIntyre KW, Shuster DJ, Gillooly KM, et al. Reduced incidence and severity of collagen-induced arthritis in interleukin-12-deficient mice. Euro J Immunol 1996; 26:2933-2938.

98. Malfait AM, Butler DM, Presky DH, Maini RN, Brennan FM, Feldman M. Blockade of IL-12 during the induction of collagen-induced arthritis (CIA) markedly attenuates the severity of the arthritis. Clin Exp Immunol 1998; 111:377-383.

99. Davidson NJ, Hudak SA, Lesley RE, Menon S, Leach MW, Rennick DM. IL-12, but not IFN-gamma, plays a major role in sustaining the chronic phase of colitis in IL-10-deficient mice. J Immunol 1998; 161:143-149.

100. Constantinescu CS, Wysocka M, Hilliard B, et al. Antibodies against IL-12 prevent superantigen-induced and spontaneous relapses of experimental autoimmune encephalomyelitis. J Immunol 1998; 161:5097-5104.

101. Butler DM, Malfait AM, Maini RN, Brennan FM, Feldman M. Anti-IL-12 and anti-TNF antibodies synergistically suppress the progression of murine collagen-induced arthritis. Euro J Immunol 1999; 29:2205-2212.

102 Sperling AI, Bluestone JA. The complexities of T-cell co-stimulation: CD28 and beyond. Immunol Rev. 1996;153:155-182.

103. McAdam AJ, Schweitzer AN, Sharpe AH. The role of B27 costimulation in activation and differentiation of CD4+ and CD8+ T cells. Immunol Rev 1998; 165:

231-247.

104. Nakajima A, Azuma M, Kodera S, et al. Preferential dependence of autoantibody production in murine lupus on CD86 costimulatory molecule. Euro J Immunol 1995; 25:3060-3069.

105. Finck BK, Linsley PS, Wofsy D. Treatment of murine lupus with CTLA4Ig. Science 1994; 265:1225-1227.

106. Abrams JR, Lebwohl MG, Guzzo CA, et al. CTLA4Ig-mediated blockade of T-cell costimulation in patients with psoriasis vulgaris. J Clin Invest 1999; 103: 1243-1252.

107. van Kooten C, Banchereau J. Functional role of CD40 and its ligand. Int Arch Allergy Immunol 1997; 113:393-399.

108. van Kooten C, Banchereau J. Functions of CD40 on B cells, dendritic cells and other cells. Curr Opin Immunol 1997; 9:330-337.

109. Aruffo A, Farrington M, Hollenbaugh D, et al. The CD40 ligand, gp39, is defective in activated T cells from patients with X-linked hyper-IgM syndrome. Cell 1993; 72:291-300.

110. Durie FH, Fava RA, Foy TM, Aruffo A, Ledbetter JA, Noelle RJ. Prevention of collagen-induced arthritis with an antibody to gp39, the ligand for CD40. Science 1993; 261:1328-1330.

111. Gerritse K, Laman JD, Noelle RJ, et al. CD40-CD40 ligand interactions in experimental allergic encephalomyelitis and multiple sclerosis. Proc Nat Acad Sci USA 1996; 93:2499-2504.

112. Balasa B, Krahl T, Patstone G, et al. CD40 ligand-CD40 interactions are necessary for the initiation of insulitis and diabetes in nonobese diabetic mice. J Immunol 1997; 159:4620-4627.

113. Mohan C, Shi Y, Laman JD, Dattta SK. Interaction between CD40 and its ligand gp39 in the development of murine lupus nephritis. J Immunol 1995; 154: 1470-1480.

114. Early GS, Zhao W, Burns CM. Anti-CD 40 ligand antibody treatment prevents the development of lupus-like nephritis in a subset of New Zealand black x New Zealand white mice. J Immunol 1996; 157:3159-3164.

115. Durie FH, Aruffo A, Ledbetter J, et al. Antibody to the ligand of CD40, gp39, blocks the occurrence of the acute and chronic forms of graft-vs-host disease. J Clin Invest 1994; 94:1333-1338.

116. Datta SK, Kalled SL. CD40-CD40 ligand interaction in autoimmune disease. Arthritis Rheum 1997; 40:1735-1745.

117. Kalled SL, Cutler AH, Datta SK, Thomas DW. Anti-CD40 ligand antibody treatment of SNF₁ mice with established nephritis: preservation of kidney function. J Immunol 1998; 160:2158-2165.

118. Weinberg AD, Wegmann KW, Funatake C, Whitham RH. Blocking OX-40/OX-40 ligand interaction in vitro and in vivo leads to decreased T cell function and amelioration of experimental allergic encephalomyelitis. J Immunol 1999; 162: 1818-1826.

119. Weinberg AD, Lemon M, Jones AJ, et al. OX-40 antibody enhances for autoantigen specific V beta 8.2+ T cells within the spinal cord of Lewis rats with autoimmune encephalomyelitis. J Neurosci Res 1996; 43:42-49.

120. Oppenheimer-Marks N, Lipsky PE. Adhesion molecules as targets for the treatment of autoimmune diseases. Clin Immunol Immunopathol 1996; 79:201-210.

121. Foster CA. VCAM-1/[alpha]4-integrin adhesion pathway: therapeutic target for allergic inflammatory disorders. J Allergy Clin Immunol 1999;98:270-277.

122. Kootstra CJ, Van Der Giezen DM, Van Krieken JHJM, De Heer E, Bruijn JA. Effective treatment of experimental lupus nephritis by combined administration of anti-CD11a and anti-CD54 antibodies. Clin Exp Immunol 1997; 108:324-332.

123. Bowen JD, Petersdorf SH, Richards TL, et al. Phase I study of a humanized anti-

CD11/CD18 monoclonal antibody in multiple sclerosis. Clin Pharmacol Ther 1998; 64: 339-346.

124. Kavanaugh AF, Davis LS, Jain RI, Nichols LA, Norris SH, Lipsky PE. A phase I/II open label study of the safety and efficacy of an anti-ICAM-1. J Rheumatol 1996; 23:1338-1344.

125. Kavanaugh AF, Davis LS, Nichols LA, et al. Treatment of refractory rheumatoid with a monoclonal antibody to intercellular adhesion molecule 1. Arthritis Rheum 1994; 37:992-999.

126. Kavanaugh AF, Schulze-Koops H, Davis LS, Lipsky PE. Repeat treatment of rheumatoid arthritis patients with a murine anti-intercellular adhesion molecule 1 monoclonal antibody. Arthritis Rheum 1997; 40:849-853.

127. Orosz CG, Ohye RG, Pelletier RP, et al. Treatment with anti-vascular cell adhesion molecule 1 monoclonal antibody induces long-term murine cardiac allograft acceptance. Transplantation 1993; 56:453-460.

128. Tsukamoto K, Yokono K, Amano K, et al. Administration of monoclonal antibodies against vascular cell adhesion molecule-1/very late antigen-4 abrogates predisposing autoimmune diabetes in NOD mice. Cell Immunol 1995; 165:193-201.

129. Yednock TA, Cannon C, Fritz LC, Sanchez-Madrid F, Steinman L, Karin N. Prevention of experimental autoimmune encephalomyelitis by antibodies against alpha 4 beta 1 integrin. Nature 1992; 356:63-66.

130. Soilu-Hänninen M, Röyttä M, Salmi A, Salonen R. Therapy with antibody against leukocyte integrin VLA-4 (CD49d) is effective and safe in virus-facilitated experimental allergic encephalomyelitis. J Neuroimmunol 1997; 72:95-105.

131. Breedveld FC. Monoclonal antibodies to CD4. Rheum Dis Clin N Amer 1998; 24:567-577.

132. Choy EH, Chikanza IC, Kingsley GH, Corrigall V, Panayi GS. Treatment of rheumatoid arthritis with single dose or weekly pulses of chimaeric anti-CD4 monoclonal antibody. Scan J Immunol 1992; 36:291-298.

133. Choy EH, Pitzalis C, Cauli A, et al. Percentage of anti-CD4 monoclonal antibody-coated lymphocytes in the rheumatoid joint is associated with clinical improvement. Implications for the development of immunotherapeutic dosing regimens. Arthritis Rheum 1996; 39:52-56.

134. Panayi GS, Choy EHS, Connolly DJA, et al. T cell hypothesis in rheumatoid arthritis (RA) tested by humanized non-depleting anti-CD4 monoclonal antibody (mAb) treatment I: suppression of disesae activity and acute phase response. Arthritis Rheum 1996; 39:S244.

135. Choy EHS, Connolly DJA, Regan T, et al. T cell hypothesis in rheumatoid arthritis (RA) tested by humanized non-depleting anti-CD4 monoclonal antibody (mAb) treatment II: clinical activity is related to pharmacodynamic effects. Arthritis Rheum 1996; 39:S244.

136 Wendling D, Racadot E, Wijdenes J, et al. A randomized, double blind, placebo controlled multicenter trial of murine anti-CD4 monoclonal antibody therapy in rheumatoid arthritis. J Rheumatol 1998; 25:1457-1461.

137. Levy R, Weisman M, Wiesenhutter C, et al. Results of a placebo-controlled, multicenter trial using a primatized non-depleting, anti-CD4 monoclonal antibody in the treatment of rheumatoid arthritis. Arthritis Rheum 1996;39:S122.

138. Choy EHS, Connolly DJA, Rapson N, Kingsley GH, Johnston JM, Panayi GS: Effect of a humanised non-depleting anti-CD4 monoclonal antibody (mAb) on synovial fluid (SF) in rheumatoid arthritis (RA). Arthritis Rheum 1997;40:S52.

139. Schulze-Koops H, Davis LS, Haverty TP, Wacholtz MC, Lipsky PE. Reduction of Th1 cell activity in the peripheral circulation of patients with rheumatoid arthritis after treatment with a non-depleting humanized monoclonal antibody to CD 4. J Rheumatol 1998; 25:2065-2076.

140. Olsen NJ, Brooks RY, Cush JJ, et al. A double-blind, placebo-controlled study

of anti-Dd5 immunoconjugate in patients with rheumatoid arthritis. Arthritis Rheum 1996; 39:1102-1108.

141. Kirkham BW, Pitzalis C, Kingsley GH, et al. Monoclonal antibody treatment in rheumatoid arthritis: the clinical and immunological effects of a CD7 monoclonal antibody. Br J Rheumatol 1991; 30:459-463.

142. Kirkham BW, Thien F, Pelton BK, et al. Chimeric CD7 monoclonal antibody therapy in rheumatoid arthritis. J Rheumatol 1992;19:1348-1352.

143. Lazarovits AI, White MJ, Karsh J. CD7-T cells in rheumatoid arthritis. Arthritis Rheum 1992; 35:615-624.

144. Choy EHS, Kingsley GH, Panayi GS. Monoclonal antibody therapy in rheumatoid arthritis. Br J Rheumatol 1998; 37:484-490.

145. Wardrop RM, Whitacre CC. Oral tolerance in the treatment of inflammatory auto-immune diseases. Inflamm Res 1999; 48:106-119.

146. Garside P, Mcl Mowat A. Mechanisms of oral tolerance. Crit Rev Immunol 1997; 17:119-137.

147. Xiao B-G, Link H. Mucosal tolerance: a two-edged sword to prevent and treat autoimmune diseases. Clin Immunol Immunopathol 1997; 85:119-128.

148. Mayer L. Oral Tolerance: new approaches, new problems. Clin Immunol 2000; 94:1-8.

149. Liblau R, Tisch R, Bercovici N, McDevitt HO. Systemic antigen in the treatment of T-cell-mediated autoimmune diseases. Immunology Today 1997; 18:599-604.

150. Karin N, Binah O, Grabie N, et al. Short peptide-based tolerogens without self-antigenic or pathogenic activity reverse autoimmune disease. J Immunol 1998; 160:5188-5194.

151. Nicholson LB, Greer JM< Sobel RA, Lees MB, Kuchroo VK. An altered peptide ligand mediates immune deviation and prevents autoimmune encephalomyelitis. Immunity 1995; 3:397-405.

152. Brocke S, Gijbels K, Allegretta M, et al. Treatment of experimental encephalomy-elitis with a peptide analogue of myelin basic protein. Nature 1996; 379:343-346.

153. Husby S, Mestecky J, Moldoveanu Z, Holland S, Elson CO. Oral tolerance in humans. T cell but not B cell tolerance after antigen feeding. J Immunol 1994; 152:4663-4670.

154. Trentham DE, Dynesius-Trentham RA, Orav EJ, et al. Effects of oral administration of type II collagen on rheumatoid arthritis. Science 1993; 261:1727-1730.

155. Nussenblatt RB, Gery I, Weiner HL, et al. Treatment of uveitis by oral administration of retinal antigens: results of a phase I/II randomized masked trial. Amer J Ophthalmol 1997; 123:583-592.

156. Weiner HL, Makin GA, Matsui M, et al. Double-blind pilot trial of oral tolerization with myelin antigens in multiple sclerosis. Science 1993; 259:1321-1324.

157. Barnett ML, Kremer JM, St. Clair EW, et al. Treatment of rheumatoid arthritis with oral type II collagen. Results of a multicenter, double-blind, placebo-con-trolled trial. Arthritis Rheum 1998; 41:290-297.

158. Fukaura H, Kent SC, Pietrusewicz MJ, Khoury SJ, Weiner HL, Hafler DA. Antigen-specific TGF-beta 1 secretion with bovine myelin oral tolerization in multiple scle-rosis. Ann NY Acad Sci 1996; 778:251-257.

159. Gold DP, Shroeder K, Goldring A, Brostoff SW, Wilson DB. T-cell receptor peptides as immunotherapy for autoimmune disease. Crit Rev Immunol. 1997;17:507-510.

160. Stinnisen P, Raus J. Autoreactive T cells in multiple sclerosis: pathogenetic role and therapeutic targeting. Acta Neurol Belgica 1999; 99:65-69.

161. McFarland HF, Hurley CK. Diversity of T-cell receptor Vα, Vβ, and CDR3 expres-sion by myelin basic protein-specific human T-cell clones. Neurology 1995; 45: 1919-1922.

162. Zhang J, Medaer R, Stinissen P, Hafler D, Raus J. MHC-restricted depletion of human myelin basic protein-reactive T cells by T cell vaccination. Science 1993;

261:1451-1454.

163. Zhang J, Raus J. Clonal depletion of human myelin basic protein-reactive T-cells by T-cell vaccination. Ann N Y Acad Sci 1995; 755:323-326.

164. Rosloniec EF, Brand DD, Whittington KB, Stuart JM, Ciubotaru M, Ward ES. Vaccination with a recombinant Vα domain of a TCR prevents the development of collagen-induced arthritis. J Immunol 1995; 155:4504-4511.

165. Iverson GM, Jones DS, Marquis D, Linnik MD, Victoria EJ. A chemically defined, toleragen-based approach for targeting anti-beta2-glycoprotein I antibodies. Lupus 1998; 2:S166-S169.

166. Jones DS, Barstad PA, Feild MJ, et al. Immunospecific reduction of antioligonucleotide antibody-forming cells with a tetrakis-oligonucleotide conjugate (LJP 394), a therapeutic candidate for the treatment of lupus nephritis. J Medicinal Chem 1995; 38:2138-2144.

15 IMMUNOTHERAPY FOR ALLERGIC DISEASES

Dale T. Umetsu and Rosemarie H. DeKruyff
Department of Pediatrics
Stanford University
Stanford, California, USA

INTRODUCTION

Allergic diseases and asthma have increased substantially in prevalence over the last two decades in industrialized countries, and constitute a major public health problem. These diseases are caused by pathological immune responses directed against generally innocuous agents such as environmental respiratory antigens or food antigens, and are characterized by immediate phase responses involving allergen-specific IgE and degranulation of mast cells, resulting in the release of several mediators, including histamine, several proteases as well as cytokines, and arachadonic acid products, including leukotrienes. More importantly, allergic responses are driven and amplified by the development of allergen-specific CD4$^+$ T cells producing high levels of Th2 cytokines (IL-4, IL-5, IL-9 and IL-13), which enhance the growth, differentiation, and recruitment of eosinophils, B cells producing IgE, as well as mast cells and basophils [1]. Together, these cells and factors produce an inflammatory process that is responsible for the symptoms of allergic disease, including urticaria, atopic dermatitis (skin manifestations of allergy), wheezing, airway hyperreactivity or asthma (pulmonary manifestations of allergy), laryngeal edema and hypotension (anaphylaxis), sneezing and nasal congestion or allergic rhinitis (upper respiratory tract), and vomiting and diarrhea or food allergy (gastro-introintestinal manifestations of allergy).

Currently, numerous pharmacologic therapies are available for allergic disease and asthma. Most of these therapies focus on neutralizing the mediators and factors produced by cells involved in allergic inflammation, or simply

A. W. Thomson (ed.), Therapeutic Immunosuppression, 385–403.
© 2001 *Kluwer Academic Publishers.*

eliminating the cell types that produce these mediators. These therapies include anti-histamines, leukotriene antagonists, and inhaled and systemic corticosteroids (and in the future, anti-IgE monoclonal antibody, soluble IL-4 receptor, and other therapies that neutralize cytokines, chemokines or adhesion molecules). Corticosteroids inhibit cytokine and chemokine production in T cells, mast cells, epithelial cells, eliminate eosinophils, inhibit the chemotaxis of cells into sites of allergic inflammation, and thus corticosteroids are extremely effective in suppressing allergic inflammation. In addition to corticosteroids, more specific immunosuppressive agents such as cyclosporin A and FK506, which inhibit cytokine production in T cells and mast cells, have been shown to be effective in the treatment of asthma and atopic dermatitis. While all of these medications are very effective in controlling the symptoms of allergic disease and asthma, in all instances, discontinuation of the medications results in the redevelopment of symptoms on reexposure to the offending allergens. Therefore, none of these drug therapies actually modifies the course of the disease or produces cure. Moreover, immunosuppressive therapies with corticosteroids or with other immunosuppressive agents have significant side effects, which limit their use in allergic disease and asthma. Even topical, inhaled corticosteroids are associated with the potential side effects, for example growth suppression in children, and glaucoma and cataracts after prolonged use. Furthermore, it is possible that corticosteroids (as well as β2 adrenergic bronchodilating agents) may indirectly increase the severity of allergic disease over extended periods of time, by reducing IL-12 production in antigen presenting cells, thereby insidiously enhancing Th2 cytokine synthesis [2,3]. Finally, therapies that focus on reducing symptoms (e.g., by neutralizing specific mediators such as histamine, IL-4, IL-13 and others) encourage patients to experience greater exposure to environmental allergen, which further strengthens the Th2 biased responses in these individuals. Therefore, other approaches to disease management must be pursued to limit the morbidity and mortality associated with allergy and asthma, and to bring about long lasting cure for these diseases.

In this review, we will discuss the rationale, goals and methodologies of immunotherapies for allergic disease and asthma. In contrast to the pharmacologic therapies for allergic disease that focus on neutralizing mediators and on temporarily reducing symptoms, immune-based therapies have the potential to modify or reverse the underlying pathological immune responses in allergy and asthma to provide long lasting cures for these problems. A major feature of this approach is the focus on antigen-specific modification of immune responses, which is possible in allergic disease because the specific antigens that cause allergic diseases (e.g., environmental allergens, such as plant pollens and dust mite allergens) have been, for the most part, identified. This contrasts with the situation in autoimmunity or in transplantation, where the specific antigens are either unknown, or differ for each individual patient. Therefore in allergic diseases, antigen-specific therapies can be developed that have the potential to induce protective immune responses that are reinforced by natural exposure to the allergen, thus conferring long-lasting protection without the need for continuous therapeutic intervention. A significant benefit of antigen-specific immunotherapies for allergic disease is that they avoid generalized immunosuppression that occurs with antigen non-specific therapies. The avoidance of significant immunosuppressive side effects is important in the treatment of allergic disease, since allergic diseases affect a large fraction of the general population, most who do not have life threatening disease. If most affected individuals are to be treated, including those without life-threatening disease, therapies must not be associated with the risk of significant harmful side effects. This differs from the situation of organ transplantation, which is often performed in the setting of life-threatening problems, and in which the use of immunosuppressive therapies that are associated with much greater risk of side effects is appropriate.

Protective immunity in allergic disease and asthma

While it is clear that Th2 driven allergen-specific immune responses are responsible for the development of the pathology in allergic disease and asthma, the specific features of immune responses that protect against allergic diseases and the therapeutic goals of immunotherapy are less clear. Nonallergic individuals, while exposed to the same allergens as allergic individuals, do not develop symptoms on exposure to allergen presumably because they are immunologically tolerant to allergen. Historically, investigators attributed the lack of symptoms in nonallergic individuals to the lack of an immune response, due to either lack of sufficient previous exposure to allergen, or to favorable immune response genes that prevented responses to various allergens. However, the clinical experience is that nonallergic individuals are indeed exposed to sufficient quantities of allergen, and these include a very broad number of antigens. This makes it unlikely that MHC immune response genes, which restrict immune responses by limiting the capacity of specific antigen peptides to bind to MHC molecules, restrict responses to so many diverse allergens. Accordingly, MHC markers have been linked to only a limited number of allergen specific responses, and these allergens have been generally minor antigens from very complex mixtures of allergen extracts [4]. Thus, immunological control of allergy is considered now to be related to broader regulatory mechanisms, for example, to immune responses that actively protect against the development of allergy or asthma. In other words, absence of allergic symptoms in normal nonallergic individuals is not due to the absence of immune responses against allergens, but rather due to active antigen-specific responses of various types that suppress the development of detrimental allergic inflammation.

Over the past ten years, there has been much interest in the role of allergen-specific Th1 cells, which produce IFN-γ and IL-2, as regulators of allergic disease and asthma. According to the Th1/Th2 paradigm proposed by Bob Coffman and Tim Mosmann, Th1 cells cross regulate Th2 cells by inhibiting the development and proliferation of Th2 cells [5]. This paradigm has been most elegantly demonstrated in a Leishmania parasite model in which Th1 cells protect against Leishmania infection, while Th2 cells are associated with dissemination of infection. This binary paradigm, in which Th1 and Th2 cells are mutually exclusive, has been extrapolated from the Leishmania model and applied to asthma, and many investigators conclude that Th1 cells protect against allergy and asthma. In this model, protection from allergy is due to the development of a different form of immunity, involving inhibitory allergen-specific Th1 cells, rather than the lack of immune responsiveness to allergens.

A significant amount of data support the idea that Th1 cells protect against allergy and asthma, but much of it is indirect. For example, investigators generated long term allergen-specific T cell clones from the peripheral blood of nonallergic individuals, and these produced Th1 cytokines, IFN-γ and IL-2 [6,7]. In addition, we and others have shown that individuals predisposed towards the production of Th1 cytokines have a reduced likelihood of developing allergic disease. Thus, individuals with strong delayed type hypersensitivity to *Mycobacteria tuberculosis* after immunization with BCG, have a reduced likelihood of developing allergy or asthma [8]. In addition, patients with multiple sclerosis, an autoimmune disease characterized by the overproduction of Th1 cytokines in myelin specific T cells were also protected from the development of allergy (Figure 1), and this correlates with an increased capacity to produce IL-12 in monocytes from these patients [9,10]. Similarly, patients with other autoimmune diseases such as rheumatoid arthritis or type 1 diabetes mellitus appeared to be protected from the development of allergy [11,12].

Additional studies that support the role of Th1-biased responses in protection against allergy and asthma include data demonstrating that administration of IL-12 intratracheally, or of IL-12 plus IL-18, inhibits allergen-induced

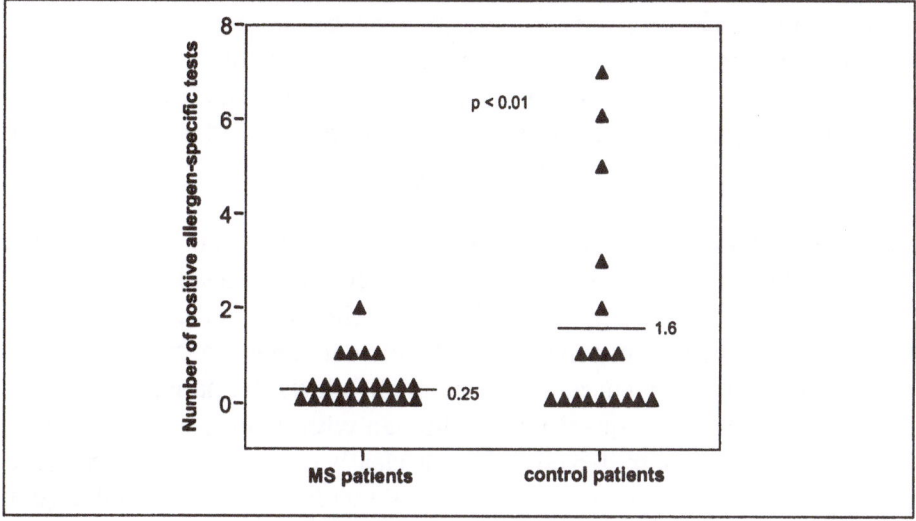

Figure 1

airway inflammation and hyperreactivity [13,14]. Both IL-12 and IL-18 are potent inducers of IFN-γ production and appear capable of preventing the development of Th2 biased inflammatory responses in the lung. IL-18 has the additional capacity to stimulate the development of CD8 cells, suggesting that IFN-γ producing CD8 cells may be important in regulating Th2 mediated diseases, as has been previously suggested [15]. Thus, protection against allergic disease and asthma is likely to involve allergen-specific Th1 biased immune responses, as well as CD8 T cells. Similarly, administration of immunostimulatory DNA sequences (ISS), which induce IL-12, TNF-α and IFN-γ production, inhibits IL-5 synthesis, eosinophilic inflammation, and the development of airway hyperresponsiveness in mice [16]. These studies indicate that methods to induce Th1 responses might be effective as therapies for suppression of the symptoms of allergic diseases.

ALLERGEN-SPECIFIC IMMUNOTHERAPIES

While the administration of IL-12, IL-18 or ISS is effective in *preventing* allergen-induced airway hyperreactivity, therapies with these cytokines and agents may be incomplete since they may not induce protective immunity that persists after discontinuation of therapy. In addition, since the effects of these cytokines when administered in vivo are not antigen-specific, they may induce unwanted Th1 biased (auto)immune responses. Therefore, a more desirable approach would be to focus on allergen-specific cells, for example by converting allergen-specific Th2 biased responses into protective and persistent immune responses, utilizing immunotherapies that induce allergen-specific immune deviation or immune modulation. This is particularly appropriate for allergic disease, since the vast majority of allergens that cause allergic disease have been identified.

Conventional allergen immunotherapy, performed by the subcutaneous injection of increasing quantities of allergen protein has been in clinical use for the treatment of allergy since 1911. This therapy appears to eliminate IgE mediated allergic responses and allergic sensitivity in an antigen-specific fashion, and upon successful completion, allows the patient to tolerate exposure to significant quantities of allergen with minimal symptoms [17]. A large number of controlled clinical trials clearly establish the clinical effectiveness of allergen immunotherapy in IgE-mediated allergic rhinitis (hay fever), allergic asthma, and Hymenoptera venom (bee sting) anaphylaxis [18]. During conventional immunotherapy for allergic rhinitis or allergic asthma, the injections are increased to a maximally tolerated level, generally 10^5 times the initial dose, equivalent to 2 to 100 μg of the major allergen. Clinical benefit occurs after several months of injections for inhalant allergy, and progressive reduction of symptoms occurs over the first 3-4 years of injection therapy. Moreover, prolonged clinical benefit with 80-90% reduction in symptoms and in medication usage is sustained following discontinuation of immunotherapy after three to four years of injections in most patients [19]. Allergen immunotherapy is effective in reducing allergic symptoms for environmental aeroallergens as well as for Hymenoptera venom anaphylaxis, reducing serious reactions from stings throughout the period of active treatment at maintenance dosage, and following discontinuation after three to five years of maintenance injections.

Mechanisms of action of allergen immunotherapy

The mechanisms by which conventional allergen immunotherapy produce its beneficial clinical effects has been studied for many years. Initially, investigators focused on the induction of blocking IgG antibodies, which were thought to bind to exogenous allergen, impeding exposure of allergen-specific IgE on the surface of mast cells or basophils to the allergen. More recently, with improved understanding of the importance of CD4 T cells in the pathogenesis of allergic disease and asthma, it has become clear that allergen immunotherapy is associated with immune deviation, with a reduction in the function of allergen-specific Th2 cells, and with the development of allergen-specific IFN-γ producing Th1 cells [20-22]. In addition, failure of conventional allergen immunotherapy is associated with the failure to reduce allergen-specific IL-4 production [23]. Whether other immunologic mechanisms also occur following successful immunotherapy, e.g., induction of CD8 regulatory cells [24] or the induction of allergen-specific IL-10 production [24a], is not yet clear. Nevertheless, conventional allergen immunotherapy is effective therapy for asthma and allergy and protects against allergy and asthma, even after the discontinuation of therapy.

Novel methodologies for allergen immunotherapy

While conventional allergen immunotherapy is unique in its capacity to induce protective immunity, it is particularly inefficient. Although conventional allergen immunotherapy effectively controls symptoms in most patients even after discontinuation of therapy, the process requires nearly 100 injections, over 3-5 years, and in addition, is associated with frequent allergic reactions, including anaphylaxis. Finally, a small number of individuals do not respond to this therapy. This inefficiency has stimulated major efforts over the past five years to improve the efficacy of allergen immunotherapy. These efforts have included the study of vaccines containing cDNA of allergens, use of immunostimulatory sequences of DNA as adjuvant, modified protein allergens, and oral administration of allergen.

a. *Naked DNA vaccination*

A large number of recent studies have demonstrated the effectiveness of genetic vaccination approach in models of infectious disease [25-27], cancer [28] and autoimmune disease [29,30]. In these models, vaccination is performed with allergen in the form of naked plasmid cDNA, which stimulates allergen-specific immune responses with a Th1 bias. CpG motifs present on the vector backbone enhance immunogenicity [31], and effectively induce IL-12, IFN-γ production and a Th1 bias. DNA vaccination has been applied to models of allergic disease and asthma, since the Th1 response is assumed to be protective in allergic disease and asthma, and capable of down modulating the Th2 biased immune responses in allergic disease and asthma. Several studies with DNA immunization strategies demonstrated its success in preventing the development of antigen-specific IgE synthesis, airway hyperresponsiveness or food-induced anaphylaxis [32-34]. The efficacy of DNA vaccination however, has varied widely, and successful reversal of *established* allergic inflammation and airway hyperreactivity with allergen cDNA vaccination has not been reported. The capacity of vaccination strategies to reverse established disease is required in order to treat patients with ongoing asthma and allergy. Preliminary studies in our laboratory suggest that combining IL-18 cDNA with allergen cDNA in a single vector may enhance the effectiveness of the DNA vaccination, and result in a potent vaccine construct that is indeed capable of reversing established airway hyperreactivity. The rationale for this approach of fusing IL-18 cDNA with OVA cDNA was based on our previous findings with protein based vaccines, using fusions of IL-12 and allergen [35] (see below).

b. Modified proteins with enhanced immunogenicity

To improve the immunogenicity of allergen and to minimize the nonspecific effects of the Th1 inducing cytokine IL-12, which can activate allergen-non-specific cells (e.g., NK cells, γδ T cells and αβ T cells) and potentially induces autoimmune disease, we generated a therapeutic construct by covalently linking allergen with IL-12 as *fusion proteins*. In these experiments, an allergen-IL-12 fusion protein increased the immunogenicity of the allergen by focusing the effects of IL-12 on antigen-specific immune cells, and minimizing the antigen-nonspecific effects of IL-12. This greatly improved the capacity of the allergen to induce Th1 biased responses and reverse established allergic responses [35]. Immunization of naïve mice with the allergen-IL-12 fusion protein induced anti-allergen IgG2a antibody and large quantities of allergen-specific IFN-γ production. The antigen-specificity of this response was dependent upon covalent linkage of antigen and IL-12, since immunization of mice with allergen and free recombinant IL-12 enhanced T cell production of IFN-γ, but the IFN-γ production was not allergen-specific. In mice with established Th2 dominated responses, vaccination with the allergen-IL-12 protein was much more effective than allergen plus free rIL-12 in increasing antigen-specific IFN-γ production, and decreasing antigen-specific IL-4 production. Moreover, administration of allergen-IL-12 increased serum anti-allergen IgG2a and significantly decreased anti-allergen IgE, presumably by localizing the IL-12 activity to sites in immune organs where allergen-specific cells were activated. Thus modification of allergen by covalently linking cytokines such as IL-12 may be an effective methodology to enhance the immunogenicity of proteins in inducing Th1 biased responses, and to treat patients with allergic disease.

c. Adjuvants for allergen immunotherapy

If Th1 responses play an important in protective responses against allergy and asthma, then vaccination with allergen plus other Th1 inducing adjuvants may be effective in the treatment of patients with allergic disease and asthma. For example, heat killed *Listeria monocytogenes* (HKL), which is

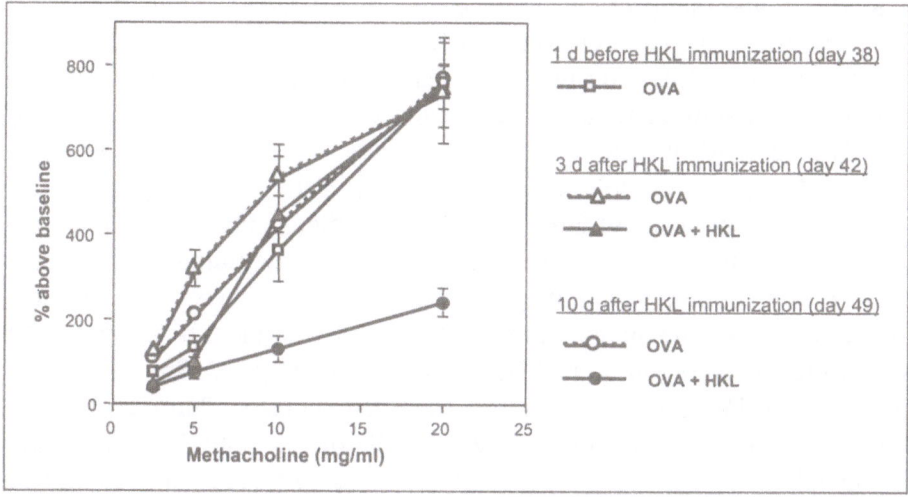

Figure 2
HKL as an adjuvant reverses established airway hyperreactivity in OVA-immu-nized BALB/c mice. BALB/c mice were sensitized with OVA intraperitoneally and intranasally. Mice then received OVA or OVA mixed with HKL (10^8 per mouse) on day 39. Airway hyperreactivity(AHR) in response to increasing concentrations of metha-choline was measured one day before, three days, and ten days after the injection of HKL. Data are expressed as percent above baseline (mean ± SEM). By day 49, 10 days after vaccination with OVA + HKL (but not with OVA alone), there was a reduction of AHR to levels observed in naïve mice [50].

potent in inducing IL-12 production in antigen presenting cells and IFN-γ in NK and CD4 T cells, when mixed with allergen and administered as a single dose, appeared to be extremely effective in converting Th2-dominated immune responses into Th1 responses. Moreover, the effect of HKL occurred in an allergen-specific manner, and was effective in reversing established airway hyperreactivity [36,37] (Figure 2). HKL as adjuvant was much more effective than Mycobacteria as adjuvant (Complete Freund's Adjuvant) [36], which has been shown to prevent the development of airway eosino-philia in animal studies [38]. The inhibitory effect on airway hyperreactivity depended on the presence of IL-12 and on CD8+ T cells, was associated with an increase of IL-18 mRNA expression, and required close physical association between HKL and the antigen. Thus, these studies demon-strate that HKL as an adjuvant very effectively promotes protective immune responses in the respiratory tract, and down-modulates ongoing Th2-domi-nated responses, and indicates that HKL as an adjuvant for immunotherapy may be clinically effective in the treatment of allergic asthma.

d. Modified allergen protein constructs with reduced allergenicity.

The recognition that allergens retain both T cell epitopes as well as B cell epitopes that bind to IgE and cause immediate responses, has prompted investigators to generate constructs with decreased "allergenicity" (IgE binding activity), but with increased "immunogenicity" (T cell activity). Theoretically, such proteins of high immunogenicity with reduced allergenicity can be given in high doses without risk of IgE-mediated immediate reactions, because they have a reduced capacity to trigger degranulation in mast cells yet are capable of inducing IFN-γ production in T cells [39]. Initially, investigators focused on generating polymers by treatment of allergen with urea, formaldehyde, glutaraldehyde or polyethylene glycol. Studies in both humans and in mice demonstrated that polymerized allergens induced immune deviation/modulation, converted allergen-specific IL-4 producing Th2 lymphocytes into allergen-specific Th1 cells, and reduced allergen-specific IgE. However, significant difficulty in producing uniform lots of these modified proteins reduced commercial interest in this idea.

More recently, other approaches to reduce allergenicity and retain immunogenicity have been undertaken. For example, investigators have generated recombinant allergens with cysteine residues removed by site directed mutagenesis. These modified allergens do not possess disulfide bonds, and therefore lack normal secondary/tertiary structure and have 100 fold reduced IgE binding activity. These modified allergens however, retain their T cell epitopes and immunogenicity, and are capable of stimulating T cells and inducing immune deviation. Another approach involves the use of *peptide fragments of allergens.* Since T cells recognize peptide fragments of antigens or allergens, generally 12-15 amino acid residues in length, such peptides, which lack tertiary structure and the capacity to bind to allergen-specific IgE and to trigger mast cell degranulation, can be administered to patients without risk of immediate reactions. As a result, peptide fragments of allergens can be administered in much larger doses (particularly on a molar basis) than possible with conventional allergen [40,41]. Initial trials utilized only one or two antigen peptides containing immunodominant epitopes, but more recent studies have used overlapping peptides from the whole allergen protein [42]. These peptides when administered in vivo, activate T cells in the absence of costimulation, and appear to result in functional inactivation or anergy in allergen-specific CD4 T cells. Several clinical studies have demonstrated the efficacy of immunotherapy with the immunodominant peptides for cat allergen and for ragweed allergen in reducing allergic symptoms on allergen challenge, though late-occurring reactions (1-6 hrs after injection) have been observed in some subjects, presumably due to activation of allergen-specific T cells. These reactions appear to decrease in frequency after 4-5 injections of peptide, presumably due to inactivation of allergen-specific CD4 T cells. In some subjects, IgE against the injected peptides develop, occasionally associated with increased immediate reactions. Peptide therapy appears to differ from other forms of immunotherapy, which induce immune deviation rather than T cell anergy. Additional studies are required to determine whether the suppressive effects are persistent over several years time.

e. Oral allergen immunotherapy

Allergen immunotherapy, performed by the administration of allergen *orally* may be an additional therapeutic method for inducing clinical tolerance to allergen in patients with allergic disease and asthma. It has become clear that oral exposure to antigens is associated with tolerance, mediated by several mechanisms. For example, high doses of oral antigen induces deletion or apoptosis in antigen-specific T cells, whereas low dose of oral antigen induces the development of regulatory cells, often associated with the production of IL-4, IL-10 and TGF-β1 [43]. Oral administration of collagen or myelin basic protein to induce regulatory cells has been proposed for the treatment of rheumatoid arthritis and multiple sclerosis, though clinical trials have provided mixed results (see Chapter 8).

In allergic disease, oral immunotherapy methods have been used for several different conditions. For example, oral therapy/desensitization methods for penicillin and other antibiotic allergy appears to be very effective, and has had widespread acceptance. The specific protocols for penicillin desensitization require dose escalation every 20-30 minutes (rush desensitization method, also effective in Hymenoptera desensitization), rather than once a week, suggesting that the mechanisms that account for the efficacy of penicillin desensitization are different from that of conventional allergen immunotherapy. In any case, oral desensitization with drugs is thought to be safe because mucosal absorption of the drug is relatively slow, and the absorbed drug is generally monomeric, functioning as haptens, and is unlikely to cross-link IgE on the surface of mast cells. Similarly, protocols for oral and sublingual/swallow methods for *aeroallergen* sensitivity have been developed, and clinical trials have demonstrated its efficacy [44]. Although further refinement of these methods and understanding of oral therapy is required for greater application in the treatment of allergic diseases and asthma, these observations indicate that oral therapy with allergen may be effective in inducing clinical tolerance to allergens.

FUTURE PROSPECTS FOR THE TREATMENT OF ALLERGIC DISEASES

Although most of the therapies designed for allergic disease and asthma are based on the Th1/Th2 paradigm and focus on enhancing "protective" allergen-specific Th1 responses, it is likely that as our understanding of allergic disease and protection from allergic disease becomes more sophisticated [45], other methodologies will emerge. For example, it is very likely that cell types in addition to Th1 are important in regulating allergic inflammation, and preventing the development of allergic inflammation, particularly in non-allergic individuals. This idea has become apparent through recent studies examining the functions of adoptively transferred Th2 and Th1 lines. We and others have recently shown that allergen-specific Th1 and Th2 cell lines are codominant, and do not necessarily inhibit the function of each other [46]. Using an adoptive transfer system, we assessed the roles of allergen-specific Th1, Th2, and Th0 cells in a mouse model of asthma, and examined the capacity of Th1 cells to counterbalance the pro-asthmatic effects of Th2 cells. Th1, Th2, and Th0 lines were transferred into lymphocyte-deficient SCID mice. OVA-specific Th2 and Th0 cells induced significant airway hyper-reactivity and inflammation. Surprisingly, Th1 cells did not attenuate Th2 cell-induced airway hyperreactivity and inflammation neither in SCID mice nor in OVA-immunized immunocompetent BALB/c mice, and in fact caused severe airway inflammation (Figure 3). These results indicate that antigen-specific Th1 cells may not protect or prevent Th2-mediated allergic disease, but rather may cause acute lung pathology [46-49]. These findings have significant implications with regard to current therapeutic goals in asthma and allergy, and suggest that conversion of Th2-dominated allergic inflammatory responses into Th1-dominated responses may be problematic.

If Th1 cells cannot regulate or down modulate Th2 effector cells, are there other cell types that might be effective in this regard? We suggest that cells producing TGF-β1 may be important for the regulation of allergic inflammation. Thus, we demonstrated that ovalbumin (OVA)-specific Th cells engineered to express latent transforming growth factor β1 (TGF-β) abolished airway hyperreactivity induced by OVA-specific Th2 effector cells in SCID and BALB/c mice [50]. These effects correlated with increased concentrations of active TGF-β in the bronchoalveolar lavage (BAL) fluid demonstrating that latent TGF-β was activated in the inflammatory environment. The inhibitory effect of TGF-β secreting Th cells was antigen-specific, and was reversed by neutralization of TGF-β. Moreover, airway inflammation, as measured by eosinophils in bronchoalveolar lavage fluid or by examination of lung histology was greatly reduced by the transfer of TGF-β1 secreting T

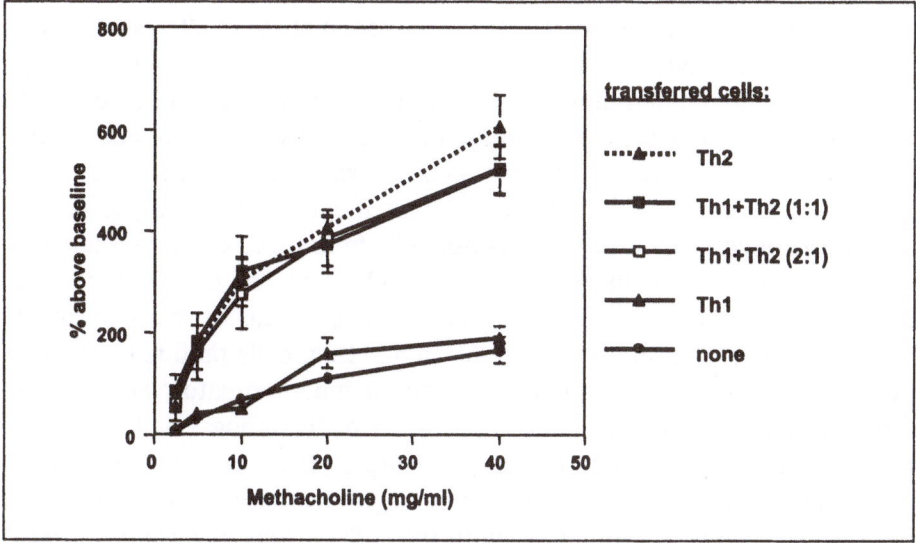

Figure 3
Th1 cells do not counterbalance airway hyperreactivity induced by Th2 cells.
SCID mice received Th1 or Th2 cells intravenously + intranasal OVA. Other SCID mice received a mixture of Th1 and Th2 cells in a ratio of 1:1 or 2:1. Airway hyperreactivity in response to inhaled methacholine was measured, and results are reported as % *above baseline* (mean ± SEM).

cells, and no increase in respiratory fibrosis was observed. These results demonstrate that T cells secreting TGF-β1 in the respiratory mucosa can indeed regulate Th2-induced airway hyperreactivity and inflammation, and suggest that TGF-β producing T cells play an important regulatory role in asthma.

We speculate that Th1 cells, TGF-β secreting T cells and possibly IL-10 secreting cells [51] play pivotal roles in regulating protective immunity in asthma, and that the production of these cytokines may be reduced in allergic and asthmatic indivdiduals. TGF-β has been shown previously to be a key immunoregulatory factor in the development of unresponsiveness to antigens in the gastrointestinal tract, an anatomic site that is closely related developmentally to the respiratory tract. For example, several investigators demonstrated that TGF-β producing Th3 cells and Tr1 cells inhibited experimental colitis [52,53], and TGF-β induced by oral tolerance inhibited subsequent tracheal esoinophilia [54]. Furthermore, TGF-β production controlled Th2-driven inflammation in chemical-induced autoimmunity [55]. These studies, as well as those showing that TGF-β regulates Th1-driven autoimmune diseases, such as EAE, uveoretinitis and collagen induced arthritis [56-61], indicate that TGF-β inhibits both Th2- as well as Th1-driven inflammation.

Thus, T cells activated to produce TGF-β may regulate both allergen-induced airway hyperreactivity as well as autoimmune diseases. Th1 cells may also regulate Th2-dominated immune responses, but may function in a different compartment and at a different stage of T cell activation. Th1 cells might act in peripheral lymphoid organs, such as lymph node and spleen, and, when present early on during the development of an immune response, may inhibit the development of Th2-effector cells from naïve or resting memory cells. However, it is unlikely that large numbers of Th1 cells function normally in the lung mucosa itself, since Th1 cells could exacerbate inflammation and cause tissue damage [46]. In addition, cells producing IL-10, a cytokine with potent anti-inflammatory and immunoregulatory activity may also effectively inhibit the development of airway inflammation [62,63]. Thus administration of IL-10 into the lungs, using replication-deficient adenovirus vectors in a murine model of airway hyperreactivity during the time of mucosal sensitization, abrogated both the cellular and physiological recall responses in vivo. These studies suggest that IL-10 may also critically regulate the development of asthma.

These studies emphasize the fact that much more work is required to more fully understand the regulation of allergic inflammation, and the mechanisms employed in nonallergic individuals that prevent the development of allergy and asthma. These mechanisms are likely to include tolerance as well as regulatory cells/suppressor cells, including CD4, CD8 cells, and regulatory Th cells secreting TGF-β or IL-10 (Th3 or Tr1 cells). In addition, mechanisms such as anergy or deletion may also be involved, as is thought to occur during gastrointestinal exposure to antigens. The lung is closely related developmentally to the gastrointestinal tract, and is part of the mucosal immune system. It is therefore very likely that the processes that occur in regulating immune responses to nonreplicating (food) antigens encountered via gastrointestinal mucosa also apply to the lung and respiratory mucosa.

Since the most effective immunotherapies for allergic diseases will be those that replicate the regulatory processes that occur in nonallergic individuals and which allow individuals to tolerate exposure to allergens without symptoms, understanding of those regulatory processes is essential for the development of curative therapies. Such therapies however, will be long lasting and not require chronic administration, since exposure to allergen should reinforce the protective immune response. Moreover, these therapies will essentially convert allergic individuals into nonallergic individuals, and produce a cure for these problems.

SUMMARY

Allergic diseases are caused by a Th2 biased inflammatory process, associated with the overproduction of Th2 lymphocytes secreting IL-4, IL-5, IL-9 and IL-13. Elimination of such inflammation occurs successfully on a daily basis in normal nonallergic individuals, but the specific mechanisms involved in preventing Th2 biased inflammation in the respiratory tract, skin and gut are poorly understood. Conventional allergen immunotherapy is a therapy that is currently available for treating allergic disease, and it appears to attenuate the underlying detrimental allergic inflammatory responses, and has the potential for altering the natural course of the disease and produce cure. Future therapies will be much more efficacious, and will be based on our developing knowledge of the mechanism of action of tolerance and immune deviation, and on replicating the processes that occur in nonallergic individuals that suppress the development of allergic inflammation. These therapies are likely to include allergen-specific methods that induce the development of tolerance, and of regulatory cells including Th1, Tr1, Th3 and CD8+ cells.

REFERENCES

1. Umetsu, D.T., and R.H. DeKruyff. 1997. Th1 and Th2 CD4+ cells in human allergic diseases. *J. Aller. Clin. Immunol.* 100:1-6.
2. Blotta, M.H., R.H. DeKruyff, and D.T. Umetsu. 1997. Corticosteroids inhibit IL-12 production in human monocytes and enhance their capacity to induce IL-4 synthesis in CD4 lymphocytes. *J. Immunol.* 158:5589-95.
3. DeKruyff, R.H., Y. Fang, and D.T. Umetsu. 1998. Corticosteroids enhance the capacity of macrophages to induce Th2 cytokine synthesis in CD4+ lymphocytes by inhibiting interleukin-12 production. *J. Immunol.* 160:2231-7.
4. Marsh, D.G., J.D. Neely, D.R. Breazeale, B. Ghosh, L.R. Freidhoff, C. Schou, and T.H. Beaty. 1995. Genetic basis of IgE responsiveness: relevance to the atopic diseases. *Intern. Arch. Aller. Immunol.* 107:25-8.
5. Mosmann, T.R., and R.L. Coffman. 1989. Th1 and Th2 cells: different patterns of lymphokine secretion lead to different functional properties. *Ann. Rev. Immunol.* 7:145-73.
6. Wierenga, E.A., M. Snoek, H.M. Jansen, J.D. Bos, R.A.W. van Lier, and M.L. Kapsenberg. 1991. Human atopen-specific types 1 and 2 T helper cell clones. *J. Immunol.* 147:2942-49.
7. Marshall, J., Y. Wen, J.S. Abrams, and D.T. Umetsu. 1993. In vitro synthesis of IL-4 by human CD4+ T cells requires repeated antigenic stimulation. *Cell. Immunol.* 152:18-34.
8. Shirakawa, T., T. Enomoto, S. Shimazu, and J.M. Hopkin. 1997. The inverse association between tuberculin responses and atopic disorder. *Science* 275:77-79.
9. Oro, A.S., T.J. Guarino, R. Driver, L. Steinman, and D.T. Umetsu. 1996. Regulation of disease susceptibility: decreased prevalence of IgE-mediated allergic disease in patients with multiple sclerosis. *J. Aller. Clin. Immunol.* 97:1402-8.

10. Tang, L., S. Benjaponpitak, R.H. DeKruyff, and D.T. Umetsu. 1998. Reduced prevalence of allergic disease in patients with multiple sclerosis is associated with enhanced IL-12 production. *J. Aller. Clin. Immunol.* 102:428-35.

11. Verhoef, C.M., J.A. van Roon, M.E. Vianen, C.A. Bruijnzeel-Koomen, F.P. Lafcber, and J.W. Biulsma. 1998. Mutual antagonism of rheumatoid arthritis and hay fever; a role for type 1/type 2 T cell balance. *Ann. Rheum. Dis.* 57:275-80.

12. Douek, I.F., N.J. Leech, H.A. Gillmor, P.J. Bingley, and E.A. Gale. 1999. Children with type-1 diabetes and their unaffected siblings have fewer symptoms of asthma. *Lancet* 353:1850.

13. Gavett, S.H., D.J. O'Hearn, X. Li, S.-K. Huang, F.D. Finkelman, and M. Wills-Karp. 1995. Interleukin 12 inhibits antigen-induced airway hyperresponsiveness, inflammation, and Th2 cytokine expression in mice. *J. Exp. Med.* 182:1527-36.

14. Hofstra, C., I. Van Ark, G. Hofman, M. Kool, F.P. Nijkamp, and A.J. Van Oosterhout. 1998. Prevention of Th2-like cell responses by coadministration of IL-12 and IL-18 is associated with inhibition of antigen-induced airway hyperresponsiveness, eosinophilia, and serum IgE levels. *J. Immunol.* 161:5054-60.

15. McMenamin, C., and P.G. Holt. 1993. The natural immune response to inhaled soluble protein antigens involves major histocompatibility complex (MHC) class I-restricted CD8+ T cell-mediated but MHC class II-restricted CD4+ T cell-dependent immune deviation resulting in selective suppression of immunoglobulin E production. *J. Exp. Med.* 178:889-99.

16. Broide, D., J. Schwarze, H. Tighe, T. Gifford, M.-D. Nguyen, S. Malek, J. Van Uden, E. Martin-Orozco, E.W. Gelfand, and E. Raz. 1998. Immunostimulatory DNA sequences inhibit IL-5, eosinophililc inflammation, and airway hyperresponsiveness in mice. *J. Immunol.* 161:7054-62.

17. Creticos, P.S. 1992. Immunotherapy with allergens. *JAMA* 268:2834-9.

18. Bousquet, J., R. Lockey, H.J. Malling, E. Alvarez-Cuesta, G.W. Canonica, M.D. Chapman, P.J. Creticos, J.M. Dayer, S.R. Durham, P. Demoly, R.J. Goldstein, T. Ishikawa, K. Ito, D. Kraft, P.H. Lambert, H. Lowenstein, U. Muller, P.S. Norman, R.E. Reisman, R. Valenta, E. Valovirta, and H. Yssel. 1998. Allergen immunotherapy: therapeutic vaccines for allergic diseases. World Health Organization. American academy of Allergy, Asthma and Immunology. *Ann. Allergy Asthma Immunol.* 81:401-5.

19. Durham, S.R., S.M. Walker, E.-M. Varga, M.R. Jacobson, F. O'Brien, W. Noble, S.J. Till, Q.A. Hamid, and K.T. Nouri-Aria. 1999. Long-term clinical efficacy of grass-pollen immunotherapy. *New Engl. J. Med.* 341:468-75.

20. Secrist, H., C.J. Chelen, Y. Wen, J.D. Marshall, and D.T. Umetsu. 1993. Allergen immunotherapy decreases interleukin 4 production in CD4+ T cells from allergic individuals. *J. Exp. Med.* 178:2123-30.

21. Varney, V.A., Q.A. Hamid, M. Gaga, S. Ying, M. Jacobson, A.J. Frew, A.B. Kay, and S.R. Durham. 1993. Influence of grass pollen immunotherapy on cellular infiltration and cytokine mRNA expression during allergen-induced late-phase cutaneous responses. *J. Clin. Invest.* 92:644-51.

22. Jutel, M., W.J. Pichler, D. Skrbic, A. Urwyler, C. Dahinden, and U.R. Muller. 1995. Bee venom immunotherapy results in decrease of IL-4 and IL-5 and increase of IFN-gamma secretion in specific allergen-stimulated T cell cultures. *J. Immunol.* 154:4187-94.

23. Benjaponpitak, S., A.S. Oro, P. Maguire, R.H. DeKruyff, and D.T. Umetsu. 1999. The kinetics of changes in cytokine production by CD4+ T cells during conventional allergen immunotherapy. *J. Aller. Clin. Immunol.* 103:468-75.

24. Rocklin, R.E., A. Sheffer, D.K. Greineder, and K.L. Melmon. 1980. Generation of antigen-specific suppressor cells during allergy desensitization. *N. Engl. J. Med.* 302:1213-19.

24a. Akdis, C.A., Blesken, T., Akdis, M., Wuthrich, B., and Blase, K. 1998. Role of interleukin 10 in specific immunotherapy. *J. Clin. Invest.* 102:98-106.

25. Ulmer, J.B., J.J. Donnelly, S.E. Parker, G.H. Rhodes, P.L. Felgner, V.J. Dwarki, S.H. Gromkowski, R.R. Deck, C.M. DeWitt, A. Friedman, and et al. 1993. Heterologous protection against influenza by injection of DNA encoding a viral protein. *Science* 259:1745-9.

26. Condon, C., S.C. Watkins, C.M. Celluzzi, K. Thompson, and L.D. Falo, Jr. 1996. DNA-based immunization by in vivo transfection of dendritic cells. *Nat Med* 2: 1122-8.

27. Tascon, R.E., M.J. Colston, S. Ragno, E. Stavropoulos, D. Gregory, and D.B. Lowrie. 1996. Vaccination against tuberculosis by DNA injection. *Nat Med* 2:888-92.

28. Syrengelas, A.D., T.T. Chen, and R. Levy. 1996. DNA immunization induces protective immunity against B-cell lymphoma. *Nat Med* 2:1038-41.

29. Waisman, A., P.J. Ruiz, D.L. Hirschberg, A. Gelman, J.R. Oksenberg, S. Brocke, F. Mor, I.R. Cohen, and L. Steinman. 1996. Suppressive vaccination with DNA encoding a variable region gene of the T-cell receptor prevents autoimmune encephalomyelitis and activates Th2 immunity. *Nat Med* 2:899-905.

30. Seder, R.A., and S. Gurunathan. 1999. DNA vaccines--designer vaccines for the 21st century. *N. Engl. J. Med.* 341:277-8.

31. Sato, Y., M. Roman, H. Tighe, D. Lee, M. Corr, M.-D. Nguyen, G.J. Silverman, M. Lotz, D.A. Carson, and E. Raz. 1996. Immunostimulatory DNA sequences necessary for effective intradermal gene immunization. *Science* 273:352-354.

32. Raz, E., H. Tighe, Y. Sato, M. Corr, J.A. Dudler, R. Roman, S.L. Swain, H.L. Spiegelberg, and D.A. Carson. 1996. Preferential induction of a Th1 immune response and inhibition of specific IgE antibody formation by plasmid DNA immunization. *Proc. Natl. Acad. Sci.* 93:5141-5.

33. Hsu, C.H., K.Y. Chua, M.H. Tao, Y.L. Lai, H.D. Wu, S.K. Huang, and K.H. Hsieh. 1996. Immunoprophylaxis of allergen-induced immunoglobulin E synthesis and airway hyperresponsiveness in vivo by genetic immunization. *Nature Medicine* 2:540-544.

34. Roy, K., H.Q. Mao, S.K. Huang, and K.W. Leong. 1999. Oral gene delivery with chitosan--DNA nanoparticles generates immunologic protection in a murine model of peanut allergy. *Nature Med.* 5:387-91.

35. Kim, T.S., R.H. DeKruyff, R. Rupper, H.T. Maecker, S. Levy, and D.T. Umetsu. 1997. An OVA-IL-12 fusion protein is more effective than OVA plus rIL-12 in inducing a Th1-dominated immune response and inhibiting antigen-specific IgE production. *J. Immunol.* 158:4137-44.

36. Yeung, V.P., R.S. Gieni, D.T. Umetsu, and R.H. DeKruyff. 1998. Heat killed Listeria monocytogenes as an adjuvant converts established Th2-dominated immune responses into Th1-dominated responses. *J. Immunol.* 161:4146-52.

37. Hansen, G., V.P. Yeung, G. Berry, D.T. Umetsu, and R.H. DeKruyff. 2000. Vaccination with heat killed listeria as adjuvant reverses established allergen-induced airway hyperreactivity and inflammation: role of CD8+ T cells and IL-18. *J. Immunol.* 164:223-30.

38. Erb, K.J., J.W. Holloway, A. Sobeck, H. Moll, and G. Le Gros. 1998. Infection of Mice with Mycobacterium bovis-Bacillus Calmette-Guérin (BCG) Suppresses Allergen-induced Airway Eosinophilia. *J. Exp. Med.* 187:561-9.

39. Secrist, H., R.H. DeKruyff, and D.T. Umetsu. 1995. Interleukin 4 production by CD4+ cells from allergic individuals is modulated by allergen concentration and antigen-presenting cell type. *J. Exp. Med.* 181:1081-90.

40. Pene, J., A. Desroches, L. Paradis, B. Lebel, M. Farce, C.F. Nicodemus, H. Yssel, and J. Bousquet. 1998. Immunotherapy with Feld 1 peptides decreases IL-4 release by peripheral blood T cells of patients allergic to cats. *J. Aller. Cliln. Immunol.* 101:571-8.

41. Maguire, P., C. Nicodemus, D. Aaronson, D. Robinson, and D.T. Umetsu. 1999.

The safety and efficacy of ALLERVAX CAT in cat allergic patients. *Clinical Immunol.* 93:222-31.

42. Kouskoff, V., S. Famiglietti, G. Lacaud, P. Lang, J.E. Rider, B.K. Kay, J.C. Cambier, and D. Nemazee. 1998. Antigens varying in affinity for the B cell receptor induce differential B lymphocyte responses. *J Exp Med* 188:1453-64.

43. Faria, A.M., and H.L. Weiner. 1999. Oral tolerance: mechanisms and therapeutic applications. *Advan. Immunol.* 73:153-264.

44. Passalacqua, G., M. Albano, A. Riccio, L. Fregonese, P. Puccinelli, S. Parmiani, and G.W. Canonica. 1999. Clinical and immunologic effects of a rush sublingual immunotherapy to Parietaria species: A double-blind, placebo-controlled trial. *J. Allergy Clin. Immunol.* 104:964-8.

45. Rolland, J., and R. O'Hehir. 1998. Immunotherapy of allergy: anergy, deletion, and immune deviation. *Curr. Opin. Immunol.* 10:640-5.

46. Hansen, G., G. Berry, R.H. DeKruyff, and D.T. Umetsu. 1999. Allergen-specific Th1 cells fail to counterbalance Th2 cell-induced airway hyperreactivity but cause severe airway inflammation. *J. Clin. Invest.* 103:175-83.

47. Cohn, L., R.J. Homer, A. Marinov, J. Rankin, and K. Bottomly. 1997. Induction of airway mucus production By T helper 2 (Th2) cells: a critical role for interleukin 4 in cell recruitment but not mucus production. J Exp Med 1997 Nov 17;186(10):1737-47. *J. Exp. Med.* 186:1737-47.

48. Li, L., Y. Xia, A. Nguyen, L. Feng, and D. Lo. 1998. Th2-induced eotaxin expression and eosinophilia coexist with Th1 responses at the effector stage of lung inflammation. *J. Immunol.* 161:3128-35.

49. Randolph, D.A., C.J. Carruthers, S.J. Szabo, K.M. Murphy, and D.D. Chaplin. 1999. Modulation of airway inflammation by passive transfer of allergen-specific Th1 and Th2 cells in a mouse model of asthma. *J. Immunol.* 162:2375-83.

50. Hansen, G., J.J. McIntire, V.P. Yeung, G. Berry, G.J. Thorbecke, L. Chen, R.H. DeKruyff, and D.T. Umetsu. 2000. CD4+ Th Cells Engineered To Produce Latent TGF-b1 Reverse Allergen-Induced Airway Hyperreactivity and Inflammation. *J. Clin. Invest.*

51. Umetsu, D.T., and R.H. DeKruyff. 1999. Interleukin-10. The missing link in asthma regulation? *Am. J. Respir. Cell Mol. Biol.* 21:562-563.

52. Chen, Y., V.K. Kuchroo, J. Inobe, D.A. Hafler, and H.L. Weiner. 1994. Regulatory T cell clones induced by oral tolerance: suppression of autoimmune encephalomyelitis. *Science* 265:1237-40.

53. Groux, H., A. O'Garra, M. Bigler, M. Rouleau, S. Antonenko, J.E. de Vries, and M.G. Roncarolo. 1997. A CD4+ T-cell subset inhibits antigen-specific T-cell responses and prevents colitis. *Nature* 389:737-42.

54. Haneda, K., K. Sano, G. Tamura, T. Sato, S. Habu, and K. Shirato. 1997. TGF-beta induced by oral tolerance ameliorates experimental tracheal eosinophilia. *J. Immunol.* 159:4484-90.

55. Bridoux, F., a. Badou, A. Saoudi, I. Bernard, E. Druet, R. Pasquier, P. Druet, and L. Pelletier. 1997. Transforming Growth Factor β (TGF-β)-dependent inhibition of T helper cell 2 (Th2)-induced autoimmunity by self-major Histocompatibility Complex (MHC) calss II-specific, regulatory CD4+ T cell lines. *J. Exp. Med.* 185:1769-75.

56. Kuruvilla, A.P., R. Shah, G.M. Hochwald, H.D. Liggitt, M.A. Palladino, and G.J. Thorbecke. 1991. Protective effect of transforming growth factor beta 1 on experimental autoimmune diseases in mice. *Proc. Natl. Acad. Sci.* 88:2918-21.

57. Thorbecke, G.J., R. Shah, C.H. Leu, A.P. Kuruvilla, A.M. Hardison, and M.A. Palladino. 1992. Involvement of endogenous tumor necrosis factor alpha and transforming growth factor beta during induction of collagen type II arthritis in mice. *Proc. Natl. Acad. Sci.* 89:7375-9.

58. Johns, L.D., K.C. Flanders, G.E. Ranges, and S. Sriram. 1991. Successful treat-

ment of experimental allergic encephalomyelitis with transforming growth factor-beta 1. *J. Immunol.* 147:1792-6.

59. Racke, M.K., B. Cannella, P. Albert, M. Sporn, C.S. Raine, and D.E. McFarlin. 1992. Evidence of endogenous regulatory function of transforming growth factor-beta 1 in experimental allergic encephalomyelitis. *Int. Immunol.* 4:615-20.

60. Neurath, M.F., I. Fuss, B.L. Kelsall, D.H. Presky, W. Waegell, and W. Strober. 1996. Experimental granulomatous colitis in mice is abrogated by induction of TGF-β-mediated oral tolerance. *J. Exp. Med.* 183:2605-16.

61. Rizzo, L.V., N.E. Miller-Rivero, C.C. Chan, B. Wiggert, R.B. Nussenblatt, and R.R. Caspi. 1994. Interleukin-2 treatment potentiates induction of oral tolerance in a murine model of autoimmunity. *J. Clin. Invest.* 94:1668-72.

62. Grunig, G., D.B. Corry, M.W. Leach, B.W. Seymour, V.P. Kurup, and D.M. Rennick. 1997. Interleukin-10 is a natural suppressor of cytokine production and inflammation in a murine model of allergic bronchopulmonary aspergillosis. *J. Exp. Med.* 185:1089-99.

63. Stampfli, M.R., M. Cwiartka, B.U. Gajewska, D. Alverez, S.A. Ritz, M.D. Inman, Z. Xing, and M. Jordana. 1999. Interleukin-10 gene transfer to the airway regulates allegic mucosal sensitization in mice. *Am. J. Resp. Cell Mol. Biol.*

16

THERAPEUTIC STRATEGIES FOR XENOTRANSPLANTATION

Jeffrey L. Platt
Transplantation Biology
Mayo Clinic
Rochester, Minnesota, USA

INTRODUCTION

The major factor limiting the clinical application of organ transplantation is the supply of human organs. This supply allows only 5-15% of transplants needed in the United States to be performed [1]. One approach to overcoming this problem is to use animals as a source of organs and tissues, that is, xenotransplantation. First attempted at the turn of the century [2], xenotransplantation seems to finally be nearing clinical application, as recent years have brought about much progress in understanding the hurdles to the clinical application of xenotransplantation and the development of novel strategies for dealing with these hurdles. This chapter will summarize the hurdles to the clinical application of xenotransplantation, and the therapeutic approaches that might be used to overcome them. Specific approaches to the control of cellular immune responses to xenotransplantation will not be given, as these approaches will be detailed elsewhere in this volume.

A Donor Species for Xenotransplantation

While it might be intuitive that the best xenogeneic donor for clinical use would be a species closely related to humans, most investigators now focus on the pig, rather than on non-human primates, as a potential source of xenografts. The reasons for using pigs number at least four. First, porcine organs are of an appropriate size for use in humans. Second, the supply of pigs, unlike the supply of primates, is unlimited. Third, pigs can be genetically engineered, whereas primates presently cannot. Fourth, the risk of zoonotic

A. W. Thomson (ed.), Therapeutic Immunosuppression, 405–426.
© 2001 *Kluwer Academic Publishers.*

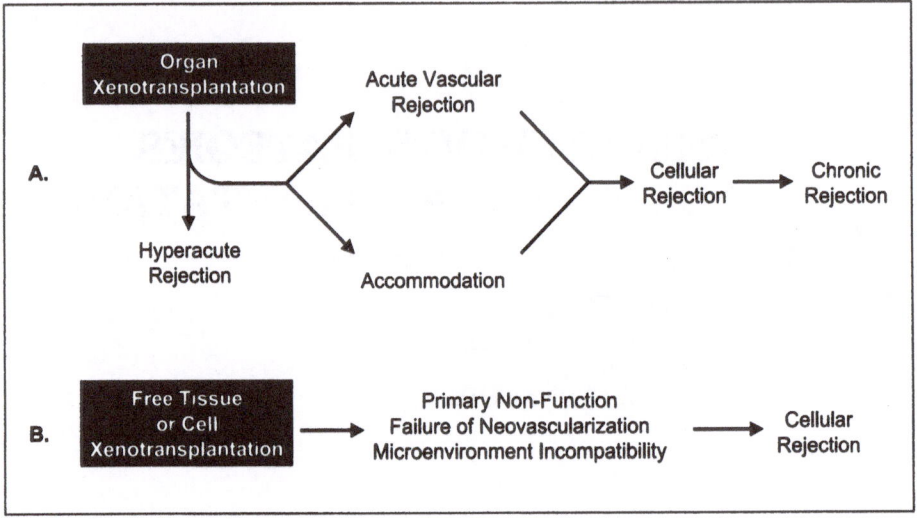

Figure 1
Biological hurdles for xenotransplantation.

(A) Organ transplantation between unmodified disparate species leads to hyperacute rejection. If hyperacute rejection is averted by depletion of xenoreactive natural antibodies or inhibition of complement system, the xenograft may be subject to acute vascular rejection, or "accommodation" may occur. If acute vascular rejection is prevented, the graft will be subject to cellular rejection or chronic rejection.

(B) Tissue or cell xenotransplants are subject to failure caused by primary nonfunction which may reflect failure of engraftment or a very rapid immune response. If primary non-function is bypassed and the tissue or cells engraft, they are then subject to cellular rejection. Humoral rejection is not usually considered a hurdle to cell transplantation because the blood vessels, of recipient origin, hinder humoral elements from reaching the graft. However, small amounts of anti-donor antibodies and complement might, in principle, impair graft function. *Adapted from Graft 1:19-24, 1998 [5].

infection from pigs is limited and more easily controlled. The hurdles to the use of pigs as a source of tissues and organs for transplantation into humans, however, are significant. The transplantation of pig organs or tissues into primates engenders severe rejection reactions, as outlined in Figure 1. There also exist certain incompatibilities between the immune and coagulation systems of pigs and primates which constitute substantive biological barriers to transplantation. Finally, while the risk of zoonosis is limited, it is still another concern, as underscored by recent studies on an endogenous retrovirus of pigs [3,4].

Table 1
Vascular Supply and Microenvironment of Xenografts.

Type of Graft	Example	Vascular Supply	Microenvironment
Isolated cells	Bone marrow hepatocytes	Recipient	Recipient
Free tissues	Skin pancreatic islets	Recipient and donor	Recipient and donor
Organ	Heart Kidney	Donor	Donor

Types of Xenografts

The biological properties of xenografts are determined, in part, by the way in which blood vessels in the graft are connected with the circulation of the recipient and by the origin of the microenvironment surrounding donor cells (Table 1).

Isolated cells, such as hepatocytes or bone marrow cells, derive their vascular supply and microenvironment entirely from the host. The "local" host growth factors, which are needed to support neovascularization or normal cellular function, might be incompatible between species. For example, transplantation of xenogeneic bone marrow is limited by the incompatibility of growth factors of cells in the donor [6]. Free tissues, such as pancreatic islets or skin, derive their vascular supply and microenvironment, in part, from the host and, in part, from the donor. To the extent that the vascular supply and microenvironment depend on the host, there is the theoretical possibility that incompatibilities across species will limit engraftment, graft function or survival. On the other hand, the presence of recipient microvasculature provides an important buffer between the immune system of the recipient and the components of the graft. In the case of pig-to-primate xenografts, this buffer would seem more important, as early trials suggest that establishment of a vascular supply allows control of rejection with conventional approaches to immunosuppression [7,8]. Organ grafts, such as kidney, heart, liver and lung, provide their own vasculature and microenvironment. Organ grafts do not depend on donor-recipient compatibility to sustain vascularization or cell function. However, the utilization of donor blood vessels allows the immune system of the recipient to act directly on the graft, with potentially devastating consequences, as discussed below.

IMMUNOLOGICAL HURDLES TO XENOTRANSPLANTATION

The sections that follow summarize the various types of xenograft rejection, the factors thought to contribute to the development of rejection and the therapeutic approaches that might be used. Because of the complexity of rejection responses, the discussion of therapeutics is necessarily limited to approaches specific to xenotransplantation. Subjects, such as control of cell mediated immune responses, ischemia- reperfusion, prevention of infection (zoonosis) and control of physiology, are not considered in detail here. The reader is referred to recent reviews for broader consideration of these subjects [9-12].

Hyperacute Rejection

A pig organ, transplanted into an unmodified, non-human primate or human, is subject to hyperacute rejection. The pathological picture of hyperacute rejection is characterized by interstitial hemorrhage and formation of platelet thrombi. These changes occur almost immediately upon perfusion of the organ by recipient blood and cause the very rapid loss of graft function.

Hyperacute rejection of pig organs, by primates, is initiated by the binding of human xenoreactive IgM to the endothelium of the porcine organ [13]. Antibody binding triggers activation of the complement system of the recipient, and it is the activation of complement on donor blood vessels that causes the dramatic manifestations of hyperacute rejection.

Xenoreactive natural antibodies and the antigens they recognize

Greater than 90% of xenoreactive antibodies that bind to porcine organs are specific for Galα1-3Gal [14-16]. This antigen is synthesized by α1,3-galactosyltransferase (α1,3GT), which exists in lower mammals and New World monkeys, but is absent in Old World monkeys, apes and humans [17]. Xenoreactive antibodies specific for Galα1-3Gal are members of a family of antibodies, which includes isohemagglutinins [18], and comprises 1% to 4% of circulating IgM [19]. Upon binding to glycoproteins and/or glycolipids bearing Galα1-3Gal on the endothelial surface, these antibodies activate complement, setting into motion a series of events leading to the destruction of the newly transplanted organ. The similarity of anti-Galα1-3Gal to other blood group antibodies suggests that at least some aspects of the immune barrier to xenotransplantation are akin to the immune barrier to transplantation across ABO blood groups [20].

Complement activation and complement regulatory proteins

Binding of xenoreactive antibodies to the endothelium of a porcine organ activates the complement system through the classical pathway [13], and the activation of complement in the xenograft is an essential step in the pathogenesis of hyperacute rejection [21]. The critical importance of complement in the pathogenesis of hyperacute rejection has been demonstrated repeatedly over the last 35 years, as every measure which effectively controls complement activation prevents hyperacute rejection.

The susceptibility of porcine organs to complement-mediated damage is not entirely a function of the binding of xenoreactive natural antibodies. The very rapid activation of complement in xenografts reflects, in part, the failure of complement regulatory proteins, expressed in the endothelium of porcine organs, to effectively control the human complement cascade [22,23]. Thus, decay accelerating factor (DAF) and membrane co-factor protein (MCP), which regulate complement activation by dissociating and degrading C3 convertase, and CD59, which prevents formation of the C8 and C9 components, function much better against homologous complement than against heterologous complement [24]. The failure of these complement regulatory proteins to control activation of the complement system of the recipient might make the xenograft more susceptible to hyperacute reaction [22]. The importance of aberrant complement control was recently demonstrated by studies in which expression of low levels of human DAF and CD59 in transgenic pigs was sufficient to prevent the hyperacute rejection of porcine organs transplanted into primates [25-28].

Which components of complement contribute to the pathogenesis of hyperacute rejection might be important for the development of therapy that would minimize the complications caused by complement inhibition. Studies in rodents suggest that terminal complement complexes may be needed for the development of hyperacute rejection, as this process does not occur in recipients deficient in C6 [29]. Although the membrane attack complex of complement is probably the most potent effector of hyperacute rejection, porcine organs transgenic for human CD59, which controls assembly of the membrane attack complex, are still subject to hyperacute rejection after transplantation into baboons [30]. This suggests that terminal complement complexes lacking C9 and, perhaps, C8, such as C5b67 complexes, can disrupt endothelial integrity [31] and might be sufficient to bring about hyperacute rejection. Thus, inhibition of complement must prevent assembly of these later complexes.

It is widely believed that nearly all porcine organ xenografts are subject to hyperacute rejection by primates. However, some reports suggest that the lung [32] and the liver [33] might resist antibody-mediated hyperacute rejection. Another recent report suggests that hyperacute rejection of porcine kidneys and hearts does not always occur in unmodified primates [28]. In considering what now appear to be exceptions to the dogma of species susceptibility to hyperacute rejection, it will be important to assure that the exception does not simply reflect a low level of xenoreactive antibodies found in young animals and humans [34], or the use of treatments which inhibit complement or prevent endothelial damage.

Prevention of hyperacute rejection

Once viewed as the most daunting hurdle to xenotransplantation, hyperacute rejection can be circumvented by various therapeutic means. The approaches which might be used to prevent hyperacute rejection of porcine organs by primates are listed in Table 2. Because hyperacute rejection emerges over a period of minutes, and destroys the graft in hours, therapeutics must be fully active in the peritransplant period.

- *Inhibition or Disruption of antibody-antigen reactions.* Given the pathogenesis of hyperacute rejection, as discussed above, a logical approach to therapy would focus first on disrupting the antibody-antigen reactions that

Table 2
Prevention of Hyperacute Rejection[†]

Approach	Standard	Method	Reference
Inhibition/depletion of xenoreactive antibody	*	Infusion of saccharide	[35]
		Immunoabsorption of anti Galα1-3Gal	[36]
Modification of antigen	*	Genetic engineering (see Figure 2)	[37]
		Breeding	[38]
Inhibition of complement		CVF	[39]
		Soluble CR1	[40]
		Anti C5	[41]
		Gammaglobulin	[42]
Regulation of complement	*	Transgenic expression of DAF/CD59 or DAF alone	
		Transgenic expression of MCP	[25]

* Preferred method
[†] Referenced here are first applications in pig-to-primate systems. More complete references will be found in the text and in reviews cited.

initiate rejection. Since the target antigen in pig-to-primate xenografts is Galα1-3Gal, such efforts should be focused on depleting or inhibiting anti-Galα1-3Gal antibodies or decreasing the expression of the antigen they recognize.

The first attempts to inhibit xenoreactive antibodies involved infusion of soluble saccharides to block antibody binding [43]. Unfortunately, this approach was not especially successful because the large amounts of sugar needed were toxic, and because the sugar used (Galα1-6Gal) would probably fail to block 30% of the xenoreactive antibodies [44]. Greater success was achieved with efforts to deplete anti-Galα1-3Gal. To deplete anti-Galα1-3Gal antibodies from xenograft recipients, Sablinski [45] and Lin [46] used columns bearing Galα1-3Gal to immunodeplete xenoreactive natural antibodies from baboons, observing that this procedure alone, without depleting complement, prevents hyperacute rejection. Plasma exchange [47] and perfusion of porcine kidneys [48] have also been used to effectively deplete antidonor antibodies. However, plasma exchange removes valuable components of blood, and organ perfusion might stimulate immune responses. Therefore, neither approach would be considered optimal today.

The use of immunoaffinity columns is usually carried out in conjunction with immunosuppressive therapy to prevent return of anti-donor antibodies. This subject will be discussed in the section on acute vascular rejection.

One potential approach for preventing the binding of xenoreactive natural antibodies involves the development of lines of pigs expressing low levels of Galα1-3Gal [38]. Various approaches to decreasing expression of Galα1-3Gal have been considered [49]. For example, decreasing antigen expression might be achieved by expression of a glycosyltransferase which can compete with α1,3galactosyltransferase for catalyzing the termination of saccharide chains. This second approach, as pursued by Sandrin [37] and Sharma [50], consists of expression of α1,2fucosyltransferase which causes synthesis of H antigen, to which humans are tolerant, in transgenic animals (Figure 2). Despite the attractiveness of genetic engineering of donors, no genetic approach to reduction of antigen expression, yet tested, has been shown to prevent hyperacute rejection, save for the complete disruption of the enzyme that synthesizes Galα1-3Gal in knockout mice [51]. Therefore, it seems likely that a successful approach will involve some combination of strategies [52].

• *Complement Inhibition.* The most reliable way to prevent hyperacute rejection involves inhibition of complement. Approaches to the inhibition

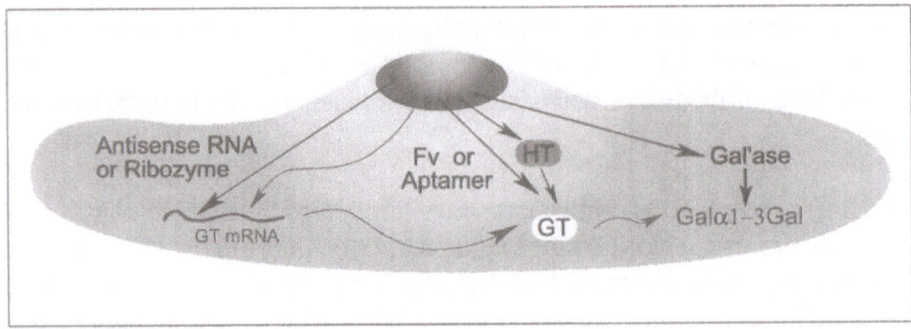

Figure 2
Some approaches to decreasing expression of α 1-3Gal by genetic engineering. Synthesis of Galα 1-3Gal is catalyzed by a α1,3-galactosyltransferase (GT). The biosynthetic pathway is shown by the curved arrows. This enzyme adds galactose residues at the termini of oligosaccharide chains. Four approaches to preventing the synthesis of the sugar are shown by the straight arrows. First, the expression of antisense RNA or a ribozyme might disrupt the structure or function of the GT mRNA. Second, introduction of a gene for an inhibitory ligand for GT, such as an appropriate Fv (an antibody-like molecule) or an aptamer (a small oligonucleotide inhibitor) might inhibit the function of the enzyme. Third, overexpression of another glycosyl transferase, such as the H transferase, which adds fucose residues, might compete with α1,3GT. This has been achieved in pigs by the overexpression of a human H transferase, resulting in the addition of fucose rather than Galα 1-3Gal to oligosaccharide side chains. Fourth, expression of a glycosidase, such as α-galactosidase, might lead to cleavage of the antigenic saccharide chains. Adapted from Nature 392 (Suppl):11-17, 1998 [5].

of complement have been reviewed in detail elsewhere [53-55]. Complement inhibitors, such as cobra venom factor (CVF) [56], soluble complement receptor type I (sCR1) [40] and gamma globulin [42] effectively prevent hyperacute rejection. Unfortunately, CVF and sCR1 may impair host defense by inhibiting C3, needed for opsonization of extracellular microorganisms. Recently, an alternative approach to complement inhibition, the administration of anti-C5 antibody, has been proposed [57]. Antibodies against C5 prevent complement mediated organ injury [41], leaving C3 intact. Although not yet tested in a hyperacute rejection model, this approach would, in principle, avert the major complication of complement inhibition.

More enduring inhibition of complement mediated injury can be achieved through the use of organs from transgenic pigs expressing human complement regulatory proteins. Expression of these proteins, such as decay accelerating factor and CD59 [22], repairs the defect in complement control discussed above, by inhibiting the activation of complement on cell surfaces. Hyperacute rejection has been prevented by expression of human DAF and

CD59 [27], DAF alone [26] or MCP (unpublished) in transgenic pigs. Expression of human CD59 alone is thought to limit tissue damage [58], but may not prevent hyperacute rejection [30].

Acute Vascular Rejection

When hyperacute rejection is averted, a xenograft is subject to rejection by a process which we have called "acute vascular rejection" [59,60] and others have called "delayed xenograft rejection" [61]. Acute vascular rejection may begin within 24 hours of reperfusion and leads to failure of the xenograft within days to weeks following transplantation. The pathologic features of acute vascular rejection of xenografts, like those of acute vascular rejection of allografts, include endothelial swelling, ischemia and thrombosis. In light of recent success in preventing hyperacute rejection, acute vascular rejection looms as the major hurdle to the enduring survival of xenografts.

Pathogenesis of Acute Vascular Rejection

The factors potentially involved in the pathogenesis of acute vascular rejection are listed in Table 3.

While the pathogenesis is a matter of controversy, there is accumulating evidence that acute vascular rejection is initiated by xenoreactive antibod-

Table 3
Factors implicated in the initiation of acute vascular rejection

Initiating Factor	Mechanism	Reference
Xenoreactive antibodies	Activation of endothelium by binding to signaling molecules such as integrins	[62]
Complement	Activation of endothelium by MAC	[63,64]
	Activation of endothelium by C5a	[65]
Macrophages	Elaboration of tissue factor	[66]
Natural killer cells	Cytotoxicity and activation of endothelial cells	[67]
Neutrophils	Oxidant mediated injury	[68]
Platelets	Activation of endothelial cells	[69]
	Secretion of vasoactive factors	[70]
Molecular incompatibility between donor and recipient	Incompatibility of thrombomodulin with recipient proteins	[60] [71]

ies. First, acute vascular rejection of xenografts and allografts is commonly associated with antibody deposits on vascular endothelium [72]. Second, the levels of xenoreactive antibodies in the blood increases following exposure to porcine tissues [73]. Third, acute vascular rejection can be induced by infusion of antidonor antibodies [74]. Fourth, depletion of antidonor antibodies, or inhibition of antibody synthesis, delays or averts acute vascular rejection [75].

Regardless of how acute vascular rejection might be initiated, many of the manifestations are thought to be caused by activation of graft endothelium [59,76]. Activation of graft endothelium induces expression of prothrombotic and inflammatory molecules, which might contribute to intravascular coagulation and inflammatory changes. For example, acute vascular rejection is associated with expression of E-selectin, P-selectin and inflammatory cytokines [76] and PAI-1 [77].

Treatment of acute vascular rejection

Some therapeutic strategies, which might be used to prevent acute vascular rejection, are listed in Table 4. Control of acute vascular rejection has proven far more difficult to achieve than control of hyperacute rejection. Thus, none of the measures discussed below are proven, except in small studies.

- *Depletion of anti donor antibodies.* Given the importance of anti-donor antibodies in the pathogenesis, the therapeutic strategies for acute vascular

Table 4
Therapeutic approaches to acute vascular rejection

Therapeutic approach	Mechanism	Reference
Column treatments	Antibody depletion	[75]
Tolerance	Decrease antibody production	[78]
Complement inhibition	Prevent endothelial cell activation and injury	[79]
Genetic engineering of antigen	Decrease antigen expression	[80]
Breeding	Decrease antigen expression	[81]
Genetic engineering of coagulation inhibitors	Prevent intravascular coagulation	[71]
Genetic engineering of signal inhibitors	Prevent endothelial cell activation	[71]
Administration of cell adhesion inhibitors	Prevent leukocyte-endothelial interaction	[68]

rejection focus especially on disrupting antibody-antigen reactions. While these strategies may overlap those described for hyperacute rejection, the effective application for acute vascular rejection requires prolonged efficacy. Thus, while one would hardly wish to consider tolerance for prevention of hyperacute rejection, tolerance might be an extremely useful way of dealing with acute vascular rejection.

One strategy for disrupting antibody-antigen reactions might involve depletion of xenoreactive antibodies, as discussed above. Efforts initially focused on removal of all immunoglobulin, as the specificity of the offending antibodies had not been defined [46]. More recently, the specific depletion of anti-Galα1-3Gal has been found to prevent acute vascular rejection [82]. One effect of antibody depletion by either means may be the induction of accommodation, as discussed below. Treatment of xenograft recipients with antibody immunoabsorption should be accompanied by treatment with immunosuppressive agents. There is very good evidence that while immunosuppression, by itself, will not greatly influence the level of xenoreactive antibodies in the circulation, the return of these antibodies, following removal from the blood, or increased production of the antibodies, following xenotransplantation, can be blunted to a certain extent by immunosuppression [83]. This impression, which has not been vigorously tested in xenotransplantation, is consistent with observations in other systems [84].

Non specific inhibition of antibody production

Inhibiting the synthesis of xenoreactive antibodies by administration of immunosuppressive agents has been attempted in rodent models, although no approach has proven clearly effective. There is some evidence that administration of leflunomide [85,86] or cyclophosphamide [87], in conjunction with other measures, might suppress production of xenoreactive antibody production. However, other mechanisms of action of these agents cannot be excluded.

Splenectomy is one potential adjunct to immunosuppressive therapy for the prevention of acute vascular rejection. While not rigorously tested following xenotransplantation, there is anecdotal evidence in xenograft models, as well as in ABO incompatible transplant models, that splenectomy blunts the humoral responses following transplantation [47,88].

• *Immunological Tolerance.* An important strategy for preventing acute vascular rejection might involve the induction of immunological tolerance. To the extent that the major antigen in acute vascular rejection is Galα1-3Gal, recent progress in inducing tolerance to that structure should be viewed as a significant step forward. Tolerance to Galα1-3Gal has been induced by the transplantation of hemotopoietic cells which express that antigen. Transplantation of Galα1-3Gal bone marrow cells into mice with targeted disruption of α1,3galactosyl transferase, the enzyme that catalyzes synthesis of Galα1-3Gal, was recently shown to prevent synthesis of anti-Galα1-3Gal antibodies [51,89]. One limitation of this approach may be the difficulty of achieving enduring engraftment of xenogeneic bone marrow. The problem of gaining engraftment of xenogeneic bone marrow might be bypassed by expressing Galα1-3Gal on autologous bone marrow cells, which can be achieved by transducing the cells with α1,3 galactosyl transferase [90]. This latter approach will not influence immune responses to other antigens carried by porcine cells.

- *Decreasing antigen expression.* A third strategy for preventing acute vascular rejection may involve the lowering of antigen expression in the xenograft, as discussed above. Various approaches to lowering antigen expression are summarized in Figure 2.

- *Inhibiting endothelial cell activation.* Given the importance of endothelial cell activation in the pathogenesis of acute vascular rejection, some have proposed intervening in this process [61]. Whether, in addition to controlling the inciting events, there will be a need to control the inflammatory and procoagulant end points associated with endothelial cell activation remains to be determined. Given the manifold pathophysiologic changes associated with endothelial cell activation, the ideal therapy would focus on an event controlling the activated state, rather than the end manifestations of that state. Since many of the proteins synthesized de novo, by activated endothelial cells, are regulated transcriptionally by NFκB, one approach might focus on the control of NFκB activation and translocation. However, inhibition of NFκB could increase susceptibility to apoptosis. Accordingly, the expression of anti-inflammatory molecules, such as hemoxygenase-1 [91,92], would seem more promising. This approach has not been tested in xenotransplant models, but experiments in cultured cells show promise [93]. Another central mechanism, controlling the activation of endothelial cells by complement, is the transcriptional activation of IL1α [94], as IL1α was shown to serve as the autocrine factor responsible for complement mediated induction of tissue factor, prostoglandins, and PAI-1 [77,95]. Limited studies in experimental animals would suggest that inhibition of IL1α can limit, but not prevent, tissue damage following xenotransplantation.

- *Accommodation.* Accommodation refers to the apparent resistance of a graft-to-humoral rejection, despite the presence of antidonor antibodies in the circulation of the recipient [22]. Such resistance to injury was originally observed in ABO-incompatible transplants after anti-donor antibodies were temporarily depleted from graft recipients. There is limited evidence that accommodation occurs in pig-to-primate xenografts [13]. Accommodation may reflect a change in antibody repertoire, a change in antigen expression on the endothelium, or an acquired resistance by the endothelium to humoral immune injury. Recent rodent studies have suggested that acquired resistance of endothelial cells may be especially important [96]. Accommodation in primates may be induced by temporary depletion of antidonor antibodies, and it is a potentially important empirical approach to dealing with acute vascular rejection, if antibody responses or antigen expression cannot be controlled.

Cellular Rejection

Increasing success in the prevention of hyperacute and acute vascular rejection brings into focus the hurdle posed by cellular immune responses to xenotransplants. The main issues to be addressed here are whether and to which extent the cellular immune response to xenotransplantation differs from the cellular immune response to allotransplantation and whether therapeutic approaches used for allotransplantation will suffice for xenotransplantation.

One potential difference between the cellular immune responses to xeno- and allotransplants is the mechanism of T cell recognition of transplanted cells. The early response to allotransplants and the response detected by the mixed leukocyte reaction in vitro is thought to involve direct recognition of allogeneic MHC molecules [97]. The human anti-porcine T cell response is similar to the allogeneic response in that human T cells can recognize porcine MHC class II antigens directly on the surface of porcine cells [98,99]. Nevertheless, in vitro responses may be impaired by defects in co-stimulation and other factors [100]. To the extent that direct recognition functions in vivo, there is the possibility of genetically engineering donors to modify or inhibit this response.

The cellular immune response to xenotransplantation might well be more intense than the cellular immune response to allotransplantation. One mechanism underlying an intense cellular immune response to xenotransplantation is that the foreign proteins in the graft will give rise to a vast repertoire of peptides and, thus, will stimulate a diverse set of recipient T cells. Another concern is that humoral immune responses to xenotransplantation might amplify cellular immune responses.

■ *Treatment of cellular rejection.* An important question for the clinical application of xenotransplantation is whether therapeutic strategies devised to control the rejection of allotransplants, as discussed elsewhere in this volume, can be applied for the control of rejection of xenotransplants. While there is, as yet, no definitive answer to that question, limited studies on the transplantation of porcine hepatocytes, in rabbits [101], and porcine organs, in non-human primates [75,102], suggest that early loss of xenografts to cellular rejection might be avoided. One therapeutic approach, which might be more effective in xenotransplantation than in allotransplantation, is the administration of anti-CD4 antibodies [103]. It is also likely that measures used to control humoral rejection, as described in the section on acute vascular rejection, will limit the intensity of cellular immune responses.

Given the potential strength of the T cell response to xenotransplantation and the potential importance of elicited antibodies, some have suggested that the success of xenotransplantation may depend on the generation of immunological tolerance [36]. One approach, discussed above, may involve the generation of mixed chimerism leading to deletion of "xenoreactive" cells [36]. A related strategy might involve the transplantation of donor thymus to allow the maturation of a mature T cell repertoire, which will not be reactive with the donor [104]. Another approach involves the manipulation of the mature T cell repertoire through the generation of microchimerism or other means so that xenoreactive cells are depleted or inhibited [105,106].

Another aspect of cellular rejection is the potential contribution of natural killer cells, the function of which might contribute to acute vascular rejection or cellular rejection [107]. There is some evidence that natural killer cells accumulate in xenografts, recognize Galα1-3Gal, and may fail to be controlled by inhibitory receptors specific for MHC class I. Recent studies have revealed non-cytotoxic mechanisms by which natural killer cells may injure xenogeneic endothelial cells, a change in morphology and endothelial cell activation [108]. Natural killer cells have been inhibited in rodent models by administration of anti-natural killer cell antibodies; however, no approaches have been reported in primates.

ZOONOSIS

One issue related to immune manipulation for xenotransplants is the issue of cross-species infection, or zoonosis. Xenotransplant recipients may be especially susceptible to zoonosis because immunosuppressive therapy leads to impairment of host defense, because the T cell repertoire may not easily recognize microbial peptides expressed in association with xenogeneic MHC molecules and because zoonotic agents might be carried at high levels in the transplanted tissues. There is also concern about the possible transmission of "new" infections from the recipient to the population as a whole. This issue was highlighted by the discovery that an endogenous porcine retrovirus might be able to infect human cells in culture [3,4]. Resistance to this virus is mediated by anti-Galα1-3Gal antibodies and complement in vitro [109]. Therefore, depletion of anti-Galα1-3Gal antibodies or inhibition of Galα1-3Gal synthesis could heighten susceptibility to infection. Furthermore, a new porcine virus, related to human hepatitis virus E, was recently reported [110]. However, it still remains to be proven whether these viruses or other "new" agents could actually infect humans, and whether such infection could lead to transmission to other individuals, or to disease. Thus far, no evidence has emerged that these agents can infect humans [111,112]. Nevertheless, the subject of zoonosis will remain of importance because genetic modifications of xenografts that lower expression of Galα1-3Gal or increase resistance to complement could allow viruses from these animals to evade immune surveillance.

CONCLUSION

The past few years have brought significant progress in defining the hurdles to xenotransplantation and progress in overcoming the immunologic and physiologic hurdles in this field. It is this author's view that the entry of xenotransplantation into the clinical area will occur as a step-by-step process. The first step involves free tissue xenografts and extracorporeal use of xenogeneic organs [7,8,113], and there is encouraging early evidence that porcine free tissue grafts may endure in a human recipient [7]. These transplants will provide insights regarding infectious disease risks and an important early opportunity to test immunosuppression strategies. The next step will involve use of xenogeneic organs as " bridge, " or temporary, transplants. Bridge transplants will not solve the problem of organ shortage, but the transplants will allow the gathering of vital information regarding the remaining immune and biological hurdles and testing of new therapies. The possibility of bridge transplants has been advanced by recent studies demonstrating prolonged function, in excess of a month, of porcine cardiac [114] and renal [26] xenografts in primates. Third, there will be the use of porcine organs as permanent replacements, but this use will probably be restricted to patients who can not receive a human organ allograft. Only with further refinements may there eventually be a fourth and final step, in which xenotransplantation is used as an alternative to allotransplantation.

Acknowledgements. *Supported by grants from the National Institutes of Health (HL52297 and HL46810).*

REFERENCES

1. Evans RW, Orians CE, Ascher NL. The potential supply of organ donors: an assessment of the efficiency of organ procurement efforts in the United States. JAMA 1992;267: 239-246.
2. Jaboulay M. De reins au pli du coude par soutures arterielles et veineuses. Lyon Med 1906;107: 575-577.
3. Patience C, Takeuchi Y, Weiss RA. Infection of human cells by an endogenous retrovirus of pigs. Nature Medicine 1997;3: 282-286.
4. Martin U, Kiessig V, Blusch JH, Haverich A, von der Helm K, Herden T et al. Expression of pig endogenous retrovirus by primary porcine endothelial cells and infection of human cells. Lancet 1998;352: 692-694.
5. Nagayasu T, Platt JL. Progress in xenotransplantation. Graft 1998;1: 19-24.
6. Kisielow P, Bluthmann H, Staerz UD, Steinmetz M, von Boehmer H. Tolerance in T-cell-receptor transgenic mice involves deletion of nonmature CD4+8+ thymocytes. Nature 1988;333: 742-746.
7. Deacon T, Schumacher J, Dinsmore J, Thomas C, Palmer P, Kott S et al. Histological evidence of fetal pig neural cell survival after transplantation into a patient with Parkinson's disease. Nature Medicine 1997;3: 350-353.
8. Groth CG, Korsgren O, Tibell A, Tollemar J, Moller E, Bolinder J et al. Transplantation of porcine fetal pancreas to diabetic patients. Lancet 1994;344: 1402-1404.
9. Platt JL. Hyperacute Xenograft Rejection. . Medical Intelligence Unit. New York: R. G. Landes, 1995.
10. Fishman J. Miniature swine as organ donors for man: Strategies for prevention of xenotransplantation associated infections. Xenotransplantation 1994;1: 47-57.
11. Chapman LE, Folks TM, Salomon DR, Patterson AP, Eggerman TE, Noguchi PD. Xenotransplantation and xenogeneic infections. New Eng. J. Med. 1995;333: 1498-1501.
12. Lin SS, Platt JL. Genetic therapies for xenotransplantation. J. Am. Coll. Surgeons 1998;186: 388-396.
13. Platt JL, Fischel RJ, Matas AJ, Reif SA, Bolman RM, Bach FH. Immunopathology of hyperacute xenograft rejection in a swine-to-primate model. Transplantation 1991;52: 214-220.
14. Good AH, Cooper DKC, Malcolm AJ, Ippolito RM, Koren E, Neethling FA et al. Identification of carbohydrate structures that bind human antiporcine antibodies: implications for discordant xenografting in humans. Transpl. Proc. 1992;24: 559-562.

15. Sandrin MS, Vaughan HA, Dabkowski PL, McKenzie IFC. Anti-pig IgM antibodies in human serum react predominantly with Galα(1,3)Gal epitopes. Proc. Natl. Acad. Sci. USA 1993;90: 11391-11395.

16. Collins BH, Parker W, Platt JL. Characterization of porcine endothelial cell determinants recognized by human natural antibodies. Xenotransplantation 1994;1: 36-46.

17. Galili U, Clark MR, Shohet SB, Buehler J, Macher BA. Evolutionary relationship between the natural anti-Gal antibody and the Gal α1-3Gal epitope in primates. Proc. Natl. Acad. Sci. USA 1987;84: 1369-1373.

18. Parker W, Yu PB, Holzknecht ZE, Lundberg-Swanson K, Buckley RH, Platt JL. Specificity and function of "natural" antibodies in immunodeficient subjects: clues to B-cell lineage and development. J. Clin. Immunol. 1997;17: 311-321.

19. Parker W, Bruno D, Holzknecht ZE, Platt JL. Xenoreactive natural antibodies: isolation and initial characterization. J. Immunol. 1994;153: 3791-3803.

20. Hammer C. Isohemagglutinins and preformed natural antibodies in xenogeneic organ transplantation. Transpl. Proc. 1987;19: 4443-4447.

21. Gewurz H, Clark DS, Cooper MD, Varco RL, Good RA. Effect of cobra venom-induced inhibition of complement activity on allograft and xenograft rejection reactions. Transplantation 1967;5: 1296-1303.

22. Platt JL, Vercellotti GM, Dalmasso AP, Matas AJ, Bolman RM, Najarian JS et al. Transplantation of discordant xenografts: a review of progress. Immunol. Today 1990;11: 450-456.

23. Dalmasso AP, Vercellotti GM, Platt JL, Bach FH. Inhibition of complement-mediated endothelial cell cytotoxicity by decay accelerating factor: Potential for prevention of xenograft hyperacute rejection. Transplantation 1991;52: 530-533.

24. Atkinson JP, Oglesby TJ, White D, Adams EA, Liszewski MK. Separation of self from non-self in the complement system: a role for membrane cofactor protein and decay accelerating factor. Clin. Exp. Immunol. 1991;86 (Supp. 1): 27-30.

25. McCurry KR, Kooyman DL, Alvarado CG, Cotterell AH, Martin MJ, Logan JS et al. Human complement regulatory proteins protect swine-to-primate cardiac xenografts from humoral injury. Nature Medicine 1995;1: 423-427.

26. Cozzi E, Yannoutsos N, Langford GA, Pino-Chavez G, Wallwork J, White DJG. Effect of transgenic expression of human decay-accelerating factor on the inhibition of hyperacute rejection of pig organs. In: Cooper DKC, Kemp E, Platt JL, White DJG, eds. Xenotransplantation: the transplantation of organs and tissues between species. 2nd ed. Berlin: Springer, 1997:665-682.

27. Byrne GW, McCurry KR, Martin MJ, McClellan SM, Platt JL, Logan JS. Transgenic pigs expressing human CD59 and decay-accelerating factor produce an intrinsic barrier to complement-mediated damage. Transplantation 1997;63: 149-155.

28. Zaidi A, Friend P, Schmoeckel M, Bhatti FNK, Tolan M, Waterworth P et al. Hyperacute rejection is not consistent after pig to primate renal xenotransplantation (abstract). 4th International Congress for Xenotransplantation. Nantes, France: World Transplantation Society, 1997:O53.

29. Brauer RB, Baldwin III WM, Daha MR, Pruitt SK, Sanfilippo F. Use of C6-deficient rats to evaluate the mechanism of hyperacute rejection of discordant cardiac xenografts. J. Immunol. 1993;151: 7240-7248.

30. Diamond LE, McCurry KR, Oldham ER, McClellan SB, Martin MJ, Platt JL et al. Characterization of transgenic pigs expressing functionally active human CD59 on cardiac endothelium. Transplantation 1996;61: 1241-1249.

31. Saadi S, Platt JL. Transient perturbation of endothelial integrity induced by antibodies and complement. J. Exp. Med. 1995;181: 21-31.

32. Kaplon RJ, Platt JL, Kwiatkowski PA, Edwards NM, Xu H, Shah AS et al. Absence of hyperacute rejection in pig-to-primate orthotopic pulmonary xenografts. Transplantation 1995;59: 410-416.

33. Calne RY, Davis DR, Pena JR, Balner H, De Vries M, Herbertson BM et al. Hepatic allografts and xenografts in primates. Lancet 1970;1: 103-106.

34. Kaplon RJ, Michler RE, Xu H, Kwiatkowski PA, Edwards NM, Platt JL. Absence of hyperacute rejection in newborn pig-to-baboon cardiac xenografts. Transplantation 1994;59: 1-6.

35. Li SF, Neethling FA, Taniguchi S, Yeh J, Kobayashi T, Ye Y et al. Glycans derived from porcine stomach mucin are effective inhibitors of natural anti-α-galactosyl antibodies in vitro and after intravenous infusion in baboons. Transplantation 1996;62: 1324-1331.

36. Sachs DH, Sablinski T. Tolerance across discordant xenogeneic barriers. Xenotransplantation 1995;2: 234-239.

37. Sandrin MS, Fodor WL, Mouhtouris E, Osman N, Cohney S, Rollins SA et al. Enzymatic remodelling of the carbohydrate surface of a xenogeneic cell substantially reduces human antibody binding and complement-mediated cytolysis. Nature Medicine 1995;1: 1261-1267.

38. Geller RL, Rubinstein P, Platt JL. Variation in expression of porcine xenogeneic antigens. Transplantation 1994;58: 272-277.

39. Leventhal JR, Dalmasso AP, Cromwell JW, Platt JL, Manivel CJ, Bolman RM et al. Prolongation of cardiac xenograft survival by depletion of complement. Transplantation 1993;55: 857-866.

40. Pruitt SK, Kirk AD, Bollinger RR, Marsh Jr HC, Collins BH, Levin JL et al. The effect of soluble complement receptor type 1 on hyperacute rejection of porcine xenografts. Transplantation 1994;57: 363-370.

41. Kroshus TJ, Rollins SA, Dalmasso AP, Elliott EA, Matis LA, Squinto SP et al. Complement inhibition with an anti-C5 monoclonal antibody prevents acute cardiac tissue injury in an ex vivo model of pig-to-human xenotransplantation . Transplantation 1995;60: 1194-1202.

42. Magee JC, Collins BH, Harland RC, Lindman BJ, Bollinger RR, Frank MM et al. Immunoglobulin prevents complement mediated hyperacute rejection in swine-to-primate xenotransplantation. J. Clin. Invest. 1995;96: 2404-2412.

43. Ye Y, Neethling FA, Niekrasz M, Koren E, Richards SV, Martin M et al. Evidence that intravenously administered α-Galactosyl carbohydrates reduce baboon serum cytotoxicity to pig kidney cells (PK15) and transplanted pig hearts. Transplantation 1994;58: 330-337.

44. Parker W, Lundberg-Swanson K, Holzknecht ZE, Lateef J, Washburn SA, Braedehoeft SJ et al. Isohemagglutinins and xenoreactive antibodies are members of a distinct family of natural antibodies. Hum. Immunol. 1996;45: 94-104.

45. Sablinski T, Latinne D, Gianello P, Bailin M, Bergen K, Colvin RB et al. Xenotransplantation of pig kidneys to nonhuman primates: I. development of the model. Xenotransplantation 1995;2: 264-270.

46. Lin SS, Kooyman DL, Daniels LJ, Daggett CW, Parker W, Lawson JH et al. The role of natural anti-Galα1-3Gal antibodies in hyperacute rejection of pig-to-baboon cardiac xenotransplants. Transplant Immunology 1997;5: 212-218.

47. Alexandre GPJ, Gianello P, Latinne D, Carlier M, Dewaele A, Van Obbergh L et al. Plasmapheresis and splenectomy in experimental renal xenotransplantation. In: Hardy MA, ed. Xenograft 25. New York, NY: Elsevier Science Publishers, 1989:259-266.

48. Cooper DKC, Human PA, Lexer G, Rose AG, Rees J, Keraan M et al. Effects of cyclosporine and antibody adsorption on pig cardiac xenograft survival in the baboon. J. Heart Transpl. 1988;7: 238-246.

49. Platt JL. New directions for organ transplantation. Nature 1998;392 (Suppl): 11-17.

50. Sharma A, Okabe JF, Birch P, Platt JL, Logan JS. Reduction in the level of gal (α1,3) gal in transgenic mice and pigs by the expression of an α(1,2) fucosyltrans-

ferase. Proc. Natl. Acad. Sci. USA 1996;93: 7190-7195.

51. Ohdan H, Yang Y-G, Shimizu A, Swenson KG, Sykes M. Mixed bone marrow chimerism induced without lethal conditioning prevents T cell- and anti-Galα1,3Gal-mediated heart graft rejection. The Journal of Clinical Investigation 1999;104: 20i-290.

52. Osman N, McKenzie IF, Ostenried K, Ioannou YA, Desnick RJ, Sandrin MS. Combined transgenic expression of alpha-galactosidase and alpha1,2-fucosyltransferase leads to optimal reduction in the major xenoepitope Galalpha(1,3)Gal. Proceedings of the National Academy of Sciences of the United States of America 1997;94: 14677-82.

53. Kalli KR, Hsu P, Fearon DT. Therapeutic uses of recombinant complement protein inhibitors. Springer Semin. Immunopathol. 1994;15: 417-431.

54. Morgan BP. Intervention in the complement system: a therapeutic strategy in inflammation. Biochem. Soc. Transactions 1995;24: 224-229.

55. Platt JL. Complement Inhibitors. In: Gallin JI, Snyderman R, Fearon DT, Haynes BF, Nathan C, eds. Inflammation: Basic Principles and Clinical Correlates. Third ed. Philadelphia: Lippincott-Raven, 1999.

56. Leventhal JR, Sakiyalak P, Witson J, Simone P, Matas AJ, Bolman RM et al. The synergistic effect of combined antibody and complement depletion on discordant cardiac xenograft survival in nonhuman primates. Transplantation 1994;57: 974-978.

57. Rollins SA, Matis LA, Springhorn JP, Setter E, Wolff DW. Monoclonal antibodies directed against human C5 and C8 block complement-mediated damage of xenogeneic cells and organs. Transplantation 1995;60: 1284-1292.

58. Kroshus TJ, Bolman RM, Dalmasso AP, Rollins SA, Guilmette ER, Williams BL et al. Expression of human CD59 in transgenic pig organs enhances organ survival in an ex vivo xenogeneic perfusion model. Transplantation 1996;61: 1513-1521.

59. Leventhal JR, Matas AJ, Sun LH, Reif S, Bolman RM, Dalmasso AP et al. The immunopathology of cardiac xenograft rejection in the guinea pig-to-rat model. Transplantation 1993;56: 1-8.

60. Parker W, Saadi S, Lin SS, Holzknecht ZE, Bustos M, Platt JL. Transplantation of discordant xenografts: a challenge revisited. Immunol. Today 1996;17: 373-378.

61. Bach FH, Winkler H, Ferran C, Hancock WW, Robson SC. Delayed xenograft rejection. Immunol. Today 1996;17: 379-384.

62. Hancock WW, Blakely ML, van der Werf W, Bach FH. Rejection of guinea pig cardiac xenografts post-cobra venom factor therapy is associated with infiltration by mononuclear cells secreting interferon-gamma and diffuse endothelial activation. Transpl. Proc. 1993;25: 2932.

63. Hong R, Horowitz S. Immunodeficiency. . Basel: S. Karger, 1977.

64. Mori N, Prager D. Transactivation of the interleukin-1α promoter by human T-cell leukemia virus type I and type II tax proteins. Blood 1996;8: 3410-3417.

65. Havele C, Bleackley RC, Paetkau V. Conversion of specific to nonspecific cytotoxic T lymphocytes. J. Immunol. 1986;137: 1448-1454.

66. Arend WP, Massoni RJ, Niemann MA, Giclas PC. Absence of induction of IL-1 production in human monocytes by complement fragments. The Journal of Immunology 1989;142: 173-178.

67. Karmann K, Min W, Fanslow WC, Pober JS. Activation and homologous desensitization of human endothelial cells by CD40 ligand, tumor necrosis factor, and interleukin 1. J. Exp. Med. 1996;184: 173-182.

68. Romano EL, Soyano A, Linares J, Lauzon GJ. Neutralization of ABO blood group antibodies by specific oligosaccharides. Transpl. Proc. 1987;14: 4426-4430.

69. Bustos M, Platt JL. Platelet-endothelial cell interactions in a xenograft model. Trans Proc 1997;29: 886.

70. Wiedmer T, Ando B, Sims PJ. Complement C5b-9-stimulated platelet secretion

is associated with a Ca2+-initiated activation of cellular protein kinases. J. Biol. Chem. 1987;262: 13674-13681.

71. Lin SS, Platt JL. The role of immunoabsorption in xenotransplantation. Submitted 1997;

72. Porter KA. Renal Transplantation. In: Heptinstall RH, ed. Pathology of the Kidney, Volume III. 4 ed. Boston, MA: Little, Brown, and Company, 1992:1799-1933.

73. Cotterell AH, Collins BH, Parker W, Harland RC, Platt JL. The humoral immune response in humans following cross-perfusion of porcine organs. Transplantation 1995;60: 861-868.

74. Perper RJ, Najarian JS. Experimental renal heterotransplantation. III. Passive transfer of transplantation immunity. Transplantation 1967;5: 514-533.

75. Lin SS, Weidner BC, Byrne GW, Diamond LE, Lawson JH, Hoopes CW et al. The role of antibodies in acute vascular rejection of pig-to-baboon cardiac transplants. J. Clin. Invest. 1998;101: 1745-1756.

76. Blakely ML, Van Der Werf WJ, Berndt MC, Dalmasso AP, Bach FH, Hancock WW. Activation of intragraft endothelial and mononuclear cells during discordant xenograft rejection. Transplantation 1994;58: 1059-1066.

77. Kalady MF, Lawson JH, Sorrell RD, Platt JL. Decreased fibrinolytic activity in porcine-to-primate cardiac xenotransplantation. Molecular Medicine 1998;4: 629-637.

78. Hellmark T, Segelmark M, Bygren P, Wieslander J. Glomerular basement membrane autoantibodies. In: Peter JB, Shoenfeld Y, eds. Autoantibodies. Amsterdam: Elsevier Science B.V., 1996:291-298.

79. Lukomska B, Winnock M, Balabaud C, Saric J, Polanski J, Olszewski WL. Human liver passenger cells suppress autologous and allogeneic blood lymphocytes proliferation. Trans Proc 1997;29: 1105-1107.

80. Karsan A, Yee E, Kaushansky K, Harlan JM. Cloning of a human bcl-2 homologue: inflammatory cytokines induce human A1 in cultured endothelial cells. Blood 1996;87: 3089-3096.

81. Iwaki Y, Terasaki PI. Primary nonfunction in human cadaver kidney transplantation: evidence for hidden hyperacute rejection. Clin. Transplant. 1987;1: 125-131.

82. Lin SS, Hanaway MJ, Gonzalez-Stawinski GV, Lau CL, Parker W, Davis RD et al. The role of anti-Galα1-3Gal antibodies in acute vascular rejection of xenotransplants and accommodations of xenografts. Transplantation. In press.

83. McCurry KR, Parker W, Cotterell AH, Weidner BC, Lin SS, Daniels LJ et al. Humoral responses in pig-to-baboon cardiac transplantation: implications for the pathogenesis and treatment of acute vascular rejection and for accommodation. Hum. Immunol. 1997;58: 91-105.

84. Mollison PL, Engelfriet CP, Contreras M. Blood transfusion in clinical medicine. London, England: Blackwell Scientific Publications, 1993.

85. Lin Y, Goebles J, Xia G, Ji P, Vandeputte M, Waer M. Induction of specific transplantation tolerance across xenogeneic barriers in the T-independent immune compartment. Nature Medicine 1998;4: 173-80.

86. Lin Y, Vandeputte M, Waer M. Suppression of T-independent IgM xenoantibody formation by leflunomide during xenografting of hamster hearts in rats. Transplantation 1998;65: 332-9.

87. Waterworth P, Cozzi M, Tolan G, Langford G, Braidley P, Chavez G et al. Pig-to-primate cardiac xenotransplantation and cyclophosphamide therapy. Transpl. Proc. 1997;29: 899-900.

88. Alexandre GPJ, Squifflet JP, De Bruyere M, Latinne D, Moriau M, Ikabu N et al. Splenectomy as a prerequisite for successful human ABO-incompatible renal transplantation. Transpl. Proc. 1985;17: 138-143.

89. Yang Y-G, deGoma E, Ohdan H, Bracy JL, Xu Y, Iacomini J et al. Tolerization

of anti-Galα1-3Gal natural antibody-forming B cells by induction of mixed chimerism. J. Exp. Med. 1998;187: 1335-1342.

90. Bracy JL, Sachs DH, Iacomini J. Inhibition of xenoreactive natural antibody production by retroviral gene therapy. Science 1998;281: 1845-1847.

91. Bach FH. Inhibition of endothelial cell function: should this be a main goal of immunosuppressive strategies? J. Heart Lung Transplant. 1997;16: 493-495.

92. Hancock WW, Buelow R, Sayegh MH, Turka LA. Antibody-induced transplant arteriosclerosis is prevented by graft expression of anti-oxidant and anti-apoptotic genes. Nature Medicine 1998;4: 1392-6.

93. Stroka DM, Badrichani AZ, Bach FH, Ferran C. Overexpression of A1, an NF-kappaB-inducible anti-apoptotic bcl gene, inhibits endothelial cell activation. Blood 1999;93: 3803-3810.

94. Saadi S, Holzknecht RA, Patte CP, Stern DM, Platt JL. Complement-mediated regulation of tissue factor activity in endothelium. J. Exp. Med. 1995;182: 1807-1814.

95. Bustos M, Coffman TM, Saadi S, Platt JL. Modulation of eicosanoid metabolism in endothelial cells in a xenograft model: role of cyclooxygenase-2. J. Clin. Invest. 1997;100: 1150-1158.

96. Bach FH, Ferran C, Hechenleitner P, Mark W, Koyamada N, Miyatake T et al. Accommodation of vascularized xenografts: expression of "protective genes" by donor endothelial cells in a host Th2 cytokine environment. Nature Medicine 1997;3: 196-204.

97. Lechler RI, Lombardi G, Batchelor JR, Reinsmoen N, Bach FH. The molecular basis of alloreactivity. Immunol. Today 1990;11: 83-88.

98. Yamada K, Sachs DH, DerSimonian H. Human anti-porcine xenogeneic T cell response. Evidence for allelic specificity of mixed leukocyte reaction and for both direct and indirect pathways of recognition. J. Immunol. 1995;155: 5249-5256.

99. Murray AG, Khodadoust MM, Pober JS, Bothwell ALM. Porcine aortic endothelial cells activate human T cells: Direct presentation of MHC antigens and costimulation by ligands for human CD2 and CD28. Immunity 1994;1: 57-63.

100. Moses RD, Winn HJ, Auchincloss Jr. H. Multiple defects in cell surface molecule interactions across species differences are responsible for diminished xenogeneic T cell responses. Transplantation 1992;53: 203-209.

101. Gunsalus JR, Brady DA, Coulter SM, Gray BM, Edge A. Reduction of serum cholesterol in watanabe rabbits by xenogeneic hepatocellular transplantation. Nature Medicine 1997;3: 48-53.

102. Bhatti FNK, Schmoeckel M, Zaidi A, Cozzi E, Chavez G, Goddard M et al. Three-month survival of HDAFF transgenic pig hearts transplanted into primates. Transpl. Proc. 1999;31: 958.

103. Pierson RN, Winn HJ, Russell PS, Auchincloss H. Xenogeneic skin graft rejection is especially dependent on CD4+ T cells. J Exp Med 1989;170: 991-996.

104. Zhao Y, Swenson K, Sergio JJ, Arn JS, Sachs DH, Sykes M. Skin graft tolerance across a discordant xenogeneic barrier. Nature Medicine 1996;2: 1211-1216.

105. Li H, Ricordi C, Demetris AJ, Kaufman CL, Korbanic C, Hronakes ML et al. Mixed xenogeneic chimerism (mouse+rat*>mouse) to induce donor-specific tolerance to sequential or simultaneous islet xenografts. Transplantation 1994;57: 592-598.

106. Starzl TE, Demetris AJ, Murase N, Ildstad S, Ricordi C, Trucco M. Cell migration, chimerism, and graft acceptance. The Lancet 1992;339: 1579-1582.

107. Inverardi L, Samaja M, Motterlini R, Mangili F, Bender JR, Pardi R. Early recognition of a discordant xenogeneic organ by human circulating lymphocytes. J. Immunol. 1992;149: 1416-1423.

108. Malyguine AM, Saadi S, Holzknecht RA, Patte CR, Sud N, Platt JL et al. Induction of procoagulant function in porcine endothelial cells by human NK cells. J. Immunol. 1997;159: 4659-4664.

109. Rother RP, Fodor WL, Springhorn JP, Birks CW, Setter E, Sandrin MS et al. A

novel mechanism of retrovirus inactivation in human serum mediated by anti-α-galactosyl natural antibody. J. Exp. Med. 1995;182: 1345-1355.

110. Meng XJ, Purcell RH, Halbur PG, Lehman JR, Webb DM, Tsareva TS et al. A novel virus in swine is closely related to the human hepatitis E virus. Proceedings of the National Academy of Sciences 1997;94: 9860-9865.

111. Heneine W, Tibell A, Switzer WM, Sandstrom P, Rosales GV, Mathews A et al. No evidence of infection with porcine endogenous retrovirus in recipients of porcine islet-cell xenografts. Lancet 1998;352: 695-699.

112. Paradis K, Langford G, Long Z, Heneine W, Sandstrom P, Switzer WM et al. Search for cross-species transmission of porcine endogenous retrovirus in patients treated with living pig tissue. Science 1999;285: 1236-1241.

113. Chari RS, Collins BH, Magee JC, Kirk AD, Harland RC, McCann RL et al. Treatment of hepatic failure with ex-vivo pig liver perfusion followed by liver transplantation. New Eng. J. Med. 1994;331: 234-237.

114. Zaidi A, Schmoeckel M, Bhatti F, Waterworth P, Tolan M, Cozzi E et al. Life-supporting pig-to-primate renal xenotransplantation using genetically modified donors. Transplantation 1998;65: 1584-1590.

17 MEDICAL COMPLICATIONS OF IMMUNOSUPPRESSION

Jerry McCauley[1] and Ron Shapiro[2]
[1] Departments of Medicine and Surgery
[2] Department of Surgery
University of Pittsburgh
Pittsburgh, Pennsylvania, USA

INTRODUCTION

Transplantation effectively owes its existence to the development of immunosuppressive agents. Loss of allografts of all types to acute rejection has become less frequent as the potency and variety of immunosuppressive agents has continued to improve. Unfortunately, the medical complications of transplantation are also largely related to these agents. Each one has been associated with well-described side effects, all of which must be anticipated and managed by the physicians caring for these patients. There is a growing recognition that patient and graft survival may be highly influenced by the side effects of these agents. Cardiovascular disease is the leading cause of death in transplant patients, and its progression may be accelerated by various immunosuppressive agents. Likewise, graft loss is largely caused by chronic allograft rejection after the first two years. The influence of hyperlipidemia and other factors may play a major role in this process. Proper management of the medical complications after transplantation may offer an important opportunity to prevent premature death and graft loss.

DRUG-RELATED COMPLICATIONS

Corticosteroids

Steroid therapy has been the mainstay of most immunosuppressive protocols. As more effective immunosuppressive agents have been developed,

A. W. Thomson (ed.), Therapeutic Immunosuppression, 427–443.
© 2001 Kluwer Academic Publishers.

Table 1 Side Effects Related to Corticosteroid Therapy	
Gastrointestinal	Peptic ulcer Gastritis Pancreatitis Perforation
Bone	Avascular necrosis Osteoporosis
Skin and soft tissues	Cushingoid appearance Acne Thin skin and easy bruisability Striae Hirsutism
Endocrine	Hyperglycemia Adrenal insufficiency
Renal	Sodium retention Hypokalemia
Eye	Cataracts Glaucoma
Neuropsychiatric	Depression Euphoria Psychosis Pseudotumor cerebri
Reproductive	Fetal growth retardation Infertility/amenorrhea
Infectious	Increased risk of common bacterial infections Increased risk of opportunistic infections
Cardiovascular	Hyperlipidemia Hypertension Accelerated atherosclerosis
Growth and Development	Growth Retardation

the dosage and associated side effects of steroid therapy have been mini-mized but not fully eliminated. The side effects of steroid therapy are well known to most physicians and are outlined in Table 1. Steroids have led to complications that range from cosmetic to life-threatening. The best known include cushingoid body habitus, pancreatitis, diabetes, and hypertension. Earlier protocols using less potent immunosuppressive agents were univer-sally fraught with severe steroid complications, since rejection was treated more frequently with high dose steroid boluses, and maintenance corticoste-roid dosages remained at very high levels, even many years after transplan-tation. During this period, steroid therapy was the major source of morbidity and infectious mortality. As newer agents are developed & utilized in trans-plant recipients, their ability to allow a reduction in steroid dosages to an absolute minimum becomes an important consideration.

Azathioprine

Azathioprine (AZA) has had a long and important role in the development of organ transplantation. The side effects of this agent also form the basis for the associated medical complications. Azathioprine may cause nausea, vomiting, and diarrhea when the drug is initiated. In the transplant setting, these symptoms are less evident, since AZA is often started peri-operatively; however, these symptoms have developed in 23% of patients treated for rheumatologic diseases [1]. Azathioprine may cause elevated hepatic trans-aminases and cholestasis. When administered chronically, it may also cause veno-occlusive disease and hepatic fibrosis. Bone marrow suppression is the most common important complication of AZA. It is usually manifested by leukopenia, anemia, and thrombocytopenia. Leukopenia is the most frequent complication and occurs in approximately 27% of patients at some time. Anemia and thrombocytopenia develop in approximately 5% of patients. In the early post-operative period, the many other potential causes of anemia and thrombocytopenia make the contribution of AZA difficult to assess. Azathioprine is a prodrug which is converted to its active metabolite, 6-mercaptopurine, by the action of glutathione in red blood cells. Hepatic xanthine oxidase and thiopurine methyltransferase are responsible for metabolism of AZA [2]. Approximately 0.3% of the population have low levels of thiopurine methyltransferase; this results in high levels of AZA and unexpected toxic side effects when the usual doses are administered. It is possible to measure enzyme levels, but at a practical level, patients can be started on the usual

Table 2 Side effects of Azathioprine	
Gastrointestinal	Hepatic dysfunction
	Anorexia, nausea and vomiting
	Diarrhea
	Cholestasis, veno-occlusive disease, fibrosis, peliosis hepatis
Bone Marrow Suppression (dose dependent)	Leukopenia
	Anemia (Megaloblastic)
	Thrombocytopenia
Skin Cancer	Squamous cell carcinoma
Decreased Fertility (temporary)	Temporarily depresses spermatogenesis and sperm viability

doses and monitored for evidence of toxicity. If excessive toxic side effects are noted, the doseage is reduced or stopped. Treatment of gout with allopurinol (a xanthine oxidase inhibitor) in patients receiving AZA may be associated with severe toxic side effects if the usual doses of AZA are continued. The most serious of the side effects is bone marrow suppression, which may be potentially lethal if not recognized. The maintenance dose of AZA is usually reduced by approximately 50% if allopurinol and AZA are co-administered. These patients must then be followed very closely to watch for neutropenia.

Mycophenolate Mofetil

Mycophenolate mofetil (MMF) is a relatively new immunosuppressive agent that inhibits the proliferation of T and B cells. Its mechanism of action involves the blockade of the enzyme inosine monophosphate dehydrogenase. Two early trials demonstrated that MMF at doses of 2 or 3 grams per day were capable of reducing the incidence of acute cellular rejection significantly, when compared to placebo (13.8%, 17%, and 38.8%, respectively) [3] or AZA (19.7%, 15.9%, and 35.5% respectively) [4]. Table 3 summarizes the side effects of MMF [3,4]. Both AZA and MMF can suppress the bone marrow and cause anemia, leukopenia, and thrombocytopenia. Although MMF given at 3 grams/day was more effective in preventing rejection, the rate of side effects and infectious complications was greater, which has led

Table 3
Side effects of MMF* compared to AZA[4] and Placebo[3]

	Placebo (%)	AZA (%)	MMF 2 Grams (%)*	MMF 3 Grams (%)*
Gastrointestinal				
Diarrhea	12.7	17	12.7, 28	15.6, 31
Abdominal pain	10.8	20	11.5, 28	11.3, 31
Nausea	2.4	20	4.2, 14	6.3, 20
Vomiting	1.2	6	2.4, 12	3.8, 16
Hematologic				
Anemia	1.8	10	4.2, 15	6.8, 9
Leukopenia	4.2	30	10.9, 19	13.8, 35
Thrombocytopenia	4.8	12	4.2, 9	3.1, 5

* MMF side effects are listed as European study group data[3] (6 month follow-up), followed by Tricontinental Study Group data[4] (12 month follow-up)

to the standard dosing of 2 grams/day. The major side effect of MMF is gastrointestinal. Diarrhea, abdominal pain, nausea, and vomiting are the most common causes of dosage reduction or cessation of MMF. Hyperbilirubinemia was reported in 1% for both MMF dosages and in 6% for AZA in the Tricontinental study. As MMF has been demonstated to be more effective than AZA without an increase in serious side effects, many programs now preferentially use MMF.

Cyclosporine and Tacrolimus

The introduction of cyclosporine (CYA) in the early 1980's ushered in a new era in transplantation, during which both renal and extrarenal transplantation became almost routine. This important agent also introduced previously unseen side effects and medical complications. Tacrolimus (TAC) has been associated with an important incremental improvement in transplantation, improving survival, further lowering steroid requirements, and allowing rescue of patients failing CYA therapy. The side effects of TAC are generally similar to CYA, with some important differences, and are listed in Table 4. Both CYA and TAC are comparably nephrotoxic and may cause acute or chronic changes. Acute CYA or TAC nephrotoxicity is due to constriction of the afferent arterioles, leading to equivalent reductions in glomerular filtration rate (GFR) and effective renal plasma flow (ERPF), and a resulting unchanged filtration fraction (FF). The spectrum of acute nephrotoxicity of these agents ranges from small changes in the serum creatinine to the rare occurrence of acute renal failure requiring hemodialysis. The histologic and functional changes of acute and chronic CYA and TAC nephrotoxicity are nearly identical [5,6,7]. Acute nephrotoxicity is typically manifested by a sudden rise in serum creatinine, in association with elevated drug blood levels. Chronic toxicity is usually associated with a persistently elevated serum creatinine, and if high drug levels are maintained, this may be progressive. The risk of nephrotoxicity has stimulated a reduction in both initial and long term dosing of CYA and TAC. This unfortunately has led to dosages which may be sub-therapeutic in CYA-treated patients (< 4-6 mg/kg/day or 150-400 ng/ml trough HPLC levels). Conversely, increasing dosages and levels chronically beyond the upper limits of these values increases the risk of chronic nephrotoxicity. The appropriate minimal effective dosage or levels for TAC have not been conclusively determined to date. However, long-term therapeutic recommended levels range between approximately 5-12 ng/ml. Whether these target levels are too high will require future study.

Most other side effects of CYA and TAC are similar, with some notable excep-

Table 4
Comparison of Toxicities of Sirolimus, Tacrolimus and Cyclosporine

Complication	Sirolimus	Tacrolimus	Cyclosporine
Nephrotoxicity	1+*	3+	3+
Neurotoxicity			
Tremors	0	3+	3+
Seizures	0	1+	1+
Insomnia	0	2+	2+
Arthralgia	2+	0	0
Hypertension	1+	2+	3+
Hyperglycemia	0	2+	2+
Hyperlipidemia	3+	1+	2+
Gingival Hyperplasia	0	0	3+
Hypertrichosis	0	0	3+
Hyperkalemia	0	3+	2+
Hypokalemia	1+	0	0
Hypophosphatemia	1+	0	0
Hyperuricemia	0	2+	2+
Hepatotoxicity	1+	1+	1+
Anorexia	0	1+	1+
Hemolytic Uremic Syndrome	0	1+	1+
Anemia	1+	0	0
Leukopenia	1+	0	0
Thrombocytopenia	3+	0	0

3+ = very common, 2+ = common, 1+ = unusual, 0= not seen, ?0=unknown but unlikely,
* nephrotoxicity noted when given with CYA

tions. The rate of post-transplant hyperglycemia has been reported to be greater with TAC in studies using relatively high doses and with target blood levels of approximately 20 ng/ml in the early post operative period. However, recent studies have shown lower rates of post-transplant diabetes mellitus under tacrolimus, and the incidence has been comparable to that reported with cyclosporine. The neurotoxicity of CYA and TAC appears to be similar. Hypertension and hyperlipidemia develop less frequently in the TAC-treated patients. Hypertrichosis and gingival hyperplasia have not been reported with the use of TAC, although alopecia has been occasionally observed.

Sirolimus (Rapamycin)

Sirolimus, previously known as rapamycin (RAPA), is a new macrocyclic lactone, which was originally isolated from the fungus Streptomyces hygroscopicus and has recently been approved by the FDA for use in transplantation. The mechanism of action of this agent is discussed in detail elsewhere in this volume. In brief, CYA and TAC both inhibit calcineurin-dependent T cell cytokine transcription; RAPA inhibits a different mechanism at the post-translational level. Sirolimus has been extensively studied in combination with CYA, and this has made isolating the side effects of the two agents rather difficult. A recent report by Groth et al used RAPA and CYA independently, which allowed an opportunity to assess the efficacy and side effects of this new agent [8]. Table 4 illustrates the relative toxicities of RAPA, TAC, and CYA. Sirolimus appears to have little or no nephrotoxicity or neurotoxicity. Arthralgia was a significant new side effect noted in the trial by Groth et al. Hyperlipidemia developed more frequently compared to CYA and (by inference) is expected to be more common than in TAC-treated patients. Instead of hyperkalemia, RAPA-treated patients developed hypokalemia. Unlike TAC or CYA, RAPA has significant effects on bone marrow elements and resulted in anemia, thrombocytopenia, and leukopenia more frequently than CYA, although these have tended not to be clinically important.

CARDIOVASCULAR COMPLICATIONS

Cardiovascular disease is the most common cause of death after transplantation. The high rate of cardiovascular disease in the renal transplant population has prompted the National Kidney Foundation's Task Force on Cardiovascular Disease in Chronic Renal Disease to call it an "epidemic" [9]. In the renal transplant population, many of the risk factors for cardiovascular disease are highly prevalent and may be influenced by many of commonly used immunosuppressive agents [10]. Hyperlipidemia is a common complication of transplantation [11,12]. Hypertriglyceridemia is most common and may occur in isolation or in association with hypercholesterolemia. Isolated hypercholesterolemia without hypertriglyceridemia may also occur. Steroid use is also associated with insulin resistance and hyperinsulinemia. These problems improve but may not completely resolve even if prednisone is tapered to low doses or discontinued. A study of cyclosporine/steroid treated patients showed that 38% of renal transplant patients had hyperlipidemia three months after transplantation; this fell to 13% by 3 years post trans-

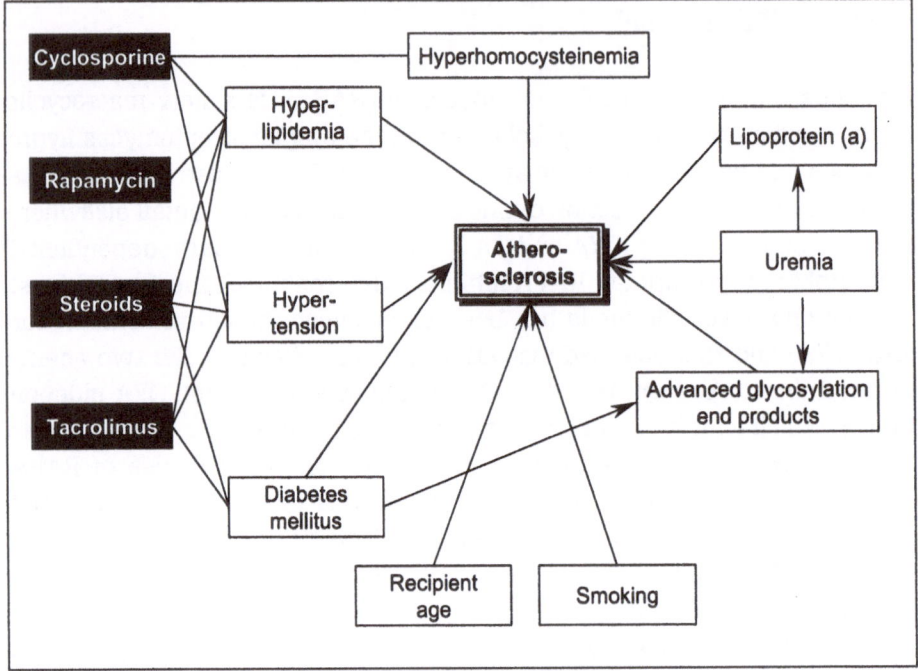

Figure 1
Risk factors for atherosclerosis in transplant recipients
The risk factors for cardiovascular disease found in the transplant recipient include hyperlipidemia, hypertension, diabetes mellitus, hyperhomocystenemia, uremia, and others (shown in white boxes). Many of these factors are exacerbated by the immuno-suppressive drugs (shown in black boxes) in current clinical use to prevent rejection. *(Reprinted with permission from UptoDate in Medicine).*

plantation [13]. The persistent abnormalities in lipid metabolism are largely related to cyclosporine, and this effect is independent of steroid dosage. In one study, total cholesterol fell with cessation of steroids, but HDL also fell to a similar degree or greater [14]. Tacrolimus has been associated with a lower rate of hyperlipidemia, and this is also independent of steroid dosage [15]. A recent report found that total serum cholesterol, LDL, & triglyceride levels were significantly lower in the TAC-treated compared to CYA-treated renal transplant recipients [16]. Steroids, CYA, and many of the other new immunosuppressive agents directly or indirectly increase the risk of atherosclerotic disease and subsequent cerebrovascular or myocardial events (Figure 1). Rapamycin (RAPA) has also been associated with hyperlipidemia when administered with CYA [16]. This appears to be a direct effect of RAPA; in a multicenter trial in which patients were randomized to CYA or RAPA, the RAPA-treated patients had higher triglyceride and total cholesterol levels at one year.

HYPERTENSION

Hypertension develops frequently after renal transplantation and has many potential etiologies (Table 5). The incidence of hypertension has been highly dependent upon the type of immunosuppressive protocol, and has increased from 40-50% in the pre-cyclosporine era to 60-70% in CYA-treated renal allograft recipients [17]. Cyclosporine and chronic rejection have been the most common causes of hypertension prior to the introduction of the more recent immunosuppressive agents [18]. Cyclosporine induces vasoconstriction of the afferent arteriole, which reduces both GFR and renal blood flow and plays an important pathophysiologic role in the development of hypertension [19]. This may be related to vasoconstricting prostaglandins and the renin-angiotensin system. Systemic vascular resistance (SVRI) also increases with CYA but apparently not with TAC. This may explain the somewhat lower rate of hypertension in TAC-treated patients [20]. Cyclosporine-induced hypertension is also in part volume dependent [17]. It worsens with measures leading to volume expansion (saline, high salt diet) and is poorly responsive to angiotensin converting enzyme inhibitors. Steroids are also a major contributor to hypertension. Their contribution to hypertension can be minimized by immunosuppressive protocols aimed at rapid tapering or discontinuation of prednisone.

Table 5 Causes of Hypertension in Renal Transplant Recipients	
Immunosuppressive Therapy	Steroids Cyclosporine Tacrolimus
Diseases in the Renal Allograft	Chronic Rejection Cyclosporine nephrotoxicity Tacrolimus nephrotoxicity Transplant renal artery stenosis Recurrent or de novo glomerulonephritis Recurrent diabetic nephropathy
High Renin Output of Native Kidneys	Renal artery stenosis in native kidneys
Recurrent Essential Hypertension	Recurrent systemic disease Transplantation of a predisposed graft

Miscellaneous	Coexistent cause of secondary hypertension
	  Primary aldosteronism
	  Pheochromocytoma
	Hypercalcemia

Adapted from Luke RG. J Am Soc Nephrol 1991;2(Suppl 1) :S37-S44	

Although hypertension generally reflects either the side effects of immuno-suppressive agents or inadequate long-term immunosuppression leading to chronic allograft nephropathy, renal artery stenosis is another potential (although less common) cause of hypertension. It can be the result of surgical complications or donor factors. Renal artery stenosis should be suspected in patients with a sudden onset of severe hypertension or worsening of stable hypertension. Another common presentation is renal insufficiency without another definable cause. Doppler ultrasonography may be helpful but may have a worrisome false positive (or, occasionally, false negative) rate, and is highly dependent upon the experience of the technician or radiologist. Other non-invasive approaches to the diagnosis might include a Captopril renal scan, but this may not be valid in the presence of CYA and may increase the risk of worsening renal function in a patient with renal artery stenosis in a solitary kidney [21]. Unsuspected renal artery stenosis in the native kidneys as a cause of post transplant hypertension probably occurs infrequently. Native nephrectomy as a cure for hypertension should be reserved for patients with well-documented disease.

The management of post transplant hypertension should be guided by the pathophysiology of hypertension. Although CYA-induced hypertension is partially mediated by hypervolemia, the use of diuretic therapy may lead to both pre-renal azotemia and the added side effects of thiazides, which include hyperglycemia and hyperlipidemia. On physiologic grounds, the preferred first line agents are probably calcium channel blockers. They vasodilate the afferent arterioles, increase renal blood flow, and induce a moderate natriuresis [22]. The dihydropyridines (nifedipine and isradipine) do not affect CYA or TAC blood levels and are very effective in lowering blood pressure. Diltiazem and verapamil increase CYA and may increase TAC blood levels. This side effect has been used to lower the total daily dosage of CYA by approximately 50%, which has represented an important savings in drug costs. Centrally acting agents (clonidine) are effective in lowering blood pressure without interfering with CYA or TAC blood levels. An added advantage, if patients can tolerate the somnolence and other side effects, is blunting of the tremors and insomnia of CYA toxicity. Excessive somnolence may develop in elderly patients and may lead to altered mental status and delirium. Alpha and beta blocking agents can also be used and do not affect CYA or TAC blood levels. Moderate to severe hypertension can often be controlled with oral agents initially (clonidine, 0.1 mg, or labetalol). Labetalol may cause hyperkalemia in patients with poor renal function, and this may be exacerbated by CYA and TAC. Short acting nifedipine (given sublingually) is no longer recommended for acute management of hypertension, since excessive lowering of the blood pressure has been associated with angina and myocardial infarction [23,24]. Long acting nifedipine, however, remains an important and effective agent in the management of post-transplant hypertension.

MALIGNANCIES AFTER TRANSPLANTATION

Malignancies develop approximately 100 times more frequently in the transplant population than in the general population [25,26]. Cancers found to be more frequent after transplantation include skin cancers, non-Hodgkin's lymphoma, Kaposi's sarcoma, in situ carcinomas of the uterine cervix, carcinomas of the vulva and perineum, renal cell carcinoma, hepatobiliary carcinomas, and sarcomas [27]. The advanced age of renal transplant recipients, pre-existing carcinoma prior to transplantation, and the increased risk of new lesions related to immunosuppression make an effective cancer surveillance program crucial. Older patients should be monitored for pulmonary, prostatic, uterine, colon, and breast cancer. Immunosuppression does not appear to increase the frequency of these lesions but may allow more rapid growth [26,27]. Non-melanotic skin and lip cancers (squamous cell) are the most common malignancies after transplantation [28]. These lesions are

Table 6
Recurrence of Pre-existing Cancers After Renal Transplantation (adapted from Penn, I. Transplantation 1993)[29]

Tumor	
Incidental renal cell cancer Testicular Cervix or Uterus Thyroid Lymphoma	Low recurrence rates (0-10%)
Body of Uterus Wilms Tumor Colon Prostate Breast	Intermediate recurrence rates (11-25%)
Bladder Sarcoma Melanoma Symptomatic Renal Cell Non-melanoma Skin Cancer Myeloma	High recurrence rates ($\geq$ 26%)

seen most frequently in areas with high sun exposure, and patients in such areas should be considered high risk. Some cancers, such as de-novo breast cancer, appear to develop at a lower frequency after transplantation.

Transplantation of patients with pre-existing cancers is becoming more common as the transplant population ages. Recurrence of pre-existing malignancies can be divided into three groups and is displayed in Table 6 [29]. The intermediate and high risk groups should be followed very closely for recurrence. The recommendations of the American Cancer Society for routine screening in asymptomatic patients should be followed in all transplant patients. All patients should have an annual skin examination to monitor for new or recurrent skin cancers, and high-risk patients should be examined more frequently. Routine digital rectal examinations should be performed annually after age 40. Sigmoidoscopy should be encouraged beginning at age 50 then every 3-5 years thereafter. Pelvic examinations and PAP smears should be performed annually in women 20-65 and earlier in sexually active teens. Routine mammograms should be performed every year in women beginning at approximately 35 years of age.

LIVER DISEASE

Liver disease after renal transplantation is an important cause of morbidity and mortality. The reported prevalence of liver disease has been reported to be 7-24% during the early post transplant period; liver disease is responsible for 8-24% of the mortality after transplantation [30,31,32]. Abnormalities in liver enzymes occur frequently after transplantation and may have many potential etiologies. Commonly used medications may cause abnormalities in liver function (Table 7) [33]. Although these specific medications have been documented to cause hepatic dysfunction, all drugs should be considered potential offenders. Cyclosporine commonly causes an isolated increase in bilirubin and/or serum transaminases. The CYA effect on hepatic enzymes is dose-dependent and responds to simple dosage reduction. Sirolimus also may cause changes in hepatic enzymes similar to CYA, but less frequently [8]. Azathioprine causes cholestatic hepatic abnormalities, and there are reported cases of veno-occlusive hepatic disease, and peliosis hepatis. Other medications can cause hepatic abnormalities that range from mild increases in transaminases to fulminant hepatic failure from hepatic necrosis. In most cases, discontinuing the medication is sufficient to correct the problem, and a liver biopsy is usually not required.

Table 7	
Commonly used agents in transplantation causing liver failure	
Agent	**Problem**
Cyclosporine Sirolimus ?	Hyperbilirubinemia, elevated transaminases
Azathioprine	Cholestasis, veno-occlusive disease, fibrosis, peliosis hepatis
Acetaminophen	Ranges from increase transaminase (chronic ingestion) to fulminant failure (overdose)
Allopurinol	Ranges from increase transaminase to hepatic necrosis, may develop vasculitis and renal failure
Anticonvulsants	Ranges from increase transaminase to hepatic necrosis
Penicillins	Increase transaminase, cholestasis, acute and chronic hepatitis
Sulfonamides	Hepatocellular necrosis, chronic liver disease
Antifungals	Ranges from increase transaminase to hepatic necrosis
Methyldopa	Increase transaminase, acute and chronic hepatitis
Hydralazine	Granulomatous hepatitis
Captopril	Cholestasis, hepatitic necrosis
Verapamil	Cholestasis and cholestasis

Hepatic dysfunction related to viral hepatitis is a growing cause of morbidity and mortality after transplantation. Hepatitis B (HBV) has long been recognized as a potential cause of liver disease and compromised patient and graft survival [34]. Vaccination for hepatitis B is now advised for all patients with end stage renal failure. The routine use of assays for hepatitis C (HCV) has revealed an increasing prevalence in dialysis patients. The importance of this virus has overshadowed even that of HBV as a cause of liver failure. HCV is now the leading cause of post-transplant liver disease [35]. Prior exposure to HCV has not been shown to impact adversely on allograft or patient survival but has been demonstrated to increase the risk of developing liver disease and sepsis [35]. It has seen estimated that as many as 25% of renal transplant patients have antibodies to HCV. Detection of subclinical hepatic dysfunction in the outpatient setting is crucial. Liver function testing should be performed in dialysis patients and in renal transplant recipients. Patients with HCV typically have an "undulating" pattern of liver function tests, with periodically elevated and normal values. Any patient with an unexplained rise in CYA or TAC blood levels should be investigated for hepatic insufficiency, which may present as a decreased ability to metabolize these agents. A liver biopsy may be required to confirm the presence of significant hepatic impairment. Interferon or ribavirin have been attempted as monotherapy for HCV patients without renal failure, with poor results, but the combination appears to be more efficacious [36,37]. Interferon treatment in renal transplant recipients has resulted in irreversible, catastrophic acute cellular rejection and is considered by most to be contraindicated in this setting [38].

HEMATOLOGIC

Hematologic complications develop for many reasons after transplantation. They may be related to immunosuppressive agents (AZA, RAPA, MMF, Tables 2, 3 & 4) or be a function of renal insufficiency or other causes. Anemia and leukopenia develop frequently. Poor renal function with associated erythropoietin deficiency is the most common cause in patients with chronic allograft nephropathy. Nutritional deficiencies such as iron, folate, and vitamin B12 should be investigated in patients with normal renal function or in those refractory to EPO. Parvovirus infection should be suspected in patients with isolated anemia without renal insufficiency or dietary deficiencies. Hemolytic anemia should prompt a search for hemolytic uremic syndrome, which may be associated with CYA or TAC (Table 3). Megaloblastic anemia and pancytopenia may be caused by AZA. Neutropenia may be due to AZA, mycophenolate, or CMV infection. Stopping or lowering the dose of the medication usually corrects neutropenia in drug-related cases, and treatment with ganciclovir is generally effective for CMV disease.

Thrombocytopenia is a side effect of several immunosuppressive agents, including AZA, RAPA, & MMF (see tables 2 and 3). It can develop with or without associated anemia or leukopenia. Other commonly used agents in transplantation causing bone marrow suppression and thrombocytopenia include trimethoprim - sulfamethoxazole, ganciclovir, and antithymocyte globulin. Hemolytic-uremic syndrome may present with severe thrombocytopenia and anemia in the absence of leukopenia. Patients with idiopathic thrombocytopenia purpura (ITP) may have an improvement in the platelet count after transplantation because of the steroids that are being administered as part of the immunosuppression. Rapid reduction in steroid dosage or withdrawal may lead to recurrence of thrombocytopenia. De novo ITP may also occur after transplantation.

Post-transplant polycythemia develops in about 15% of renal transplant patients. Venesection has been the standard therapy until recently. Angiotensin converting enzyme inhibitors reliably reduce the hematocrit and are now the standard of care for polycythemia after renal transplantation. However, these agents may cause de novo anemia or exacerbate pre-existing anemia, particularly in those with chronic allograft nephropathy.

SKIN AND SOFT TISSUES

Non-malignant abnormalities of the skin are some of the most common complications after transplantation. Acne is a well-known side effect of steroids, as is increased bruising and fragility. Hirsutism and gingival hyperplasia became common after the introduction of CYA. Gingival hyperplasia related to CYA may be exacerbated by poor oral hygiene. Nifedipine and other agents may also cause gingival hyperplasia. Warts due to human papilloma virus (HPV) are frequent. Common warts on the hands (HPV2,4), plantar warts (HPV1), and flat warts (HPV 3,10) may develop and proliferate rapidly even many years after transplantation.

METABOLIC

Many metabolic derangements develop after transplantation and may be related to immunosuppression (Table 3), other medications, or longstanding renal failure. Renal osteodystrophy develops in patients with chronic renal failure and end stage renal disease because of poor control of serum phosphate. Hyperparathyroidism persisting beyond one year, with evidence of hypercalcemia, hypophosphatemia, and increased bone activity (increased alkaline phosphatase) may require parathyroidectomy. Hyperkalemia is a common complication of CYA and TAC therapy, and hypokalemia may develop with RAPA. The reduction in potassium excretion may be due to decreased aldosterone, NA-K ATPase, or other undefined tubular defects. Hyperkalemia may also be due to iatrogenic causes, such as injudicious replacement of potassium in patients with poor renal function. Florinef has been useful in controlling the hyperkalemia of TAC. Both TAC and CYA cause hypomagnesemia, which is probably related to urinary magnesium wasting. In most cases hyperkalemia and hypomagnesemia improve after a reduction in dosage. Post transplant diabetes mellitus (PTDM) develops in 4-20% of renal transplant patients [39]. The most commonly used immunosuppressive agents (steroids, CYA, and TAC) are all diabetogenic. AZA, MMF, and RAPA have not been associated with hyperglycemia. Steroids may induce insulin resistance in addition to changes in glucose uptake, insulin receptors, and insulin production. Proposed mechanisms for CYA and

TAC include decreased insulin secretion, increased insulin resistance, and a toxic effect on beta cells. Dosage reduction or discontinuation of the above agents may improve blood sugars and allow many patients to stop insulin therapy or oral hypoglycemic agents.

REFERENCES

1. Weinshilboum, RM, Sladek, SL. Mercaptopurine pharmacogenetics: Monogenic inheritance of erythrocyte thiopurine methyl transferase activity. Am J Hum Genet 1980; 32:651.
2. Lennard, L, Van Loon, JA, Weinshilboum, RM. Pharmacogenetics of acute azathioprine toxicity: Relationship to thiopurine, methyl transferase, genetic polymorphism. Clin Pharmacol Ther 1989; 46:149.
3. European Mycophenolate Mofetil Cooperative Study Group. Placebo-controlled study of mycophenolate mofetil combined with cyclopsorin and corticosteroids for prevention of Acute Rejection. Lancet 1995;345(8961):1321
4. The Tricontinental Mycophenolate Mofetil Renal Transplantation Study Group. A blinded, randomized clinical trial of mycophenolate mofetil for the prevention of acute rejection in cadaveric renal transplantation. Transplantation 1996;61(7): 1029
5. McCauley J. The nephrotoxicity of FK 506 as compared with cyclosporine. Curr Opin Nephrol Hyperten 1993;2:662-66
6. Puschett JB, Greenberg A, Holley J, McCauley J. The spectrum of cyclosporine nephrotoxicity. Am J Nephrol 1990;10:296-309
7. Randhawa P, Shapiro R, Jordan M, Starzl T. The histologic changes associated with allograft rejection and drug toxicity in renal transplant recipients maintained on FK 506: Clinical significance and comparison with cyclosporine. Am J Surg Pathol 1993;17:
8. Groth, CG, Backman, L, Morales, J-M, et al. Sirolimus (rapamycin)-based therapy in human renal transplantation. Transplantation 1999; 67:1036.
9. Levey AS, Breto JA, Coronado BE, et al. Controlling the epidemic of cardiovascular disease in chronic renal disease. What do we know? What do we need to know? Where do we go from here? Am J Kidney Dis 1996;27:347-354.
10. Danovitch GH. The Epidemic of Cardiovascular Disease in Chronic Renal Disease: A challenge to the Transplant Physician. Graft 1999;2:S108-112.
11. Arnadottir, M, Berg, AL. Treatment of hyperlipidemia in renal transplant recipients. Transplantation 1997; 63:339.
12. Hricik, DE. Posttransplant hyperlipidemia: The treatment dilemma. Am J Kidney Dis 1994; 23:766.
13. Vathsala, A, Weinberg, RB, Schoenberg, L, et al. Lipid abnormalities in cyclosporine-prednisone-treated renal transplant recipients. Transplantation 1989; 48:37.
14. Hricik, DE, Bartucci, MR, Mayes, JT, Schulak, JA. The effects of steroid withdrawal on the lipoprotein profiles of cyclosporine-treated kidney and kidney-pancreas transplant recipients. Transplantation 1992; 54:868.
15. Satterthwaite, R, Aswad, S, Sunga, V, et al. Incidence of new-onset hypercholesterolemia in renal transplant patients treated with FK506 or cyclosporine. Transplantation 1998; 65:446.
16. Murgia, MG, Jordan, S, Kahan, BD. The side effect profile of sirolimus: A phase I study in quiescent cyclosporine-prednisone-treated renal transplant patients.

Kidney Int 1996; 49:209.

17. First RM, Neylan JF, Rocher LL, Tejani A. hypertension after renal transplantation. J Am Soc Nephrol 1994;4:S30-S36

18. Luke RG. Pathophysiology and treatment of posttransplant hypertension. J Am Soc Nephrol 1991;2(Suppl 1):S37-S44

19. Curtis JJ, Luke RG, Dubovsky E, et al. Cyclosporine in therapeutic doses increases renal allograft vascular resistance. Lancet 1986;2:447-479

20. McCauley, J.; Fung, J.; Jain, A.; Todo, S., and Starzl, T. E. The effects of FK 506 on renal function after liver transplantation. Transplant Proc. 1990 Feb; 22(1):17-20.

21. Laslow DA, Curtiss JJ. Post-transplant hypertension . Am J Hypertens 1990;3; 721-725

22. Curtis JJ. Hypertension following kidney transplantation. Am J Kid Dis 1994;23(3): 471-475

23. The Sixth Report of the Joint National Committee on Detection, Evaluation, and Diagnosis of High Blood Pressure (JNC VI). Arch Intern Med 1997; 157:2413.

24. Grossman, E, Messerli, FH, Grodzicki, T, Kowey, P. Should a moratorium be placed on sublingual nifedipine capsules for hypertensive emergencies or pseudoemergencies? JAMA 1996; 276:1328.

25. Penn, I. Cancers complicating organ transplantation. N Engl J Med 1990;323: 1767.

26. Barret W, First MR, Aron BS, Penn I. Clinical course of malignancies in renal tansplant recipients. Cancer 1993;72(7):2186-2189

27. Penn, I. The changing patterns of posttransplant malignancies. Transplant Proc 1991;23:1101.

28. Penn I. Occurrence of cancers in immunocompromised organ transplant recipients. Clinical Transplants 1990, P Terasaki ed. UCLA Tissue Typing laboratory, Los Angeles CA

29. Penn I. The effect of immunosuppression on pre-existing cancers. Tranplantation 1993;55:742-747

30. Weir MR, Kirkman RL, Strom TB, et al. Liver disease in recipients of long surviving renal allografts. Kidney Int 1985;28:839-844

31. Pereira BJ. Hepatitis C in organ transplantation: its significance and influence on transplantation policies. Curr Opin Nephrol Hyperten 1993;2:912-922

32. Braun WE. Nephrology Forum: Long term complications of renal transplantation. Kidney Int 1990;37:1363-1378

33. Bass NM, Ockner RK. Drug Induced Liver Disease. Hepatology: A Textbook of Liver Disease. Ed: Zakim D, Boyer TD, WB Saunders Co, Philadelphia, 1990

34. Parfrey PS, Forbes RDC, Hutchinson TA, Kenick S, et al. The impact of renal transplantation on the course of hepatitis B liver disease. Transplantation 1985;39: 610-615

35. Periera BJG, Wright TL, Schmid CH, et al. The impact of pretransplantation hepatitis C infection on the outcome of renal transplantation. Transplantation 1995; 60:799-805

36. Bodenheimer, H, Lindsay, KL, Davis, GL, et al. Tolerance and efficacy of oral ribavirin treatment of chronic hepatitis C: A multicenter trial. Hepatology 1997; 26:473.

37. Schalm, SW, Weiland, O, Hansen, BE, et al. Interferon-ribavirin for chronic hepatitis C with and without cirrhosis: Analysis of individual patient data of six controlled studies. Gastroenterology 1999; 117:408.

38. Magnone M, Holley JL, Shapiro R, Scantlebury V, McCauley J, Jordan M, Vivas C, Starzl T, Johnson JP . Interferon-alpha-induced acute renal allograft rejection. Transplantation 59(7):1068-70, 1995 Apr.

39. Jindal RM. Posttransplant diabetes mellitus: A review. Transplantation 1994;58: 1289-1298

18

NEUROLOGICAL COMPLICATIONS OF IMMUNOSUPPRESSIVE AGENTS

Benjamin H. Eidelman and Ron Shapiro
Department of Neurology and Department of Surgery
University of Pittsburgh
Pittsburgh, Pennsylvania, USA

INTRODUCTION

The majority of immunosuppressive agents used to prevent rejection in organ transplant recipients are neurotoxic and can impact upon the function of structures throughout the nervous system. The clinical manifestations can be quite diverse.

This section will discuss the neurological complications of the most commonly used agents in solid organ transplantation, particularly cyclosporine (CyA) and tacrolimus (TAC, formerly FK 506), and sirolimus (rapamycin), but also including a brief discussion of mycophenolate mofetil, corticosteroids, and muromonab CD3 (OKT3).

MECHANISMS OF ACTION OF CYA AND TACROLIMUS

The actions of CyA and tacrolimus are mediated by their respective immunophilins [1], which, by binding to calcineurin, inhibit its phosphatase activity.[2] This results in an impairment of intracellular signaling mechanisms, in particular impacting upon the function of the nuclear factor of activated T cells (NF-AT). In the absence of phosphatase activity, this factor is unable to unable to translocate to the nucleus, and IL-2 gene transcription cannot take place.[3] Other genes whose transcriptional control is also influenced by these immunosuppressive agents have been identified.[4]

A. W. Thomson (ed.), Therapeutic Immunosuppression, 445–457.

Inhibition of calcineurin phosphatase activity impacts upon the phosphory-lation of other proteins that are also calcineurin substrates, and both tacro-limus and CyA have been demonstrated to inhibit nitric oxide synthetase (NOS) activity, which is essential to the formation of nitric oxide. This in turn appears to result in the blocking of N-methyl-D-aspartate (NMDA), a sub-type of glutamate receptors. [5] Inhibition of NOS has been demonstrated to have a neuroprotective effect against neural damage caused by ischemia.[6] Tacrolimus has also been described to modulate neurotransmitter release[7], again through an effect on nitric oxide. Through inhibition of calcineurin, tacrolimus and CyA may exhibit widespread and divergent effects through-out the central nervous system. There are also additional mechanisms which could be operative. High concentrations of immunophilins exist in the ner-vous system and actually exceed levels found in the immune system.[8] These immunosuppressive agents may have a direct influence upon the immunophilins themselves.[9] The latter have important actions in the form of peptidyl-prolyl-cis-trans isomerase activity (PPIase). Such activity can be directly inhibited by the respective binding immunosuppressive agent. [10] Disruption of such function could potentially alter intracellular systems and thus disrupt cell function.

Immunophilins within the nervous system appear to be of structural and functional importance. By binding to their respective immunophilin, immu-nosuppressive agents may disrupt these functions, and this could poten-tially contribute to neurotoxicity, although the exact mechanisms have yet to be defined.

CLINICAL NEUROTOXICITY OF CYA AND TACROLIMUS

These two agents, which may be termed immunophilin-binding immunosup-pressive agents, have similar neurotoxicity [11], and thus will be discussed together. Differences as they arise will be highlighted. Traditionally, the ner-vous system is divided into central and peripheral components. This pro-vides a convenient method of classification of the neurotoxic effects of the immunophilin-binding agents.

Table 1
Major neurological complications of Tacrolimus and CyA

A. Central Nervous System
1. Encephalopathy
2. Akinetic Mutism
3. Seizures
4. Disorders of Speech
5. Reversible Posterior of Leukoencephalopathy
6. Cerebellar Swelling
7. Basal Ganglion Syndromes
8. Motor Dysfunction
    a. hemiplegia
    b. quadriparesis
9. Neuropathy
10. Myopathy

CENTRAL NERVOUS SYSTEM COMPLICATIONS (see table 1)

Encephalopathy

This entity may occur as a complication of both CyA [12,13] and tacrolimus [14] and is often characterized by disorientation and delusional thinking. When less overt, the patient may become withdrawn and appear depressed. Later, the level of consciousness may decline. The patient may lapse into coma. In some instances, loss of consciousness may occur without an intervening period of confusion. Additional features may include seizures [13], cortical blindness [15], and focal motor disturbances.[13] Encephalopathy is usually an early manifestation of immunosuppression-induced toxicity in that it is most commonly encountered immediately after transplantation and often responds to reduction or cessation of the immunosuppressive agent. In some instances, disturbances of cognitive function may persist for a prolonged period of time after the drug is withdrawn. Pre-existing hepatic encephalopathy appears to predispose to the development of this complication.[14,16]

Akinetic Mutism

This complication is common to CyA [17,18] and tacrolimus [14,19]and is usually another early post-transplant complication. The affected individual may initially appear to be in coma, then seemingly recovers but does not improve beyond a state of appearing alert. There is no attempt to communicate. The subject does not react to verbal stimuli and while painful stimuli may evoke facial grimacing and posturing of the extremities, there is no vocal response. Frontal release signs may be prominent. The condition is usually reversible, and improvement tends to occur after withdrawal or a decrease in the dose of the immunosuppressive agent. While this complication may occur with either CyA or tacrolimus, "cross reactivity" seemingly does not develop and substituting one agent for the other or decreasing the dose of the immuno-suppressive agent is the usual method of treatment. Recovery may be pro-tracted but may be accelerated by removing the patient from the intensive care environment and subjecting the individual to the much more varied existence of a rehabilitation setting. This raises the possibility that sensory deprivation may play some role in perpetuating a state of reduced respon-siveness.

The pathophysiology of immunosuppression-induced akinetic mutism is unknown, but a similar state may be encountered in vascular lesions, inter-rupting the mesencephalic-frontal pathways.[20] It is thus possible that CyA and tacrolimus may in some manner inhibit this system.

Seizures

Seizures may complicate the use of CyA [12,21,22] and tacrolimus [14,19], and while these may occur in isolation, they may often be a component of the encephalopathic syndrome mentioned above.[13] They often occur soon after the immunosuppressive agent has been introduced [21] and are not necessarily reflective of structural disease, often having an excellent progno-sis.[21]

Disorders of Speech

Disorders of speech or language are rare but disturbing complications of transplantation, and have been well-described by Bronster et al.[23] As with liver transplant subjects receiving CyA, this syndrome has also been reported as a complication of tacrolimus.[24,19] Dysarthria is the first mani-festation. The patient then rapidly develops further difficulties with commu-nication and eventually may be unable to communicate verbally. In the most severe instances, the patient may be mute and can only utter a few primitive sounds. There is usually no accompanying receptive aphasia and the ability to write is largely preserved. A severe apraxia of the lips and tongue appears to be at the root of the disorder. Other focal signs are generally absent. Consciousness is preserved, and the individual may often be extremely frustrated by an inability to speak. CT and MRI studies are usually unrevealing. Patients tend to improve after the immunosuppressive agent is withdrawn, but recovery is often protracted. The pathophysiology of this complication is unknown. Severe dysarthria occurring in association with generalized tremulousness has also been described as a complication of tacrolimus.[25]

The Reversible Posterior Leukoencephalopathic Syndrome

White matter abnormalities in the occipital region with accompanying clinical disturbances characterize this syndrome.[26] In some instances, occipital white matter abnormalities may be part of a more generalized encephalopathy.[13] Clinical features include headaches, altered level of consciousness, and visual hallucinations.[27]

In severe instances cortical blindness may also be evident.[15] White matter abnormalities, often focal to the occipital region, are the usual findings on the MRI studies, and these often resolve after the immunosuppressive agent has been withdrawn.[26,28,29] The condition is not always associated with an elevated immunosuppressive drug level. Biopsies of the affected areas have been carried out and histologic examination in one patient revealed demyelination.[26] The mechanism for development of this complication remains unknown, and similar radiological findings have been described in other conditions.[30] A variety of mechanisms for the development of this complication have been postulated [30], and these include a direct toxic effect of the immunosuppressive agent, a disturbed blood-brain barrier, and a toxic vasculopathy.

FOCAL CENTRAL NERVOUS SYSTEM SYNDROMES

Deficits attributable to localized abnormalities within the central nervous system have also been described as complications of CyA and tacrolimus.

Cerebellar Syndromes

The first of these are cerebellar syndromes. Disturbances of cerebellar function have been reported by a number of authors [31,32], and descriptions indicate a clinical syndrome dominated by cerebellar dysfunction, but confusion and motor dysfunction are also present. A case of isolated cerebellar swelling, however, has been reported as a complication of CyA therapy.[33] The patient presented with an acute onset of headache, accompanied by nausea and vomiting and rapidly lost consciousness. Imaging studies revealed marked swelling of the cerebellar hemispheres, so much so that surgical intervention was required. After decompression, the patient made an uneventful recovery. A biopsy specimen was obtained at the time of surgery, and histologic examination revealed non-specific edema and loss of purkinge cells. Similar findings have not been described with tacrolimus.

Focal Motor Deficits

Pure motor syndromes have been described as complications of both tacrolimus and CyA therapy. Hemiplegia [13] and quadriparesis [31,32] have been described. While these focal abnormalities may occur as the sole manifestation of immunosuppressive-induced toxicity, such abnormalities may at times also occur as a component of a more diffuse encephalopathic type of presentation.[34] Brain imaging studies may reveal abnormalities which correlate with the motor deficits.[11,13,26,29]

Movement Disorders

Involuntary movements are common complications of the immunophilin-binding immunosuppressive agents. Various movement disorders have been described, and these may include:

a. tremors of the limbs,
b. involuntary facial movements,
c. Parkinson-like syndromes.

a. *Tremors of the Extremities*
   Tremors of the limbs are extremely prominent side effects of the immunophilin-binding agents.[12,14] The disturbance of movement is most marked in the early days following transplantation and often recedes over the course of time. Tremors may involve the upper limbs, and both

postural and action types of tremor may be evident. The former are most obvious when the hands are held in an outstretched position, at which time the rhythmic oscillation of the limbs may be evident. This tremor may continue as the subject engages in voluntary movements and at times can become quite disabling. The tremor may abate as the hands are allowed to settle into a position of rest. In extreme cases the tremor may spread proximally and may involve the trunk and head. Such symptoms tend to become worse under conditions of anxiety and stress. The movement disorder is often self-limiting, disappearing or becoming much less severe over the course of time. Pharmacological agents such as Propranolol and Clonazepam may be quite helpful in reducing the severity of these tremors.

b. Facio-Lingual Dyskinesia

These abnormal movements, which are largely confined to the face and tongue, have been described by a number of authors. Tongue tremulousness was described by Wijdicks[12], and dystonic movements of the tongue and pharyngeal musculature, causing impaired speech, have also been reported.[25] Blepharospasm, characterized by frequent blinking and involuntary closure of the eyelids on exposure to light, has also been described as a complication of CyA[25], but this may also be seen as a prominent component of the akinetic mutism that may occur with tacrolimus.[14]   .

c. Parkinson-like State

A reduction in spontaneous motor activity (similar to that seen in Parkinson's disease) may occur in the original phase of immunosuppressive-induced encephalopathy [13], and may also be a component of the akinetic mutism syndrome.[14] A Parkinson syndrome as a complication of tacrolimus has been reported by Meuller et al.[34] This occurred in the context of an organic brain syndrome. Thus, while motor features similar to those seen in Parkinson's disease may appear as a component of an encephalopathic-like state, they have usually been described as a compound of a more generalized neurologic disorder.

Headache

Headaches are a frequent complication of the immunophilin-binding immunosuppressive agents. These may be mild but at times can be quite intense.[35] The pathophysiology of such headaches is not entirely understood. CyA has been shown to enhance the effect of the sympathetic nervous system[36], and this possibly could be a contributing factor. The stress of transplantation itself may induce headaches, particularly in individuals who are prone to develop headaches. In some instances, headache may be severe enough to warrant the consideration of an alternative immunosuppressive agent.[37]

Insomnia

Insomnia has been prominent in patients receiving tacrolimus-based immunosuppression.[38,39] This frequent complication is typically seen early in the post-transplant phase and improves over time. Rarely, insomnia may be a persistent phenomenon.

Other Disorders

There are other infrequent but troublesome side effects, which may include tinnitus, dizziness, and photophobia.[39] These in general are transient in nature, but dizziness can sometimes be a persistent and troublesome symptom.

PERIPHERAL NERVOUS SYSTEM COMPLICATIONS

These include neuropathy and myopathy.

Neuropathy

Patients frequently develop sensory symptoms after these immunosuppressive agents have been introduced. These may take the form of burning, tingling, and numbness, and tend to be most marked distally. In many instances, there are few if any accompanying clinical abnormalities, and EMG studies may also be negative. It is presumed that the presentation relates to a subclinical neuropathy, but definitive evidence of this is lacking. There are, however, case reports which indicate that both axonal and demyelinating neuropathy may occur with either CyA [13,49] or tacrolimus.[41,42] Acute onset and generalized weakness occurring as a result of widespread axonal neuropathy has been attributed to tacrolimus.[43] In this instance EMG study revealed an axonal type of dysfunction which improved after withdrawing the agent.

Myopathy

Weakness of acute onset attributable to myopathy has been reported with both tacrolimus[44,45] and CyA.[46,38,39]

The mechanisms for these toxic neuropathic and myopathic disturbances have not been fully elucidated. Immune-mediated mechanisms have been postulated, although it is possible that direct toxic effects on peripheral neural structures may also be responsible.[42]

SIROLIMUS (RAPAMYCIN)

Sirolimus (Rapamycin) is the newest of the immunophilin-binding immuno-suppressive agents. As with CyA and tacrolimus, this macrocyclic lactone interacts with a binding immunophilin (FKBP). Sirolimus, however, acts at a latter stage (the so-called mTOR, or mammalian target of rapamycin) in the activation process and blocks cytokine-mediated signal transduction path-ways.[47] It thus acts independently of Ca^2-dependent pathways.

Sirolimus is potent immunosuppressive agent, but has only seen limited clin-ical use, largely in the realm of renal transplantation. Clinical studies have revealed few neurological complications.[48] In one study, tremor was the only nervous system complication reported. Watson and his co-workers [49], in a series of 50 renal transplant patients, described two neurological events of seizure and encephalopathy. Both of these occurred in subjects co-immu-nosuppressed with CyA, and withdrawal of the latter agent resulted in improvement, suggesting that the neurotoxicity was a CyA-induced compli-cation.

Sirolimus has thus far been used on relatively few patients. It may take larger studies to determine the full extent of the neurotoxicity of this agent.

NEUROLOGICAL COMPLICATIONS OF OTHER IMMUNOSUPPRESSIVE AGENTS

Muromonab-CO3 (OKT3)

The most common side effect associated with the use of this murine mono-clonal antibody is an aseptic meningitis, which usually develops within the first 3-4 days after initiation of treatment. The clinical features are typical of any meningitis and are characterized by headache, nuchal rigidity, and fever.[50] CSF examination usually reveals a lymphocytic pleiocytosis.[50] An encephalopathic-like syndrome may also occur, but this is somewhat less common.[51] The features largely relate to impairment of conscious-ness, and the patient may become lethargic or even comatose. Myoclonic activity and seizures may also develop. Cerebral edema may be evident on imaging studies, and the CSF may also show increased protein in the pleio-cytosis. Patients invariably recover, although the course may be somewhat protracted.[52]

Corticosteroids

Acute neurological side effects are largely of the neuropsychiatric-type.[53] Prompt recognition of this particular complication is essential, as the symp-toms will abate once the appropriate adjustments in therapy have been made. Chronic steroid therapy may be accompanied by a myopathy [54] char-acterized by proximal weakness, most obvious in the lower limbs. Weak-ness is profound, and EMG changes may be quite subtle. Improvement in strength will often occur after steroid withdrawal, but it may take many months before strength begins to return.

Mycophenolate Mofetil

This relatively new immunosuppressive has increasingly been used as an adjunctive agent in transplantation. There are, thus far, no reports of signifi-cant neurological side effects. There are, however, indications that move-ment disorders may be associated with its use (personal observation). Again, the true neurotoxic profile may only emerge once mycophenolate mofetil has been used in a large number of patients.

REFERENCES

1. Schreiber SL, Crabtree GR. The mechanism of action of cyclosporin A and FK 506. Immunol Today 1992;13:136-142.
2. Liu J, Farmer JDJ, Lane WS, Friedman J, Weissman I, Schreiber SL. Calcineurin is a common target of cyclosporin-cyclosporin A and FKBP-FK506 complexes. Cell 1991;66:807-815.
3. Flanagan WM, Corthesy B, Bram RJ, Crabtree GR. Nuclear association of a T-cell transcription factor blocked by FK-506 and cyclosporin A. Nature 1991;352: 803-807.
4. Ruhlmann A and Nordheim A. Effects of the immunosuppressive drugs CyA and FK506 on intracellular signalling and gene regulation. Immunobiol 1997;198: 192-206.
5. Dawson TM, Steiner JP, Dawson VL, Dinerman JL, Uhl GR, Snyder SH. Immuno-suppressant FK 506, enhances phosphenylation of nitric oxide synthetase and protects against glutamate toxicity. Proc Natl Acad Sci USA 1993;90:9808-9812.
6. Dawson VL, Dawson TM, London ED, Bredt DS, Snyder SH. Nitric oxide medi-ates glutamate neurotoxicity in primary cortical culture. Proc Natl Acad Sci USA 1991;88:6368-6371.
7. Steiner JP, Dawson TM, Fotuhi M, et al. High brain densities of the immunophilin FKBP colocalized with calcineurin. Nature 1992;358:584-586.
8. Steiner JP, Dawson TM, Fotuhi M, Synder SH. Immunophilin regulation of neu-rotransmitter release. Molecular Medicine 1996;2:325-333.
9. Synder SH, Sabatim DM, Lai MM, Steiner JP, Hamilton GS, Suzdak PD. Neural action of the immunophilin ligands. T. PS 1998; 19:21-25.
10. Steinmann B, Bruckner P. Superti-Furga A. Cyclosporin A slows collagen triple-helix formation in vivo: indirect evidence for physiologic role of peptidyl-prolyl-cis-tran-isomerase. J. Biol. Chem 1991; 266:1299-303.
11. Freise CE, Rowley H, Lake J, Herbert M, Ascher NL, Roberts JP. Similar clinical presentation of neurotoxicity following FK506 and cyclosporine in a liver trans-plant recipient. Transplant Proc 1991;23:3173-3174.
12. Wijdicks EFM, Wiesner RH, Krom RAF. Neurotoxicity in liver transplant recipi-ents with cyclosporine immunosuppression. Neurology 1995;45:1962-64.
13. deGroen PC, Aksamit AJ, Rakela J, Forbes GS, Krom RAF. Central nervous system toxicity after liver transplantation: the role of cyclosporine and choles-terol. N Engl J Med 1987;317:861-866.
14. Eidelman BH, Abu-Elmagd K, Wilson J, et al. Neurological complications of FK 506. Transplant Proc 1991;23:3175-3178.
15. Rubin AM, Kang H. Cerebral blindness and encephalopathy with cyclosporin A toxicity. Neurology 1987;37:1072-1076.
16. deGroen PC, Wiesner RH, Krom RAF. Advanced liver failure predisposes to cyclo-sporine-induced central nervous system symptoms after liver transplantation. Transplant Proc 1989;21:2456.
17. Bird GLA, Meadows J, Goka J, Polson R, Williams R. Cyclosporin-associated aki-netic mutism and extrapyramidal syndrome after liver transplantation. J Neurol Neurosurg Psychiatry 1990;53:1068-1071.
18. Valldeoriola F, Graus F, Rimola A, et al. Cyclosporine-associated mutism in liver transplant patients. Neurology 1996;46:252-254.
19. Wijdicks EFM, Wiesner RH, Dahlke LJ, Krom RAF. FK 506-induced neurotoxicity in liver transplantation. Am Neurol 1994;35:498-501.
20. Miller Fischer C. Abulia. In: Bogousslavsky J, Caplan L. editors. Stroke Syn-dromes. Cambridge: Cambridge University Press, 1995:182-187.
21. Wijdicks EFM, Plevak DJ, Wiesner RH, Steers JL. Causes and outcome of sei-

zures in liver transplant recipients. Neurology 1996;47:1523-1525.

22. Appleton RE, Farrell K, Teal P, Hashimoto SA, Wong PKH. Complex partial status epilepticus associated with cyclosporin A therapy. J Neurol Neurosurg Psychiatry 1989;52:1068-1071.

23. Bronster DJ, Boccagni P, O'Rourke M, Emre S, Schwartz M, Miller C. Loss of speech after orthotopic transplantation. Transpl Int 1995;8:234-237.

24. Boeve BF, Kimmel DW, Aronson AE, deGroen PC. Dysathria and apraxia of speech associated with FK 506 (tacrolimus). Mayo Clin Proc 1996;71:969-972.

25. Reichard A, Eidelman BH. Cyclosporin A-induced dysarthria and tremulousness. Neurology 1989;39(Suppl 1):208.

26. Small SL, Fukui M, Bramblett GT, Eidelman BH. Immunosuppression-induced leukoencephalopathy from tacrolimus (FK 506). Ann Neurol 1996;40:575-580.

27. Noll RB, Kulkarni R. Complex visual hallucinations and cyclosporine. Arch Neurol 1984;41:329-330.

28. Thyagarajan GK, Cobanglu A, Johnston W. FK 506-induced fulminant leukoencephalopathy after single lung transplant. Ann Thorac Surg 1997;64:1461-1464.

29. Idilman R, DeMaria N, Kugelmas M, Colantoni A, Van Thiel D. Immunosuppressive drug-induced leukoencephalopathy in patients with liver transplant. Eur J Gastroenterol Hepatol 1998;10:433-436.

30. Hinchey J, Chaves C, Appignani B, et al. A reversible posterior leukoencephalopathy syndrome. N Engl J Med 1996;334:494-500.

31. Atkinson K, Biggs J, Darveniza P, Boland J, Concannon A, Dodds A. Spinal cord and cerebellar-like syndromes associated with the use of cyclosporine in human recipients of allogenic marrow transplants. Transplant Proc 1985;17:1673-1675.

32. Stein DP, Lederman RJ, Vogt DP, Carey WD, Broughan TA. Neurological complications following liver transplantation. Ann Neurol 1992;31:644-649.

33. Nussbaum ES, Maxwell RE, Bitterman PB, Hertz MI, Bula W, Latchaw RE. Cyclosporine A toxicity presenting with acute cerebellar edema and brainstem compression. J Neurosurg 1995;82:1068-1070.

34. Mueller AR, Platz K-P, Bechstein W-O, et al. Neurotoxicity after orthotopic liver transplantation. Transplantation 1994;58:155-169.

35. Steiger MJ, Farrah T, Rolles K, Harvey P, Burroughs AK. Cyclosporine induced headaches. J Neurol Neurosurg Psychiatry 1994;57:1258-1259.

36. Grobecker HF, Riebel K, Wellenhofer T. Cyclosporine A-induced hypertension in SHR and WKY: role of the sympatho-adrenal system. Clin Exp Pharmacol Physiol 1995;22(Suppl 1):S94-95.

37. Rozen TD, Wijdicks EF, Hay JE. Treatment - refractory cyclosporine-related headache: relief with conversion to FK-506. Neurology 1996;47:1347.

38. Fung J, Abu-Elmagd K, Jain A et al. A randomized trial of primary liver transplantation under immunosuppression with FK 506 vs. cyclosporine. Transplant Proc 1991;23:2977-83.

39. Fung JJ, Todo S, Tzakis A, Demetris A, Jain A, Abu-Elmagd K. Conversion of liver allograft receipients from cyclosporine to FK 506 based immunosuppression: benefits and pitfalls. Transplant Proc 1991;23:3105-3108.

40. Berden JHM, Hoitsma AJ, Merx JL, Keyser A. Severe central nervous system toxicity associated with cyclosporine. Lancet 1985;1:219-20.

41. Wilson JR, Conwit RA, Eidelman BH, Starzl T, Abu-Elmagd K. Sensorimotor neuropathy resembling CIDP in patients receiving FK 506. Muscle and Nerve 1994;17:528-532.

42. Bronster DJ, Yanover P, Stein J, Scelsa S, Miller CM, Sheiner PA. Demyelinating sensorimotor polyneuropathy after administration of FK 506. Transplantation 1995;59:1066-1068.

43. Ayres RCS, Dousset B, Wixon S, Buckels J, McMaster JAC, Mayer P. Peripheral neurotoxicity with tacrolimus. Lancet 1994;343:862-863.

44. Hibi S, Misawa A, Tamai M et al. Severe rhabdomyolysis associated with tacrolimus. Lancet 1995;346:702-703.
45. Campellone JV, Lacomis D, Kramer DJ, Van Cott AC, Giuliani MJ. Acute myopathy after liver transplantation. Neurology 1998;50:46-53.
46. Chassagne P, Meggad O, Moore N, Leloet X, Deshayes P. Myopathy as a possible side effect of Cyclosporine. Lancet 1989;2:1104.
47. Segal SN. Rapamune (Sirolimus, Rapamycin): An overview and mechanism of action. Ther Drug Monit 1995;17:660-665.
48. Groth CG, Backman L, Morales JM et al. Sirolimus (Rapamycine) based therapy in human renal transplantation. Similar efficacy and different toxicity compared with cyclosporine. Transplantation 1999;67:1036-1042.
49. Watson CJ, Friend PJ, Jamieson NV et al. Sirolimus: A potent new immunosuppressant for liver transplantation. Transplantation 1999;67:505-509.
50. Adair JC, Woodley SL, O'Connell JB, et al. Aseptic meningitis following cardiac transplantation: clinical characteristics and relationship to immunosuppressive regimen. Neurology 1991;41:249-252.
51. Shihab FS, Barry JM, Norman DJ. Encephalopathy following the use of OKT3 in renal allograft transplantation. Transplant Proc 1993;25:31-34.
52. Heyman R, Eidelman BH. Aseptic meningitis transplant patients treated with OKT3. Neurology 1988;38:205.
53. Lewis DA, Smith RE. Steroid-induced neuropsychiatric syndromes: a report of 14 cases and a review of the literature. J Affective Disord 1983;5:319-332.
54. Khalali AA, Edwards RHT, Gohil K. Corticosteroid myopathy: a clinical and pathological study. Clin Endocrinol 1983;18:155-166.

19 INFECTIOUS COMPLICATIONS IN ORGAN TRANSPLANT RECIPIENTS

Shimon Kusne[1] and Ron Shapiro[2]
[1] *Departments of Medicine and Surgery*
[2] *Department of Surgery*
University of Pittsburgh
Pittsburgh, Pennsylvania, USA

In this section, the general principles of infectious complications in transplant recipients will be reviewed, and the diseases associated with specific pathogens and their management will be discussed. While prophylaxis against the more common organisms has generally been employed, in recent years the concept of preemptive therapy has been introduced, with the goal of providing more selective prevention of disease. There has been significant progress made in the development of new and sensitive diagnostic methods, e.g. the introduction of PCR techniques. These new modalities offer the promise of allowing clinicians to diagnose infectious complications early and to intervene before infection becomes symptomatic.

GENERAL PRINCIPLES

Diagnosis of infection

Signs and symptoms of infection can be mild in the transplant recipient receiving immunosuppressive agents. Obvious signs and symptoms may be totally absent; an example is peritonitis without a temperature elevation and without a significant elevation in the white count. Therefore, clinical suspicion and clinical assessment are important. Empiric antimicrobial therapy may be administered initially, but an effort should be made to establish an accurate diagnosis, so that specific treatment can ultimately be administered. Unnecessary anti-microbial therapy may encourage the emergence of resistant organisms, and clinicians should try to limit antimicrobial cover-

A. W. Thomson (ed.), Therapeutic Immunosuppression, 459–501.
© 2001 *Kluwer Academic Publishers.*

age and base their choices on susceptibility testing.

Risk factors for infection

The most important factors which are directly associated with the emergence of infectious complications after organ transplantation include surgical problems and mechanical factors, the immunosuppressive state of the patient, and exposure to infectious agents. Bacterial and fungal infections usually occur during the first month after organ transplantation. At this stage, technical factors related to the operation may play an important role in the development of infection. Therefore, it is important to understand the technical aspects of the transplant in the assessment of the patient for infectious complications. For example, in a patient who has had a recent pancreas transplantation, it would be crucial to know if exocrine drainage was to the bladder or to the GI tract. In the case of peritonitis caused by an anastomotic leak, the content of the material would be different, and therefore the anti-microbial agents utilized might be different.

The type and intensity of the immunosuppressive regimen are also important to know. Certain immunosuppressive agents have been associated with higher infection rates and with particular infectious agents.

Lastly, it is important to determine during the recipient evaluation if there has been any exposure to infectious agents. The exposure may have occurred recently or remotely. A patient may have been exposed recently to resistant bacteria in the ICU or a few weeks previously to a child with varicella. The patient may have lived in or may have visited parts of the world where certain infections are endemic. A patient may have had exposure to *Mycobacterium tuberculosis* or *Histoplasma capsulatum* in the remote past, and after transplantation, on immunosuppression, reactivation may occur and cause symptomatic disease, i.e. tuberculosis or histoplasmosis.

Timing of infection

Knowing the typical timing for the occurrence of infectious complications after transplantation can be useful. Certain pathogens will almost never appear in the early postoperative course. It is therefore important to be familiar with these time frames in order to make a reasonable assessment of the probability of a specific infection at a given interval after transplantation. Infections that occur in the immediate postoperative course are usually associated with the surgical procedure. Most bacterial and fungal infections after liver transplantation occur within the first two months after surgery. Most CMV infections occur in the second month after transplantation; therefore, in a patient who develops a fever 10 days after liver or kidney transplantation, it will most likely not be related to CMV.

BACTERIAL DISEASES

The most important bacterial infections after organ transplantation originate at the site of transplantation and occur relatively close in time to the transplant operation (see General Principles). For example, after liver transplantation, the abdomen becomes the first "suspect" when infection is a consideration. Infections may include infected fluid collections near the allograft, peritonitis, cholangitis, or intrahepatic abscess. Immediately after transplantation, the patient may be exposed in the hospital to various bacteria and may develop a nosocomial infection. Therefore, good infection control practices are important. A patient may be initially colonized with resistant organisms and may then develop invasive disease because of postoperative complications and immunosuppression. An example would be an infection with vancomycin-resistant *Enterococcus*, which has emerged in recent years as a significant pathogen in many hospitals around the country. It is believed that the emergence of resistant organisms is related to the nonselective use of antibiotics and consequent selection of resistant strains. Most authors have identified indiscriminate use of vancomycin as an important risk factor for the emergence and spread of VRE in many hospitals. After the patient is discharged from the hospital, he/she may still be exposed to pathogens and develop community acquired infections.

Vancomycin-Resistant Enterococcus (VRE)

The pathogen
Enterococcus is a common colonizer of the gastrointestinal tract. Vancomycin is a glycopeptide antibiotic which interferes with the synthesis of the bacterial cell wall by binding to D-alanine-alanine in the cell wall. VRE has instead D-alanine-lactate in the cell wall, so that vancomycin cannot bind to the cell wall, and cell wall synthesis is uninterrupted. There are three main phenotypes in VRE; the first is VAN-A with high resistance to both vancomycin and teicoplanin, another glycopeptide. The second phenotype is VAN-B, in which the bacteria is resistant to vancomycin but sensitive to teicoplanin.

The third phenotype is VAN-C, which has a low degree of resistance to vancomycin. While VAN-B and VAN-C are chromosome-mediated, VAN-A is plasmid-mediated. Resistance to vancomycin can occur in the two important clinical species, *Enterococcus faecalis* and *Enterococcus faecium*.

Diagnosis

The isolation of VRE is carried out in the microbiology laboratory. Hospitals should screen their *Enterococcus* isolates for vancomycin resistance. Transmission between patients can be ascertained in the hospital by molecular diagnostic techniques, such as pulse-field gel electrophoresis. PCR can be useful in epidemiological investigations and can detect the three phenotypes.

Clinical

Over the last decade, there has been an increase in infectious complications from Gram positive bacteria in transplant recipients. Vancomycin-resistant *Enterococcus*, especially *Enterococcus faecium*, has emerged as a significant pathogen. Although it was originally thought not to be very virulent, it is now recognized as one associated with significant morbidity and mortality in transplant recipients.

A study was performed comparing the outcomes in adult liver transplant recipients who developed bacteremia with vancomycin-resistant (VREF) or vancomycin-sensitive isolates of *Enterococcus faecium*. Mortality in the hospital was higher in patients with VREF, with longer hospitalization and recurrent infections [1]. In a time-matched case control study in adult liver transplant recipients, VREF bacteremia occurred at a median of 10 days after liver transplantation and was associated with a high mortality [2]. Risk factors which were found to be associated with bacteremia included significant hypotension at the time of the transplant, primary non-function of the allograft, and isolation of VREF in other sites [2]. VREF was isolated from these sites a median of 10 days before bacteremia occurred [2]. VRE often behaves like an "opportunistic pathogen"; it is often merely a colonizer, but when the patient is very ill with multiple organ system failure, including renal and respiratory failure, it becomes an "invasive" pathogen. A particularly difficult clinical problem is VRE peritonitis after liver transplantation.

Management

In 1994 the CDC published recommendations to limit the spread of VRE in hospitals. These recommendations included education of the hospital personnel, laboratory screening for resistance, using gowns and gloves when colonized or infected patients are being examined, cohorting, and careful use of vancomycin [3]. Compliance with strict infection control rules has been shown to be effective in reducing transmission of VRE in wards where VRE was endemic [4]. The importance of hand washing in limiting the spread of resistant organisms in any hospital setting is critical.

As a general rule, treatment of VRE is more likely to be successful when surgical drainage is possible. Chloramphenicol and doxycycline have been used to treat VRE infection, with mixed results. Nitrofurantoin has been used successfully for simple urinary tract infections. More recently, the treatment of VRE infection has been affected by the development of new antibacterial agents active against resistant gram-positive bacteria. The first antibiotic belonging to the family of streptogramins, quinupristin/dalfopristin (Synercid) was recently approved in the US. This new antibiotic is active against *E. faecium* but not against *E. faecalis*. The antibiotic inhibits bacterial protein synthesis at the level of the ribosome, but is only bacteriostatic. Another promising drug, which also inhibits bacterial protein synthesis, is linezolid, which belongs to the oxazolidinone family [5].

Listeria

The pathogen
Listeria monocytogenes is a gram-positive aerobic bacteria, which is motile at room temperature. Although the bacteria is a rod, it may appear in the shape of a coccus and a rod, "cocco-bacillary" on the gram stain. The bacteria has been cultured from animals and plants, and can be cultured in the stool of individuals who are carriers.

Diagnosis
The diagnosis of listeriosis is usually made based on microbiologic culture of blood or cerebrospinal fluid (CSF). In cases of *Listeria* meningitis, a gram stain of the CSF may show gram positive bacteria. Brain parenchymal disease may be demonstrated by CT or MRI.

Clinical
Listeria is an important organism to remember in the differential diagnosis of a transplant recipient who presents with meningitis (together with cryptococcal meningitis). Most of the literature regarding listeriosis comes from kidney transplant recipients. Certain foods have been associated with fecal colonization of *Listeria* and with acute disease. In one study, fecal colonization was found in 2.3% of kidney transplant recipients or patients on home hemodialysis [6]. This study and others found a correlation of increased colo-

nization with consumption of certain types of dry cheese [6]. When *Listeria* infection occurs in a cluster of patients, an epidemiologic investigation is performed, to find a possible association with certain foods or close contacts among affected patients. *Listeria monocytogenes* usually presents as bacterial meningitis or as bacteremia. *Listeria* may cause parenchymal brain lesions, and there are also cases in the literature of non-immunosupressed patients presenting with brain stem lesions. Progressive multifocal leukoencephalopathy secondary to listeria has been reported in kidney transplant recipients [7]. A review of the literature in 1982 described 102 reported cases of listeriosis in kidney transplant recipients; 50% presented with meningitis, and 30% had primary bacteremia with *Listeria monocytogenes* [8]. The overall mortality was 36% [8]. In a more recent series, the incidence of listeriosis was higher in kidney transplant recipients and in HIV-positive patients compared to other patients [9]. Less common presentations in the literature have included acute hepatitis in liver transplant recipients [10], myocarditis after heart transplantation [11], recurrent abortion after kidney transplantation [12], endophthalmitis in renal transplantation [13], pneumonia, and joint infection.

Management
The treatment of *Listeria monocytogenes* is with the combination of penicillin or ampicillin and gentamicin. When *Listeria* meningitis is being treated, up to 12 gm/day of ampicillin is given. In patients who are allergic to penicillin, trimethoprim-sulfamethoxazole has been used successfully [14].

Legionella

The pathogen
Legionella is an aquatic gram negative rod. To culture this organism, the microbiology laboratory uses a special media called BCYE, which is buffered charcoal yeast extract agar.

Diagnosis
The symptoms of Legionnaire's disease are in general similar to those associated with pneumonia caused by other pathogens. The patient presents with fever and lung infiltrates and will usually have a non-productive cough. It is important to include *Legionella* in the differential diagnosis in this setting. Not all laboratories will culture this bacteria unless it has been specifically requested by the clinician. Patients may have a non-productive cough, which makes the diagnosis more difficult. Special media are required for growth of this bacteria, and it can be easily missed on a gram stain by

inexperienced individuals. Rapid diagnosis is usually obtained in respiratory secretions by the Direct Fluorescence Antibody stain (DFA). There is a Urinary Antigen test available in some hospitals that utilizes a radioimmunoassay (RIA). This test is very sensitive but will detect only *Legionella pneumophila* serogroup 1. Therefore, if hospitals have other *Legionella* serogroups in their water supply, they will be missed by this test. *Legionella* serologic testing is also available and requires serial testing to show an increase in titers. Molecular diagnostic techniques have been able to show an association between the clinical isolates and the environmental isolates, usually in the hospital water supply, and have confirmed nosocomial acquisition.

Clinical

Legionellosis is an important nosocomial infection in transplant recipients, because it has been associated with contamination of the water supply in hospitals, and therefore can be prevented if infection control measures are adequate. Nosocomial cases are usually defined based on the incubation time of the organism, which is between 2 and 10 days. Patients who have spent more than 10 days in the hospital before developing pneumonia most likely have nosocomially-acquired disease. Transmission of this bacteria occurs by inhalation of the organism or possibly by aspiration of contaminated water. Usually a lung infiltrate is seen on chest X ray, which confirms the diagnosis of pneumonia (Legionnaire's disease), but some patients may present with a febrile illness without radiographic changes [15]. It is believed that the main defense mechanism against *Legionella* is cell-mediated immunity, which explains why transplant recipients are at increased risk for legionellosis. Most cases reported in immunosuppressed patients are secondary to *Legionella pneumophilia* or *Legionella micdadei*, and both have been associated with a high mortality. We found less severe disease and reduced mortality from *Legionella* pneumonia in transplant recipients, when compared with other patients [16]. The most important factors which affected outcomes were nosocomial acquisition and lung complications [16]. Nosocomial transmission of legionellosis which occurred in a transplant center but was not recognized has been reported [17]. Over a 9 year period there were 25 patients with legionellosis, and 18 cases occurred in transplant recipients, with a mortality of 48% [17]. The authors demonstrated that almost all their *Legionella* isolates were identical to environmental ones [17].

Management

Since nosocomial legionellosis may occur, hospitals should check their water supply for growth of *Legionella* in their water. Unfortunately, there are no accepted guidelines. It is unclear how frequently water should be checked, and whether it should be routinely done in all hospitals, even if no cases of nosocomial legionellosis have been described. The methods that are used to treat water in hospitals include hyperchlorination, increasing the water temperature, UV light, and more recently copper-silver ionization.

Treatment of *Legionella* pneumonia historically has been with high dose erythromycin, 4 gm a day. The newer macrolides, such as azithromycin are also active against *Legionella*. In transplant recipients, because of the interaction of macrolides with the immunosuppressive agents tacrolimus and cyclosporine, which is associated with a dramatic increase in immunosuppressive drug levels, quinolones have been used preferentially. Both ciprofloxacin, ofloxacin, and other quinolones are effective in the treatment of *Legionella*.

Nocardia

The pathogen
Nocardia is a gram positive aerobic bacteria which is found in the environment and especially in the soil. It produces filaments, and they form true branches, ie branches produce secondary branches, (in contrast with actinomyces, which also produces filaments, but is an anaerobic bacteria and does not produce true branches).

Diagnosis
Nocardia is suspected when the gram stain of a body fluid, such as an aspirate of an abscess or bronchial secretions, shows filamentous bacteria with a positive modified acid fast stain. Confirmation is made by microbiologic culture. The most frequently encountered species is *Nocardia asteroides*, but other species, like *Nocardia brasiliensis*, can also be seen.

Clinical
The bacteria may be found in dust. There have been clusters of nocardiosis, and in one series there were 7 cases, possibly caused by dispersed dust, which were diagnosed in a liver unit [18]. Usually, patients develop pneumonia, and the organism can then disseminate to the CNS and lead to brain abscesses. *Nocardia* can be inoculated accidentally into the skin through a sharp object from the environment and cause a local infection, which may then disseminate. Transplant recipients, like other immunosuppressed patients, may present with multiple subcutaneous abscesses secondary to hematogenous spread [19]. Typically, it is considered a late infection after

transplantation. In one series, it occurred in 3.7% of liver transplant recipients who were more than 3.5 years post-transplantation, and was associated with a mortality of 43% [20]. In the lung, it may present as consolidation, pleural effusion, cavitation, or nodules [21].

Management

Nocardia is usually treated with a long course of antibiotics, because it tends to relapse if it is not treated long enough. Transplant recipients are usually treated for 6-12 months. It is important to obtain an accurate diagnosis of the species and susceptibility testing, because different species of Nocardia have diverse susceptibility patterns. Within the Nocardia asteroides group, one species tends to be relatively more resistant to antibiotics, Nocardia farcinica. In addition, although Nocardia is usually sensitive to sulfa drugs, there are reports of sulfa resistance leading to treatment failure [22]. Antibiotics used for the treatment of Nocardia include amikacin, ceftriaxone, cefotaxime, imipenem, and minocycline. A combination of antibiotics is usually given, based on susceptibility testing. Nocardia brain abscesses are treated with antibiotics and drainage. Trimethoprim-sulfamethoxazole, which is used for PCP prophylaxis, may also provide effective prophylaxis against Nocardia.

Mycobacterium Tuberculosis (MTB)

The pathogen

Mycobacterim tuberculosis (MTB) is an acid-fast bacteria and is the main cause of tuberculosis (TB).

Diagnosis

When pulmonary TB is a clinical consideration, an acid fast stain is usually ordered on respiratory secretions, such as sputum and bronchoalveolar fluid. The culture may take weeks to become positive. In recent years there have been new methods introduced for the rapid diagnosis of TB. The use of radiometric BACTEC systems and DNA probes have made the diagnosis of TB much more rapid. Other techniques, such as PCR, may have a more important diagnostic role in the future, once issues of sensitivity, specificity, and standardization are established. Molecular diagnostic techniques like Restriction Fragment Length Polymorphism (RFLP) can be helpful in an epidemiological investigation, because they can prove or disprove transmission between patients.

Clinical

Mycobacterial disease should be considered in the differential diagnosis of transplant recipients who present with fever of unclear etiology. The transplant recipient should be investigated regarding possible exposure to tuberculosis, including a travel history to endemic areas. Most cases of tuberculosis in transplant recipients are secondary to reactivation of old tuberculous lesions.

We reviewed our experience with MTB infections in our adult liver transplant recipients. Between 1983 and 1994 we encountered 14 cases of MTB infection, an incidence of 0.5% [23]. When we compared the demographic characteristics of these patients to randomly selected controls, we found that the most important risk factor for development of MTB infection was being from a foreign country endemic for TB [23]. The clinical presentation of the 14 patients included pneumonia (7), miliary TB (2), pleural TB (1), and tuberculous lymphadenitis (4). Eight of 14 patients had developed hepatic granulomas, which were diagnosed on liver biopsy, and 10 of 14 patients had recurrent fevers before the diagnosis was made [23]. The overall mortality in this group was 50%; 5 (36%) patients died directly of tuberculosis. Of the 14 cases with tuberculosis, in 7 patients the original treatment had to be modified because of hepatotoxicity. Of the 14 MTB isolates, one was resistant to isoniazid and ethambutol, and another isolate was resistant only to ethambutol [23].

In our adult kidney transplant recipients, we experienced a nosocomial outbreak of MTB related to a kidney transplant recipient transmitting MTB to five other patients, 4 of whom were kidney transplant recipients [24]. There was a delay in placement of the index case in respiratory isolation, related to the difficulty in making the diagnosis, as the index case presented with chest pain and a normal chest x-ray. Transmission between the index case and the secondary cases was confirmed by DNA amplification using Restriction Fragment Length Polymorphism (RFLP) [24]. The incubation period was between 5 and 11 weeks. Transplant recipients may progress very rapidly to develop widespread pulmonary TB after exposure, most likely related to their immunosuppressed condition.

The worldwide increase in resistant TB is of concern. An increase in resistant TB among transplant recipients could have devastating consequences. According to a recent survey, the prevalence of resistance to at least one of commonly used agents (isoniazid, ethambutol, pyrazinamide, rifampin) was 12.6%, and the prevalence of multi-drug resistance (MDR) was 2.2% [138]. The concern of transmission of resistant TB is illustrated by a report of a highly resistant TB strain (W), which was the cause of nosocomial outbreaks in New York, and has spread to other areas [139].

Management

Clinicians should have a high index of suspicion when patients are admitted to the hospital with an atypical presentation of pneumonia, because of the risk of nosocomial transmission of MTB. If mycobacterial infection is a consideration, patients should be placed promptly in respiratory isolation until it can be ruled out. It is better to be overcautious than to have to deal with secondary cases of MTB.

In our program, isoniazid (INH) prophylaxis is routinely given to PPD-positive transplant recipients. Adult liver, kidney, and pancreas transplant patients receive 6 months of INH prophylaxis after transplantation when liver function is stable. Patients who have received prophylaxis in the past usually are given another course of prophylaxis because of the risk of reactivation. It is important to keep in mind that many candidates for transplantation are anergic. In fact, over 60% of 1065 candidates evaluated for liver transplantation were anergic [27]. While the incidence of PPD positivity was 7% in American-born candidates, it was 20% in candidates born in foreign countries [27]. With the increase in resistant TB, particularly the multi-drug resistant (MDR) mycobacteria, INH may not be sufficient for prophylaxis. If the chance of resistance is very high, some authors recommend prophylaxis with pyrazinamide and a quinolone.

Clinicians who treat transplant recipients with active TB should keep in mind the possibility of resistant TB. It is now recommended to start the treatment of tuberculosis with four anti-TB drugs until the mycobacteria susceptibility testing is completed. The initial anti-TB drug combination usually includes isoniazid, rifampin, pyrazinamide, and ethambutol. In addition, immunosuppression is usually discontinued.

VIRAL DISEASES

CMV is the most common viral infection in organ transplantation. It has also been linked with the development of chronic rejection, particularly in cardiac transplant recipients. The prevention of infection with antiviral drug prophylaxis has been attempted; more recently, the use of preemptive therapy has been described. New drugs active against CMV have been developed. At the same time, there has also been the (admittedly still rare) emergence of antiviral drug resistance. Many other viruses can infect the transplant recipient, some of them quite commonly, such as Herpes simplex virus (HSV). Some viruses have recently received more attention in transplant recipients, like HHV6, the cause of roseola, and HHV8, which has been associated with Kaposi's sarcoma. The hepatotrophic viruses, hepatitis B (HBV) and hepatitis C (HCV), will also be discussed in this section, because of their high prevalence among transplant recipients. In the last decade, end stage liver disease secondary to HCV has become one of the most frequent indications for liver transplantation.

Cytomegalovirus

The Pathogen
CMV is a Herpesviridae virus.

Diagnosis
When CMV infection occurs in a sero-negative recipient, it is considered a primary infection, while infection occurring in sero-positive recipient is either a reactivation or a superinfection with a different strain. Because transplant recipients frequently shed CMV in their bodily secretions, it is important to differentiate between asymptomatic and symptomatic infection. The latter is also called CMV disease. There are strict definitions of CMV disease. The two main categories include CMV syndrome (presumptive disease), which is manifested by unexplained fever and leukopenia, with viremia, and invasive disease (proven disease) which is established by pathologic changes (viral inclusion bodies) in a specific organ, together with signs and symptoms. For example, the diagnosis of CMV hepatitis requires liver function abnormalities together with a liver biopsy showing viral inclusion bodies [28, 29].

The timing of CMV diagnosis is crucial. Traditional viral culture consists of placement of body fluids in human fibroblasts and watching the fibroblasts for cytopathic effect. This obsolete diagnostic modality can take many weeks. Therefore, more rapid methods have been developed to help make the diagnosis in a more timely manner. The Shell-vial culture uses a monoclonal antibody stain against the p72 protein. Staining of the fibroblasts with this method will usually take about 72 hours. More recently, very sensitive techniques have been developed for the early diagnosis of CMV. The CMV antigenemia (pp65) test uses a monoclonal antibody staining against the pp65 lower matrix phosphoprotein of leukocytes [30, 31]. The result is reported as the number of positively staining leukocytes per 200,000 cells. This test can be completed in 5 hours. Other extremely sensitive tests include the use of PCR. There is ongoing debate in the literature regarding the usefulness of PCR, since the test may be too sensitive, and it may be unclear how to interpret a positive test in a completely asymptomatic patient.

Clinical

In solid organ transplantation, high-risk patients are those who are sero-negative prior to transplantation and receive an organ from a sero-positive donor. The virus in this case is transmitted with blood or the transplanted organ. Another category at significant risk is the patient who is sero-positive before transplantation and who receives anti-lymphocyte agents (OKT3 or ATG) for the treatment of rejection. A sero-negative recipient who gets an organ from sero-negative donor is at low risk, but these patients can still acquire CMV infection from a blood transfusion. After organ transplantation, almost all high risk recipients will develop CMV infection, and are at risk to develop symptomatic CMV. Because of lack of availability of donors, it is not feasible to match donors to their recipients according to CMV serology (except perhaps for intestinal transplantation, where the number of potential recipients is small).

Management

The most frequently used drug for the treatment of CMV disease is ganciclovir (DHPG). It is an acyclic nucleoside analogue that inhibits viral replication. In order to be active, the drug needs to be converted to the triphosphate form. The initial phosphorylation is controlled by the CMV virus enzyme (viral protein kinase), and the subsequent phosphorylation steps are controlled by cellular enzymes. The viral protein kinase is controlled by a gene (UL97) in the CMV genetic material. Mutation in this gene may cause resistance of the virus to ganciclovir [32]. Another mutation that can lead to development of resistant CMV involves the gene that controls the viral DNA polymerase [33].

Foscarnet (Trisodium Phosphonoformate) is an inorganic pyrophosphate analogue that inhibits CMV replication by a direct inhibition of the viral DNA polymerase. Because of its nephrotoxicity, it has been used only as a second-line drug in transplant recipients.

The use of immune globulin together with ganciclovir was reported to be effective in treatment of CMV pneumonia in BMT recipients [34]. Other authors have not found any benefit with this combination [35].

There are two strategies that clinicians use in order to prevent CMV disease in transplant recipients. The first method is prophylaxis, in which all transplant recipients are given an antiviral agent immediately after the transplant operation in order to prevent CMV disease. With the second, preemptive therapy, patients are monitored by a sensitive test, and only when the virus is detected is an antiviral agent administered [36]. Because the method of detection is very sensitive, the virus is detected early, and therapy is initiated and the virus eradicated before it causes symptomatic infection (disease). This method targets only a selected group of the population, those patients that are more likely to develop disease. This method requires close monitoring of the patients by the sensitive laboratory test and therefore may be difficult to implement routinely.

Trials of CMV prophylaxis in adult liver transplant patients have shown that prophylaxis is an effective method of prevention in both sero-positive individuals and in high risk recipients [37]. We have also successfully used preemptive therapy in adult liver transplant recipients [38]. The patients are monitored after transplantation with the pp65 antigenemia test. Treatment with intravenous ganciclovir is initiated once the virus is detected using this test. Sero-negative recipients are started on the drug at the first positive result (i.e. an antigenemia of 1), and sero-positive patients are started on it if their count is of at least 10 per 200,000 leukocytes. Following these rules, the overall incidence of CMV disease in adult liver transplant recipients decreased significantly, to 5-8%. Additional prospective trials are needed to determine the optimal method of CMV disease prevention in the various solid organ recipient populations.

Human Herpesvirus-6 (HHV-6)

The Pathogen
HHV-6 belongs to the herpes family, and was isolated for the first time from peripheral blood lymphocytes. There have been two variants of the virus, A and B. Variant B is thought to be the cause of roseola (exanthem subitum) in small children. The transmission of this virus occurs by secretions from the respiratory tract. It is known from serologic studies that by age 3, most of the population is seropositive. There are also some data in bone marrow transplantation that suggest transmission of virus through blood products. It is believed that the primary target of the virus is CD4+ lymphocytes.

Clinical
There have been various reports of clinical syndromes associated with

HHV-6, including exanthem subitum in children, and possibly encephalitis, febrile convulsions, mononucleosis syndrome, and even multiple sclerosis. Some of these associations are controversial.

In BMT patients HHV-6 was reported to be associated with a rash, viremia, acute and chronic marrow suppression [39] (mainly leukopenia, but also thrombocytopenia and anemia), and mental status changes, with neurological deficits and meningoencephalitis [40]. Some authors claimed an association with the initiation or exacerbation of GVHD. In recent years there have been many reports of the virus affecting solid organ transplant recipients, usually with variant B. Singh reported in 1995 a liver transplant recipient with variant B HHV6, who developed thrombocytopenia, encephalopathy, and a rash [41]. Between 31% to 55% of patients develop an HHV6 infection after solid organ transplantation about 2 to 4 weeks postoperatively [42]. Some authors have found association between HHV6 and CMV in transplant recipients [43, 44, 45]. When we prospectively followed liver transplant recipients, HHV6 viremia was a predictor of invasive fungal infection and was associated with encephalopathy of unclear etiology [46]. It is possible, although not established, that the virus, like CMV, has immunomodulatory properties.

Diagnosis
The viral DNA can be detected by PCR testing, but is of limited value to clinicians because most or all the population is seropositive, and a positive PCR may not be clinically significant. More useful to the clinician is viral isolation by culture, but the culture is technically demanding, and very slow to grow. There is a rapid shell vial culture on MRC-5 cells, but only a few centers are able to provide this test.

Management
HHV-6 shares a similar antiviral susceptibility with CMV, and in general the antivirals that are active against CMV are also active against HHV-6. Susceptibility antiviral testing has shown that both ganciclovir and foscarnet have good anti-viral activity against HHV-6 [47], and both agents have been used successfully [48, 49].

Varicella-zoster virus (VZV)

The Pathogen
VZV is a member of the Herpesviridae; by age 20, more than 90% of the population is seropositive.

Diagnosis

The diagnosis is usually easy to make on a clinical basis, and the virus can be cultured in the Virology laboratory. Tzanck smear of fluid taken from a vesicle will show giant cells, suggestive of herpes infection.

Clinical

Varicella (chickenpox) is the primary disease and zoster (shingles) is a reactivation. Patients with impaired cellular immunity are more prone to infection. Zoster usually follows the course of a single dermatome, but immunocompromised patients may have involvement of multiple dermatomes, and the virus may disseminate to internal organs. Interestingly, there are cases reported of VZV of the internal viscera without skin lesions. Higher levels of immunosuppression are associated with an increased incidence of VZV infection. Mycophenolate mofetil has been reported by some authors to be associated with an increased incidence of VZV [50].

Management

The antivirals that are usually active against herpes simplex virus, mainly acyclovir, are also active against VZV. With severe dermatomal disease, acyclovir should be administered intravenously for 7-10 days, before conversion to oral acyclovir. In uncomplicated dermatomal disease, oral acyclovir may be given. Acyclovir is a very efficient propylactic agent for both HSV and VZV infection [51]. Other drugs which show activity against VZV are valacyclovir and famcyclovir. Both antivirals have a significantly higher bioavailability compared to acyclovir [52]. Like acyclovir, in order to be activated they need to be phosphorylated by a viral enzyme called thymidine kinase, but resistance may develop in virus mutants which lack this enzyme [53]. In cases of resistance, foscarnet is used.

There have been some reports of the use of varicella vaccine, which is a live attenuated vaccine, in transplant recipients. When it was administered to children after BMT, it was well tolerated and was quite effective in preventing VZV infection, with a follow up of two years [54]. Seventy-six percent of children undergoing renal transplantation who received the varicella vaccine pre-transplant still had a positive antibody titer two years after transplantation [55]. VZIG has been given to varicella negative patients within 72-96 hours of exposure to the virus, but may not be protective, and therefore some authorities recommend pre-transplant vaccination of transplant candidates [56]. Acyclovir, given for prevention after exposure to chickenpox within families, was effective in the prevention of secondary cases [57, 58], and may have a role after exposure of transplant recipients to VZV.

Epstein-Barr virus (EBV)

The Pathogen

The virus belongs to the Herpesviridae family. It is usually transmitted by saliva ("kissing disease"), but in transplant recipients, it may be transmitted also by the organ or by blood products. The response to EBV in the normal host is complex. It involves interferon production, antibody production, and CD4+/CD8+ response. At the end of this process, there are EBV-specific CD8+ cytotoxic T-lymphocytes (CTL's), which are able to control the proliferation of B-cells infected with EBV. These cells are non-functioning in transplant recipients, because of the immunosuppressive agents which are administered for the prevention of rejection, and this can allow the EBV-infected B-cells to expand, leading to Post Transplant Lymphoproliferative Disorder (PTLD). Most, but not all PTLD syndromes are associated with EBV.

Diagnosis

Serologic testing for EBV can be helpful, because it shows whether the patient was sero-negative pre-transplantation and has developed an IgM (consistent with an acute infection), or whether he was sero-positive and has reactivated the virus. In this case there will be a significant rise in the IgG titer, usually a 4-fold increase in viral-capsid-antigen (VCA). However, the presence of IgG is not necessarily predictive of protective immunity. In recent years, quantitative EBV/PCR analysis has been extremely helpful in the early diagnosis of EBV infection, before it progresses to become PTLD. Pathologic examination of biopsy material can show findings consistent with PTLD, and viral antigen in tissue may be shown by in situ hybridization (EBER). Different authors have distinguished among the polyclonal and monomorphous histopathologies and have conventionally associated a more benign course to the polyclonal and a more malignant course to monomorphous types, but this may in fact not be true. In some instances, the morphology of the lesion may be helpful to clinicians in predicting the behavior of the tumor and whether it is going to respond to manipulation of the immune system [59].

Clinical

The virus causes Infectious Mononucleosis in the normal host. Most of the adult population is sero-positive. Only about 5% are seronegative. Although there is a well-established association between EBV and PTLD, the virus has been found also in other tumors. In PTLD, there is proliferation of lymphocytes in various organs, and in some cases there is a malignant transformation, leading to the development of a B-cell lymphoma. PTLD occurs in about 1-3% of solid organ transplant recipients. The main risk factors are increased immunosuppression, specifically OKT3, and EBV seronegativity of the transplant recipient [60]. The incidence of PTLD may vary also with the different organs, the highest incidence being in the small bowel transplant recipients. The site of the PTLD can be in nodal locations, such as the oropharyngeal and cervical area, with tonsillar swelling and lymphadenopathy, the allograft, the bone marrow, or the gastrointestinal tract, but at times is limited to non-accessible sites, such as the retroperitoneum or extranodal areas.

Management

Starzl showed that marked diminution or discontinuation of immunosuppressive agents may lead to regression of PTLD [61]. Patients are taken off cyclosporine or tacrolimus and maintained on low dose steroids, usually 5 mg of prednisone per day. Some antivirals like acyclovir, ganciclovir, and foscarnet inhibit the virus in vitro. These antivirals have been used together with reduction of immunosuppression. Preemptive therapy was used by Green et al. by monitoring the number of EBV viral copies in the circulation and initiating antiviral agents and intravenous immunoglobulin to prevent the occurrence of PTLD [62]. EBV PCR can be detected in the blood many months before the diagnosis of PTLD is made [63]. The use of antivirals for EBV lymphomas is controversial. EBV thymidine kinase does not phosphorylate acyclovir or ganciclovir the way herpes simplex or herpes zoster does [64]. This initial phosphorylation by viral thymidine kinase is needed in order to activate these antivirals. Some monoclonal non-Hodgkin's lymphomas do not carry the gene which make them susceptible to these antiviral agents [65]. In BMT patients, the identified risk factors for PTLD are depletion of T-cells and occurrence of GVHD [66]. Rooney et al. [67, 68] successfully used donor derived CD4 and CD8 T-cell lines for prevention and treatment of PTLD. These lines contain EBV-specific cytotoxic T-lymphocytes (CTL's). Other authors have used anti-B cell monoclonal antibodies and obtained remission [69]. We and others have used successfully lymphokine activated killer cells [70, 71]. Some EBV-associated lymphomas do not respond to antivirals or manipulation of the immune system and continue to progress. These tumors are treated with chemotherapy, with mixed results.

Parvovirus B19

The Pathogen

Parvovirus is a small single-stranded DNA virus, and is the cause of Fifth disease (erythema infectiosum). The virus is acquired during early childhood, usually between 5 and 15 years of age. The seroprevalence among adults, according to various series, is between 30% and 60%. In the normal host, after the first infection occurs, lifelong immunity is acquired. It is believed that the P antigen on the red cell is a necessary receptor for the virus to infect the red cells [72].

Diagnosis

The viral DNA may be detected in the blood and in the bone marrow by PCR. Typically the bone marrow biopsy shows giant pronormoblasts with viral inclusions, and the reticulocyte count is very low. There are special B-19-specific monoclonal antibody stains available which may confirm the presence of the virus in the bone marrow. Serologic tests are also available (RIA and ELISA), and a positive IgM is consistent with acute B-19 infection, while a positive IgG would mean past infection.

Clinical

The virus can be transmitted by blood products, including platelets and clotting factor concentrates [73, 74], but the respiratory route is the most common means of transmission. It can cause epidemics in schools. Its DNA has been found in circulating cells in the blood [75]. Parvovirus B19 has been associated not only with Fifth disease but also with hydrops fetalis, red cell aplasia, and chronic anemia (and possible pancytopenia) in immunosuppressed patients, including transplant recipients. We have seen transplant recipients who develop recurrent anemia over 3-5 years after their transplant operation. They have a persistent B19 infection, and the virus may be detected in blood and their marrow for an extended period of time. Between 1994 and 1997, we have seen 8 patients after solid organ transplantation who developed B19-induced red cell aplasia, for an overall incidence of 0.5%. Four of them developed at least one recurrent episode of anemia. Rarely, it can cause myocarditis after heart transplantation, and the viral DNA has been found in myocardial cells [76].

Management

No antivirals are effective against Parvovirus B19. Intravenous immunoglobulin preparations (IVIG) have been used to treat the red cell aplasia. The mechanism of action is unclear but may involve blocking of some cellular receptors. The dose is 0.4-1.0 gm/kg/day. Relapses of B19 anemia are treated with additional courses of IVIG [77].

Polyoma virus

The Pathogen

Polyoma is a DNA virus and includes the following three viruses: 1. BK virus, which can be found commonly in childhood, 2. JC virus, found later in childhood and which can cause progressive multifocal leukoencephalopathy (PML), mostly in AIDS patients, and 3. Simian virus 40 (SV40) which was reported to cause a similar syndrome in macaques.

Diagnosis

Viral culture is available but the growth of the virus is very slow. Cytology can show large cells with inclusions in kidney biopsies and in the urine. Electron microscopy and PCR testing are also available. The correlation between the various tests to detect this virus and the particular clinical syndromes is still not defined. Although polyomavirus is quite prevalent in the general population, clinicians do not routinely screen for this virus in transplantation, and the incidence may be underestimated in transplant recipients [78]. Some authors advocate the routine search for polyomavirus in biopsies and urine of kidney recipients [79].

Clinical

BK virus has been associated with ureteral strictures after kidney transplantation. The virus may present with a rising serum creatinine, and a biopsy will show interstitial nephritis and tubulitis with intranuclear inclusion bodies; the pathology has been confused with rejection. There are reports of hemorrhagic cystitis after BMT secondary to polyomavirus. Early occurrence of this infection after BMT (before day 100) has been associated with reduced survival. Polyoma virus has been the focus of renewed attention, mostly in kidney transplant recipients. Infection may occur either by reactivation or by transmission from the donor [80]. This infection is important because it has been frequently confused with rejection and treated with increased immunosuppression, with unfavorable results. In a series of twenty-two patients from our institution [81], BKV was the most prevalent virus but co-infection with JC virus was also seen. Graft loss was the ultimate outcome in 67% of patients who had an increase in their immunosuppression [81]; reduction of immunosuppression was associated with graft salvage in some cases. Polyomavirus has been more prevalent in patients who have had repeated rejection episodes and have received intensive immunosuppression [82]. Some authors found an association between polyomavirus and treatment with mycophenolate mofetil [83]. According to some authors [84], up to 20% of kidney recipients excrete polyomavirus in their urine, and most infections with BK virus are reactivation, while most JC virus infections are primary [84]. More recently, the DNA of simian virus 40 (SV40), the third member of the polyomavirus family, was found in kidney allografts of three children [85].

Management

No antivirals are active against polyomavirus, and the only option is to reduce the level of immunosuppression. Some clinicians have treated this virus with reduction of immunosuppression and administration of immune globulin, with mixed results. Rimantidine has been used anecdotally, with unclear benefit. Cidofovir has been suggested as a therapeutic agent, but is profoundly nephrotoxic.

Hepatitis C virus (HCV)

The pathogen

HCV is an enveloped RNA virus which has been said to be related to the Flaviviridae family. The virus contain 6 genotypes but is very heterogenous genetically (quasispecies), and because of the constant change, it can escape the immune system [86].

Diagnosis

There are two general methods to diagnose HCV. The first is with serologic studies for antibodies against certain protein components of the virus, and the second is by detection of the actual circulating viral genomes. The antibodies are tested by two techniques, the Enzyme Linked Immunosorbent Assay (ELISA) or the Recombinant Immunoblot Assay (RIBA). These techniques are becoming more sensitive over time, and have evolved from the first generation tests to the second and third generation. The viral genome of HCV RNA can be found in blood by PCR. This method is considered very sensitive. Quantitation of the virus can be done by another technique called branched chain DNA or b-DNA. Although this method can quantitate the virus, it is not as sensitive as the qualitative PCR technique. The viral genome can also be detected in biopsy material. Transplant recipients may not form antibodies after exposure to HCV, or the formation of antibodies may be delayed [87]. Therefore, tests which detect the viral genome are the preferable method of diagnosis.

Clinical

Hepatitis C has become one of the most common indications for liver transplantation. It is estimated that about 4 millions Americans are infected with this virus. About 80% will develop chronic infection, and a significant proportion will progress to cirrhosis. With the advances made in the detection of hepatitis C viral genome, we know that the virus can be almost always be detected after liver transplantation, but histologically-proven hepatitis and cirrhosis are not necessarily seen. In one study, allograft HCV hepatitis and cirrhosis occurred in 51% and 9%, respectively [88], and genotype 1b was associated with severe hepatitis and cirrhosis [88]. Other authors found an association between genotype 1b and the development of graft cirrhosis after liver transplantation [89]. Still others found no association between particular genotypes and overall survival or development of cirrhosis after liver transplantation [90]. Short term graft and patient survival after organ transplantation (especially kidney transplantation) is quite good, in HCV seropositive recipients, and the use of an organ from an HCV positive donor seems not to be associated with worse outcomes (in HCV seropositive recipients).

The importance of the quasispecies variants in clinical progression after transplantation is controversial. Immunosuppression causes an increase in genetic diversity and may be important in the development of severe cholestatic hepatitis after liver transplantation [91]. Response of hepatitis C to interferon treatment may be controlled by NS5A gene, but this is also unclear [92].

Management

Not all transplant centers in the US accept donors from HCV positive donors for transplantation. We accept livers and kidneys from seropositive donors, for transplantation into HCV seropositive recipients. In some cases where the short term risk of dying from liver failure or heart failure is substantial, physicians and patients have accepted seropositive organs for seronegative patients.

Treatment for hepatitis C is usually with combination of interferon-alfa and ribavirin for 12 months. The usual dose of interferon is 3 million units, 3 times a week, by subcutaneous injection. Ribavirin is given orally 1200 mg a day, in patients who are at least 75 kg. Prior to initiation of treatment, the patient has to be carefully evaluated by physicians who are experienced with HCV. Candidates for transplantation may be treated before transplantation. Treatment of patients after kidney transplantation has been associated with acute cellular rejection. There is at least theoretically a risk of rejection also in other organs. A liver biopsy is important in order to assess whether there are signs of cirrhosis in the liver. Base-line liver function tests, especially ALT are important. Monitoring during treatment is usually done by serial LFT's and quantitative PCR. A high viral load (1-2 million copies), and certain genotypes (1b) may be associated with less favourable response to treatment. A favorable response is usually obtained after six months of treatment, with disappearance of the viral genome from the blood.

In adult liver transplantation with recurrence of HCV after transplantation, we usually do not start treatment unless there are histological changes suggestive of hepatitis. The reason for this practice is the high recurrence rate of HCV after discontinuation of treatment and the fact that not all patients respond to these agents. In addition, the drugs available for treatment are not benign agents and have significant side effects. Patients receiving interferon usually complain of flu-like symptoms and occasionally depression. Ribavirin can cause hemolytic anemia in up to 10% of patients. Currently we do not use these agents for prophylaxis, only for treatment. Prospective trials are needed to assess regimens for the treatment and prophylaxis of HCV in organ transplantation.

Hepatitis B virus (HBV)

The pathogen

Hepatitis B is a DNA virus which belongs to the Hepadnaviridae. It was found in animals that, in order to replicate, the virus needs to undergo reverse transcription, and from RNA it becomes DNA. The virus is shaped like a ball, and the two main structures are the inside proteins (HBcAg) and the outside protein (HBsAg), which surround the core like an envelope. The DNA of the virus and the enzyme DNA polymerase are found in the core of this structure. The e antigen (HBeAg) is a non structural protein which can be found when the virus is replicating, and its presence is associated with a high degree of infectivity. The presence of HBsAb is a sign of immunity to the virus.

Diagnosis

Serologic testing can determine the presence of the virus and whether it is in an acute or chronic stage based on the presence of the various antigens or the antibodies against them. Recent HBV hepatitis may be diagnosed by a positive antibody to the core protein (IgM anti-HBc) even when HBsAg is not found. There are cases of HBV transmitted from donors who were HBsAg negative and HBcAb positive, with a negative HBcAb IgM (the latter usually indicates that the infection is not recent). This has happened more frequently in liver transplantation, compared with other organs [93].

Different authors have tried to quantify the degree of activity of the virus and its infectivity. The virus is said to be in a "replicative state" when there is evidence of DNA, DNA polymerase, and often the presence of HBeAg. Liver enzymes are usually elevated, especially ALT. The virus is said to be in a non-replicative state when these tests are negative and the liver enzymes are not high. PCR techniques are available for detection of HBV in blood. Quantitation by branched DNA (bDNA) is also available but is usually used for research. This test can detect the virus in up to 100% of patients who are HBeAg+ and up to 30% of HBeAg- patients with chronic HBV infection [94].

Clinical

Most recipients after liver transplantation for HBV-associated liver disease have recurrence of HBV. Therefore, many centers do not perform liver transplantation for this indication. Of the patients who undergo liver transplantation for HBV, the prognosis is better if they have fulminant HBV infection or if they are also infected with the delta virus [95]. Most centers do not perform liver transplantation in recipients with evidence of viral replication, ie HBeAg+ or DNA positivity, because of a very high recurrence rate and poor outcome. Recent data, however, have suggested that a long course of Hepatitis B Immune Globulin (HBIG) after liver transplantation is associated with favorable outcomes. Although most published data are in liver transplant recipients, there is a literature showing a high incidence of cirrhosis in non-liver transplant recipients who acquired HBV infection (HBsAg+) before or after transplantation. Whether the new anti-hepatitis agents will have an impact on this progression is not yet known.

Management

Because of the potential of transmission of HBV from donors who are HBcAb+, we usually follow the following guidelines in our institution: the liver or kidney is offered to recipients who are HBsAb+, and prophylaxis is not given, since the surface antibody positivity is protective. In the absence of an appropriate HBcAb+ recipient, the liver would then be offered to a HBcAb+ recipient who is HBsAb-, together with HBIG and lamivudine prophylaxis; the kidneys would not be used. In our experience, naive recipients can get infected with HBV even if their donors are HBcAb+ and HBsAb+ [96]. At present naive patients who get a liver from HBcAb+ donor in our institution receive combination of HBIG and lamivudine. The results were recently published and appear to be promising [97].

Because the recurrence rate of HBV in the liver after liver transplantation has been very high, many centers stopped offering transplantation for end stage liver disease secondary to HBV. However, in light of recently improved outcomes, liver transplantation can be offered to HBsAg+ recipients who do not have evidence of viral replication, followed by long term prophylaxis with HBIG. We usually use intravenous HBIG 10,000 IU/kg in the anhepatic phase, and then the same dose every month for 6 doses. This is followed by 1500 IU/kg1M q month for 18 months. Monitoring of HbsAB is usually done to maintain a protective titer of 100 IU/kg. HBIG treatment has been associated with mutations in the a-determinant of the surface viral gene and in the polymerase gene. This occurs most likely as a result of immune pressure and viral selection. These mutations have been associated with failure of HBIG in 19% after 3 years [98].

Lamivudine is an antiviral agent which inhibits HBV replication. It has been used as an inhibitor of reverse transcriptase in HIV patients. It is given orally daily at 100-150 mg/day. In a multi-center trial, it cleared HBV DNA in 60% of patients after treatment with 100 mg per day for 52 weeks after liver transplantation [99]. There was also normalization of ALT and histologic improvement [99]. Resistance to lamivudine may occur during treatment and is related to polymerase mutations [100].

There are still a number of unresolved questions, including some reports of the inhibition of HBV DNA, with clinical improvement, after the administration of other antiviral agents, such as ganciclovir and famcyclovir, in transplant recipients [101, 102].

FUNGAL INFECTION

Fungal infections are associated with a high mortality in organ transplantation. One of the main reasons is that the diagnosis of invasive fungal infection is usually made very late in the course of the infection, after the fungus has disseminated. Many diagnoses are being still made at autopsy. Symptoms and signs of invasive fungal infection can be very mild and may not even be associated with a rise in temperature. The diagnostic tools for fungal infections have poor sensitivity and specificity. Therefore, fungal infections may go undetected until they are far advanced.

In a recent survey of invasive fungal infections at the University of Pittsburgh Medical Center (UPMC) between 1989 and 1992, we found an incidence of 6.6% among 834 adults who had undergone primary liver transplantation. These infections included candidiasis (65%), aspergillosis (16%), cryptococcosis (16%) and others (2%). The overall fungal-related mortality was 54.5%. These infections usually occurred in patients who had a technically difficult transplant, who had a long ICU stay, and who received long courses of antibiotic treatments. In one study, predictors of fungal infections after liver transplantation were a high serum creatinine, retransplantation, long operative time, and early fungal colonization [103].

Candida

The pathogen
Candida is a yeast; it colonizes the human GI tract and skin. Therefore, the presence of *Candida* in a culture does not necessarily imply *Candida*-related disease. The most prevalent species is *Candida albicans*, although other *Candida* species are also seen. Certain *Candida* species, such as *Candida krusei*, and *Candida glabrata* (*Torulopsis glabrata*), have become more prevalent in association with the routine use of fluconazole prophylaxis.

Clinical
The most common fungal infection after organ transplantation is candidiasis; it is associated with high morbidity and mortality. *Candida* usually colonizes mucosal surfaces and may cause superficial mucositis. *Candida* is a known colonizer of the bowel and in liver transplant recipients may cause abdominal infections.

Liver transplant recipients have had the highest risk of development of fungal infections (up to 40%), particularly candidiasis. This is related to many factors, including the surgery itself, which can be long and complicated, colonization with candida, and the use of multiple antibiotics. We have cultured the alimentary tract of liver transplant candidates and found that 100% of the patients were colonized [104]. Colonization was identified as predictor of infection, together with severity of illness in critically ill patients [105]. In our survey of candidemia in adult liver transplant recipients, we had an incidence of 1.4%, with an associated mortality of 70% [106]. The factors which were found to be associated with the occurrence of candidemia in our study were the administration of multiple intravenous antibiotics and hyperglycemia [106].

There have been reports of *Candida* infections causing mycotic pseudoaneurysms of the arterial suture line; these can rupture and cause major hemorrhage and even death after organ transplantation. Rupture of the renal artery after kidney transplantation [107], and rupture of the aorta after heart [108] or heart-lung [109] transplantation have been reported.

Diagnosis

Because candida is a known colonizer of mucosal surfaces and the skin, it is necessary to differentiate between colonization and invasive disease. Thrush, or oral mucositis, is not considered invasive disease. Invasive candidiasis is diagnosed by the histologic demonstration of tissue invasion or a positive culture of ordinarily sterile fluids. Disseminated disease is defined by the presence of candida in multiple organs. A positive blood culture (Candidemia) is considered invasive disease by most authors.

The sensitivity of commercial blood cultures is only around 50%. Much better are the Lysis centrifugation system, or Isolator bottles [110]. There have been some reports of *Candida* detection by enolase antigenemia testing [111] or by PCR, but their clinical utility has not yet been defined.

Management

Amphotericin B is the drug of choice for most fungal infections in transplant patients. More recently, the liposomal amphotericin preparations have been used, with reduced nephrotoxiciy compared to conventional amphotericin. The triazoles, especially fluconazole, have been used mostly for prophylaxis. However, fluconazole has been associated with the emergence of possibly resistant *Candida* species, such as *Candida krusei* and *Candida glabrata*. The use of fluconazole in transplant recipients also interferes with the metabolism of the calcineurin inhibitor immunosuppressive agents, such as cyclosporin and tacrolimus, and may lead to nephrotoxicity secondary to high levels of these agents, when their dosage is not reduced appropriately.

Aspergillus

The pathogen

Aspergillus is a filamentous fungus which has been associated with construction, usually secondary to spore dispersal into the environment. In tissue, *Aspergillus* is recognized by the presence of branching hyphae (at a 45 degree angle), with abundant septae.

Clinical

Aspergillus is the second most frequent fungal infection in transplant patients. The mortality associated with invasive aspergillosis is very high and approaches 100% in transplant recipients. In one study based on consecutive autopsies from a single hospital, liver transplant recipients and those with hematological malignancies were at highest risk for this infection [112]. The most common species causing disease in transplant patients are *Asper-*

gillus fumigatus and *Aspergillus flavus*. The spores of the fungus are inhaled and may cause pneumonia, and tend to invade blood vessels, leading to infarcts and cavitary lesions, and frequently may disseminate to the CNS. Most brain abscesses in transplant recipients are fungal in origin, and are most commonly aspergillus species. Aspergillus can invade the blood vessels in the brain and cause ischemic and hemorrhagic infarcts, and patients usually present with mental status changes [113]. When we reviewed our experience with invasive pulmonary aspergillosis at UPMC between 1981 and 1990 in adult liver transplant recipients, we found an incidence of 1.5%. Of 29 patients with *Aspergillus* pneumonia, only 23 (79%) had a positive culture of respiratory secretions [114]. *Aspergillus* wound infections can be very difficult to eradicate in transplant recipients, despite aggressive debridement, and may look like necrotizing fasciitis [115].

Diagnosis

Pathologically, the hyphae may look very similar to many other invasive fungi, and therefore the only reliable diagnosis is by culture. Once the fungus has been found in respiratory secretions, it is difficult to tell if the fungus is colonizing the airway or if it represents an invasive lung infection. It is important to evaluate the patient carefully in order to answer this question. Some authors have calculated the positive predictive value of positive respiratory tract cultures for invasive aspergillosis and found it to be 58% in solid organ transplant recipients [116]. It is usually accepted that multiple positive respiratory cultures are associated with invasive disease, and at least 3 sputum cultures should be submitted [116].

Radiologically, on CT scan there are round lesions which have a low attenuation area around them, the "halo sign". This is considered a relatively early sign of pulmonary aspergillosis. Unfortunately, this may be not early in the clinical course of the patient, and dissemination may have already occurred. In recent years there have been reports of the early diagnosis of aspergillosis by serum PCR [117] and by detection of *Aspergillus* galactomannan antigen in the circulation [118].

Management

Two antifungals which have been contributed to the management of aspergillosis in organ transplantation are the liposomal amphotericin preparations and oral itraconazole. Amphotericin remains the drug of choice for treatment of aspergillosis. The liposomal agents allow high dosing, usually up to 5 mg/kg/day, with relatively less nephrotoxicity. It is still unclear whether these agents are more efficacious than conventional amphotericin. There are no randomized trials comparing these agents with amphotericin, only historical controls. Oral itraconazole has been successfully used in some cases of pulmonary aspergillosis. The oral itraconazole solution has a better bio-availability than the oral capsules. The intravenous preparation has been recently approved for use in this country, but there are not enough data yet to assess its utility. In one study from Greece, amphotericin B was more effective than intravenous itraconazole in a limited number of heart transplant recipients with pulmonary aspergillosis [119].

There have been reports of successful treatment of invasive pulmonary aspergillosis with the combination of antifungals and surgical resection in neutropenic patients [120]. Native lung pneumonectomy has been performed in a lung transplant recipient with invasive native lung aspergillosis [121].

As a general rule effective prophylactic agents for *Candidida* infections, such as fluconazole, are not efficacious in the prevention of aspergillosis. There are only a few reports in the literature of prophylaxis trials using liposomal amphotericin in transplant recipients. In one double-blind, placebo-controlled study, AmBisome 1mg/kg/day was given for 5 days after liver transplantation with no fungal infections seen in the first month, compared to 16% in the placebo arm (one case of aspergillosis) [122]. In another prophylaxis study, 1 mg/kg/day of AmBisome was given for 7 days in liver transplant recipients, and 3(5%) of 58 patients developed invasive aspergillosis [123].

Cryptococcus

The pathogen
Cryptococcus is a round yeast which has been associated with bird excrements. Human disease has been associated mostly with *Cryptococcus neoformans*. Most isolates have a polysaccharide capsule which is believed to contribute to the yeast's virulence. The yeast is inhaled and in the normal host may cause a self-limited pneumonitis. From the respiratory tract, the yeast can disseminate to the central nervous system and cause meningitis.

Clinical
Infection usually occurs months or years after organ transplantation, presenting usually as meningitis or pneumonia. Between 1989 and 1998 we encountered 41 cases in solid organ transplant recipients [124]. They included pneumonia (14 cases), meningitis (9 cases), disseminated cryptococcosis (14 cases), and other sites of involvement (4 cases). Cryptococcosis occurred

more frequently among heart transplant recipients, compared with other organ recipients. The mortality associated with cryptococcosis was 22%. The diagnosis was made a median of 11.8 months after transplantation. Meningitis may present with low grade fever and headache, confusion, or seizures; signs of meningeal irritation are not very common [125, 126]. Some cases are diagnosed as pneumonia or lung nodules. We have seen patients who had resection of a lung nodule to confirm metastatic cancer in the lung, and were found to have *Cryptococcus*. There have been cases of disseminated cryptococcosis which presented with cellulitis not responding to antibiotic treatment or necrotizing fasciitis [127]. Biopsy may show necrotizing vasculitis [128]. Whenever *Cryptococcus* is recovered from one site, it is always necessary to look for dissemination in other sites.

Diagnosis

The diagnosis is usually made by culture of the organism or by obtaining a positive cryptococcal antigen in serum or CSF. Although the *Cryptococcus* antigen is usually positive in meningitis or in cases of disseminated disease, this is not always the case in pulmonary disease. We have seen cases of histologically proven pulmonary cryptococcosis with a negative cryptococcal antigen. Although theoretically *Cryptococcus* may be a colonizer in the respiratory tract, in organ transplantation it should be regarded as invasive and treated.

Management

Cryptococcosis is usually treated with the combination of amphotericin B and flucytosine (5FC). The two agents are synergistic. Treatment is usually for 6 weeks and is followed by a long course (usually 6 months) of maintenance treatment with oral fluconazole. The purpose at the onset of treatment is to obtain killing of the organism, and amphotericin B is cidal to the fungus. The experience with the treatment of AIDS patients with cryptococcal meningitis has taught us how to treat this disease in organ transplant recipients. Intensive initial antifungal therapy is important in AIDS patients with cryptococcal meningitis [129]. Fluconazole was reported to be a better agent compared to itraconazole for maintenance in AIDS patients with cryptococcal meningitis [130]. In this population, 5FC used during the first two weeks of treatment of cryptococcal meningitis was associated with a lower relapse rate [130]. In a few difficult cases, we have utilized instillation of amphotericin B into the CSF through an Omaya catheter, with mixed results. Serum and CSF cryptococcal antigen are monitored during treatment. Usually it is desirable to see a four-fold decrease in the level of the cryptococcal antigen, but many times the decrease in titers occurs very slowly, over many months. Clinicians therefore need to assess the clinical response using more than just one variable. The use of amphotericin often leads to nephrotoxicity, which limits the dose and duration of treatment. The liposomal amphotericin preparations have therefore been used preferentially [131]. The combination of fluconazole and 5FC was also found to be synergistic and was used successfully in one report to treat a patient with disseminated cryptococcosis [132].

PROTOZOAL INFECTION

The incidence of protozoal infections in the western world is relatively low, and therefore the problem is not very common after organ transplantation. Nevertheless, clinicians should be aware of the possibility. With successfully transplanted patients travelling so much, and transplantation being increasingly performed in third world countries, the likelihood of seeing tropical diseases, including infections caused by protozoal pathogens, is increasing steadily. Living unrelated kidney transplants are being done now in developing countries. A case report to illustrate this point is a 28 year old Taiwanese, who received a living unrelated kidney transplantation in India and developed malaria [133]. Twenty days after his transplant he developed high fevers, and his blood smear demonstrated Plasmodium vivax organisms [133]. Only two infections will be summarized here, *Pneumocystis carinii* pneumonia (PCP) and Toxoplasmosis.

Pneumocystis

The pathogen
Pneumocystis carinii has been considered to be a protozoal organism, but in recent years some investigators have argued, based on DNA studies, that *Pneumocytis* is not really a protozoan but a fungus [134].

Clinical
PCP usually presents as a bilateral interstitial pneumonia with hypoxemia, and occurs 3-6 months after transplantation. In one series after heart transplantation, hypoxemia occurred in 63%, and patients were febrile in 89% [135]. The association with CMV infection has been seen in many series. Radiological findings are similar in both CMV and PCP. With the introduction of trimethoprim-sulfamethoxazole prophylaxis, the incidence of PCP has decreased dramatically in all centers. Prior to the routine use of prophylaxis, the reported incidence of PCP was about 10% [136]. The infection is much

more common in heart-lung or lung recipients not receiving prophylaxis [137]. The only cases of PCP that have occurred in recent years in our institution have been in patients who did not take their medication. Recurrence of PCP is not common but may occur [138]. Transmission between patients does not occur, although according to one report there was a cluster of PCP in kidney transplant recipients, which was transmitted from AIDS patients [139].

Diagnosis
The diagnosis of PCP is usually made by bronchoalveolar lavage using a silver stain, which shows the cell wall of the organism. Also available are immunofluorescence techniques, and most recently DNA amplification techniques [140, 141]. Rarely, an open lung biopsy is required to make the diagnosis of PCP [142].

Management
Treatment of PCP is with intravenous trimethoprim-sulfamethoxazole or with intravenous pentamidine. Steroids are added in moderate or severe hypoxemia in AIDS patients, and also in transplant recipients [143]. There is synergy between dapsone and trimethoprim - sulfanethoxazole or pentamidine, and combination treatment has been used [144], although trimethoprim-sulfamethoxazole is usually given for severe cases, and is considered the drug of choice.

Prophylaxis for PCP is usually given with trimethoprim-sulfamethoxazole, and a single strength tablet daily for the first 6-12 months and 3 times a week thereafter is used successfully to prevent PCP. Although most cases of PCP occur within one year of transplantation, the risk of PCP is still substantial after one year, especially in lung transplant recipients [145]. Transplant recipients who cannot take sulfa are usually given dapsone, 100 mg po qd, or inhalational pentamidine, 300mg once a month [146]. Aerosolized pentamidine is associated, rarely, with severe bronchospasm [147]. Dapsone may cause hypoxemia secondary to methemoglobinemia [148]. Atovaquone suspension, 1500mg a day, was found to be equivalent to pentamidine for prevention of PCP in HIV patients [149, 150].

Toxoplasma

The pathogen
Toxoplasma gondii is a protozoan parasite which is intracellular and can affect transplant recipients.

Clinical

While the normal host usually develops a febrile illness or lymphadenopathy after infection with this organism, the immunocompromised host may develop visceral disease with pneumonitis, meningitis, and necrotizing encephalitis, or myocarditis and sometimes dissemination to multiple organs. Most of the clinical experience comes from heart transplant recipients, because the organism can be transmitted in the myocardium of the allograft. The risk of development of clinical toxoplasmosis is mostly in seronegative transplant recipients who receive a heart from seropositive donor. This was illustrated by Luft et al. [151]. Of 31 seronegative individuals, 4 received a heart from seropositive donor, and three of them developed serious toxoplasmosis, while ten of the remaining 19 patients had a rise in their titer without any clinical disease [151]. Although clinical toxoplasmosis secondary to reactivation may occur, it is not common [152]. There are also rare cases of clinical toxoplasmosis reported in seronegative heart recipients of organs from seronegative donors [153]. The risk for development of toxoplasmosis after kidney and liver transplantation is much lower than after heart transplantation, but may still occur; therefore, in the right clinical setting, toxoplasmosis should be considered as a possibility [154, 155].

Diagnosis

The diagnosis of toxoplasmosis is usually made by serological methods with compatible clinical presentation. The most reliable serological test is the Sabin-Feldman dye test, which is not done routinely. Other tests have variable sensitivity and specificity. Histology will show the toxoplasma cysts. In endomyocardial biopsies after heart transplantation, it can be sometimes confused with rejection because of infiltration with mononuclear cells [156]. The organism can grow in fibroblasts in viral culture, and a cytopathic plaque can be seen. PCR techniques may be useful to clinicians in the future and could replace the other methods [157].

Management

Treatment of acute toxoplasmosis is usually with a combination of two agents, pyrimethamine and a sulfonamide (usually sulfadiazine). These two agents act synergistically against *Toxoplasma gondii*. Prophylactic therapy is given for 6 weeks to seronegative patients after heart transplantation with a seropositive donor. Pyrimethamine is usually used with or without sulfonamide, and folic acid or folinic acid is given to reduce marrow suppression caused by pyrimethamine. Hakim et al. showed the beneficial effect of this prophylaxis; clinical toxoplasmosis occurred in 4 of seven positive donor/negative recipient cases not receiving prophylaxis, while no patient developed toxoplasmosis among seven patients who received prophylaxis

[158]. Some authors feel that in areas of low prevalence of toxoplasma sero-positivity, there is really no need for routine serologic testing for toxoplasma in heart recipients, and the prophylaxis given for *Pneumocystis carinii* pneumonia is probably sufficient also to prevent toxoplasmosis [159].

SUMMARY

More patients are undergoing organ transplantation, with reduced morbidity and mortality. The reasons for these better outcomes are multifactorial. There have been improvements made in terms of surgical techniques, better immunosuppressive regimens, and better management of complications, including infections. The discovery of new anti-infective agents and the use of better diagnostic tools have allowed clinicians to diagnose infections relatively early and to treat them promptly, sometimes at a subclinical stage. Sound clinical judgment and decision-making based on experience, using a team approach, remain the most important factors in the progress that has been achieved.

REFERENCES

1. Differences in outcomes for patients with bacteremia due to vancomycin- resistant Enterococcus faecium or vancomycin-susceptible E. faecium. Linden PK; Pasculle AW; Manez R; Kramer DJ; Fung JJ; Pinna AD; et al. Clin Infect Dis 1996 Apr;22(4):663-70

2. Risk Factors Associated with Vancomycin Resistant Enterococcus faecium (VREF) Bacteremia in Liver Transplant Recipients (abstract). Kusne S., Molmenti E., Krystofiak S., Rakela J., Fung J. The 37th Interscience Conference on Antimicrobial Agents and Chemotherapy, Toronto, Canada, September 1997.

3. Recommendations for preventing the spread of vancomycin resistance. Centers for Disease Control and Prevention. MMWR 1994;59:25758-25763

4. Infection-control measures reduce transmission of vancomycin-resistant enterococci in an ending endemic setting. Montecalvo MA; Jarvis WR; Uman J; Shay DK; Petrullo C; Rodney K; et al. Ann Intern Med 1999 Aug 17;131(4):269-72

5. Use of linezolid, an oxazolidinone, in the treatment of multidrug-resistant gram-positive bacterial infections. Chien JW; Kucia ML; Salata RA. Clin Infet Dis 2000 Jan;30(1):146-51

6. Listeria faecal carriage by renal transplant recipients, haemodialysis patients and patients in general practice: its relation to season, drug therapy, foreign travel, animal exposure and diet. MacGowan AP; Marshall RJ; MacKay IM; Reeves DS. Epidemiol Infect 1991 Feb;106(1):157-66

7. Two cases of progressive multifocal leukoencephalopathy after renal transplantation. Reznik M; Halleux J; Urbain E; Mouchette R; Castermans P; Beaujean M. Acta Neuropathol Suppl (Berl) 1981;7:189-91

8. Listeriosis in renal transplant recipients: report of an outbreak and review of 102 cases. Stamm AM; Dismukes WE; Simmons BP; Cobbs CG; Elliot A; Budrich P; et al. Rev Infect Dis 1982 May-Jun;4(3):665-82

9. Report of 24 cases of Listeria monocytogenes infection at the University of Miami Medical Center. Qayyum QJ; Scerpella EG; Moreno JN; Fischl MA. Rev Invest Clin 1997 Jul-Aug;49(4):265-70

10. Listeria monocytogenes hepatitis in a liver transplant recipient: a case report and review of the literature. Bourgeois N; Jacobs F; Tavares ML; Rickaert F; Deprez C; Liesnard C; et al. J Hepatol 1993 Jul;18(3):284-9

11. Listerial myocarditis in cardiac transplantation. Stamm AM; Smith SH; Kirklin JK; McGiffin DC. Rev Infect Dis 1990 Sep-Oct;12(5):820-3

12. Listeriosis and recurrent abortion in renal transplant recipient. Dick JP; Palframann A; Hamilton DV. J Infect 1988 May;16(3):273-7

13. Listeria monocytogenes endophthalmitis in a renal-transplant patient receiving cyclosporin. Algan M; Jonon B; George JL; Lion C; Kessler M; Burdin JC. Ophthalmologica 1990:201(1):23-7

14. Treatment of Listeria monocytogenes infection with trimethoprim-sulfamethoxazole: case report and review of the literature. Spitzer PG; Hammer SM; Karchmer AW. Rev Infect Dis 1986 May-Jun;8(3):427-30

15. Legionellosis in heart transplant recipients. Horbach I; Fehrenbach FJ. Infection 1990 Nov-Dec;18(6):361-3

16. Epidemiology of legionella pneumonia and factors associated with legionella-related mortality at a tertiary care center. Tkatch LS; Kusne S; Irish WD; Krystofiak S; Wing E. Clin Infect Dis 1998 Dec;27(6):1479-86

17. More then 10 years of unrecognized nosocomial transmission of legionnaires' disease among transplant patients. Kool JL; Fiore AE; Kioski CM; Brown EW; Benson RF; Pruckler JM; et al. Infect Control Hosp Epidemiol 1998 Dec;19(12): 898-904

18. Epidemiology, bacteriology and control of an outbreak of Nocardia asteroides infection on a liver unit. Sahathevan M; Harvey FA; Forbes G; O;Grady J; Gimson A; Bragman S; et al. J Hosp Infect 1991 Jun;18 Suppl A:473-80

19. Disseminated subcutaneous Nocardia asteroides abscesses in a patient after bone marrow transplantation. Hodohara K; Fujiyama Y; Hiramitu Y; Sumiyoshi K; Kitoh K; Hosoda S; et al. Bone Marrow Transplant 1993 Apr;11(4):341-3

20. Nocardiosis in liver ttransplantation: variation in presentation, diagnosis and therapy. Forbes GM; Harvey FA; Philpott-Howard JN; O'Grady JG; Jensen RD; Sahathevan M; et al. J Infect 1990 Jan;20(1):11-9

21. Nocardia infection in patients with liver transplants or chronic liver disease: radiologic findings. Raby N; Forbes G; Williams R. Radiology 1990 Mar;174(3Pt1): 713-6

22. Trimethoprin/sulfamethoxazole-resistant Nocardia asteroides causing multiple hepatic abscesses. Successful treatment with ampicillin, amikacin, and limited computed tomography-guided needle aspiration. Cockerill FR 3d; Edson RS; Roberts GD; Waldorf JC. Am J Med 1984 Sep;77(3):558-60

23. Foreign born is the most important risk factor for Tuberculosis infection in adult liver transplant recipients (abstract). Wada S., Kusne S., Fung J., Rakela J. The 36th Interscience Conference on Antimicrobial Agents and Chemotherapy, New Orleans, September 1996.

24. Nosocomial outbreak of tunerculosis in a renal transplant unit: application of a new technique for restriction fragment length polymorphism analysis of Mycobaterium tuberculosis isolates. Jereb JA; Burwen DR; Dooley SW; Haas WH; Crawford JT; Geiter LJ; et al. J Infect Dis 1993 Nov;168(5):1219-24

25. Global surveillance for antituberculosis-drug resistance, 1994-1997. World Health Organization-International Union against Tuberculosis and Lung Disease Work-

ing Group on Anti-Tuberculosis Drug Resistance Surveillance. Pablos-Mendez A; Raviglione MC; Laszlo A; Binkin N; Rieder HL; Bustreo F; et al. N Engl J Med 1998 Jun 4;338(23):1641-9

26. Spread of strain W, a highly drug-resistant strain of Mycobaterium tuberculosis, across the United States. Agerton TB; Valway SE; Blinkhorn RJ; Shilkret KL; Reves R; Schluter WW; et al. Clin Infect Dis 1999 Jul;29(1):85-92;discussion 93-5

27. Anergy panel and purified protein derivative(PPD) skin testing are poor tuberculosis(TB) screening method in adult liver transplant candidates (abstract). Kusne S., Irish W., Geary K., Ondick L., Rakela J., Fung J. The 35th Interscience Conference on Antimicrobial Agents and Chemotherapy, San Francisco, September, 1995.

28. Workshop on CMV disease; definitions, clinical severity scores, and new syndromes. Ljungman P., Plotkin SA. Scand J Infect Dis Suppl 1995: 99: 87-89.

29. Definitions of cytomegalovirus infection and disease, page 233-237. Ljungman P., Griffiths P. In Multidisciplinary approach to understanding cytomegalovirus desease. S Michelson and AS Plotkin eds. Elsevier Science Publishers, 1993.

30. Nuclear expression of the lower matrix protein of human cytomegalovirus in peripheral blood leukocytes of immunocompromised viraemic patients. Revello MG, Percivalle E, Matteo AD, Morini F, Gerna G. Journal of General Virology 1992: 73: 437-442.

31. Direct detection of cytomegalovirus in peripheral blood leukocytes -- a review of the antigenemia assay and polymerase chain reaction. The TH, Van Der Ploeg M, Van Den Berg AP, Vlieger AM, Van Der Giessen M, Van Son WJ. Transplantation 1992: 54: 193-198.

32. Human cytomegalovirus UL97 open reading frame encodes a protein that phosphorylates the antiviral nucleoside analogue ganciclovir. Littler E, Stuart AD, Chee MS. Nature 1992: 358: 160-164.

33. A point mutation in the human cytomegalovirus DNA polymerase gene confers resistance to ganciclovir and phosphonylmethoxyalkyl derivatives. Sullivan V, Biron KK, Talarico C, Stanat SC, Davis M, Pozzi LM, et al. Antimicrobial Agents and chemotherapy 1993: 37: 19-25.

34. Treatment of cytomegalovirus pneumonia with ganciclovir and intravenous cytomegalovirus immunoglobulin in patients with bone marrow transplants. Reed EC, Bowden RA, Dandliker PS, Lilleby KE, Meyers JD. Annals of Internal Medicine 1988: Nov 15: 783-788.

35. Treatment of interstitial pneumonitis due to cytomegalovirus with ganciclovir and intravenous immune globulin: Experience of European Bone Marrow Transplant Group. Ljungman P, et al. Clinical Infectious Diseases 1992: 14: 831-835.

36. Preemptive therapy in immunocompromised hosts. Rubin RH. The New England Journal of Medicine 1991: 324: 1057-1059.

37. Randomised trial of efficacy and safety of oral ganciclovir in the prevention of cytomegaloviurs disease in liver-transplant recipients. Gane E, Saliba F, Valdecasas GJC, O'grady J, Pescovitz MD, Lyman S, et al. The Lancet 1997: 350: 1729-1733.

38. CMV PP65 antigenemia monitoring as a guide for preemptive therapy: A cost effective strategy for prevention of CMV disease in adult liver transplant recipients. Kusne S, Grossi P, Irish W, St.George K, Rinaldo C, Rakela J, et al. Transplantation, 1999, October;68(8): 1125-1131.

39. Human herpesvirus-6 (HHV-6) infection in allogeneic bone marrow transplant recipients; evidence of a marrow-suppressive role for HHV-6 in vivo. Drobyski WR; Dunne WM; Burd EM; Knox KK; Ash RC; Horowitz MM; et al. J Infect Dis 1993 Mar;167(3):735-9

40. Human herpesvirus-6 meningoencephalitis in a recipient of an unrelated allo-

geneic bone marrow transplantation. Rieux C; Gautheret-Dejean A; Challine-Lehmann D; Kirch C; Agut H; Vernant JP. Transplantation 1998 May 27;65(10): 1408-11

41. Variant B human herpesvirus-6 associated febrile dermatosis with thrombocytopenia and encephalopathy in a liver transplant recipient. Singh H; Carrigan DR; Gayowski T; Singh J; Marino IR. Transplantation 1995 Dec 15;60(11):1355-7

42. Human herpesvirus-6 in trasplantation: an emerging pathogan. Singh H; Carrigan DR. Ann Intern Med 1996 Jun 15;124(12):1065-71

43. Seroconversion to human herpevirus 6 following liver transplantation is a marker of cytomegalovirus disease. Dockrell DH; Prada J; Jones MF; Patel R; Badley AD; Harmsen WS, et al. J Infect Dis 1997 Nov; 176(5):1135-40

44. Cytomegalovirus and human herpesvirus 6 both cause viral disease after renal transplantation. Ratnamohan VM; Chapman J; Howse H; Bovington K; Roberston P; Byth K; et al. Transplantation 1998 Oct 15;66(7):877-82

45. Human herpesvirus 6 reactivation is associated with cytomegalovirus infection and syndromes in kidney transplant recipients at risk for primary cytomegalovirus infection. DesJardin JA, Gibbons L, Cho E, Supran SE, Falagas ME, Werner BG, et al. J Infect Dis 1998;178(6):1783-6

46. Clinical relevance of human Herpesvirus-6 in liver transplant recipients: role of pathogenesis of fungal infections, neurologic complications, and impact on outcome. Rogers J; Singh N; Carrigan DR; Rohal S; Kusne S; Knox KK. Transplantation 2000, in press.

47. Susceptiblity of human herpesvirus 6 to antivirals in vitro. Burns WH; Sandford GR. J Infect Dis 1990 Sep;162(3):634-7

48. Human herpes virus-6 encephalitis after bone marrow transplantation: successful treatmeent with ganciclovir. Mookerjee BP; Vogelsang G. Bone Marrow Transplant 1997 Nov;20(10):905-6

49. Human herpesvirus 6 DNA in cerebrospinal fluid specimens from allogeneic bone marrow transplant patients; does it have clinical significance? Wang FZ; Linde A; Hagglund H; Testa M; Locasciulli A; Ljungman P. Clin Infect Dis 1999 Mar;28(3):562-8

50. Disseminated varicella infection in pediatric renal transplant recipients treated with mycophenolate mofetil. Rothwell WS; Gloor JM; Morgenstern BZ; Milliner DS. Transplantation 1999 Jul 15;68(1):158-61

51. Acyclovir and renal transplantation. Pettersson E; Eklund B; Hockerstedt K; Salmela K; Ahonen J. Scand J Infect Dis Suppl 1985;47:145-8

52. Famciclovir: review of clinical efficacy and safety. Cirelli R; Herne K; McCrary M; Lee P; Tyring SK. Antiviral Res 1996 Mar;29(2-3):141-51

53. Current pharmacological approaches to the therapy of varicella zoster virus infections: a guide to treatment. Snoeck R; Andrei G; De Clercq E. Drugs 1999 Feb;57(2):187-206

54. Varicella vaccination in children after bone marrow transplantion. Sauebrei A: Prager J; Hengst U; Zintl F; Wutzler P. Bone Marrow Tranplant 1997 Sep;20(5): 381-3

55. Attenuated varicella virus vaccine in children with renal tranplants. Zamora I; Simon JM; Da Silva ME; Piqueras AI. Pediatr Nephrol 1994 Apr;8(2):190-2

56. Varicella in pediatric renal transplant recipients. Lynfield R; Herrin JT; Rubin RH. Pediatrics 1992 Aug;90(2 Pt 1):216-20

57. Persistence of protective immunity after postexposure prophylaxis of varicella with oral aciclovir in the family setting. Yoshikawa T; Suga S; Kozawa T; Kawaguchi S; Asano Y. Arch Dis Child 1998 Jan;78(1):61-3

58. Varicella-zoster virus-specific cellular immunity in subjects given acyclovir after household chicken pox exposure. Kumagai T; Kamada M; Igarashi C; Yuri K; Furukawa H; Chiba S; et al. J Infect Dis 1999 Sep;180(3):834-7

59. The morphologic and molecular genetic categories of posttransplantation lymphoproliferative disorders are clinically relevant. Chadburn A; Chen JM; Hsu DT; Frizzera G; Cesarman E; Garrett TJ; et al. Cancer 1998 May:15;82(10): 1978-87

60. Pretransplantation assessment of the risk of lymphoproliferative disorder. Walker RC; Marshall WF; Strickler JG; Wiesner RH; Velosa JA; Habermann TM; et al. Clin Infect Dis 1995 May;20(5):1346-53

61. Reversibility of lymphomas and lymphoproliferative lesions developing under cyclosporin-steroid therapy. Starzl TE; Nalesnik MA; Porter KA; Ho M; Iwatsuki S; Griffith BP; et al. Lancent 1984 Mar 17;1(8377):583-7

62. Serial measurement of Esptein-Barr viral load in periperal blood pediatric liver transplant recipients during treatment for posttransplant lymphoproliferative disease. Green M; Cacciarelli TV; Mazariegos GV; Sigurdsson L; Qu L; Rowe DT. Tranplantation 1998 Dec 27;66(12):1641-4

63. Detection of Epstein-Barr virus DNA in sera from transplant recipients with lymphoproliferative disorders. Limaye AP; Huang ML; Atienza EE; Ferrenberg JM; Corey L. J Clin Microbiol 1999 Apr;37(4):1113-6

64. The Epstein-Barr virus thymidine kinase does not phosphorylate ganciclovir or acyclovir and demonstrates a narrow substrate specifity compared to the herpes smplex virus 1 thymidine kinase. Gustafson EA; Chillemi AC; Sage DR; Fingeroth JD. Antimicrob Agents Chemother 1998 Nov;42(11):2923-31

65. Arginine butyrate-induced susceptibility to ganciclovir in an Epstein-Barr virus associated lymphoma. Mentzer SJ; Fingeroth J; Reilly JJ; Perrine SP; Faller DV. Blood Cells Mol Dis 1998 June:24(2):114-23

66. Lymphoproliferative disorders following allergeneic bone marrow transplantation: the Vancouver experience. Micallef IN; Chhanabhai M; Gascoyne RD; Shepherd JD; Fung HC; Nantel SH; et al. Bone Marrow Transplant 1998 Nov;22(10):981-7

67. Use of gene-modified virus-specific T lymphocytes to control Epstein-Barr virus-related lymphoproliferation. Rooney CM; Smith CA; Ng CY; Loftin S; Li C; Krance RA; et al. Lancet 1995 Jan 7;345(8941):9-13

68. Infusion of cytotoxic T cells for the prevention and treatment of Epstein-Barr virus-induced lymphoma in allogeneic transplant recipients. Rooney CM; Smith CA; Ng CY; Loftin SK; Sixbey JW; Gan Y; et al. Blood 1998 Sep 1;92(5):1549-55

69. Anti-B-cell monoclonal antibodies in the treatment of severe B-cell lymphoproliferative sundrome following bone marrow and organ transplantation. Fischer A; Blanche S; Le Bidois J; Bordigoni P; Garnier JL; Niaudet P; et al. N Engl J Med 1991 May 23;324(21):1451-6

70. Autologous lymphokine-activated killer cell therapy of Epstein-Barr virus-positive and negative lymphoproliferative disorders arising in organ transplant recipients. Nalesnik MA; Rao AS; Furukawa H; Pham S; Zeevi A; Fung JJ, et al. Transplantation 1997 May;63(9): 1200-5.

71. Effective treatment of high-grade lymphoproliferative disorder after renal transplantation using autologous lymphocyte activated killer cell therapy. Li PK; Tsang K; Szeto CC; Wong TY; To KF; Leung CB. Am J Kidney Dis 1998 Nov;32(5): 813-9

72. Resistance to parvovirus B19 infection due to lack of virus receptor (erythocyte P antigen). Brown KE; Hibbs JR; Gallinella G; Anderson SM; Lehman ED; McCarthy P; et al. N Engl J Med 1994 Apr 28;330(17):1192-6

73. Chronic anemia due to parvovirus B19 infection in a bone marrow transplant patient after platelet transfusion. Cohen BJ; Beard S; Knowles WA; Ellis JS; Joske D; Goldman JM; et al. Transfusion 1997 Sep;37(9):947-52

74. Transfusion-transmitted disease. Lee CA. Baillieres Clin Haematol 1996 Jun;9(2): 369-94

75. B19 Parvovirus replicates in circulating cells of acutely infected patients. Kurtzman GJ; Gascon P; Caras M; Cohen B; Young NS. Blood 1988 May;71(5):1448-54

76. Parvovirus B19 infection associated with myocarditis following adult cardiac transplantation. Heegaard ED; Eiskjaer H; Baandrup U; Hornsleth A. Scand J Infect Dis 1998;30(6):607-10

77. Parvovirus B19 infection-related complications in renal transplant recicpients: treatment with intravenous immunoglobulin. Moudgil A; Shidban H; Nast CC; Bagga A; Aswad S; Graham SL; et al. Transplantation 1997 Dec 27;64(12):1847-50

78. Post-transplantation polyomavirus infections. Boubenider S; Hiesse C; Marchand S; Hafi A; Kriaa F; Charpentier B. J Nephrol 1999 Jan-Feb;12(1):24-9

79. Human polyma virus in renal allograft biopsies: morphological findings and correlation with urine cytology. Drachenberg CB; Beskow CO; Cangro CB; Bourquin PM; Simsir A; Fink J; et al. Hum Pathol 1999 Aug;30(8):970-7

80. A serological investigation of BK virus and JC virus infections in recipients of renal allografts. Andrews CA; Shah KV; Daniel RW; Hirsch MS; Rubin RH. J Infect Dis 1988 Jul;158(1)176-81

81. Human polyoma virus-associated interstitial nephritis in the allograft kidney. Randhawa PS; Finklestein S; Scantlebury V; Shapiro R; Vivas C; Jordan M; et al. Transplantation 1999 Jan 15;67(1):103-9

82. Polyomavirus disease under new immunosuppressive drugs: a cause of renal graft dysfunction and graft loss. Binet I; Nickeleit V; Hirsch HH; Prince O; Dalquen P; Gudat F; et al. Transplantation 1999 Mar 27;67(6):918-22

83. Diagnosis and management of BK polyomavirus interstitial nephritis in renal transplant recipients. Howell DN; Smith SR; Butterly DW; Klassen PS; Krigman HR; Burchette JL Jr; et al. Transplantation 1999 Nov 15;68(9):1279-88

84. Human polyoma virus infections with JC virus and BK virus in renal transplant patients. Hogan TF; Borden EC; McBain JA; Padgett BL; Walker DL. Ann Intern Med 1980 Mar;92(3):373-8

85. Molecular evidence of simian virus 40 infections in children. Butel JS; Arrington AS; Wong C; Lednicky JA; Finegold MJ. J Infect Dis 1999 Sep;180(3):884-7

86. The hepatitis C virus; overview. Purcell R. Hepatology 1997 Sep;26(3 Suppl 1):11S-14S

87. Serologic responses to hepatitis C virus is solid organ transplant recipients. Preiksaitis JK; Cockfield SM; Fenton JM; Burton NI; Chui LW. Transplantation 1997 Dec 27;64(12):1775-80

88. Pretransplant virological markers hepatitis C virus genotype and viremia level are not helpful in predicting individual outcome after orthotopic liver transplantation. Berg T; Hopf U; Bechstein WO; Muller AR; Fukumoto T; Neuhaus R; et al. Transplantation 1998 July;66(2): 225-228.

89. High incidence of allograft cirrhosis in hepatitis C virus genotype 1b infection following transplantation: relationship with rejection episodes. Prieto M; Berenguer M; Rayon JM; Cordoba J; Arguello L; Carrasco D; et al. Hepatology 1999 Jan;29(1):250-6

90. The influence of hepatitis C virus genotypes on the outcome of liver transplantation. Vargas HE; Laskus T; Wang LF; Radkowski M; Poutous A; Lee R; et al. Liver Transpl Surg 1998 Jan;4(1):22-7

91. Evolution of hepatitis C virus quasispecies in patients with severe cholestatic hepatitis after liver transplantation. Pessoa MG; Bzowej N; Berenguer M; Phung Y; Kim M; Ferrel L; et al. Hepatology 1999 Dec;30(6):1513-20

92. The non-structural 5A protein of hepatitis C virus. Pawlotsky JM; Germanidis G. J Viral Hepat 1999 Sep;6(5):343-356

93. The risk of transmission of hepatitis B from HBsAg(-), HBcAb(+), HBIgM(-) organ

donors. Wachs ME; Amend WJ; Ascher NL; Bretan PN; Emond J; Lake JR; et al. Transplantation 1995 Jan 27;59(2):230-4

94. Quantitation of HBV DNA in human serum using a branched DNA (bDNA) signal amplification assay. Hendricks DA; Stowe BJ; Hoo BS; Kolberg J; Irvine BD; Neuwald PD; et al. Am J Clin Pathol 1995 Nov;104(5):537-46

95. Liver Transplantation in European patients with the hepatitis B surface antigen. Samuel D; Muller R; Alexander G; Fassati L; Ducot B; Benhamou JP; et al. N Engl J Med 1993 Dec 16;329(25):1842-7

96. Infectivity of hepatic allografts with antibodies to hepatitis B virus. Dodson SF; Issa S; Araya V; Gayowski T; Pinna A; Eghtesad B; et al. Transplantation 1997 Dec 15;64(11):1582-4

97. Prevention of de novo hepatitis B infection in recipients of hepatic allografts from anti-HBc positive donors. Dodson SF; Bonham CA; Geller DA; Cacciarelli TV; Rakela J; Fung JJ; et al. Transplantation 1999 Oct 15;68(7):1058-61

98. Incidence and clinical consequences of surface and polymerase gene mutations in liver transplant recipients on hepatitis B immunoglobulin. Terrault NA; Zhou S; McCory RW; Pruett TL; Lake JR; Roberts JP; et al. Hepatology 1998 Aug; 28(2):555-61

99. Multicenter study of lamivudine therapy for hepatitis B after liver transplantation. Lamivudine Transplant Group. Perrillo R; Rakela J; Dienstag J; Levy G; Martin P; Wright T; et al. Hepatology 1999 May;29(5):1581-6

100. Outcome of lamivudine resistant hepatitis B virus infection in the liver transplant recipent. Mutimer D; Pillay D; Shields P; Cane P; Ratcliffe D; Martin B; et al. Gut 2000 Jan 46(1):107-13

101. Famciclover treatment of chronic hepatitis B in heart transplant recipients: a prospective trial. Wedemeyer H; Boker KH; Pethig K; Petzold DR; Flemming P; Tillmann HL; et al. Transplantation 1999 Nov 27;68(10):1503-11

102. Long term ganciclovir therapy for hepatitis B virus infection after liver transplantation. Roche B; Samuel D; Gigou M; Feray C; Virot V; Majno P; et al. J Hepatol 1999 Oct;31(4):584-92

103. Risk factors for invasive fungal infections complicating orthotopic liver transplantation. Collins LA; Samore MH; Roberts MS; Luzzati R; Jenkins RL; Lewis WD. J Infect Dis 1994 Sep;170(3):644-52

104. Candida Carriage in the alimentary tract of liver transplant candidates. Kusne S; Tobin D; Pasculle AW; Van Thiel DH; Ho M; Starzl TE. Transplantation 1994 Feb;57(3):398-402

105. Candida colonization and subsequent infections in critically ill surgical patients. Pittet D; Monod M; Suter PM; Frenk E; Auckenthaler R. Ann Surg 1994 Dec;220(6):751-8

106. Factors associataed with the development of candidemia and candidemia related death among liver transplant recipients. Neito-Rodriguez JA; Kusne S; Manez R; Irish W; Linden P; Magnone M; et al. Ann Surg 1996 Jan;223(1):70-6

107. "True" mycotic aneurysm of a renal artery allograft. Potti A; Danielson B; Sen K. Am J Kidney Dis 1998 Jan;31(1):E3

108. Successful outcome after massive bleeding in a heart transplant recipient with mycotic aortitis. Case report. Berggren H; Berglin E; Kjellman U; Mantovani V; Nilsson B. Scand J Thorac Cardiovasc Surg 1994;28(1):45-7

109. Management of mycotic rupture of the ascending aorta after heart-lung transplantation. Albes J; Haverich A; Freihorst J; von der Hardt H; Manthey-Stiers F. Ann Thorac Surg 1990 Dec;50(6):982-3

110. Evaluation of lysis-centrifugation system for recovery of yeasts and filamentous fungi from blood. Bille J; Stockman L; Roberts GD; Horstmeier CD; Ilstrup DM. J Clin Microbiol 1983 Sep;18(3):469-71

111. Detection of circulating candida enolase by immunoassay in patients with cancer

and invasive candidiasis. Walsh TJ; Hathorn JW; Sobel JD; Merz WG; Sanchez V; Maret SM; et al. N Engl J Med 1991 Apr 11;324(15):1026-31

112. 10 year review of invasive aspergillosis detected at necropsy. Boon AP; O'Brien D; Adams DH. J Clin Pathol 1991 Jun;44(6):452-4

113. CNS aspergillosis in organ transplantation: a clinicopathological study. Torre-Cisneros J; Lopez OL; Kusne S; Martinez AJ; Starzl TE; Simmons RL; et al. J Neurosurg Psychiatry 1993 Feb;56(2):188-93

114. Factors associated with invasive lung aspergillosis and the significance of positive Aspergerillus culture after liver transplantation. Kusne S; Torre-Cisneros J; Manez R; Irish W; Martin M; Fung J; et al. J Infect Dis 1992 Dec;166(6):1379-83

115. Surgical wound infection by Aspergillus fumigatus in liver transplant recipients. Pla MP; Berenguer J; Arzuaga JA; Banares R; Polo JR; Bouza E. Diagn Micrrobiol Infect Dis 1992 Nov-Dec;15(8):703-6

116. The use of respiratory-tract cultures in the diagnosis of invasive pulmonary aspergillosis. Horvath JA; Dummer S. Am J Med 1996 Feb;100(2):171-8

117. Evaluation of PCR for detection of DNA specific for Aspergillus species in sera of patients with various forms of pulmonary aspergillosis. Yamakami Y; Hashimoto A; Yamagata E; Kamberi P; Karashima R; Nagai H; et al. J Clin Microbiol 1998 Dec;36(12):3619-23

118. Serial monitoring of Aspergillus antigen in the early diagnosis of invasive aspergillosis. Preliminary investigations with two examples. Verweij PE; Dompeling EC; Donnelly JP; Schattenberg AV; Meis JF. Infection 1997 Mar-Apr;25(2):86-9

119. Itraconazole for the treatment of pulmonary aspergillosis in heart transplant recipients. Nanas JN; Saroglou G; Anastasiou-Nana MI; Kostis EB; Petrochilou-Paschou VP; Kontoyannis DA; et al. Clin Transplant 1998 Feb;12(1):30-4

120. Surgical management of invasive pulmonary aspergillosis in neutropenic patients. Bernard A; Caillot D; Couallier JF; Casasnovas O; Guy H; Favre JP. Ann Thorac Surg 1997 Nov;64(5):1441-7

121. Native lung pneumonectomy for invasive pulmonary aspergillosis following lung transplantation: a case resport. Sandur S; Gordon SM; Mehta AC; Maurer JR. J Heart Lung Transplant 1999 Aug;18(8):810-3

122. Liposomal amphotericin B prevents invasive fungal infections in liver transplant recipients. A randomized, placebo-controlled study. Tollemar J; Hockerstedt K; Ericzon BG; Jalanko H; Ringden O. Transplantation 1995 Jan 15;59(1):45-50

123. Systemic mycoses during prophylactical use of liposomal amphotericin B (ambisome) after liver transplantation. Lorf T; Braun F; Ruchel R; Muller A; Sattler B; Ringe B. Mycoses 1999 Apr;42(1-2):47-53

124. The epidemiology of cryptococcal infection in solid organ transplantation (abstract). Kusne S, Madariaga J, McCurry K, Kormos R, Fung J. The 17th Annual Scientific Meeting of The American Society of Transplant Physicians, Chicago, May 1998.

125. Cryptococcosis in a renal unit. Kong NC; Shaariah W; Morad Z; Suleiman AB; Wong YH. Aust N Z J Med 1990 Oct;20(5):645-9

126. Cryptococcal meningitis after liver transplantation. Jabbour N; Reyes J; Kusne S; Martin M; Fung J. Transplantation 1996 Jan 15;61(1):146-9

127. Risk factors in necrotizing fasciitis: a case involving Cryptococcus neoformans. Marcus JR; Hussong JW; Gonzalez C; Dumanian GA. Ann Plast Surg 1998 Jan;40(1):80-3

128. Disseminated cryptococcosis presenting as cellulitis with necrotizing vasculitis. Shrader SK; Watts JC; Dancik JA; Band JD. J Clin Microbiol 1986 Nov;24(5):860-2

129. Early mycological treatment failure in AIDS-associated cryptococcal meningitis. Robinson PA; Bauer M; Leal MA: Evans SG; Holtom PD; Diamond DA; et al. Clin Infect Dis 1999 Jan;28(1):82-92

130. A comparison of itraconazole versus fluconazole as maintenance therapy for AIDS-associated cryptococcal meningitis. National Institute of Allergy and Infectious Diseases Mycoses Study Group. Saag MS; Cloud GA; Graybill JR; Sobel JD; Tuazon CU; Johnson PC; et al. Clin Infect Dis 1999 Feb;28(2):291-6

131. Successful treatment of cryptococcal meningitis with amphotericin B colloidal dispersion: report of four cases. Valero G; Graybill JR. Antimicrob Agents Chemother 1995 Nov;39(11):2588-90

132. Successful treatment of disseminated cryptococcosis in a liver transplant recipient with fluconazole and flucytosine, an all oral regimen. Singh N; Gayowski T; Marino IR. Transpl Int 1998;11(1):63-5

133. Malaria infection in kidney transplant recipients. Lee PC; Lee PY; Lei HY; Chen FF; Tseng JY; Ching YT. Transplant Proc 1994 Aug;26(4):2099-100

134. Pneumocystis carinii pneumonia: the status of Pneumocystis biochemistry. Kaneshiro ES. Int J Parasitol 1998 Jan;28(1):65-84

135. Pneumocystis carinii infection in heart transplant recipients. Efficacy of a weekend prophylaxis schedule. Munoz P; Munoz RM; Palomo J; Rodriguez-Creixems M; Munoz R; Bouza E. Medicine (Baltimore) 1997 Nov;76(6):415-22

136. Pneumocystis carinii pneumonia in renal transplant recipients. Branten AJ; Beckers PJ; Tiggeler RG; Hoitsma AJ. Nephrol Dial Transplant 1995;10(7):1194-7

137. Trimethoprin-sulfamethoxazole prophylaxis for Pneumocystis carinii infections in heart-lung and lung transplantation- how effective and for how long? Kramer MR; Stoehr C; Lewiston NJ; Starnes VA; Theodore J. Transplantation 1992 Mar;53(3):586-9

138. Pneumocystis carinii pneumonia in heart transplant recipients. Grossi P; Ippoliti GB; Goggi C; Cremaschi P; Scaglia M; Minoli L. Infection 1993 Mar-Apr;21(2): 75-9

139. Transmission of Pneumocystis carinii from AIDS patients to other immunsuppressed patients: a cluster of Pneumocystis carinii pneumonia in renal transplant recipients. Chave JP; David S; Wauters JP; Van Melle G; Francioli P. AIDS 1991 Aug;5(8):927-32

140. Comparison of DNA amplification and immunofluorescence for detecting Pneumocystis carinii in patients receiving immunosuppressive therapy. Leigh TR; Wakefield AE; Peters SE; Hopkin JM; Collins JV. Transplantation 1992 Sep;54(3): 468-70

141. Diagnosis of Pneumocystis carinii pneumonia: immunofluorescence staining, simple PCR or nPCR. Khan MA; Farrag N; Butcher P. J Infect 1999 Jul;39(1): 77-80

142. Bronchiolitis obliterans organizing pneumonia associated with Pneumocystis carinii infection in a liver transplant patient receiving tacrolimus. Kleindienst R; Fend F; Prior C; Margreiter R; Vogel W. Clin Transplant 1999 Feb;13(1Pt1):65-7

143. Pneumocystis carinii pneumonia. Schliep TC; Yarrish RL. Semin Respir Infect 1999 Dec;14(4):333-43

144. Use of dapsone in the prevention and treatment of Pneumocystis carinii pneumonia: a review. Hughes WT. Clin Infect Dis 1998 Jul;27(1):191-204

145. Should prophylaxis for Pneumocystis carinii pneumonia in solid organ transplant recipients ever be discontinued? Gordon SM; LaRosa SP; Kalmadi S; Arroliga AC; Avery RK; Truesdell-LaRosa L; et al. Clin Infect Dis 1999 Feb;28(2):240-6

146. Utility of inhaled penatmidine prophylaxis in lung transplant recipients. Nathan SD; Ross DJ; Zakowski P; Kass RM; Koerner SK. Chest 1994 Feb;105(2):417-20

147. Aerosolized pentamidine as alternative primary prophylaxis against Pneumocystis carinii pneumonia in adult hepatic and renal transplant recipients. Saukkonen K; Garland R; Koziel H. Chest 1996 May;109(5):1250-5

148. Dapsone-induced methemoglobinemia. Ward KE; McCarthy MW. Ann Pharmacother 1998 May;32(5):549-53

149. Atovaquone suspension compared with aeosolized pentamidine for prevention of Pneumocystis carinii pneumonia in human immunodeficiency virus-infected subjects intolerant of trimethoprim or sulfonamides. Chan C; Montaner J; Lefebvre EA; Morey G; Dohn M; McIvor RA; et al. J Infect Dis 1999 Aug;180(2):369-76

150. Atovaquone compared with dapsone for the prevention of Pneumocystis carinii pneumonia in patients with HIV infection who cannot tolerate trimethoprim, sulfonamides, or both. Community Program for Clinical Research on AIDS and the AIDS Clinical Trials Group. El-Sadr WM; Murphy RL; Yurik TM; Luskin-Hawk R; Cheung TW; Balfour HH JR; et al. N Engl J Med 1998 Dec 24;339(36):1889-95

151. Primary and reactivated toxoplasma infection in patients with cardiac transplants. Clinical spectrum and problems in diagnosis in a defined population. Luft BJ; Naot Y; Araujo FG; Stinson EB; Remington JS. Ann Intern Med 1983 Jul;99(1):27-31

152. Toxoplasmosis in heart transplant recipients. Gallino A; Maggiorini M; Kiowski W; Martin X; Wunderli W; Schneider J; et al. Eur J Clin Microbiol Infect Dis 1996 May;15(5):389-93

153. Cytomegalovirus infections and toxoplasmosis in heart transplant recipients in Sweden. Andersson R; Sandberg T; Berglin E; Jeansson S. Scand J Infect Dis 1992;24(4):411-7

154. Transmission of Toxoplasma gondii infection by liver transplantation. Mayes JT; O'Conner BJ; Avery R; Castellani W; Carey W. Clin Infect Dis 1995Sep;21(3):511-5

155. Transmission of Toxoplasmosis by renal transplant. Mejia G; Leiderman E; Builes M; Henao J; Arbelaez M; Arango JL; et al. Am J Kidney Dis 1983 May;2(6):615-7

156. Toxoplasmosis of donor and recipient hearts after heterotopic cardiac transplantation. Rose AG; Uys CJ; Novitsky D; Cooper DK; Barnard CN. Arch Pathol Lab Med 1983 Jul;107(7):368-73

157. Diagnosis of toxoplasma infection in cardiac transplant recipients using polymerase chain reaction. Holliman R; Johnson J; Savva D; Cary N; Wreghitt T. J Clin Pathol 1992 Oct;45(10):931-2

158. Toxoplasmosis in cardiac transplantation. Hakim M, Esmore D, Wallwork J, English TA, Wreghitt T. Br Med J 1986 Apr;292(6528): 1108

159. Outcome of Toxoplasma gondii mismatches in heart transplant recipients over a period of 8 years. Orr KE; Gould FK; Short G; Dark JH; Hilton CJ; Corris PA; et al. J Infect 1994 Nov;29(3):249-53

Index

Immunology and Medicine Series

Kluwer Academic Publishers – Dordrecht / Boston / London